Prevention's FIRM UP *in* 3 WEEKS

Prevention's

FIRM UP *in* 3 WEEKS

Lose Your Belly and Burn Fat Fast—The Prevention Way!

Michele Stanten
Senior Fitness Editor, Prevention Magazine

With Selene Yeager; Carol Krucoff; Tracy Gensler, R.D.; and Kristine Napier, R.D.

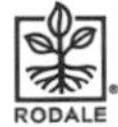
RODALE

Printed in the United States of America
Rodale Inc. makes every effort to use acid-free ♾, recycled paper ♲.

Book design by Carol Angstadt
Interior photographs by Mitch Mandel/Rodale Images, except for photographs on page 401 (by Hilmar).
Footprint illustrations on pages 364 and 365 by John Sterling Ruth

Library of Congress Cataloging-in-Publication Data

Stanten, Michele.
Prevention's firm up in 3 weeks : lose your belly and burn fat fast—the prevention way! / Michele Stanten, with Selene Yeager . . . [et al.].
p. cm.
Includes index.
ISBN-13 978–1–57954–939–8 hardcover
ISBN-10 1–57954–939–X hardcover
ISBN-13 978–1–57954–940–4 paperback
ISBN-10 1–57954–940–3 paperback
1. Weight loss. 2. Reducing exercises. I. Title: Firm up in 3 weeks. II. Yeager, Selene. III. Title.
RM222.2.S743 2004
613.7'12—dc22 2004007642

Distributed to the book trade by Holtzbrinck Publishers

2 4 6 8 10 9 7 5 3 1 hardcover
2 4 6 8 10 9 7 5 3 1 paperback

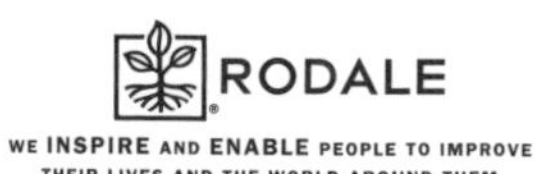

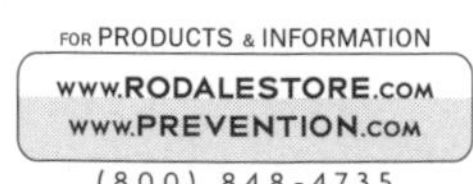

About *Prevention* Health Books

The editors of *Prevention* Health Books are dedicated to providing you with authoritative, trustworthy, and innovative advice for a healthy, active lifestyle. In all of our books, our goal is to keep you thoroughly informed about the latest breakthroughs in natural healing, medical research, alternative health, herbs, nutrition, fitness, and weight loss. We cut through the confusion of today's conflicting health reports to deliver clear, concise, and definitive health information that you can trust. And we explain in practical terms what each new breakthrough means to you, so you can take immediate, practical steps to improve your health and well-being.

Every recommendation in *Prevention* Health Books is based upon reliable sources, including interviews with qualified health authorities. In addition, we retain top-level health practitioners who serve on our board of advisors. *Prevention* Health Books are thoroughly fact-checked for accuracy, and we make every effort to verify recommendations, dosages, and cautions.

The advice in this book will help keep you well-informed about your personal choices in health care—to help you lead a happier, healthier, and longer life.

Notice

This book is intended as a reference volume only, not as a medical manual. The information given here is designed to help you make informed decisions about your health. It is not intended as a substitute for any treatment that may have been prescribed by your doctor. If you suspect that you have a medical problem, we urge you to seek competent medical help, especially before starting a diet or exercise program, increasing your exercise intensity, or changing the type of exercise or diet you follow. If you're not accustomed to exercising, ask your doctor's guidance before beginning an exercise program.

Mention of specific companies, organizations, or authorities in this book does not imply endorsement by the publisher, nor does mention of specific companies, organizations, or authorities imply that they endorse this book.

Internet addresses and telephone numbers given in this book were accurate at the time it went to press.

CONTENTS

FOREWORD

You may not be able to judge a book by its cover, but you most certainly can judge a book by its author. Michele Stanten is one of the most authoritative individuals in the field of fitness and weight loss, as well as one of the most proficient writers in the journalistic profession. Over the past 10 years, I have been privileged to serve as a consultant to Michele in her role as fitness editor for *Prevention* magazine. During this time, I have been continually impressed with her breadth and depth of knowledge in the areas of health, fitness, exercise, and weight loss. Michele is tireless in researching her topics, examining all of the relevant information, interviewing the sources, and checking with her consultants before writing her insightful and interesting fitness columns that have so positively impacted the lives of *Prevention* readers.

I can assure you that this book is written with the same degree of care, competence, and precision, as well as a comprehensiveness that is most unusual for a single text. As you perform Michele's fitness programs, you will realize that she is the master of exercise innovation and training progression. As you follow her nutritional recommendations, you will see that she is unmatched in developing palatable and practical plans for healthy eating and successful fat loss.

Michele is most impressive, however, in her sound understanding of the muscle and metabolism connection that is the key to losing fat, reshaping your body, and maintaining an ideal body weight. Her safe, sensible, and time-efficient muscle-conditioning programs are unequaled in effectiveness and variety, and her personalized training progressions are appropriate for women of all fitness levels.

If there is a book in the weight-loss arena that can actually do what it claims to do, this is it. As you read and apply the information that Michele presents so clearly in these pages, you should quickly experience excellent results that will reinforce both her recommendations and your efforts in applying them.

WAYNE L. WESTCOTT, Ph.D.

Fitness Research Director, South Shore YMCA, Quincy, Massachusetts

Fitness Consultant and Advisor, Prevention *Magazine*

ACKNOWLEDGMENTS

I never realized the amount of work that goes into writing a book. To everyone who helped to make this book possible (and there are many), I owe you big time.

Selene Yeager and Carol Krucoff, my cowriters and fitness buddies, thanks for all your hard work under some crazy deadlines and circumstances.

Tracy Gensler, R.D., for developing delicious recipes and meals, and Regina Ragone, R.D., and Kristine Napier, R.D., for your advice and experience in developing the diet plan.

Wayne Westcott, Ph.D., for everything that you've taught me about fitness and exercise during the past 10 years. It is always a pleasure to work with you.

Ellen Phillips, my editor, for your guidance, wisdom, and reassurance. Karen Neely, for your meticulous copyediting.

Carol Angstadt, for creating a great-looking, easy-to-use design.

And finally to my family: My parents, Rosalie and Gary, who pitched in whenever needed. My son, Jacob, for always making me smile and reminding me of what's really important in life. And most of all, to my husband, Andrew, for taking care of me when I didn't have the time to do it myself. Thanks for picking up the slack . . . and the dry cleaning, the groceries, and lots of takeout. You're simply the best. I could never have done this without you. I love you.

INTRODUCTION

Welcome! I'm so glad you've chosen this book to help you get into shape. Whether you're already exercising or just getting off the couch, you're about to discover the amazing power that exercise has to help you look and feel more energized, more confident, more relaxed—and more beautiful.

This program is based on my more than 10 years of experience as an editor of *Prevention* magazine and as a certified fitness instructor. Every day I review the latest scientific research in the exercise and weight-loss fields, and every day I read letters and e-mails from readers just like you who are trying to lose weight, get firm, eat better, and be healthier. Everyone wants to see results—and no one wants to wait. With that in mind, I took the latest research findings and turned them into a comprehensive program that will get you results—fast. But it's not one of those quick fixes that promises quick results but then leaves you to slide right back into your previous shape. What you learn and achieve in this 3-week program will lay the foundation for a lifetime of fitness.

Prevention's Firm Up in 3 Weeks Program is based on three major components.

- Strength-training workouts that firm all your major muscle groups in a variety of ways
- Walking workouts that crank up your calorie burn
- A diet plan that won't leave you feeling deprived—but *will* help you take off pounds and inches

And there are three workout levels, so you can find the one that's right for your current fitness level.

Every day, you'll get detailed exercise instructions, a daily meal plan, advice on maximizing your efforts, and tips to help you stay motivated—all in one spot.

For the best possible results, follow all the components. But if that's not possible, you'll find several options for customizing the program to meet your needs and schedule, such as Must-Do Moves for the days you don't have time to complete an entire workout or Mix-and-Match Meals if you want more variety in the eating plan.

So what are you waiting for? Let's firm up fast!

MICHELE STANTEN
Senior Fitness Editor, Prevention *Magazine*

PART 1

THE FIRM UP FOCUS

CHAPTER 1

Firm Up in 3 Weeks: The Premise, the Promise, the Program

Almost 2 years after I gave birth to my son, Jacob (and before I developed the Firm Up in 3 Weeks Program), I still couldn't button or zip some of my favorite pants and skirts. I'd lost the pregnancy pounds, but something happened to the shape of my body. It seemed that the little bit of curve I'd had in my chest prebaby had migrated down to my waist and hips postbaby. So even though I weighed the same, I had to go up a size in some clothes. From all the letters I'd received from *Prevention* magazine readers and the frequent cries of woe from the women I'd talked to, I knew I wasn't alone.

Even if you haven't had children, shape-shifting is a fairly common phenomenon for women, occurring as we age. The scale may be holding steady, and your eating and exercising habits may not have changed, but your waistline is growing, your clothes feel tighter, and some parts are looking flabbier. A primary culprit behind this softening up as we age is a loss of muscle mass. Not only is this a major threat to our figures, but it also threatens our health. The good news is that you can do something about it.

Whether you're still battling those postpregnancy pounds or new ones that are making an appearance along with hot flashes, *Prevention*'s Firm Up in 3 Weeks Program is the answer to your body woes. The results are fast and unmistakable: You'll see them in the mirror, feel them in your clothes, appreciate them in your soaring energy, and love them in the compliments you'll receive. I know I have!

Success: Week by Week

YOU MAY BE wondering if you can *really* firm up in just 3 weeks. If you've never trained with weights before, you'll be surprised at how quickly your body responds. If you're following the complete Firm Up in 3 Weeks Program, you can expect to see these results.

- After week 1: You'll increase the amount of weight you're lifting, feel more confident, and have more energy.
- After week 2: You'll get firmer, especially in the arms and calves, so your clothes fit better and you'll feel stronger.
- After week 3: You'll drop 3 to 6 pounds, lose several inches, and feel great.

METABOLISM MELTDOWN

Usually in your thirties, or even as early as your twenties if you're really inactive, you start to lose muscle mass, which is what fuels your body's metabolism. Metabolism is all the work your body does that requires calories (energy): staying alive, thinking, breathing, and moving your muscles. And it plays a major role in how much you weigh, especially with each passing birthday. Sometime in your thirties, your resting metabolic rate—the number of calories you burn each day just to stay alive—starts slowing down by about 5 percent every decade. That means if you eat about 1,800 calories a day and fit into size 10s when you're 35, you'll be shopping for 12s when you're 45, even if you're eating the same number of calories. By the time you're 55 . . . well, you get the idea.

The culprit behind this decline in calorie burn is the same one responsible for the softening up of your figure: muscle loss. Every pound of muscle you lose can decrease the number of calories you burn by as many as 30 a day. In your late thirties and during your forties, you lose about ½ pound of muscle a year, a loss that can double once you hit menopause (blame it on lack of activity and just plain aging). If you're not

careful, by the time you're 65, it's possible to have lost half of your muscle mass and see your metabolism slowed by 200 to 300 calories a day.

But the scale usually tells a different story. Instead of inching down a pound a year as you lose muscle, it usually inches up about a pound a year—which means you're replacing 1 firm, compact, calorie-burning pound of muscle with 2 pounds of soft, lumpy fat every year. No wonder your clothes are getting tighter, you're looking flabbier, and you're having a harder time losing weight.

This muscle-for-fat swap—called creeping obesity—is common as we grow older. And extra fat puts you at more risk for deadly diseases, including heart disease, diabetes, and some types of cancer. But a growing body of research shows that it doesn't have to happen.

A FOUNTAIN OF YOUTH

The truth is, most of the undesirable changes we chalk up to getting older—waning strength, a flabby physique, failing health, a faulty memory, a dowager's hump—happen because most of us

Best Belly Flatteners

TO COME UP with the very best tummy-toning moves, researchers at San Diego State University asked 31 people, both occasional and daily exercisers ages 20 to 45, to perform 13 exercises that target the midsection. While the volunteers were performing the exercises, the researchers measured the work of the abdominals (specifically, the rectus abdominis, which runs the length of your torso and is the "workhorse" muscle of the body, and the obliques, which are muscles that lie along the sides of the abdominal cavity that rotate your body and stabilize the pelvis). They then compared how each exercise stacked up against the traditional crunch.

The top-ranking home exercise, the bicycle maneuver, was up to 2½ times more effective at working the obliques and at least 50 percent better at strengthening the rectus abdominis compared with the traditional crunch. Other winning moves included the long-arm crunch and the crunch on a stability ball (also known as an inflatable exercise ball and a Swiss ball). Unlike many abdominal exercises, these two crunches isolate the ab muscles specifically, rather than relying on the hip flexors at the front of the hip to help out with the move, says lead researcher Peter Francis, Ph.D., director of the biomechanics lab at San Diego State University.

These and other belly-flattening moves are an important part of the Firm Up Action Plan. You'll find out how to do them as you move through the three weekly chapters that are the heart of the program. And in just 3 weeks, you'll notice a tighter midsection, and your jeans will be easier to button.

move less as we get older. This is actually *great* news, because it's so easy to fix. Get moving now, and you can help slow, stop, or even reverse many of these changes. Exercise is the closest thing we have to a Fountain of Youth.

As the senior fitness editor of *Prevention* magazine and a certified fitness instructor for more than 10 years, I am constantly reviewing the latest research on exercise, talking to the leading experts, and seeing firsthand what exercise can do for women, including myself. And now I'd like to share with you the best of all that I've discovered. I've used all that experience and expertise to develop *Prevention*'s Firm Up in 3 Weeks Program.

It may sound like a crash diet or exercise program, but it's not. Many people who want to lose weight or firm up want to do it quickly—often in time for a wedding or reunion. Even if you're not looking for a quick fix, you're very motivated at the beginning. Think about New Year's resolutions. Every January, health club memberships jump by 65 percent, according to the International Health, Racquet, and Sportsclub Association. The parking lots are so crowded that you have to drive around waiting for an empty space, and then you even have to wait to get on most of the equipment. But usually by early to mid-February, you can park in the front row and hop right on the treadmill.

Prevention's Firm Up in 3 Weeks Program takes advantage of this initial burst of motivation and makes sure that you'll see results in just 3 weeks, so you'll be inspired to stick with it. I *know* this approach works, because I've seen it happen with high-protein, low-carb diets such as Atkins and South Beach. The first 2 weeks of these diets are very restrictive, but people see quick results, so they are motivated to continue.

The Firm Up Program is a jumping-off point. It gets you started, gets you results, and gives you the tools you need to continue living a healthy, active life.

THE FIRM UP ACTION PLAN

High-intensity workouts are the secret to dropping pounds and inches quickly. But don't panic and think, "No way!" A high-intensity workout doesn't necessarily mean that you have to run for miles or take an hour-long Spinning class. Intensity is relative. What's high intensity for someone who's unfit may be low intensity for someone who's moderately fit. So no matter what your fitness level, you can get a high-intensity workout just by pushing yourself out of your comfort zone—and the Firm Up Program will show you how to do it safely. The results will definitely be worth it.

High-intensity exercise can burn 25 to 75 percent more calories than low-intensity exercise. For example, cycling at a leisurely pace for ½ hour burns about 200 calories, while cycling vigorously for the same amount of time burns nearly 350. And the benefits continue even after you stop exercising. After a high-intensity bout of activity, the number of calories that you're burning can stay elevated for up to 15 hours, which means that you could burn an extra 75 calories a day.

As you become fitter, moderate-intensity activities will become easier. You'll be able to do more for the same amount of time and effort—meaning that you'll burn even more calories. For example, if you start out by walking 2 miles in an hour, you'll burn about 160 calories. But as you get fit, you'll be able to walk 3 miles in an hour for the same effort, and you'll burn 50 percent more calories.

And research shows that the fitter you are, the more calories you burn while digesting food. It appears that active women's muscles need fuel faster, so their bodies work harder, burning more calories, to absorb what they eat. Which is more great news!

Intensity doesn't apply only to aerobic activities. When you're strength training, you can burn up to three times as many calories and do fewer repetitions by using a heavier weight.

In addition to bouts of high-intensity exercise, the Firm Up Program also incorporates another training principle, called periodization. If you want to change your body for the better, you have to change your workout—often. That's the idea behind periodization training. Vary the types of exercises you do and the order in which you do them, the weight you use and the number of repetitions you lift, even how often you exercise and how frequently you rest, and your muscles will soon reward you with increased strength and shape. In one study, researchers followed 24 women through a 6-month resistance-training program. The multiple-set, periodized group lost 7 percent of their body fat and gained more than 7 pounds of beautifully toned muscle. That was more than double the results of women doing a single-set routine.

The Firm Up in 3 Weeks Program applies these two training principles—intensity and periodization—to two popular types of exercise—strength training and walking—to help you shift your body's calorie-burning engines into overdrive and firm up fast. I've used them all to help me get back into my favorite skirts and pants and firm up after 4 months of sitting on my butt and writing this book!

STRENGTH TRAINING FOR A GREAT SHAPE

Strength training, working your muscles against resistance such as a dumbbell, is the key to halting muscle loss and to keeping your metabolism in high gear. (For more on the benefits of this type of workout, see chapter 9, Strength Training: The Firm Up Secret Weapon, beginning on page 357.) The Firm Up Program combines two types of strength-building workouts: traditional weight lifting using dumbbells, and core training using your own body weight and isometric muscle contractions (holding a specific position for a certain amount of time).

The weight-lifting workouts target your arms, legs, shoulders, chest, and upper back, while the core workouts focus on your abs, lower back, hips, and buttocks. You'll be doing each workout three times a week. During the 3-week program, the routine will change (the periodization principle), requiring you to perform different exercises, to do more or fewer reps, to vary the speed of reps, and to lift heavier weights (the intensity

You *Won't* Get Big and Bulky!

IF ALL THIS talk of gaining pounds of muscle from strength training is making you nervous, relax. If you're over 40, you've been losing muscle for years now, so in most cases, you're just replacing what was once there (back when you were younger and slimmer).

Muscle is much more compact than fat, so those extra pounds will look sleeker, smaller, and firmer. And you won't bulk up. Women don't have enough of the male hormones such as testosterone to allow their muscles to get big and bulky. If you're still seeing visions of female bodybuilders, picture this: Most of them spend about 4 hours a day at the gym, follow very strict diets, and in many cases still need a little artificial steroid boost. On the Firm Up Program, you'll just lose fat, get firm, and look great!

principle). This mixing things up will keep your muscles working, and it will really challenge them so they'll get strong and firm up fast.

And to really crank up the fat burn, you'll be doing three sets of each strength-training exercise. When researchers from the University of Maryland in College Park compared 17 women performing one set of resistance exercises with 18 women doing three sets, they found that, while both groups had similar strength gains, the three-set group had a 25 percent drop in body fat, compared with 16 percent in the one-set group. Lifting weights demands a lot of calories, and when you perform three sets, that calorie burn can increase threefold, which is significant for burning fat.

WALKING YOUR WAY TO FITNESS

If there's a single perfect exercise, it's probably walking. It's easy, convenient, and inexpensive. Nearly anybody can do it at any skill level, from Grandma to the kids. You can do it almost anywhere, anytime. Plus, it has the lowest dropout rate and injury rate of all exercise programs. That's why it's a key component of the Firm Up Program.

Granted, other forms of exercise, like running, bicycling, and swimming, may burn more calories per minute. But studies have shown that people who take up walking actually stick with it, while those who pursue other activities tend to give up after the first few months. One of the reasons may be that it makes you feel so good. We all know that exercise can boost your mood and your sense of well-being. But compared to other exercisers, who feel better *after* a workout, walkers report feeling better *during* the actual exercise. By choosing an activity than makes you feel good while you do it, not just after you're through, you'll be more likely to stick with it.

Despite all those benefits, every month I get e-mails or letters from women saying: "I walk

every day, but I'm not losing any weight." Because walking is such a comfortable, familiar activity, and most of us don't like to push ourselves, you may not be walking at a high enough intensity to get the results you want. That's why the Firm Up Walking Plan incorporates higher-intensity speed and interval walks along with easier, more moderate walks.

By sneaking short, high-intensity bouts of activity into your regular walk, you won't feel as though you're killing yourself, you'll reduce your risk of an injury, and you'll burn more calories, so you firm up fast. In one study, a group of exercisers worked out 5 days a week at their target heart rates for up to 45 minutes. A second group exercised the same amount of time, only they did intervals, alternately increasing their intensity just five beats above their target heart rates, then slowing down to five beats below. After 10 weeks, the interval group lost more than three

Get Firm *and* Disease-Free

SURE, LOOKING AND feeling good are great reasons to try the Firm Up in 3 Weeks Program. But the program's benefits are more than skin deep. It can help you beat disease, too. Here are just a few examples of how exercise helps you reduce your risk of, or helps you relieve, six common health conditions.

Diabetes. In the Finnish Diabetes Prevention Study, the people who exercised the most—up to 4 hours a week—dropped their risk of diabetes by 80 percent, even if they didn't lose any weight.

Cancer. You can cut your risk of getting or dying from colon cancer by 50 percent if you get at least 30 minutes of activity most days, according to the American Cancer Society.

Heart disease. A Harvard University study showed that women who walked at a 3-miles-per-hour or faster pace at least 3 hours a week reduced their risk of heart disease by 40 percent.

Osteoporosis. You can start to lose bone as early as your midthirties. As you get older, this bone loss speeds up, dropping as much as a precipitous 20 percent in the 5 to 7 years following menopause. But in one study, postmenopausal women increased their bone density by lifting weights just twice a week for a year.

Arthritis. Exercise can reduce pain, cut your need for medications, and help you avoid joint-replacement surgery in the future. Some studies also show that aerobic exercise, such as walking, can decrease inflammation in some joints.

Depression. Studies have shown that as little as 10 minutes of exercise can boost energy and reduce tension for up to an hour afterward. And less than 1 hour a week of brisk activity can relieve major depression as well as antidepressants do—and the effect is long-lasting.

times the weight lost by the continuous exercisers. This type of training also helps beat boredom and fatigue.

A FIRM BODY DOESN'T LIVE ON EXERCISE ALONE

Exercise just isn't enough to firm you up and help you stay that way. Your eating style–that is, your diet plan–is just as important as your exercise routine. That's why the Firm Up Program makes eating–what, when, and how much–an integral part of your 3-week program.

Does what you eat really make that big a difference? I'll answer that question with a simple math exercise: If you weigh 130 pounds and ride a stationary bike for 30 minutes at a moderate pace (one that *really* makes you sweat), you burn 173 calories. Not knowing that number, though, you feel entitled to a piece of apple pie–which weighs in at a whopping 410 calories. Not only did you *not* burn off the pie, but you also gained an extra 237 calories!

That's the obvious reason why eating the wrong foods–or too much of *any* food–can derail your efforts to firm up. But the not-so-obvious reason to avoid overeating may be at least as critical in keeping you healthfully trim: Overindulging, even in healthy foods, may make it harder to burn fat. Preliminary research on animals suggests that chronically overindulging may desensitize fat cells to epinephrine, a hormone that is released during exercise and normally signals fat cells to empty their contents. So no matter how hard you exercise, you may not be able to burn fat efficiently if you overindulge too often.

Now, notice that I didn't say *never* indulge. In fact, the Firm Up Eating Plan allows for a daily indulgence. This meal plan limits calories without leaving you feeling hungry or deprived. It focuses on high-fiber whole grains, beans, fruits, and veggies to fill you up; low-saturated-fat proteins such as lean meats, poultry, fish, and eggs to keep you satisfied longer; and low-fat dairy foods to boost your calcium intake, which has been shown to help make losing weight and staying slim easier.

I've made sure that all the recipes are fast and easy to make, so you're not tempted to skip this vital part of the program because it's just too much work. (There are even suggestions for fast-food and restaurant meals that fall within the plan, so you can stay focused on firming up even when you're shopping or eating out with your spouse or family.) Best of all, there are lots of choices. You can follow the daily meal plans in the weekly chapters (3, 4, and 5) or choose from the meals and snacks in chapter 7, Mix-and-Match Meals, to create your own menus.

FIRM UP YOUR ATTITUDE

It all comes down to this: Any exercise and diet plan you embark on can succeed or fail because of your attitude, not just because of your food or exercise choices. So throughout this book, I focus on firming up your attitude and motivation as well as your body. You'll find real-life success stories to inspire you, tons of tips to help you

stay in the Firm Up mindset, and chapters specially geared toward pumping up your attitude and boosting your motivation.

FIRM UP FOR LIFE

What happens *after* you've finished the 3-week program? To stay firm, you have to keep working–doing the weight-resistance exercises, walking, watching your calories. So I've devoted an entire section of this book (part 5, Firm Up and Beyond) to keeping you on track for lifetime firmness.

In this section, you'll find my Stay Firm Plan, advice on how to get back into firming up if you've "fallen off the wagon" (it happens to everyone now and then), and ways to avoid boredom and enjoy your path to firmness forever.

Real-Life Success Story

Six months before her wedding, Lisa (Getz) Trollinger of Allentown, Pennsylvania, started shopping for her dress. "I was mortified to discover that the only size that fit well was a 16," she says. When she found a style she liked, she ordered it two sizes too small. That same week, she committed herself to getting in shape by following the *Prevention* program.

In just 3 weeks, she lost nearly 4 pounds and 2½ inches. "Two months later, my size 12 wedding dress arrived. I still couldn't quite get it buttoned, and I knew the salesperson thought I'd set my expectations too high," she says. "But when I tried it on again a month before the wedding—my dress had to be taken in!"

"Imagine starting a strength-training program at age 45—after being sedentary and overweight—and going from 168 pounds to 144 pounds in 6 months! I looked and felt fabulous on my wedding day."

And 6 years later, Lisa has lost another 6 pounds and easily maintains her new figure. "This program showed me how simple and effective strength training is. I never would have thought I could lift weights," she says. "Now I lift 2 or 3 days a week. It energizes me, maintains my muscle tone, and keeps my weight steady, even though I love bread and butter. The only tools you need to stay young are some dumbbells."

PART 2

THE FIRM UP ACTION PLAN

CHAPTER 2

Let's Get Started

I recommend starting the Firm Up Program on a Sunday. For most of us, weekends tend to allow us a little more flexibility in our schedules. So there's a better chance that you'll have time on Saturday to go food shopping and pick up anything else you might need (like a new pair of walking shoes or dumbbells), you'll be less likely to skip your first workout, and you'll feel great on Monday morning for having accomplished the first day of the program. But keep in mind that this program has to fit into your life if it's going to work for you. So get started when it feels right for you.

Read on for the five to-do items that you'll need to take care of before you start.

TO-DO #1: GET YOUR GROCERIES

Review the first week's meal plans in chapter 3. The meal plans and grocery lists are based on eating 1,700 calories a day—that includes breakfast, lunch, dinner, two healthy snacks, and one indulgent treat each day. If you want to cut more calories (we don't recommend going below 1,500), see page 312 in chapter 6, The Science behind the Firm Up Eating Plan, for healthy ways to do that. If you don't like a particular meal, you can make a substitution. (Review chapter 7, Mix-and-Match Meals, for lots of healthy low-cal alternatives.) Just remember, if you alter the meal plans, make sure you adjust the grocery list. And then go shopping and stock up on a week's worth of meals.

You'll also notice some vitamins on the first week's grocery list. As added nutritional insurance, we recommend that you take a daily multivitamin/mineral supplement that contains 100 percent of the Daily Value (DV) of most nutrients, plus take 100 to 500 milligrams of vitamin C and 500 milligrams of calcium if you're under 50. Take two 500-milligram doses of calcium (for example, morning and evening) if you're 50 or older.

HOW TO CHOOSE YOUR INGREDIENTS AT THE GROCERY STORE

Your first trip to stock up on ingredients may involve some extra time. You'll be reading labels and comparing brands to find the specific items. Return grocery trips should be a whiz, however, as you become familiar with the products. Some of your first-week grocery items that are canned or frozen will take you through the second- and third-week menus.

Skim through all the recipes first. Decide what you want to have when given a choice (for example, an apple versus a pear). If you don't like the suggested meal or snack, go ahead and nix it from your list. Be sure to cross off the ingredients from your grocery list, too! Simply substitute another meal or snack from chapter 7, Mix-and-Match Meals.

Here are some tips to make your Firm Up food shopping a success. For some specific brand recommendations, see page 321 in chapter 7, Mix-and-Match Meals.

- Before your first trip to the grocery store, take a quick inventory of what you already have on hand. You can probably eliminate a few things from your grocery list, such as black pepper and vanilla extract. Don't fret over the exact sizes of the items as specified on the grocery list. For example, if your can of black beans is 16 ounces and the grocery list calls for a 15½-ounce can, you have basically the same amount. Choose the closest possible size to what is specified and move on. If you feel better changing your grocery list to reflect subtle differences in amounts (particularly if you are sending someone else to the store), please do so.
- When choosing dairy products, be sure to note the product expiration date. You'll be shocked at what you may find if you're not careful. I once

Time-Saving Tips for Healthy Meal Preps

YOU'VE WORKED LATE, you're starving and exhausted, and all you want to do is kick up your heels and have dinner waiting for you. You arrive home and realize that the meat needs to be defrosted before you can even start dinner. Before you eat the leg off the table (and everything in your cupboard), quickly scan the suggested dinners in the three weekly chapters (3, 4, and 5) and chapter 7, Mix-and-Match Meals, and choose something that requires little prep. Or better yet, plan ahead by using some of these easy tips for defrosting your frozen items. You'll soon learn that a little planning goes a long way in simplifying your life.

- Thaw frozen berries in the refrigerator the night before or, to thaw quickly, use the defrost feature on your microwave.
- For the softest, bakery-fresh bread, store it in the freezer in a tightly sealed plastic bag. Transfer the bread you need to a new sealed plastic bag and thaw on the counter the night before. Or you can defrost each serving in your microwave. You'll be amazed at how long your bread will last, and you'll be able to savor every last soft crumb.
- Always defrost frozen meat or fish in the refrigerator—*never* in the sink or out on the counter. Once your meat has camped out in your refrigerator for 3 days, cook it, or you must throw it out, since significant bacterial growth occurs beyond this time frame. You may defrost your frozen meat in your microwave as well, but watch it carefully because it may start cooking.
- If you use part of a can of soup or vegetable broth for a recipe, pour the remainder immediately into an ice cube tray and freeze for future use.

purchased cottage cheese that was more than 2 months old–yuck! Taking a moment now to check the dates may save you a lot of hassle later.

- Choose canned products–including canned tomatoes, tomato paste, and vegetables–that are labeled "no salt added" or "lower sodium." For canned soups, choose "low-sodium for sodium-restricted diets" whenever possible. A "light" or "less-sodium" soup is still very high in sodium. The "low-sodium for sodium-restricted diets" soups used in these recipes can usually be found in the "special diet" aisle of your grocery store. Your jar of spaghetti sauce should provide no more than 400 milligrams of sodium per ½-cup serving.
- Look for canned fruit packed in juice or water. "Lite" varieties have some added sugar.
- You'll notice that some recipes call for rinsing your canned products. To do this, you put the food in a colander and rinse with cold water for 2 or 3 minutes to remove some of the excess sodium. Canned beans, vegetables, tuna, and

fruits will taste better when rinsed before adding them to the recipe. Be sure to let all of the water drain off before continuing with the recipe.

- Try farmer's cheese, because it has less saturated fat than 50%-reduced-fat cream cheese.

TO-DO #2: GEAR UP

Here's what you'll need for the exercise portion of the program. Make sure you have everything before you get started.

- A good pair of walking shoes and socks (for details on what to look for, see page 364)

Q&A WHEN TO EXERCISE

Q. What's the best time of day to exercise?

A. It varies from one person to the next. You need to pick a time when you are most willing and able to exercise. You need to fit your workouts into your life when it's most convenient for you—otherwise, other things will always bump exercise off your schedule. I'm not a morning person, so I'll always pick my bed over my sneakers before 9:00 A.M. For me, lunchtime is perfect for getting in my strength-training workout. It's quick and low-sweat, so I don't have to shower. And since I'm a night owl, I hit the pavement or treadmill after I put my son to bed. There's no significant impact on the calories you burn or how quickly you'll see results based on the time of day you exercise. What matters most is that you just do it.

- Dumbbells (see page 22 to determine the appropriate level for you)
  - Level 1: 3-, 5-, and 10-pound
  - Level 2: 5-, 8-, and 12-pound
  - Level 3: 5-, 8-, 10-, and 15-pound

These are general guidelines. You should use an amount of weight that allows you to perform the recommended number of reps while using good form, with the last rep or two being very difficult to complete. If you can crank out the recommended number of reps and still feel as if you could keep going, you need a heavier weight. When you increase to a heavier weight, if you're unable to complete an entire set with the heavier weight, do as many as possible and then finish the set with a lighter weight. Eventually, you'll be able to do the entire set with the heavier weight, and you'll save yourself the clutter and expense of buying sets of dumbbells in 1-pound increments.

TO-DO #3: SCHEDULE YOUR WORKOUTS

Make your workouts part of your regular daily schedule. Below is an overview of the program; the workouts should take no more than an hour a day. You'll learn how to do each set of exercises in the three weekly chapters that follow.

If a 7-day workout schedule feels daunting, I've included suggestions on page 21 on how you can fit your workouts into 3 or 5 days a week. Pick the one workout schedule that fits your lifestyle best–and get going!

7-DAY WORKOUT SCHEDULE

	Aerobic	Strength
Sunday	Easy walk	Basic weights
Monday	Interval walk	Core training
Tuesday	Easy walk	High-rep weights*
Wednesday	Interval walk	Core training
Thursday	Easy walk	Heavy weights*
Friday	Speed walk	Core training
Saturday	Long walk	Rest

*For week 1, do a basic weight workout instead.

THE WORKOUT COMPONENTS

What's the difference between an easy walk and an interval walk, you ask? Or basic weights and high-rep weights? Here's what this program's all about.

The Walks

Easy walk. This doesn't mean you're strolling along. It's "easy" because you don't have to think about anything or push yourself to go faster or farther. Just get out there and walk at a moderate pace, as if you had to get somewhere. You should be breathing a little harder but still be able to carry on a conversation.

Interval walk. On these days, you'll be picking up the pace for short periods of time,

How Hard Should You Work?

MOST EXERCISE SHOULD feel like you're working between levels 5 and 7 on a scale of 1 to 10. For interval training, you want to pick up the intensity to a level 8 or 9 for short periods of time. Below are descriptions of how each level should feel.

Level 1: watching TV

Level 2: light housecleaning

Level 3: puttering around the yard

Level 4: window shopping

Level 5: strolling and chatting with a friend

Level 6: walking purposefully, but talking is still easy

Level 7: rushing to an appointment, conversation limited to short sentences

Level 8: speeding because you're about to miss the bus, only yes or no responses are possible

Level 9: running to catch the bus as it pulls away; not doable for more than 90 seconds

Level 10: sprinting after the bus when you realize you left your purse on it; after 30 seconds forget it

from 30 seconds to 3 minutes. In between, you'll slow down to a moderate pace to catch your breath and then speed back up. These bursts of speed will kick up your calorie burn more than you if continued walking at the same pace.

During the moderate phase of the walk, you should feel as if you're working at an effort of 6 or 7 (based on a perceived-exertion scale of 1 to 10, with 1 being no effort). For the speed phase, you want to push yourself so that you feel as if you're at an 8 or 9. At this rate, it should be difficult for you to carry on a conversation.

Speed walk. After warming up for 5 minutes, you'll need to pick a route that will take you about 10 minutes to complete if you're walking at a fast pace. This might be a loop around your neighborhood, or you could walk out 5 minutes and then turn around and walk back. If you choose the latter option, note where you turned around, because you'll want to use that same turnaround point for future weeks. Each week, you should push yourself to go a little faster so that you cover the same distance in less time.

Long walk. This is your endurance workout. After warming up, walk at a pace you can sustain for the recommended time. It's okay if you slow down a little as you go, but start at the same pace you use for your easy walks. Focus on walking for the allotted time, not on how fast you're going.

The Weights

Basic weights. All the weight routines use dumbbells and target your arms, shoulders, chest, upper back, legs, and butt. For this workout, you'll be using weights that you can lift for 10 to 12 repetitions at a time. These are slow reps: about 3 seconds to lift, pause for a second, and then lower for 3 seconds.

Core training. This workout will specifically target your abs, lower back, hips, and buttocks. These muscles make up your core and are important for maintaining good posture. You won't need dumbbells for this workout. Instead, you'll be working against your own body weight and holding poses in isometric contractions.

High-rep weights. This workout is similar to the basic weight routine, but you'll be doing more repetitions. It won't take you any longer, though. You'll be alternating basic reps with quick reps, called pulses, which are done in a shorter range of motion. Start with the same amount of weight as you use for the basic workout. If it feels too heavy as you're doing the reps, switch to a lighter weight in the middle of your set and then finish the set.

Heavy weights. Start with a heavier weight for this workout; you'll need to complete only four to six reps of each exercise. The exercises are grouped in pairs, two exercises for each major body part. Generally, the first exercise will isolate a specific muscle, and then the second exercise will target the entire muscle group. This way of working your muscles will more effectively fatigue them, which is the key to building strength and muscle more quickly. In later weeks and in the higher-level workouts, you'll also be adding some jumps to up the intensity, improve agility, and build more bone.

FITTING IN FIRMING UP

This is a pretty ambitious workout schedule, and it's guaranteed to get you the best results in only 3 weeks. But as you know, life happens. Working late, chauffeuring the kids to dance class and soccer practice, dealing with home repairs, and a myriad of other distractions can make it impossible to fit in all the workouts, despite your best intentions. No problem. The workout is designed to be flexible. Here are some options.

- You can break up the aerobic and strength workouts. Do one in the morning and the other at lunch or in the evening.
- If you can't commit to exercising every day, aim for 5 days a week. You can skip one core workout, the heavy-weight workout, an easy walk, and the speed walk. If you do that, rearrange your remaining workouts to the days of the week that work best for you. See the example above.
- If you can only commit to 3 days a week, stick with the Sunday, Monday, and Tuesday workouts and spread them throughout the week. See the example at right.
- If you commit to the daily routine, and then some days you find that you just don't have time to do the entire workout, at least do the highlighted Must-Do Moves. Each day, the exercises that will give you the most bang for your buck will be noted so that you never have to think it's all or nothing.

Just remember that as you decrease your workouts, it will take longer for you to see results.

5-DAY WORKOUT SCHEDULE

	Aerobic	Strength
Sunday	Easy walk	Basic weights
Monday	Interval walk	Core training
Tuesday	–	–
Wednesday	Interval walk	Core training
Thursday	Easy walk	High-rep weights*
Friday	–	–
Saturday	Long walk	Rest

*For week 1, do a basic weight workout instead.

3-DAY WORKOUT SCHEDULE

	Aerobic	Strength
Sunday	–	–
Monday	Easy walk	Basic weights
Tuesday	–	–
Wednesday	Interval walk	Core training
Thursday	–	–
Friday	–	–
Saturday	Easy walk	High-rep weights*

*For week 1, do a basic weight workout instead.

TO-DO #4: CHOOSE A WORKOUT LEVEL

Review the workouts in the next chapter, Week 1, to determine your level. The workouts are broken into three levels. Level 1 is right for you if you're just starting out or are a sporadic exerciser. Level 2 is the place to start if you've been exercising once or twice a week for the past 3 months but haven't been very consistent. And Level 3 is most appropriate if you have been exercising regularly, 3 to 5 days a week, for at least 3 months.

You don't have to follow the same level for all parts of the program. For instance, if you walk regularly but are new to strength training, you may want to do Level 2 or 3 for the walking workouts and Level 1 for the strength workouts. Unless you have been lifting weights regularly for at least a month, it's best to start with Level 1 for the strength-training portion of the program.

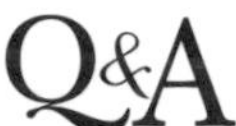

FOOD AND EXERCISE

Q. Should I eat before I exercise?

A. Probably. Too many women exercise on empty, hoping they'll burn more calories and lose more weight. In reality, you don't perform as well and can't lift as much or go as fast when you're not well-fueled, so the workout is less effective. If it's been more than 2 or 3 hours since your last meal, eat a snack (or part of one), such as a banana, an energy bar, or a bagel with peanut butter, about 30 minutes before exercising. And drink a tall glass of water.

TO-DO #5: CHOOSE YOUR REWARDS

One final thing before you start: Write down three weekly rewards. You can put them right into the plan on days 7, 14, and 21; there's a space for them (see pages 114, 210, and 306). Choose something that you can look forward to, something that will inspire you. Start small–maybe a manicure or pedicure–and build up to something really indulgent, like a day at a spa, to reward yourself for completing the program.

Finished your five to-dos? Then it's time to get started on week 1!

CHAPTER 3

Week 1

Are you ready to start firming up? Three weeks from today, you'll see wonderful results: a flatter belly, toned arms (take that sleeveless dress back out of storage), firmer thighs, and a tauter butt. You'll have lost weight and inches of flab. Your clothes will look and feel fabulous again. And so will you!

Grocery List

Photocopy this list and take it with you to the store. You can stock up on everything you need to make the first week's Firm Up meals and snacks, so all the ingredients will be at hand when you need them. This list is longer than subsequent ones because you'll be buying nonperishable items for all 3 weeks. So future shopping trips will be a whiz. For some specific brand recommendations, see page 321 in chapter 7, Mix-and-Match Meals.

Produce Aisle

- ☐ Choose: 3 apples *or* 1 apple and 2 pears
- ☐ 1 pint blueberries
- ☐ 1 large bag baby carrots
- ☐ 3 stalks celery
- ☐ 1 small jar minced garlic or 1 bunch (8 to 10 cloves) fresh garlic
- ☐ 1 bunch (12 ounces) grapes (red or green)
- ☐ Choose: 2 small honeydews *or* 2 small cantaloupes
- ☐ 1 bag romaine lettuce
- ☐ 1 small carton mushrooms
- ☐ 1 orange
- ☐ 1 red or green pepper
- ☐ 1 small bunch scallions (green onions)—if desired
- ☐ 2 (9-ounce) bags baby spinach (ready-to-microwave bag)
- ☐ 1 tomato
- ☐ 1 pint cherry or grape tomatoes (if desired)
- ☐ 1 small green or yellow zucchini

Dairy Aisle

- ☐ 1 package Lender's refrigerated 2½- to 3-ounce honey wheat bagels
- ☐ 1 (4-ounce) package farmer's cheese (look for brands with 50 calories per ounce, such as Friendship or Andrulis) *or* a 4-ounce tub reduced-fat cream cheese (any variety)
- ☐ 1 small tub trans-fat-free margarine
- ☐ 1 small canister grated Parmesan cheese
- ☐ 1 (8-ounce) block 50% reduced-fat cheese (any flavor)
- ☐ 1 (8-ounce) package 2% milk reduced-fat shredded cheese (any flavor)
- ☐ 1 dozen eggs (option: choose "omega-3" eggs such as Eggland's Best to save 60 milligrams cholesterol and 0.5 gram saturated fat per egg) *or* 2 cartons Egg Beaters (for fat-free eggs)
- ☐ 1 gallon plus 1 quart fat-free milk
- ☐ 1 small package fat-free pudding cups (any flavor)
- ☐ 1 package low-fat ravioli (such as Buitoni Light Four-Cheese Ravioli)
- ☐ 1 Yoplait Nouriche smoothie

☐ 4 (8-ounce) containers fat-free yogurt (120 calories or less per cup)

Canned Fruit/Vegetables/Beans/Soup Aisle

☐ 1 package (6 single-serving containers) unsweetened applesauce (such as Mott's Healthy Harvest or Mott's Natural Style)

☐ 1 package dried apricot halves

☐ 1 (15-ounce) can chickpeas (garbanzo beans)

☐ 2 (15½-ounce) cans vegetarian chili (look for 400 milligrams sodium per serving or less, 170 calories per 1-cup serving; Natural Touch Low-Fat Vegetarian Chili is a good choice)

☐ 1 package dried, sweetened cranberries

☐ 2 (4-ounce) cans fruit cocktail (packed in juice or water; suggest Del Monte Fruit Naturals or Dole FruitBowls)

☐ 1 small container honey

☐ 2 (4-ounce) cans mandarin oranges (packed in juice or water)

☐ 2 (2¼-ounce) cans sliced mushrooms

☐ 1 (4-ounce) can pear halves (packed in juice or water)

☐ 1 package Sunsweet dried plums

☐ 8 ounces seedless unsweetened raisins

☐ 1 (8-ounce) can Campbell's Healthy Request Chicken Noodle soup

☐ 2 (8-ounce) cans Campbell's Healthy Request Cream of Mushroom soup

☐ 2 (8-ounce) cans reduced-sodium tomato soup

☐ 1 (8-ounce) can stewed tomatoes (no salt added)

☐ 1 package dried tropical fruit mix

Crackers/Snacks/Cereals/Pasta Aisle

☐ 1 small package quick-cooking barley

☐ 1 (14-ounce) box Cheerios cereal

☐ 1 (14-ounce) box shredded wheat cereal

☐ 1 small box Wasa crispbreads

☐ 1 package regular graham crackers

☐ 1 small box low-fat granola (without raisins; suggest Healthy Choice brand)

☐ 1 small package Hostess Blueberry Mini Muffins

☐ 1 small box plain instant oatmeal packets

☐ 2 (16-ounce) boxes pasta (any variety)

☐ 1 box mini bags Orville Redenbacher's Movie Theater Butter popcorn

☐ 1 (1¼-ounce) bag potato chips (any variety)

☐ 1 small box instant brown rice

☐ 1 small box rice pilaf (suggest Uncle Ben's Chicken and Harvest Vegetable Pilaf)

☐ 2 (16-ounce) jars spaghetti sauce (look for 400 milligrams sodium or less per ½-cup serving)

Bread Aisle

- [ ] 1 loaf whole grain bread (look for 80 calories and at least 2 grams fiber per slice)
- [ ] 1 whole wheat French baguette
- [ ] 1 small package whole grain hamburger rolls (4 rolls; look for 160 calories and at least 2 grams fiber per roll)
- [ ] 1 large Neapolitan-style pizza crust (plain—avoid crusts flavored with added olive oil, cheese, and so forth)

Deli/Meat Aisle

- [ ] 1 (6-ounce) can chicken breast meat (packed in water)
- [ ] 1-pound package chicken breasts (four 4-ounce breasts)
- [ ] 8 ounces salmon
- [ ] 12 ounces round, sirloin, or flank steak
- [ ] 1 (6-ounce) can white-meat tuna packed in water
- [ ] 1 pound ground turkey breast meat

Condiments Aisle

- [ ] 1 large jar almond butter
- [ ] 1 small jar all-fruit-style apricot preserves
- [ ] 1 small canister Italian-style bread crumbs
- [ ] 1 small bottle instant coffee or brew-variety coffee
- [ ] 1 small jar horseradish spread (if desired)
- [ ] 1 small bottle ketchup
- [ ] 1 small bottle maple syrup
- [ ] 1 small jar light mayonnaise
- [ ] 1 small jar horseradish mustard or Dijon/spicy brown mustard
- [ ] 1 (4-ounce) bottle olive oil
- [ ] 1 (2¼-ounce) can sliced black olives
- [ ] 1 large jar smooth or chunky peanut butter
- [ ] 1 (4-ounce) jar roasted red peppers (if desired)
- [ ] Choice: 1 (8-ounce) bottle light salad dressing (any flavor) *or* 1 (8-ounce) bottle full-fat salad dressing (any flavor)
- [ ] 1 small bottle Russian-style salad dressing
- [ ] 1 (4-ounce) bottle balsamic vinegar
- [ ] 1 (4-ounce) bottle white wine vinegar
- [ ] 1 small bottle white cooking wine

Frozen-Food Aisle

- [ ] 1 (16-ounce) package frozen berries (strawberries, raspberries, blackberries or mixture)
- [ ] 1 (16-ounce) package broccoli florets
- [ ] 1 Don Miguel's Lean Olé! or Amy's burrito (270 to 290 calories)
- [ ] 1 small box crinkle-cut carrots
- [ ] 1 (10-ounce) box cauliflower florets

- ☐ 1 Lean Cuisine Chicken Enchilada Suiza or Smart Ones Fajita Chicken Supreme or Amy's Black Bean Enchilada Whole Meal (270 to 290 calories)
- ☐ 1 Lean Cuisine Everyday Favorites Chicken Fettuccini (270 to 290 calories)
- ☐ 1 small box green beans
- ☐ 1 pint Healthy Choice ice cream (any variety) or Edy's regular chocolate or coffee ice cream or Baskin-Robbins Cherries Jubilee
- ☐ 1 package Silhouette ice cream sandwiches (any variety)
- ☐ 1 Uncle Ben's Mexican-Style Rice Bowl Beef Fajita or Lean Cuisine Café Classics Southern Beef Tips (270 to 300 calories)
- ☐ 1 small bag shoestring-style fries (suggest Ore-Ida)
- ☐ 1 (10-ounce) box snow peas
- ☐ 2 (16-ounce) bags spinach (chopped or cut-leaf)
- ☐ 2 (10-ounce) boxes spinach (chopped or cut-leaf)
- ☐ 1 box veggie burgers (look for 120 calories or less per burger)
- ☐ 1 box low-fat frozen waffles (170 calories per 2-waffle serving; look for whole grain)
- ☐ 1 small container light whipped topping

Nuts/Baking/Spices Aisle

- ☐ 1 large package whole shelled almonds (any variety)
- ☐ 1 small spice bottle or tin dried basil
- ☐ 1 small spice bottle or tin black pepper
- ☐ 1 (8-ounce) package mini chocolate chips
- ☐ 1 small bottle or jar chocolate syrup
- ☐ 1 small bottle coconut extract
- ☐ 1 small can nonstick olive oil cooking spray
- ☐ 1 small spice bottle or tin ground coriander (if desired)
- ☐ 1 small spice bottle or tin ground cumin (if desired)
- ☐ 1 small box or package granulated sugar
- ☐ 1 small bottle maple extract (if desired)
- ☐ 1 small spice bottle or tin onion powder
- ☐ 1 large jar dry-roasted peanuts
- ☐ 1 small package pistachios
- ☐ 1 small bottle salt
- ☐ 1 small package soy nuts (about ½ ounce)
- ☐ 1 small bottle vanilla extract
- ☐ 1 large package chopped walnuts

Other/Checkout Aisle

- ☐ 1 small box chocolate-covered raisins or chocolate-covered peanuts
- ☐ 1 (1½-ounce) bag Crispy M&Ms
- ☐ 2 Luna bars (any flavor)
- ☐ 1 small bottle wine (any variety)

FIRM UP / DAY 1

Four Moves to Wake You Up

Every morning, get your body ready for a more active lifestyle with this easy 5-minute, in-bed stretch routine. It will loosen up your muscles and get your blood flowing before you even hit the shower. It's a great way to start the day–not just today, but every day, especially while you're on the Firm Up in 3 Weeks Program.

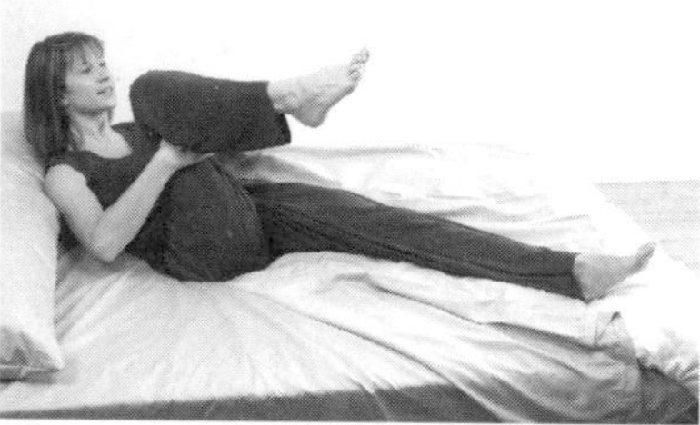

KNEE TO CHEST. Lying on your back with your legs straight, lift your right leg and grasp it with both hands behind your thigh. Gently pull your knee toward your chest until you feel a slight stretch in the back of your thigh. Hold in this position for three deep breaths. Then without letting go of your leg, lift your head and bring your forehead toward your knee. Hold for three deep breaths, then slowly return to the starting position. Repeat with your left leg. Do three times for each leg.

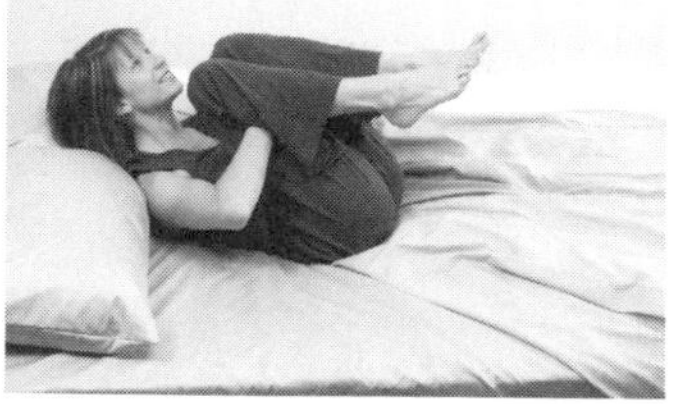

KNEE HUG. Bring both knees in toward your chest, wrapping your arms behind your thighs. Hold in this position for three deep breaths. Then without letting go of your legs, lift your head and bring your forehead toward your knees. Hold for three deep breaths, then slowly release. Do three times.

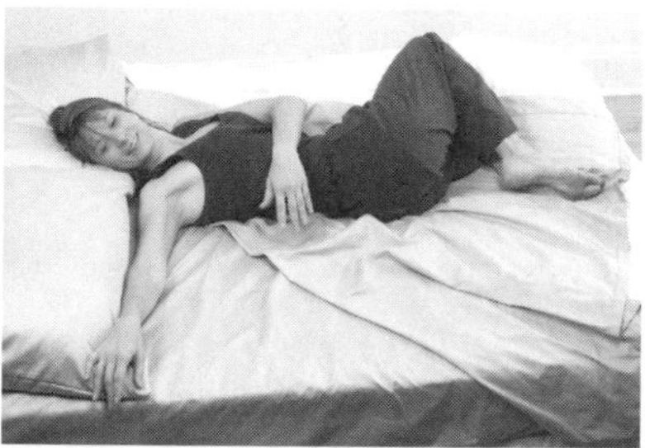

SPINE TWIST. Lie on your back with your knees bent, your feet flat on the bed, and your arms at your sides. Slowly lower your knees to the left, your arms to the right, and look to your right. (You'll have to nudge your spouse out of the way for this one.) Go only as far as comfortable and keep your shoulders down on the bed and your upper body relaxed. Hold for three deep breaths, then slowly return to the starting position. Repeat in opposite directions. Do three stretches to each side.

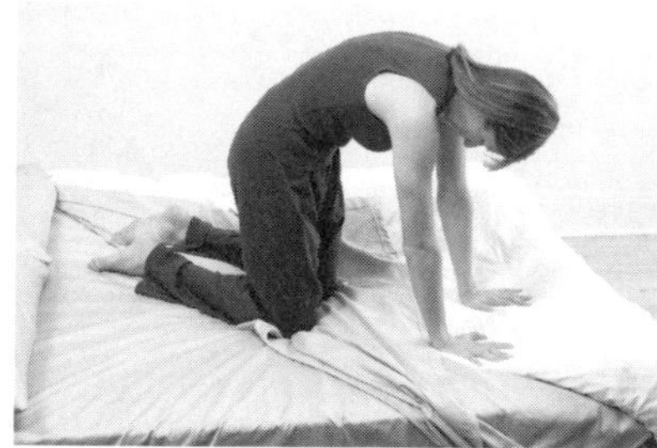

CAT STRETCH. Kneel on all fours. (If your bed is really soft, you may prefer doing this one on the floor.) Pulling your belly toward your spine, drop your head, and round your back. Hold for three deep breaths. Slowly release, dropping your belly toward the floor, arching your back, and looking up toward the ceiling. Hold in this position for three deep breaths, then return to the starting position. Do three times.

Meal Plan

Most of these recipes are custom designed to make 1 serving–no fuss, no muss; just fix, eat, and go! If a recipe makes more than 1 serving, it's noted below. Save that extra serving for another meal, or share it with your spouse or your walking buddy.

Breakfast

Toast and Eggs: Scramble 1 egg and 1 egg white (use omega-3 eggs if you're watching your cholesterol) or ½ cup Egg Beaters in a nonstick skillet coated with cooking spray. (If you'd like, scramble with ¼ cup mushrooms and 1 teaspoon chopped scallions.) Serve with 1 slice whole grain toast spread with 1 teaspoon trans-fat-free margarine, 1 cup fruit salad, and 1 cup fat-free milk.

Healthy Snack

Fruit with Toasted Nuts: Serve 2 cups cut fruit (such as honeydew) with 1½ tablespoons toasted chopped nuts (any variety).

Lunch

Chicken Salad: Makes 2 servings. Mix a 6-ounce can chicken breast meat with 2 teaspoons horseradish spread, 2 tablespoons light mayonnaise, ½ cup finely chopped celery, 10 sliced baby carrots, and 7 halved grapes. Spread half of the mixture on 1 toasted whole grain hamburger roll. Serve with 1 cup fat-free milk.

Healthy Snack

Raisin-Nut Cluster: Mix ½ cup raisins with ½ cup chopped walnuts, 3 tablespoons honey, and 1½ teaspoons maple extract. Spoon the mixture into 4 small paper or plastic cups, and top each cup with ½ teaspoon granulated sugar. Freeze and serve slightly thawed. Makes 4 servings; have one today and save the rest.

Dinner

Salmon with Parmesan Spinach: Makes 2 servings. Microwave a 9-ounce microwave-ready bag (2 cups cooked) fresh baby spinach (such as Ready Pac brand) according to package directions, about 3 minutes. Carefully remove the hot spinach from the bag. Divide into 2 microwave-safe bowls. In each bowl, add ½ cup (3 ounces) cooked salmon or ½ cup (about 3 ounces) cooked chicken strips. Top each bowl with 3 tablespoons Parmesan cheese. Microwave each bowl for 30 to 45 seconds, until the cheese begins to melt. Accompany each serving with 2 slices whole wheat French bread (each slice about the size of your palm).

Indulgent Treat

Graham Crackers with Chocolate and Peanut Butter: Preheat the toaster oven to 250°F. Set out 4 graham cracker squares (2½-inch size). Spread 1 tablespoon mini chocolate chips on 2 squares. Bake for 4 to 6 minutes. Let cool for 1 to 2 minutes. Spread the remaining 2 squares with 1 tablespoon peanut butter. Press one of each together and enjoy.

Nutrient analysis: 1,721 calories, 102 g protein, 194 g carbohydrates, 63 g total fat, 14 g saturated fat, 352 mg cholesterol, 32 g dietary fiber, 1,830 mg sodium, 1,118 mg calcium

The Workout

Level 1

Easy Walk: 20 Minutes

- 5-minute warmup: Walk 2 to 2½ miles per hour, or 95 to 100 steps per minute.
- 10-minute moderate walk: Increase your speed to 2½ to 3 miles per hour, 100 to 115 steps per minute, or a pace that lets you comfortably carry on a conversation.
- 5-minute cooldown: Slow down to 2 to 2½ miles per hour, or 95 to 100 steps per minute.

Basic Strength Training: 20 Minutes

- Do 10 to 12 reps of each exercise. Repeat the sequence of exercises three times.
- To warm up, do not use weights the first time through, and for the squat exercise, only go partway down.

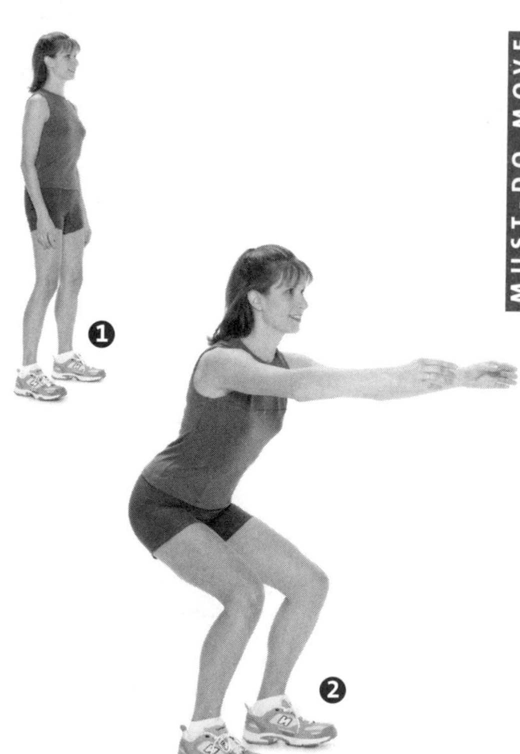

MUST-DO MOVE

Squat

Starting position: Stand with your feet about shoulder width apart, arms at your sides.

Movement: Keeping your back straight, lower yourself, bending from your knees and hips as though you're sitting down, as you inhale. Let your arms come out in front of you to help you balance. Stop just before your thighs are parallel to the floor. Hold for a second and then exhale as you slowly stand back up.

Technique: Don't let your knees move forward over your toes. Don't round your back.

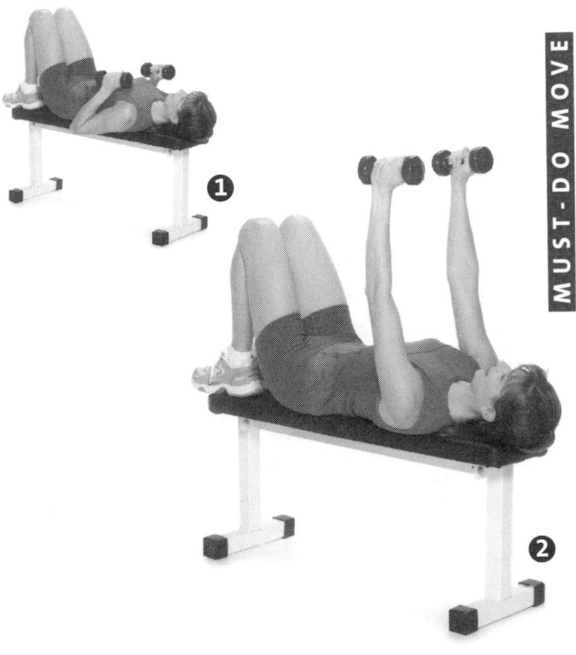

MUST-DO MOVE

Parallel Chest Press

Starting position: Lying on the floor (or on a bench), hold dumbbells parallel and just above your shoulders; your elbows should be pointing toward your feet.

Movement: Exhale as you press the dumbbells straight up over your chest, extending your arms. Hold for a second and then inhale as you slowly lower them.

Technique: Don't press the dumbbells back toward your head or forward toward your feet: They should go straight up and down. Don't arch your back.

Alternate position: If it's uncomfortable to have your feet on the bench, you can place them on the floor. Make sure your back doesn't arch in that position.

MUST-DO MOVE

Seated Bent-Over Row

Starting position: Sit on the edge of a chair with your feet hip width apart and hold a dumbbell in each hand. Keep your back flat and lean forward, bending at the hips so that the dumbbells are hanging at arm's length down by your calves, palms facing each other.

Movement: Bending your elbows back and squeezing your shoulder blades, lift the weights toward your ribs as you exhale. Hold for a second and then inhale as you slowly lower them.

Technique: Don't arch your back. Don't raise your torso as you lift the dumbbells.

Alternate move: If you have back problems, do the rows one arm at a time and place the forearm of your other arm across your thighs for extra support.

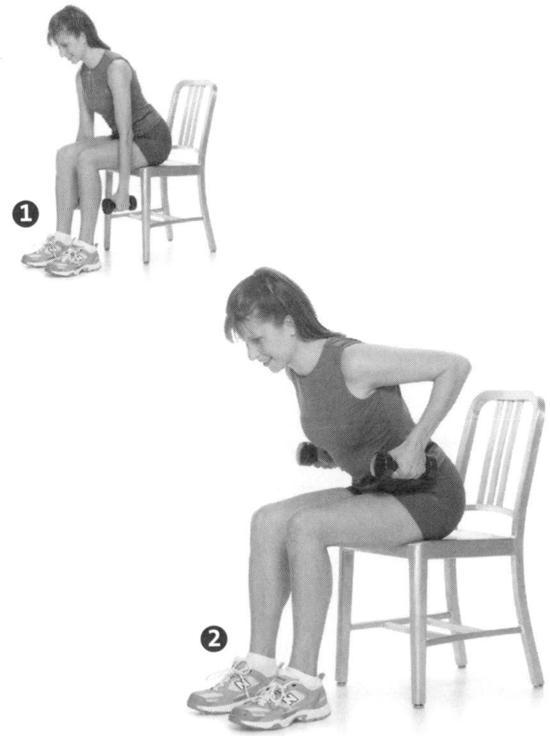

continued

The Workout

Level 1 *continued*

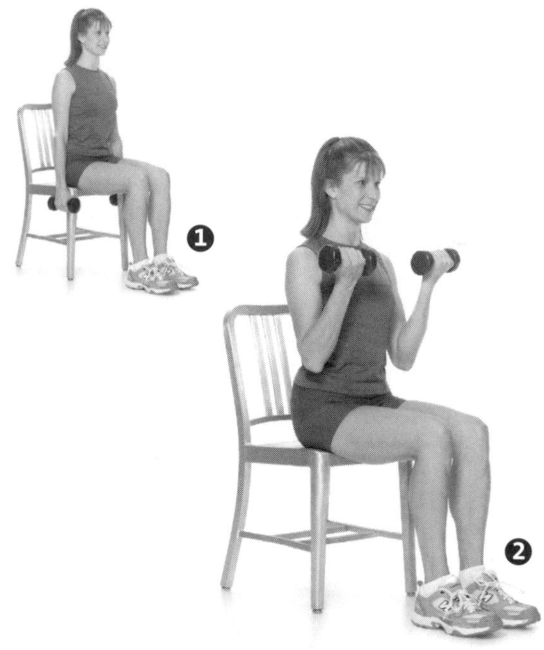

Seated Biceps Curl with a Twist

Starting position: Sit on the edge of a chair with your feet hip width apart and hold dumbbells at your sides, your palms facing in.

Movement: Bending your elbows and turning your wrists upward, lift the dumbbells toward your shoulders as you exhale. Stop when the dumbbells are at chest height, palms facing your body. Hold for a second and then inhale as you slowly lower them.

Technique: Don't move your upper arms.

Seated Triceps Kickback with a Twist

Starting position: Sit on the edge of a chair with your feet hip width apart and hold a dumbbell in each hand. Keep your back flat and lean forward, bending at the hips. Bend your arms at about 90-degree angles with your dumbbells at about hip height.

Movement: Without moving your upper arms, press the dumbbells back as you exhale, extending your arms and turning your wrists so that your palms face the ceiling. Hold for a second and then inhale as you slowly lower them.

Technique: Don't move from your shoulders. Don't raise your torso as you lift the dumbbells.

Alternate move: If you have back problems, do the kickbacks one arm at a time and place the forearm of your other arm across your thighs for extra support.

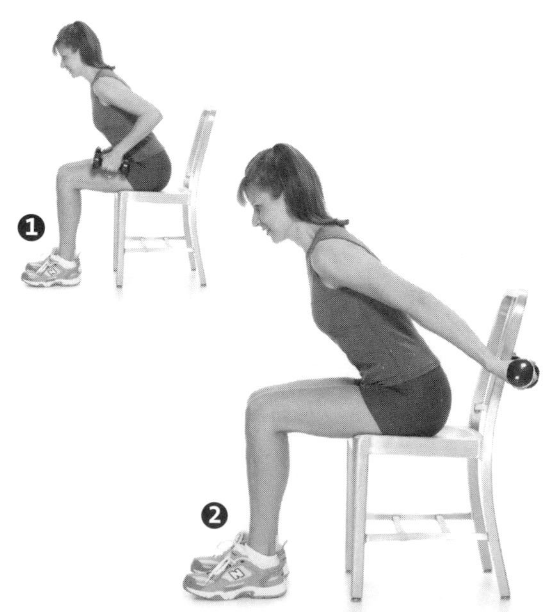

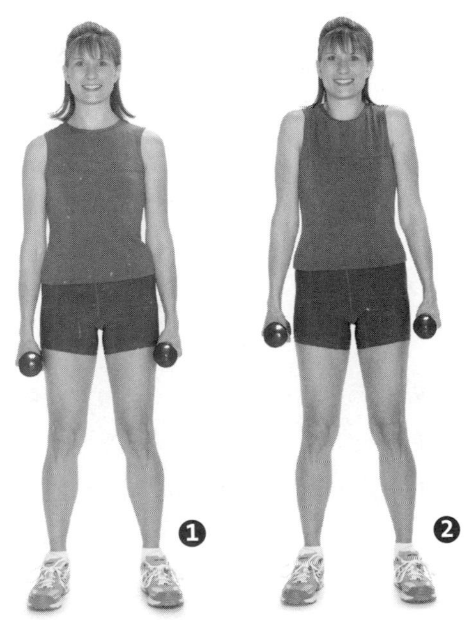

Shoulder Shrug

Starting position: Stand with your feet shoulder width apart, knees bent slightly. Hold a dumbbell in each hand with your arms at your sides, palms facing in.

Movement: Exhale as you slowly lift your shoulders up toward your ears as high as possible. Hold for a second and then inhale as you slowly lower them.

Technique: Don't bend your elbows. Don't use your arms to lift.

FIRM UP TIPS

ENERGY BOOSTER	HAVE FUN!
Drink more water. It has no calories and no nutritional value, but you wouldn't last long—or have much energy—without water. If your body is even ½ cup shy of the amount it normally needs, your physical and mental energy will dip sharply. Keep that from happening by making sure to drink at least eight glasses of water per day (more if you're exercising).	*Rediscover childhood favorites. Dust off your bike—pedaling around town can blast off 400-plus calories in an hour. Or pick up a Frisbee. You don't have to wait until your next picnic to throw one around. A half-hour of tossing and catching works off 100 calories.*

The Workout
Level 2

Easy Walk: 20 Minutes

- 5-minute warmup: Walk 2½ to 3 miles per hour, or 100 to 115 steps per minute.
- 10-minute moderate walk: Increase your speed to 3 to 3½ miles per hour, 115 to 125 steps per minute, or a pace that lets you comfortably carry on a conversation.
- 5-minute cooldown: Slow down to 2½ to 3 miles per hour, or 100 to 115 steps per minute.

Basic Strength Training: 30 Minutes

- Do 10 to 12 reps of each exercise. Repeat the sequence of exercises three times.
- To warm up, use lighter weights, or none at all, the first time through, and for the squat and lunge exercises, only go partway down.

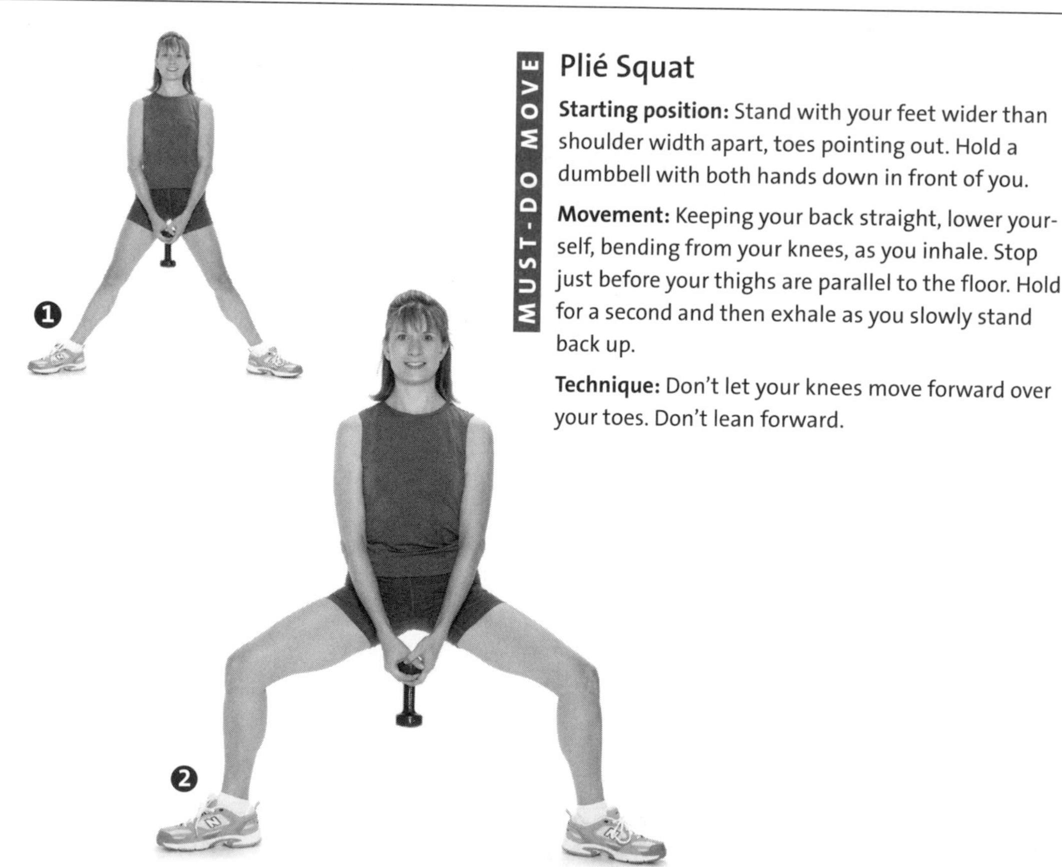

MUST-DO MOVE

Plié Squat

Starting position: Stand with your feet wider than shoulder width apart, toes pointing out. Hold a dumbbell with both hands down in front of you.

Movement: Keeping your back straight, lower yourself, bending from your knees, as you inhale. Stop just before your thighs are parallel to the floor. Hold for a second and then exhale as you slowly stand back up.

Technique: Don't let your knees move forward over your toes. Don't lean forward.

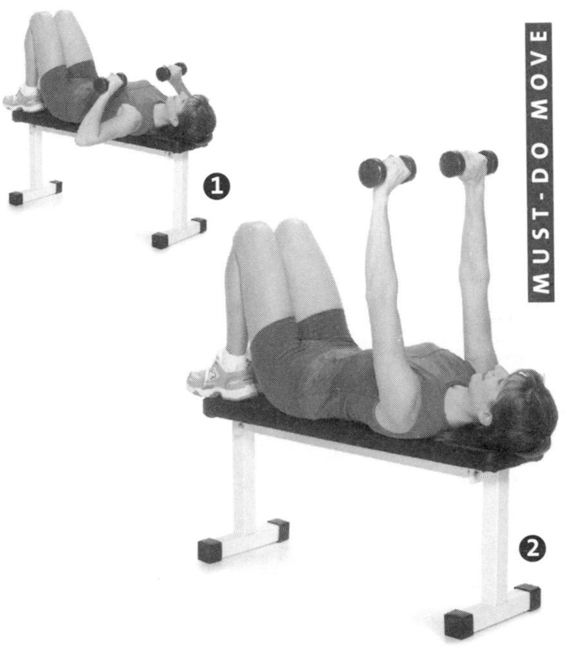

MUST-DO MOVE

Chest Press

Starting position: Lie on the floor (or on a bench) and hold dumbbells end to end, just above your shoulders. Your elbows should be pointing out to the sides.

Movement: Exhale as you press the dumbbells straight up over your chest, extending your arms. Hold for a second and then inhale as you slowly lower them.

Technique: Don't press the dumbbells back toward your head or forward toward your feet: They should go straight up and down. Don't arch your back.

Alternate position: If it's uncomfortable to have your feet on the bench, you can place them on the floor. Make sure your back doesn't arch in that position.

MUST-DO MOVE

Bent-Over Row

Starting position: Stand with your feet shoulder width apart, knees bent slightly. Hold a dumbbell in each hand with your arms at your sides. Keep your back flat and lean forward, bending at the hips so that the dumbbells are hanging at arm's length in front of you, palms facing each other.

Movement: Bending your elbows back and squeezing your shoulder blades, lift the weights toward your ribs as you exhale, until your elbows are higher than your back. Hold for a second and then inhale as you slowly lower them.

Technique: Don't arch your back. Don't pull your shoulders up toward your ears. Don't raise your torso as you lift the dumbbells.

Alternate move: If you have back problems, support yourself with one hand on a chair and do the rows one arm at a time.

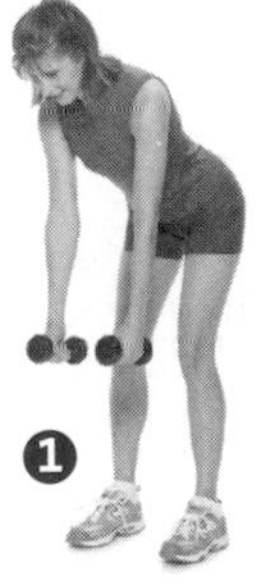

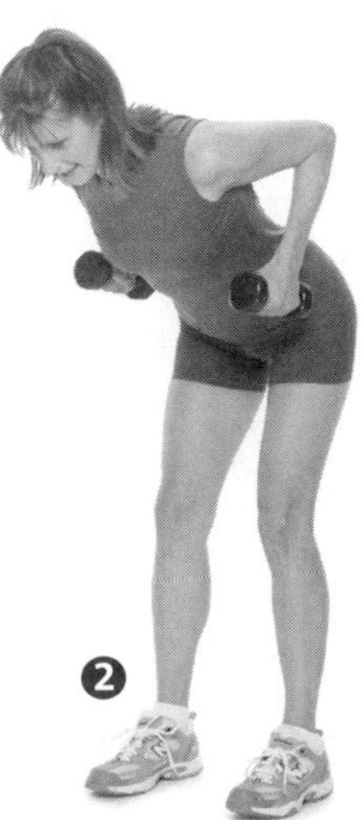

continued

The Workout

Level 2 *continued*

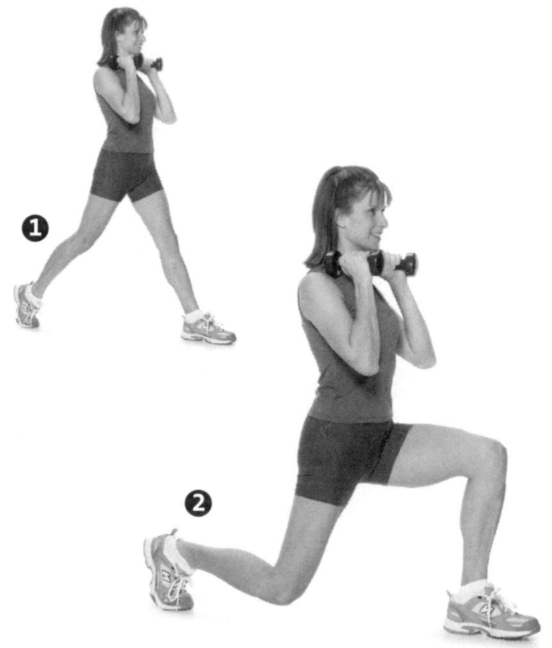

Lunge

Starting position: Stand with your feet 2 to 3 feet apart and your left foot in front of your right. Hold a dumbbell in each hand, either at shoulder height or at your sides.

Movement: Inhale as you bend your left knee and lower your body straight down until your left knee is bent 90 degrees and your right knee nearly touches the floor. Your rear heel will come off the floor. Hold for a second and then exhale as you slowly push yourself back up to the starting position. Finish all of your repetitions, then repeat the exercise with your right foot in front of your left.

Technique: Don't lean forward. Don't let your front knee move forward over your toes.

Biceps Curl

Starting position: Stand with your feet shoulder width apart, knees bent slightly. Hold a dumbbell in each hand with your palms facing forward.

Movement: Bending your elbows, lift the dumbbells toward your shoulders as you exhale. Stop when the dumbbells are at chest height, palms facing your body. Hold for a second and then inhale as you slowly lower them.

Technique: Don't move your upper arms.

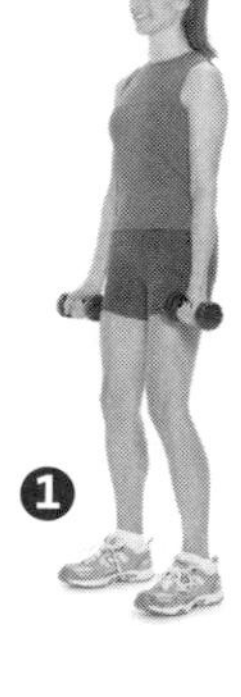

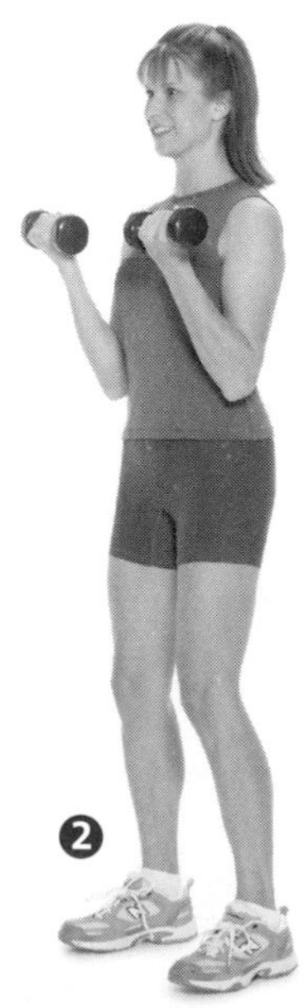

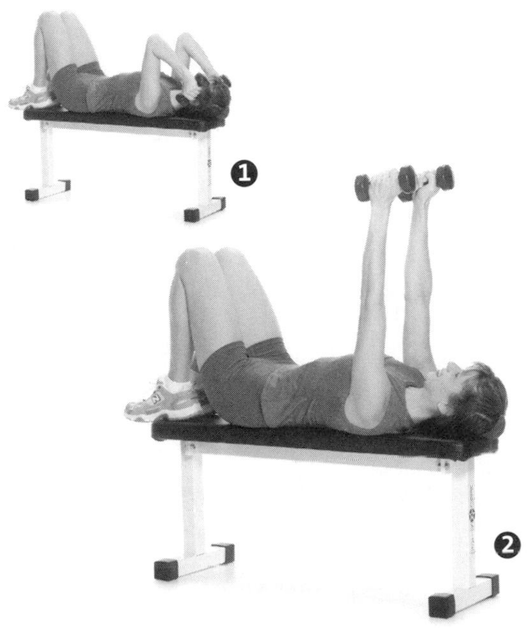

Lying Triceps Extension

Starting position: Lie face up on the floor (or on a bench). Hold a dumbbell in each hand over your chest. Bend your arms so that your elbows are pointing toward the ceiling and the dumbbells are by your ears.

Movement: Without moving your upper arms, press the weights up over your chest as you exhale. Hold for a second and then inhale as you slowly lower them.

Technique: Don't move from your shoulders. Don't arch your back.

Alternate position: If it's uncomfortable to have your feet on the bench, you can place them on the floor. Make sure your back doesn't arch in that position.

Lateral Raise

Starting position: Stand with your feet shoulder width apart, knees bent slightly. Hold a dumbbell in each hand with your arms at your sides, palms facing in, and elbows bent slightly.

Movement: Exhale as you slowly raise the dumbbells out to the sides until they are at about shoulder height. Hold for a second and then inhale as you slowly lower them.

Technique: Don't lift your shoulders. Don't lift higher than shoulder height.

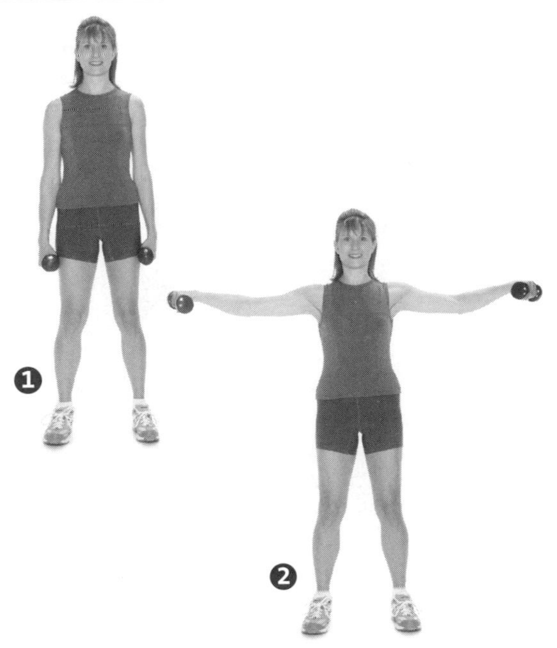

The Workout

Level 3

Easy Walk: 20 Minutes

- 5-minute warmup: Walk 2½ to 3 miles per hour, or 100 to 115 steps per minute.
- 10-minute moderate walk: Increase your speed to 3½ to 4 miles per hour, 125 to 135 steps per minute, or a pace that lets you comfortably carry on a conversation.
- 5-minute cooldown: Slow down to 2½ to 3 miles per hour, or 100 to 115 steps per minute.

Basic Strength Training: 40 Minutes

- Do 10 to 12 reps of each exercise. Repeat the sequence of exercises three times.
- To warm up, use lighter weights, or none at all, the first time through, and for the squat and lunge exercises, only go partway down.

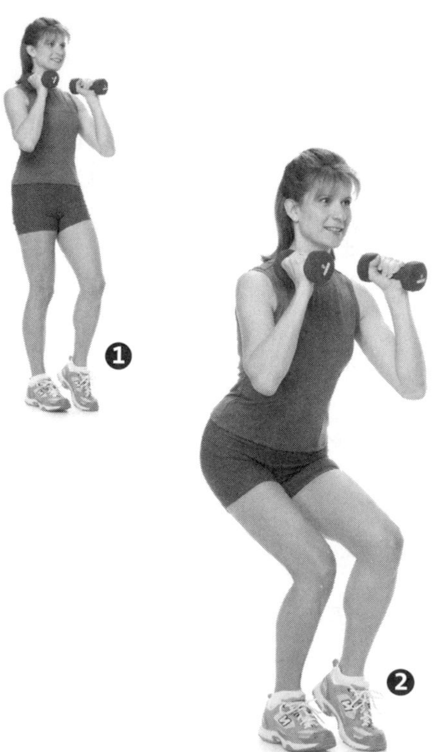

MUST-DO MOVE

One-Leg Squat

Starting position: Hold dumbbells in each hand at shoulder height or down at your sides. Shift your weight to your right foot and lift your left foot off the floor so that only your toes are lightly touching for balance.

Movement: As you inhale, bend your right knee and lean forward slightly from your hips, lowering yourself as if you were sitting in a chair. Go as low as comfortable, but don't go past your right thigh being parallel to the floor. Hold for a second and then exhale as you slowly stand back up. Do the recommended number of reps and then switch legs.

Technique: Don't let your working knee come forward past your toes.

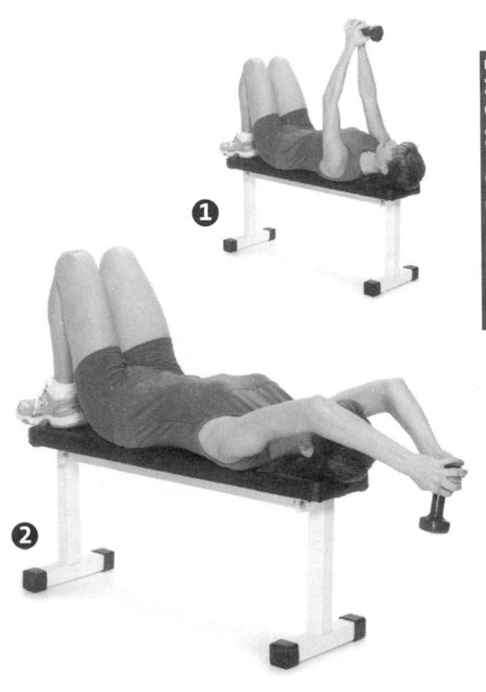

MUST-DO MOVE

Pullover

Starting position: Lie face up on the floor (or on a bench). Grasp a dumbbell with both hands and hold it above your chest with your elbows bent slightly.

Movement: Inhale as you lower the dumbbell backward over your head as far as comfortably possible without bending your elbows any farther than at the start. Hold for a second and then exhale as you slowly raise it to the starting position.

Technique: Don't arch your back. Don't bend your elbows to lower the weight.

Alternate position: If it's uncomfortable to have your feet on the bench, you can place them on the floor. Make sure your back doesn't arch in that position.

MUST-DO MOVE

Wide Bent-Over Row

Starting position: Stand with your feet shoulder width apart, knees bent slightly. Hold a dumbbell in each hand with your arms at your sides. Keep your back flat and lean forward, bending at the hips so that the dumbbells are hanging at arm's length in front of you, palms facing you.

Movement: Bending your elbows out to the sides and squeezing your shoulder blades, lift the dumbbells toward your ribs as you exhale, until your elbows are higher than your back. Hold for a second and then inhale as you slowly lower them.

Technique: Don't arch your back. Don't pull your shoulders up toward your ears. Don't raise your torso as you lift the dumbbells.

Alternate move: If you have back problems, support yourself with one hand on a chair and do the rows one arm at a time.

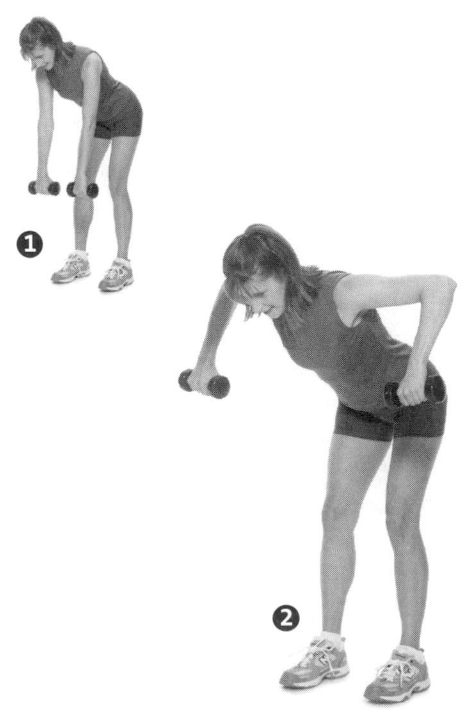

continued

The Workout

Level 3 *continued*

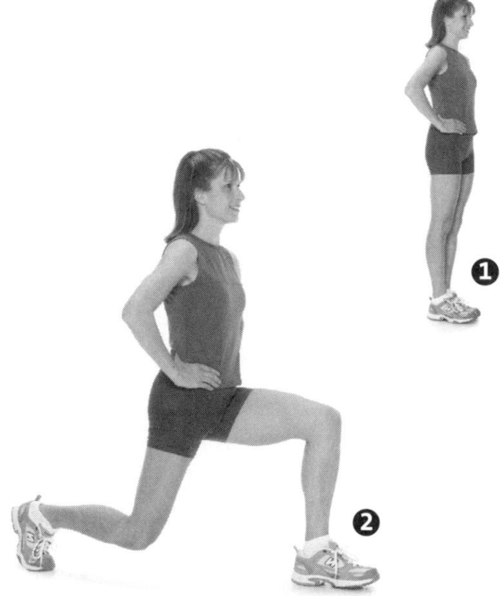

Back Lunge (no weights)

Starting position: Stand with your feet together and place your hands on your hips.

Movement: Step your right foot back 2 to 3 feet. Inhale as you bend your left knee and lower your body straight down until your left knee is bent 90 degrees and your right knee nearly touches the floor. Your rear heel will come off the floor. Hold for a second and then exhale as you push yourself back up, bringing your right foot in. Finish all of your repetitions, then repeat the exercise stepping your left foot back.

Technique: Don't lean forward. Don't let your front knee move forward over your toes.

Biceps Curl

Starting position: Stand with your feet shoulder width apart, knees bent slightly. Hold a dumbbell in each hand with your palms facing forward.

Movement: Bending your elbows, lift the dumbbells toward your shoulders as you exhale. Stop when the dumbbells are at chest height, palms facing your body. Hold for a second and then inhale as you slowly lower them.

Technique: Don't move your upper arms.

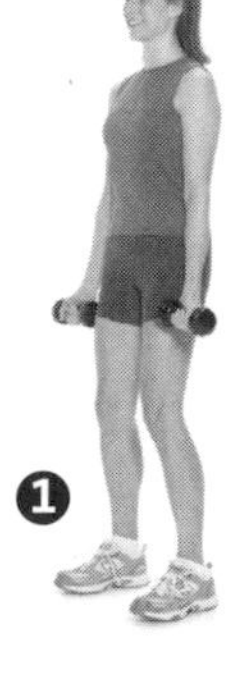

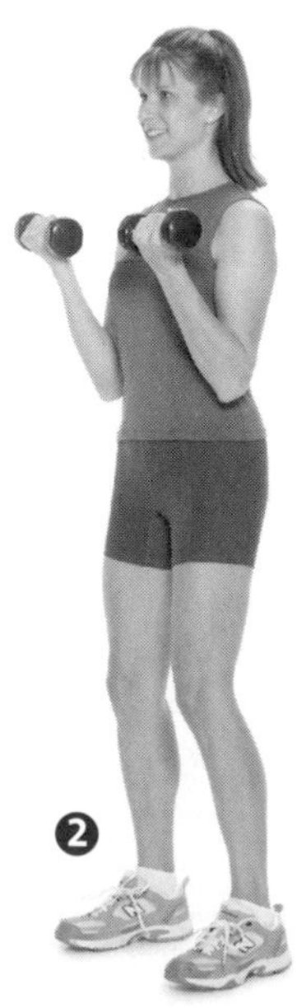

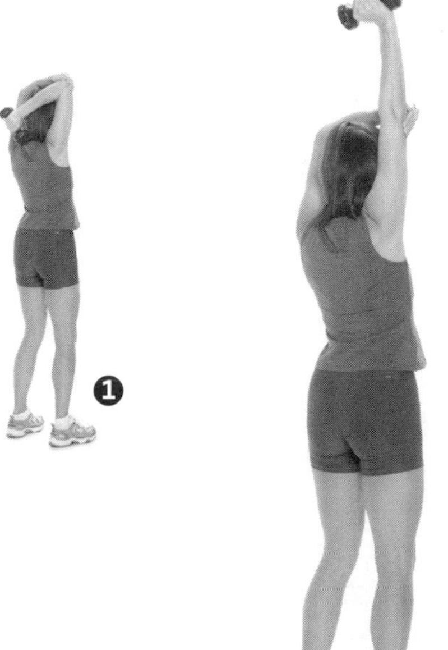

Overhead Triceps Extension

Starting position: Stand with your feet shoulder width apart and knees bent slightly. Hold a dumbbell in your right hand and lift it up over your head. Bend your elbow so that it is pointing toward the ceiling and the dumbbell is behind your head. Place your left hand on your right elbow for support.

Movement: Exhale as you extend your right arm and lift the dumbbell over your head. Hold for a second and then inhale as you slowly lower it. Do the recommended number of reps and then repeat with your left arm.

Technique: Don't lift your shoulders up toward your ears. Don't bend your wrist.

Overhead Press

Starting position: Stand with your feet shoulder width apart and knees bent slightly. Hold a dumbbell in each hand at shoulder height with your palms facing forward and elbows pointing out to the sides.

Movement: Exhale as you slowly press the dumbbells straight up overhead. Hold for a second and then inhale as you slowly lower them.

Technique: Don't arch your back. Don't lift the dumbbells forward or back.

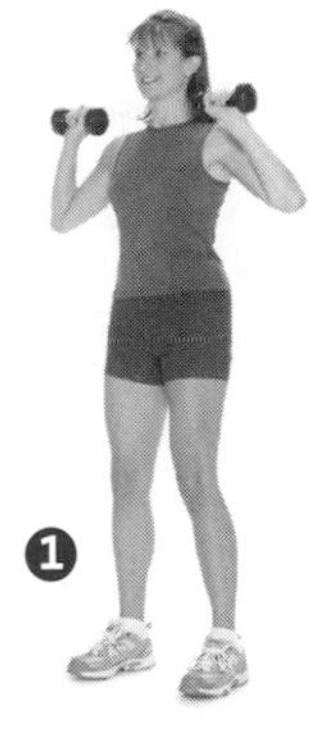

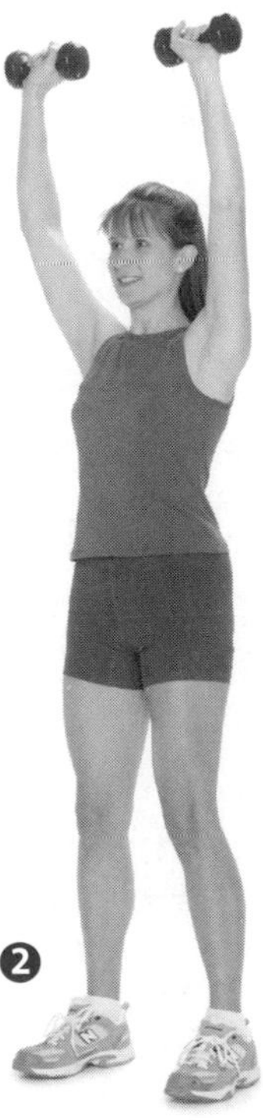

FIRM UP / DAY 2

Gear Up for Walking

One of the great things about walking for exercise is you don't need a lot of equipment, just a good pair of walking shoes. For advice on how to find the right fit, see chapter 10, Walk Off Pounds and Inches. But that's not all that's important when it comes to walking shoes. To keep your feet, knees, and back healthy and injury-free, you need to replace your walking shoes regularly—every 500 to 700 miles. Beyond that distance, even if the shoes don't look worn-out, their shock-absorbing capacity is no longer as good as it used to be. (If you tend to have foot or joint problems, you may need to replace them more frequently—every 300 to 500 miles.)

If you didn't buy a new pair before you started the Firm Up Program and if you're not sure how long you've had your current pair of shoes, set them on a table and examine them from the heel. Does the heel show any signs of wear? Does the upper look as though it has been pushed toward one side by your foot? If you answer yes to either question, it's definitely time to invest in a new pair.

When you buy new shoes, mark the date inside your shoes, in your logbook, or on a calendar. Then, as you rack up miles, you'll know when you need a new pair. Or if you consistently walk, say, 3 miles, 5 days a week (or 15 miles per week), you can mark the "expiration date" of your current shoes on your calendar.

Ideally, you should have two pairs of walking shoes rather than just one. That way, you can allow each pair to dry out completely after each use, minimizing foot odor and creating a less hospitable environment for bacteria and fungi. Plus, when you buy a new pair, you can switch between them and an old pair—one that has already formed to your feet. Your feet will appreciate it!

FIRM UP TIP

ENERGY BOOSTER

Make pleasure a priority every day. It doesn't have to take a lot of time or money. Give yourself time for a 10-minute phone call to a friend you love. Take 5 minutes to cuddle with your spouse. Pet your dog. Rent a funny movie.

Meal Plan

Most of these recipes are custom designed to make 1 serving–no fuss, no muss; just fix, eat, and go! If a recipe makes more than 1 serving, it's noted below. Save that extra serving for another meal, or share it with your spouse or your walking buddy.

Breakfast

Cheerios and Blueberries: Top 1 cup Cheerios (or 100 calories' worth of other whole grain "O"-type cereal) with ½ cup fresh or ¼ cup frozen blueberries, 2 tablespoons chopped almonds, and 1 cup fat-free milk. Drink all the milk.

Healthy Snack

Crackers and Almond Butter: Top 1 Wasa crispbread with 2 teaspoons almond butter. Serve with 1 cup fat-free milk.

Lunch

Bean Burrito: Microwave according to package directions Amy's Bean and Rice Burrito, Amy's Bean and Cheese Burrito, Don Miguel's Lean Olé! Bean and Rice Burrito, or Don Miguel's Chicken and Black Bean Burrito (check the labels for 260 to 280 calories and 6 to 9 grams of fat). Serve with 1 cup celery sticks stuffed with 2 tablespoons reduced-fat cream cheese.

Healthy Snack

Raisin-Nut Cluster: Have 1 serving from Sunday.

Dinner

Beef and Barley in the Slow Cooker: Makes 3 servings. Combine in a slow cooker 12 ounces round, sirloin, or flank steak cut into 1-inch pieces with ½ cup quick barley, 1 can Campbell's Healthy Request Cream of Mushroom soup, 1 cup water, 1½ cups sliced mushrooms (fresh, frozen, or canned), 1½ cups frozen carrots, ½ teaspoon salt, ¼ teaspoon black pepper, and ½ teaspoon dried thyme. Mix well, cover, and cook on low for 7 to 8 hours.

Indulgent Treat

M&Ms: Have a 1½-ounce bag Crispy M&Ms.

Nutrient analysis: 1,705 calories, 73 g protein, 230 g carbohydrates, 60 g total fat, 17 g saturated fat, 111 mg cholesterol, 28 g dietary fiber, 2,126 mg sodium, 1,001 mg calcium

FIRM UP TIP

ON YOUR PLATE

Eat more fruit. In a 12-week study of 35 overweight women, those who ate three pears or apples a day lost 30 percent more weight than women who ate a similar diet minus the added fruit. Researchers believe that fruit's high-fiber, low-calorie combo helps curb overeating because the fiber leaves you feeling fuller on fewer calories.

The Workout

Level 1

Interval Walk: About 30 Minutes

- 5-minute warmup: Walk 2 to 2½ miles per hour, or 95 to 100 steps per minute.
- 4-minute moderate pace: Increase your speed to about 3 miles per hour, or about 115 steps per minute.
- 30-second speedup: Pick up your pace even more to about 3½ miles per hour, or about 125 steps per minute.
- Repeat moderate and speedup intervals four times.
- 5-minute cooldown: Slow down to 2 to 2½ miles per hour, or 95 to 100 steps per minute.

Core Training: 10 Minutes

- Do the exercise sequence one time.

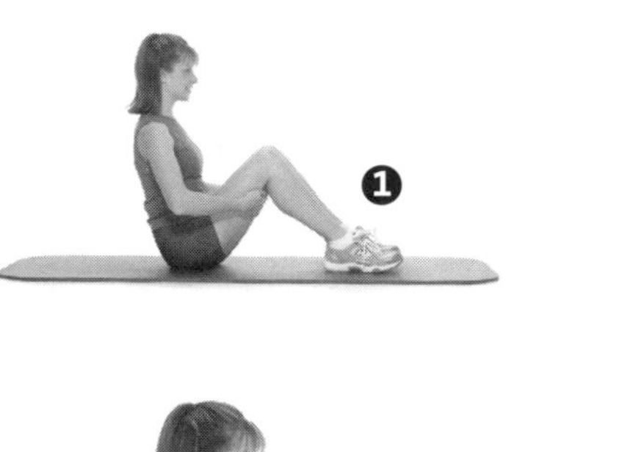

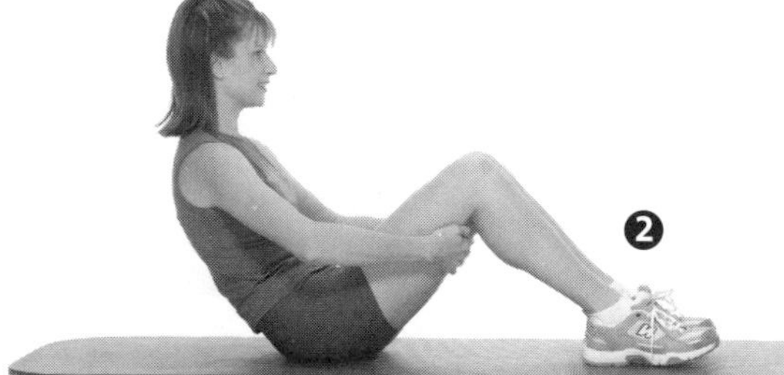

Two-Hand Roll-Down

Starting position: Sit on the floor with your knees bent and your feet flat. Place your hands behind your thighs.

Movement: Using your abs, slowly roll down 2 to 3 inches, one vertebra at a time, as you inhale. Hold for a second and then exhale as you slowly roll back up. Do eight reps.

Technique: Your abs should be powering the move. Don't move quickly.

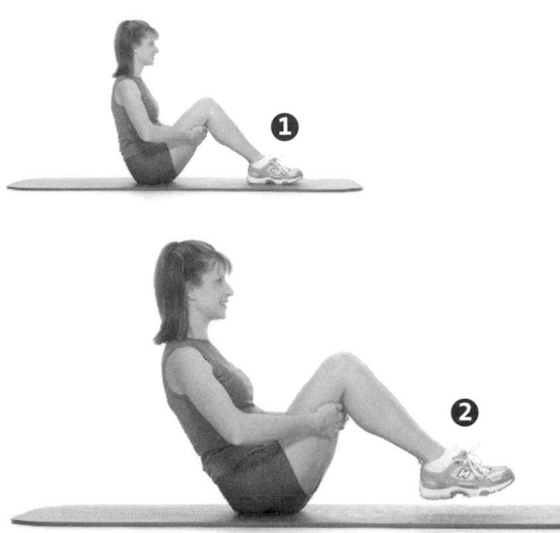

Holding Balance

Starting position: Sit on the floor with your knees bent and your feet flat. Place your hands behind your thighs.

Movement: Lift your feet off the floor slightly and balance on your "sitting bones" (the ones in your derriere). Hold for three slow breaths and then relax. Do one time only.

Technique: Keep your abs tight and the rest of your body relaxed, especially your shoulders.

MUST-DO MOVE

Easy Ab Crunch

Starting position: Lie on your back with your knees bent, feet flat on the floor, and arms at your sides, palms facing down.

Movement: Using your abs, slowly raise your head, shoulders, and upper back about 45 degrees off the floor as you exhale. Think of shortening the distance between your ribs and pelvis. Hold for a second and then inhale as you slowly lower yourself. Do eight reps.

Technique: Don't pull your chin to your chest. Don't arch your back.

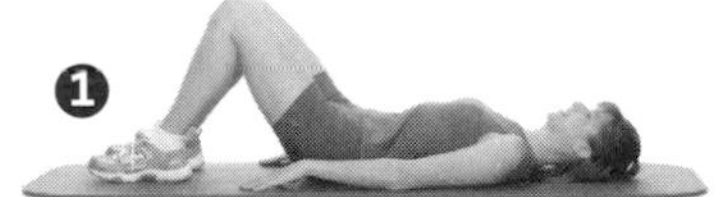

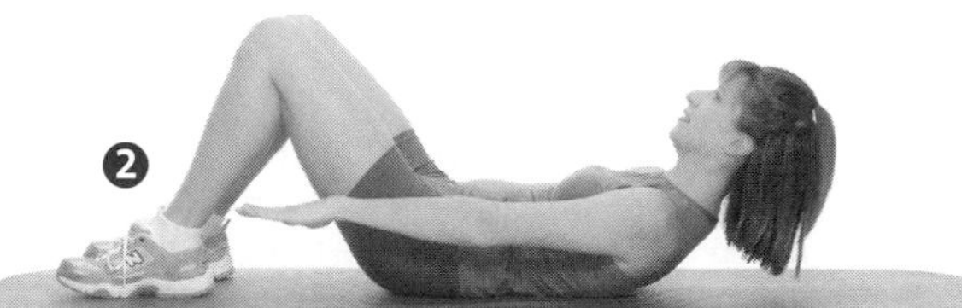

continued

The Workout

Level 1 *continued*

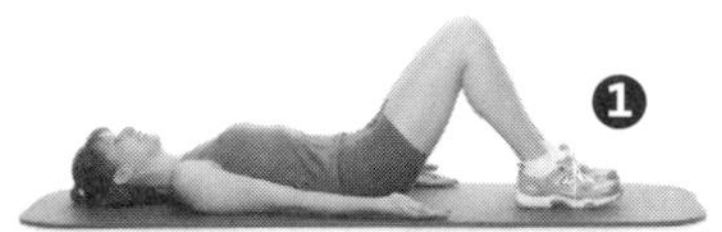

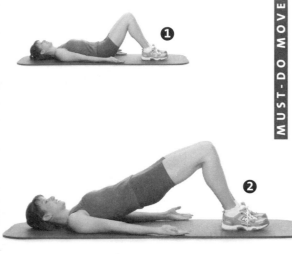

MUST-DO MOVE

Bridge

Starting position: Lie on your back with your knees bent, feet flat on the floor, and arms at your sides, with palms facing up.

Movement: Contracting your abs, buttocks, and lower back, press into your feet and lift your butt, hips, and back off the floor as you exhale, to form a straight line from your shoulders to your knees. Hold for three slow breaths and then relax. Do one time only.

Technique: Don't lift too high—your upper back and shoulders should remain on the floor. Don't bend at the waist or hips. Don't let your knees fall inward or outward.

MUST-DO MOVE

Knee Plank

Starting position: Lie facedown with your knees bent so that your feet are in the air. Your elbows should be under your shoulders and your forearms and palms on the floor.

Movement: Contracting your abs and back, press into your forearms as you exhale and lift your pelvis off the floor so that your back and thighs form a straight line. Hold for three breaths and then relax. Do one time only.

Technique: Don't lift your head up or let it drop. Don't bend at the waist. Don't arch your back.

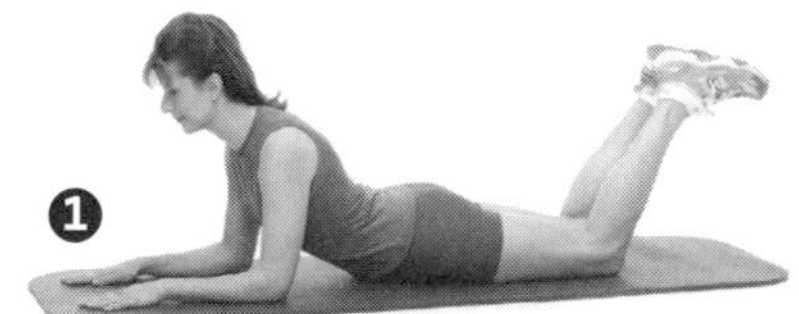

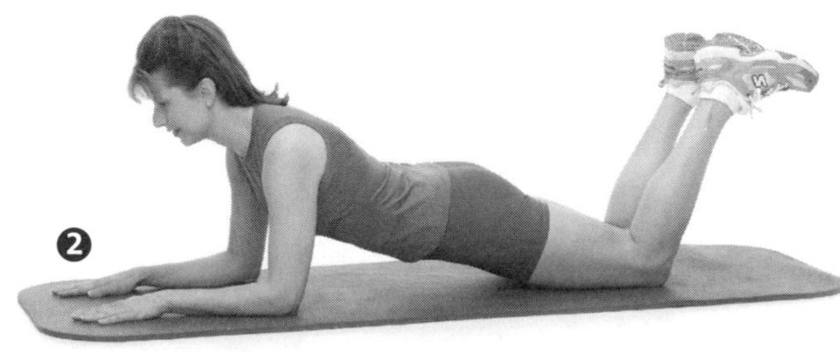

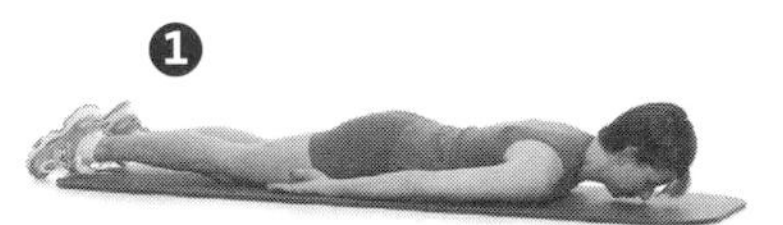

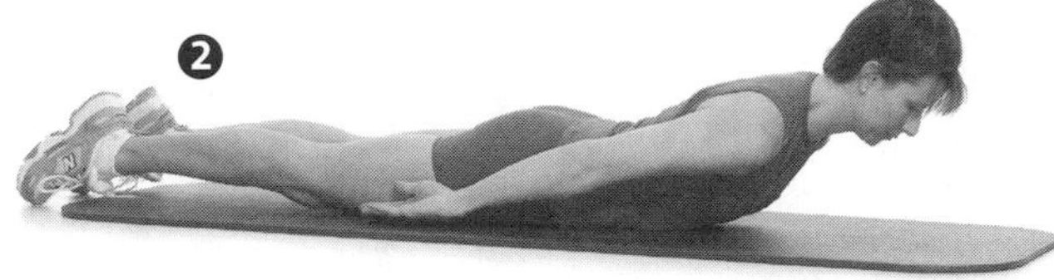

Chest Lift

Starting position: Lie facedown on the floor with your arms at your sides and palms facing up.

Movement: Exhale as you lift your head and chest 5 to 6 inches off the floor. Hold for a second and then inhale as you slowly lower yourself. Do eight reps.

Technique: Don't look up. Don't lift too high.

FIRM UP TIP

MIND OVER MATTER

Focus on the essentials when you're overwhelmed. It's 10:00 P.M., and you still have to clean up the kitchen, fold the laundry, unload the dishwasher, pay the bills, and iron clothes. Just do what is absolutely necessary, such as ironing clothes for the next day or paying the bills if they're due. The rest can wait until tomorrow.

The Workout

Level 2

Interval Walk: About 30 Minutes

- 5-minute warmup: Walk 2½ to 3 miles per hour, or 100 to 115 steps per minute.
- 3-minute moderate pace: Increase your speed to about 3½ miles per hour, or about 125 steps per minute.
- 90-second speedup: Pick up your pace even more to about 4 miles per hour, or about 135 steps per minute.
- Repeat moderate and speedup intervals four times.
- 5-minute cooldown: Slow down to 2½ to 3 miles per hour, or 100 to 115 steps per minute.

Core Training: 10 Minutes

- Do the exercise sequence one time.

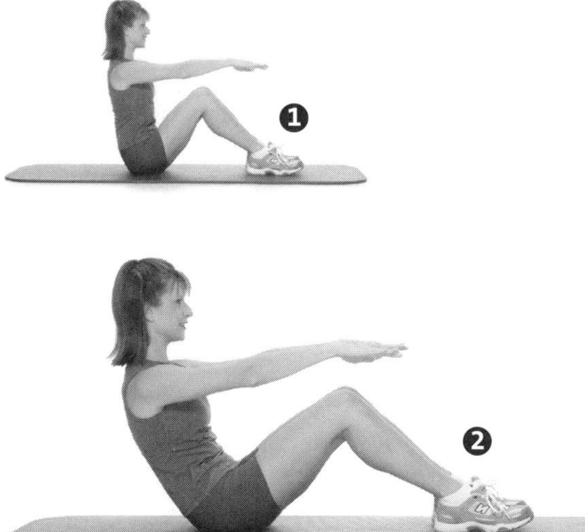

Roll-Down

Starting position: Sit on the floor with your knees bent and your feet flat. Hold your arms straight out in front of you, parallel to the floor.

Movement: Using your abs, slowly roll down 3 to 4 inches, one vertebra at a time, as you inhale. Hold for a second and then exhale as you slowly roll back up. Do eight reps.

Technique: Your abs should be powering the move. Don't move quickly.

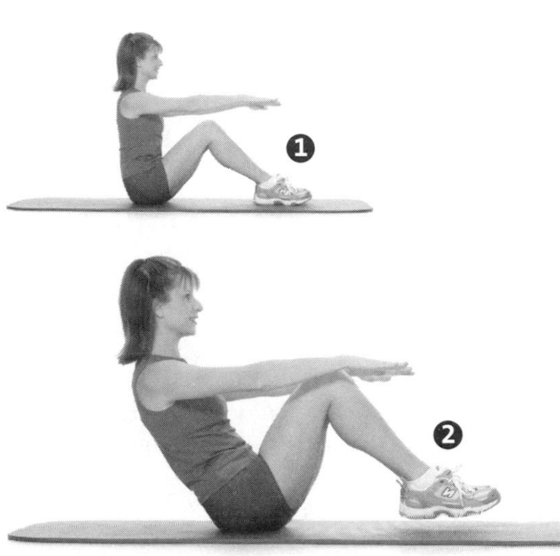

Partial Balance

Starting position: Sit on the floor with your knees bent and your feet flat. Hold your arms straight out in front of you, parallel to the floor.

Movement: Lift your feet off the floor slightly and balance on your "sitting bones" (the ones in your derriere). Hold for four breaths and then relax. Do one time only.

Technique: Keep your abs tight and the rest of your body relaxed, especially your shoulders.

MUST-DO MOVE

Ab Crunch

Starting position: Lie on your back with your knees bent, feet flat on the floor, and hands behind your head.

Movement: Using your abs, slowly raise your head, shoulders, and upper back about 45 degrees off the floor as you exhale. Think of shortening the distance between your ribs and pelvis. Hold for a second and then inhale as you slowly lower yourself. Do eight reps.

Technique: Don't pull your chin to your chest. Don't arch your back.

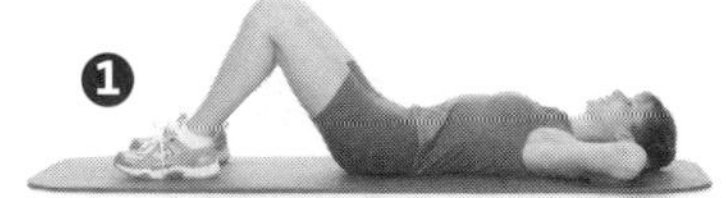

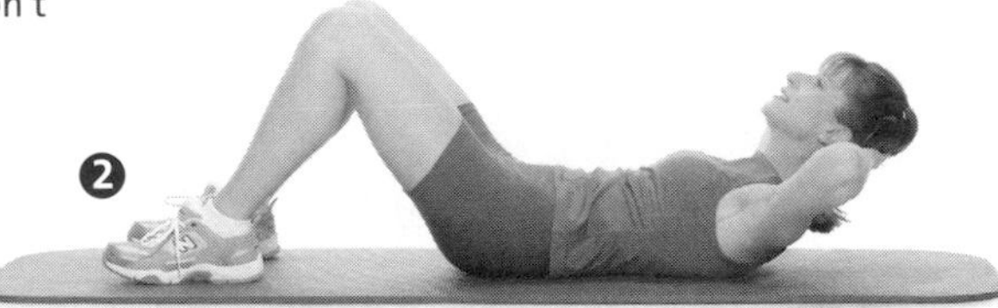

continued

The Workout

Level 2 *continued*

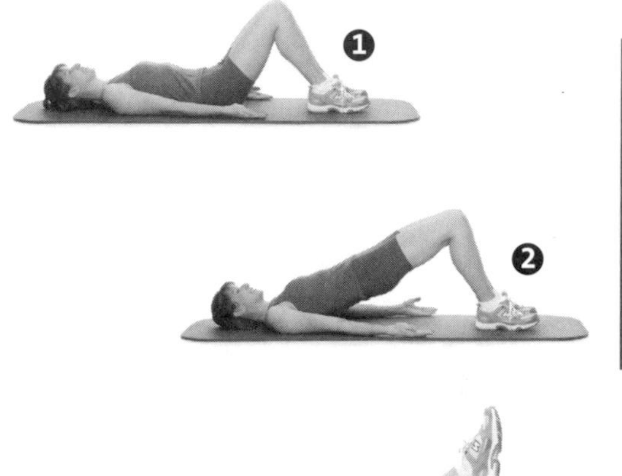

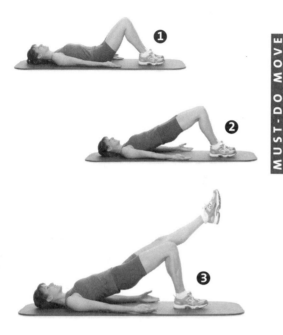

MUST-DO MOVE

Bridge with Leg Lift

Starting position: Lie on your back with your knees bent, feet flat on the floor, and arms at your sides, palms facing up.

Movement: Contracting your abs, buttocks, and lower back, press into your feet and lift your butt, hips, and back off the floor as you exhale, to form a straight line from your shoulders to your knees. Lift one foot off the floor and extend that leg. Hold for two breaths and then lower your foot. Lift the other foot up and hold for two breaths. Lower your foot and return to the starting position. Do one time only.

Technique: Don't lift too high—your upper back and shoulders should remain on the floor. Don't bend at the waist or hips. Don't let your knees fall inward or outward.

MUST-DO MOVE

Plank

Starting position: Lie facedown with your feet flexed and toes tucked. Your elbows should be under your shoulders and your forearms and palms on the floor.

Movement: Contracting your abs and back, press into your forearms as you exhale and lift your pelvis and legs off the floor so that your back and legs form a straight line. Hold for four breaths and then relax. Do one time only.

Technique: Don't lift your head up or let it drop. Don't bend at the waist or hips. Don't let your belly drop toward the floor.

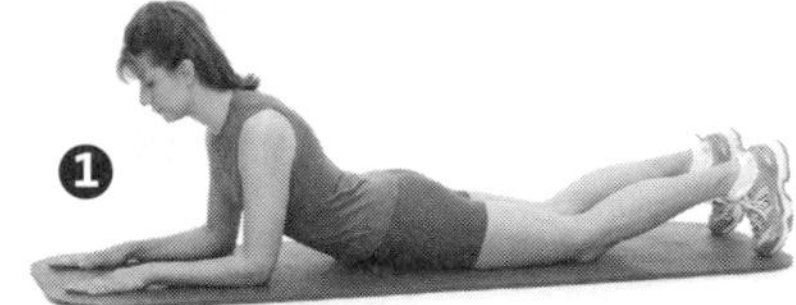

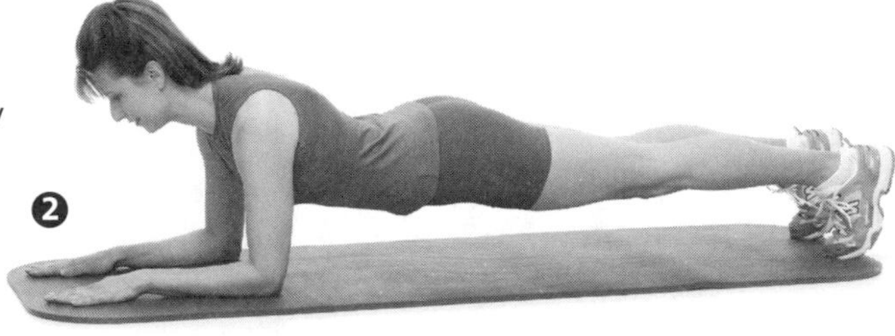

❶

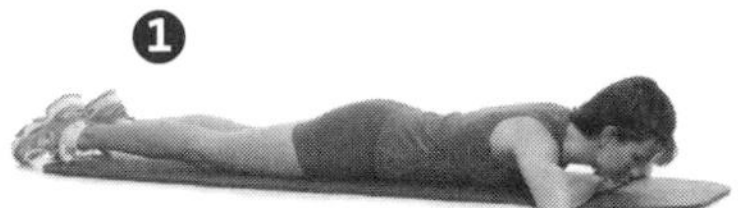

❷

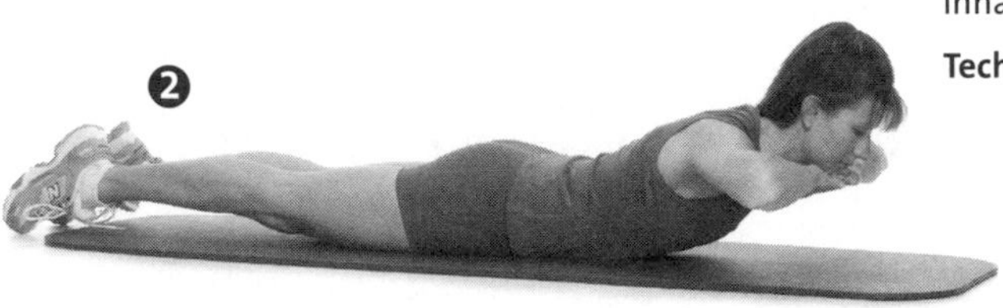

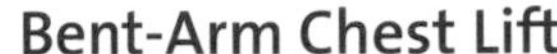

Bent-Arm Chest Lift

Starting position: Lie facedown on the floor with your hands under your chin.

Movement: Exhale as you lift your head and chest 5 to 6 inches off the floor. Hold for a second and then inhale as you slowly lower yourself. Do eight reps.

Technique: Don't lift too high.

FIRM UP TIP

FIT FACT

The treadmill can be as mood-altering as some illegal drugs! In a study of 20 healthy men, British researchers found that those who ran on a treadmill for 30 minutes produced 77 percent more phenylethylamine—a natural mood-lifting chemical similar to amphetamine—than those who stayed sedentary. And the effect lasted for 24 hours.

The Workout

Level 3

Interval Walk: About 30 Minutes

- 5-minute warmup: Walk 2½ to 3 miles per hour, or 100 to 115 steps per minute.
- 2-minute moderate pace: Increase your speed to about 4 miles per hour, or about 135 steps per minute.
- 2-minute speedup: Pick up your pace even more to about 4½ miles per hour, or about 145 steps per minute.
- Repeat moderate and speedup intervals five times.
- 5-minute cooldown: Slow down to 2½ to 3 miles per hour, or 100 to 115 steps per minute.

Core Training: 10 Minutes

- Do the exercise sequence one time.

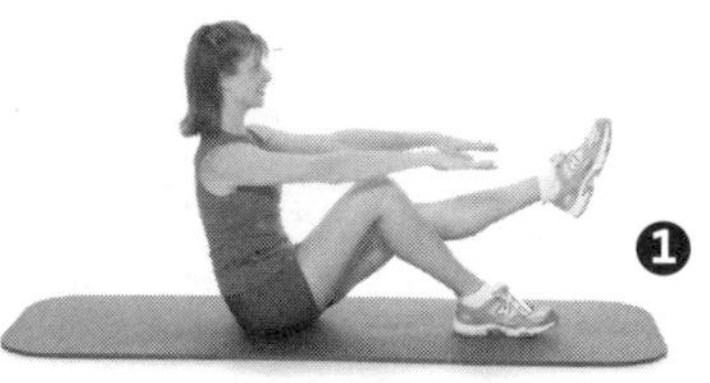

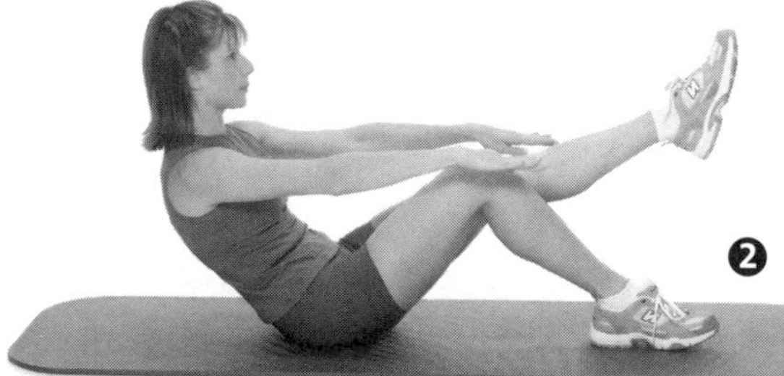

One-Leg Roll-Down

Starting position: Sit on the floor with your knees bent and your feet flat. Lift your left foot off the floor and extend your left leg. Hold your arms straight out in front of you, parallel to the floor.

Movement: Using your abs, slowly roll down 4 to 5 inches, one vertebra at a time, as you inhale. Hold for a second and then exhale as you slowly roll back up. Do four reps, switch legs, and do four more reps.

Technique: Your abs should be powering the move. Don't move quickly.

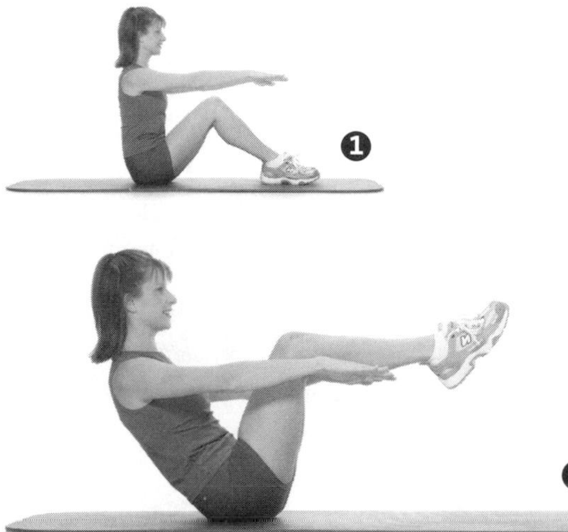

Full Balance

Starting position: Sit on the floor with your knees bent and your feet flat. Hold your arms straight out in front of you, parallel to the floor.

Movement: Lift your feet so that your calves are parallel to the floor, and balance on your "sitting bones" (the ones in your derriere). Hold for five breaths and then relax. Do one time only.

Technique: Keep your abs tight and the rest of your body relaxed, especially your shoulders.

MUST-DO MOVE

Legs-Up Ab Crunch

Starting position: Lie on your back with your legs in the air and your hands behind your head.

Movement: Using your abs, slowly raise your head, shoulders, and upper back about 45 degrees off the floor as you exhale. Think of shortening the distance between your ribs and pelvis. Hold for a second and then inhale as you slowly lower yourself. Do eight reps.

Technique: Don't pull your chin to your chest.

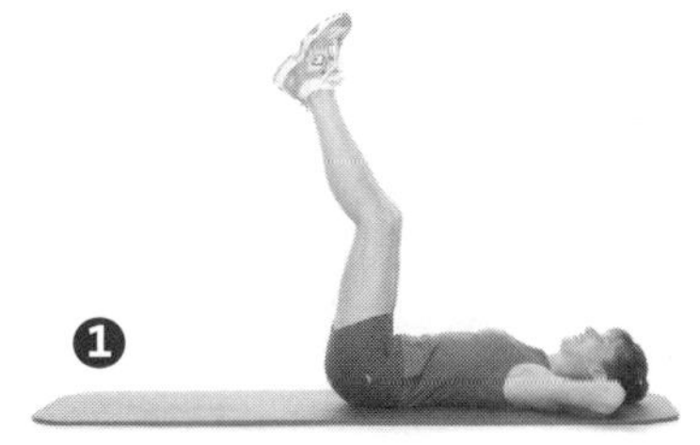

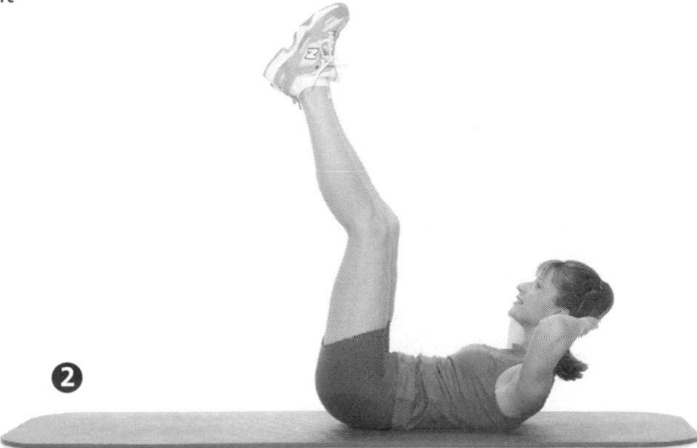

continued

The Workout

Level 3 *continued*

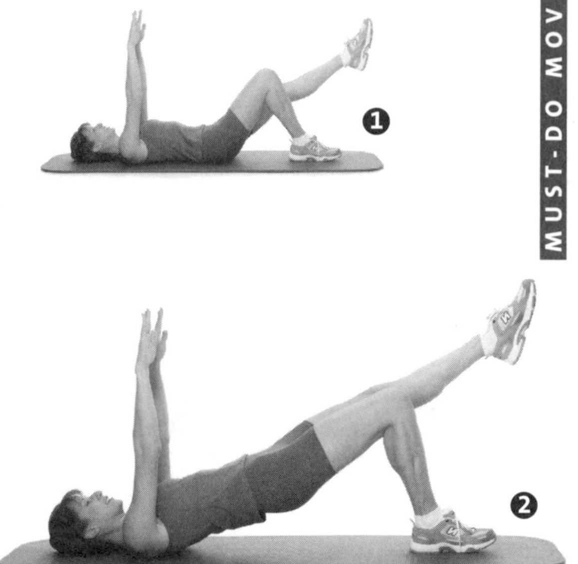

MUST-DO MOVE

One-Leg Bridge with Arms Up

Starting position: Lie on your back with your knees bent, feet flat on the floor, and arms extended over your chest. Lift your left foot off the floor and extend your left leg.

Movement: Contracting your abs, buttocks, and lower back, press into your right foot and lift your butt, hips, and back off the floor as you exhale, to form a straight line from your shoulders to your knees. Hold for three breaths and then lower yourself. Repeat with your right leg extended. Do one time only with each leg.

Technique: Don't lift too high—your upper back and shoulders should remain on the floor. Don't bend at the waist or hips. Don't let your knees fall inward or outward.

MUST-DO MOVE

Plank with Leg Lift

Starting position: Lie facedown with your feet flexed and toes tucked. Your elbows should be under your shoulders and your forearms and palms on the floor.

Movement: Contracting your abs and back, press into your hands and forearms as you exhale and lift your pelvis and legs off the floor so that your back and legs form a straight line. Lift your left foot off the floor, hold for three breaths, and then relax. Repeat by lifting your right foot off the floor. Do one time only with each leg.

Technique: Don't lift your head up or let it drop. Don't bend at the waist or hips. Don't let your belly drop toward the floor.

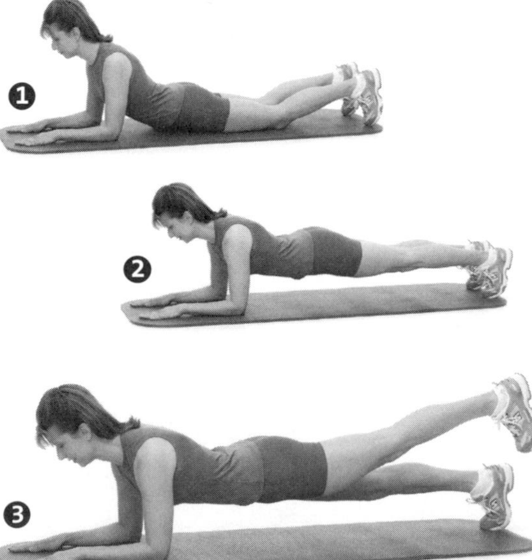

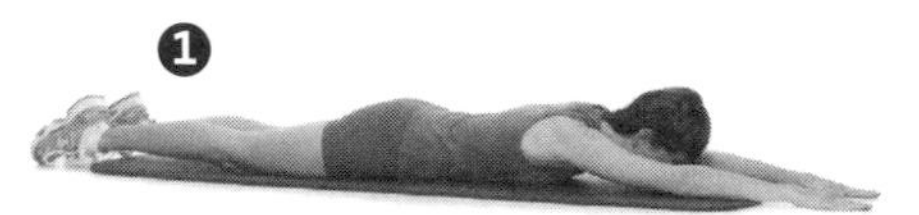

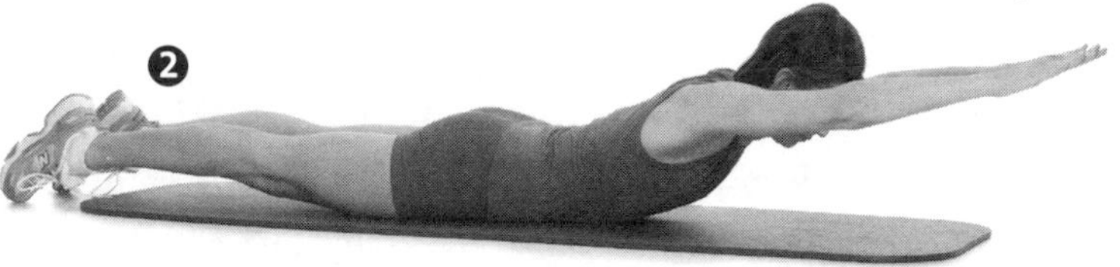

Extended Chest Lift

Starting position: Lie facedown on the floor with your arms extended overhead.

Movement: Exhale as you lift your arms, head, and chest 5 to 6 inches off the floor. Hold for a second and then inhale as you slowly lower yourself. Do eight reps.

Technique: Don't lift too high.

FIRM UP TIP

MIND OVER MATTER

Write your worries down. Review them for just 15 minutes a day—if you must! We can't control whether a terrorist is cooking up a threat or whether it will rain at rush hour, but we can control how much time we spend worrying. Each time a worry pops into your mind, jot it down, place it in an envelope, then forget about it. At the end of the day, give yourself 15 minutes to review your worry notes. You'll learn two things: One, you can control how much time you spend worrying, and two, worry is repetitive—a little goes a long way.

FIRM UP / DAY 3

Think Yourself Thinner

When you're trying to get in shape, your mind can be both your best friend and your worst enemy. At a moment's notice, the strong inner voice that encouraged you to exercise or cut back on fat can turn cruel, undermining your weight-loss efforts with negative emotions and an endless stream of criticism. You tend to achieve what you focus on, so when negativity gets you down, you need to fight back–fast.

Muzzle that inner critic. A friend who constantly told you how fat you looked probably wouldn't be your friend for very long. So if you wouldn't put up with that kind of abuse from others, don't put up with it from yourself. Every time you hear your inner critic, stop what you're doing. Then think of something to encourage yourself, just as you'd try to encourage a friend. Say to yourself, "Okay, my body isn't as thin and fit as I'd like, but I'm working on it. I'm making progress."

Banish all-or-nothing thinking. Just because you don't have 45 minutes to work out doesn't mean that you should skip exercising entirely. After I had my son, I had to tell myself this over and over again. My workouts became more casual. Forget changing into exercise clothes; I'd just slip on my sneakers for a quick walk around the block with Jacob on my shoulders. Or I'd go up and down the steps an extra time whenever I used them at work. Doing something is better than doing nothing. That's why every day in the Firm Up Action Plan, we give you quickie workout options for those days when you just don't have time for the whole thing.

FIRM UP TIP

ON YOUR PLATE

Eat slowly for the first 10 minutes of a meal. Do this, and your brain will help you lose weight. High-tech images of the brains of 21 adults showed that 10 minutes after they started eating a meal, their brains turned off their appetite switches. At that point, the urge to continue eating lessens. So learn to pace yourself for 10 minutes instead of wolfing down your food, and you'll find yourself satisfied with a smaller meal.

Meal Plan

Most of these recipes are custom designed to make 1 serving–no fuss, no muss; just fix, eat, and go! If a recipe makes more than 1 serving, it's noted below. Save that extra serving for another meal, or share it with your spouse or your walking buddy.

Breakfast

Waffle with Peanut Butter: Toast 1 frozen whole grain waffle. Spread with 1½ tablespoons peanut butter. Serve with 1 cup fruit of your choice and ½ cup fat-free milk.

Healthy Snack

Nutty Yogurt: Top 8 ounces (1 cup) fat-free yogurt (any flavor–check the label for no more than 120 calories per cup) with 2 tablespoons chopped walnuts.

Lunch

Subway Sandwiches: Order a 6-inch Subway Veggie Delite on wheat bread with 2 servings (4 triangles) cheese of any type and 1 tablespoon light mayo, honey mustard, or Southwest dressing. Ask them to stuff your sandwich with veggies, such as tomatoes and peppers. Or have the Subway Deli Tuna, Ham, Roast Beef, or Turkey Breast Sandwich ("deli" sandwiches are on smaller rolls than subs) with a Veggie Delite salad, and use 1 tablespoon fat-free Italian dressing.

Indulgent Treat

Silhouette Ice Cream Sandwich: Serve 1 Silhouette ice cream sandwich with a 2½-inch graham cracker square topped with 2 teaspoons peanut butter.

Dinner

Pasta and Turkey Meatballs: Prepare 1 cup cooked pasta (any type). Simmer 3 (1-ounce) turkey meatballs in a nonstick skillet containing ½ inch water (replenish the water if needed during cooking). Top with ¼ cup spaghetti sauce, and serve with ⅔ cup cooked green beans.

To make turkey meatballs, combine 1 pound ground turkey breast meat with ⅓ cup Italian-style bread crumbs and 1 egg and mix thoroughly. (This makes 12 meatballs, about 1¾ inches in diameter each. Save 3 for tomorrow and freeze extras in a tightly sealed plastic bag for future meals.)

Healthy Snack

Pudding and Fruit: Have 1 ready-to-serve fat-free pudding cup (any flavor). Serve with ¾ cup blueberries.

Nutrient analysis: 1,629 calories, 92 g protein, 223 g carbohydrates, 44 g total fat, 7 g saturated fat, 128 mg cholesterol, 29 g dietary fiber, 2,764 mg sodium, 1,227 mg calcium

FIRM UP TIP

GET FIRM FASTER

Declare this no-TV Tuesday. One day a week, turn off the TV and computer. Fill that time by playing with the kids or dancing the night away. Once you see how good you feel, it may become a habit.

The Workout

Level 1

Easy Walk: 20 Minutes

- 5-minute warmup: Walk 2 to 2½ miles per hour, or 95 to 100 steps per minute.
- 10-minute moderate walk: Increase your speed to 2½ to 3 miles per hour, 100 to 115 steps per minute, or a pace that lets you comfortably carry on a conversation.
- 5-minute cooldown: Slow down to 2 to 2½ miles per hour, or 95 to 100 steps per minute.

Basic Strength Training: 20 Minutes

- Do 10 to 12 reps of each exercise. Repeat the sequence of exercises three times.
- To warm up, don't use weights the first time through, and for the squat exercise, only go partway down.

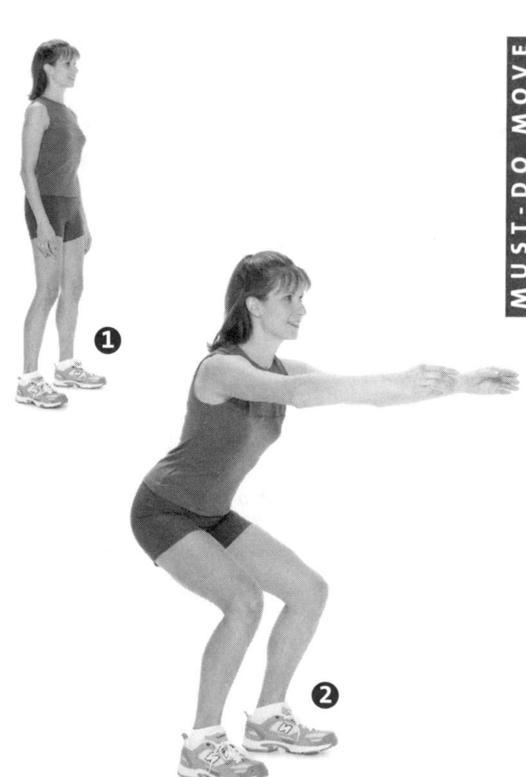

MUST-DO MOVE

Squat

Starting position: Stand with your feet about shoulder width apart, arms at your sides.

Movement: Keeping your back straight, lower yourself, bending from your knees and hips as though you're sitting down, as you inhale. Let your arms come out in front of you to help you balance. Stop just before your thighs are parallel to the floor. Hold for a second and then exhale as you slowly stand back up.

Technique: Don't let your knees move forward over your toes. Don't round your back.

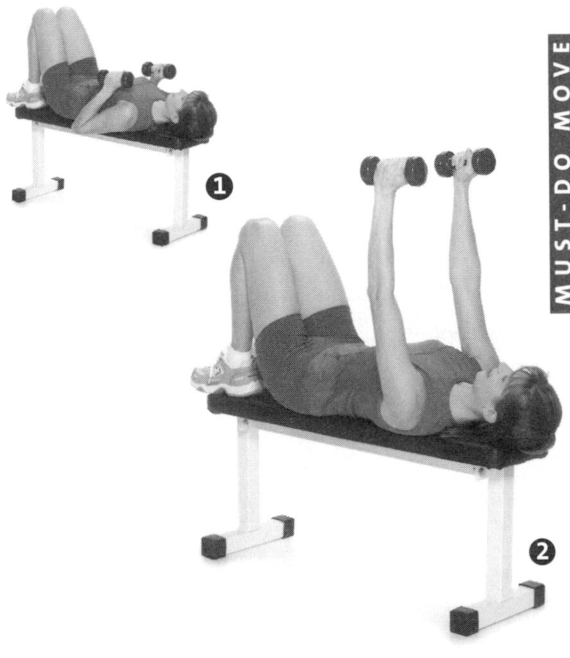

MUST-DO MOVE

Parallel Chest Press

Starting position: Lying on the floor (or on a bench), hold dumbbells parallel and just above your shoulders; your elbows should be pointing toward your feet.

Movement: Exhale as you press the dumbbells straight up over your chest, extending your arms. Hold for a second and then inhale as you slowly lower them.

Technique: Don't press the dumbbells back toward your head or forward toward your feet: They should go straight up and down. Don't arch your back.

Alternate position: If it's uncomfortable to have your feet on the bench, you can place them on the floor. Make sure your back doesn't arch in that position.

MUST-DO MOVE

Seated Bent-Over Row

Starting position: Sit on the edge of a chair with your feet hip width apart and hold a dumbbell in each hand. Keep your back flat and lean forward, bending at the hips so that the dumbbells are hanging at arm's length down by your calves, palms facing each other.

Movement: Bending your elbows back and squeezing your shoulder blades, lift the weights toward your ribs as you exhale. Hold for a second and then inhale as you slowly lower them.

Technique: Don't arch your back. Don't raise your torso as you lift the dumbbells.

Alternate move: If you have back problems, do the rows one arm at a time and place the forearm of your other arm across your thighs for extra support.

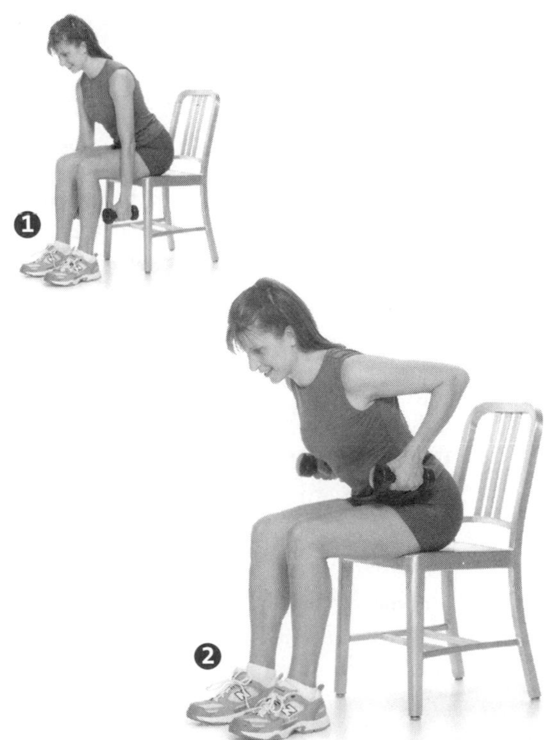

continued

The Workout

Level 1 *continued*

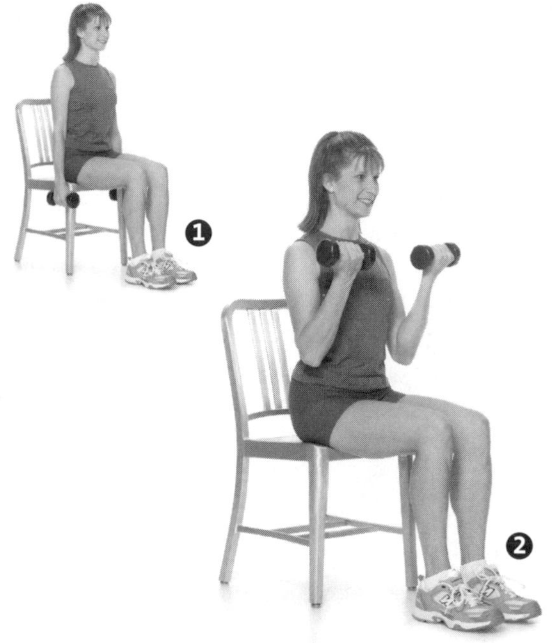

Seated Biceps Curl with a Twist

Starting position: Sit on the edge of a chair with your feet hip width apart and hold dumbbells at your sides, your palms facing in.

Movement: Bending your elbows and turning your wrists upward, lift the dumbbells toward your shoulders as you exhale. Stop when the dumbbells are at chest height, palms facing your body. Hold for a second and then inhale as you slowly lower them.

Technique: Don't move your upper arms.

Seated Triceps Kickback with a Twist

Starting position: Sit on the edge of a chair with your feet hip width apart and hold a dumbbell in each hand. Keep your back flat and lean forward, bending at the hips. Bend your arms at about 90-degree angles with your dumbbells at about hip height.

Movement: Without moving your upper arms, press the dumbbells back as you exhale, extending your arms and turning your wrists so that your palms face the ceiling. Hold for a second and then inhale as you slowly lower them.

Technique: Don't move from your shoulders. Don't raise your torso as you lift the dumbbells.

Alternate move: If you have back problems, do the kickbacks one arm at a time and place the forearm of your other arm across your thighs for extra support.

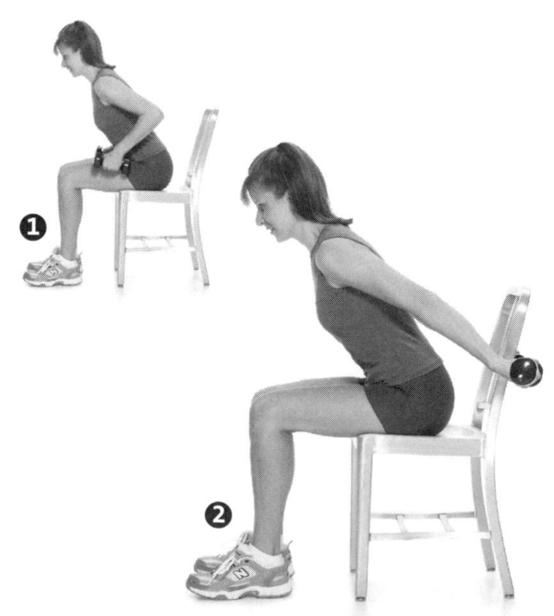

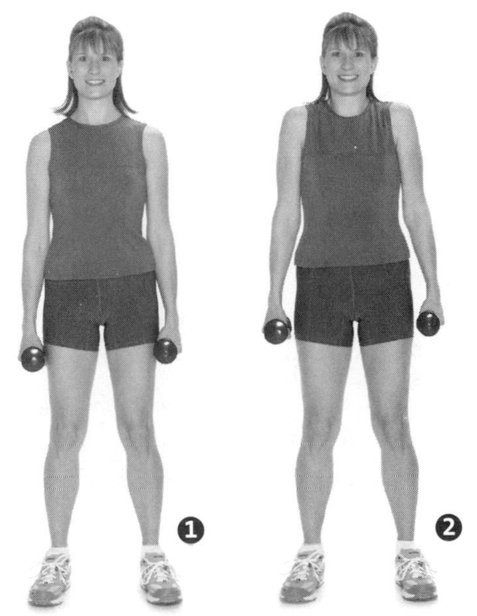

Shoulder Shrug

Starting position: Stand with your feet shoulder width apart, knees bent slightly. Hold a dumbbell in each hand with your arms at your sides, palms facing in.

Movement: Exhale as you slowly lift your shoulders up toward your ears as high as possible. Hold for a second and then inhale as you slowly lower them.

Technique: Don't bend your elbows. Don't use your arms to lift.

FIRM UP TIPS

ENERGY BOOSTER	FIT FACT
Replace your morning cup of joe with a bracing mug of peppermint tea. Whether you use the fresh herb or tea bags, let the tea steep for 10 minutes before drinking. As it steeps, breathe in the steam from the tea—the powerful peppermint aroma is a proven pick-me-up.	*On average, inactive Americans spend approximately $330 a year more on health-care expenses than their more active counterparts. The figure jumps to a whopping $1,053 for people with health conditions that limit their physical activity.*

The Workout

Level 2

Easy Walk: 20 Minutes

- 5-minute warmup: Walk 2½ to 3 miles per hour, or 100 to 115 steps per minute.
- 10-minute moderate walk: Increase your speed to 3 to 3½ miles per hour, 115 to 125 steps per minute, or a pace that lets you comfortably carry on a conversation.
- 5-minute cooldown: Slow down to 2½ to 3 miles per hour, or 100 to 115 steps per minute.

Basic Strength Training: 30 Minutes

- Do 10 to 12 reps of each exercise. Repeat the sequence of exercises three times.
- To warm up, use lighter weights, or none at all, the first time through, and for the squat and lunge exercises, only go partway down.

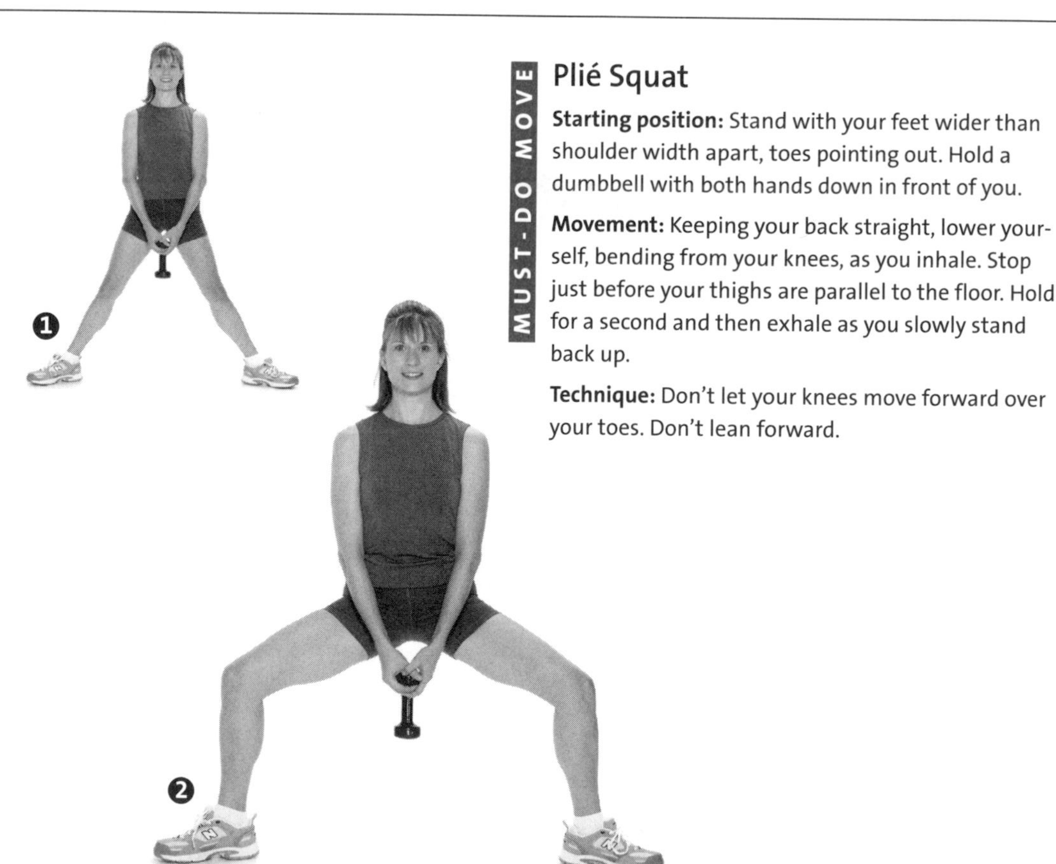

MUST-DO MOVE

Plié Squat

Starting position: Stand with your feet wider than shoulder width apart, toes pointing out. Hold a dumbbell with both hands down in front of you.

Movement: Keeping your back straight, lower yourself, bending from your knees, as you inhale. Stop just before your thighs are parallel to the floor. Hold for a second and then exhale as you slowly stand back up.

Technique: Don't let your knees move forward over your toes. Don't lean forward.

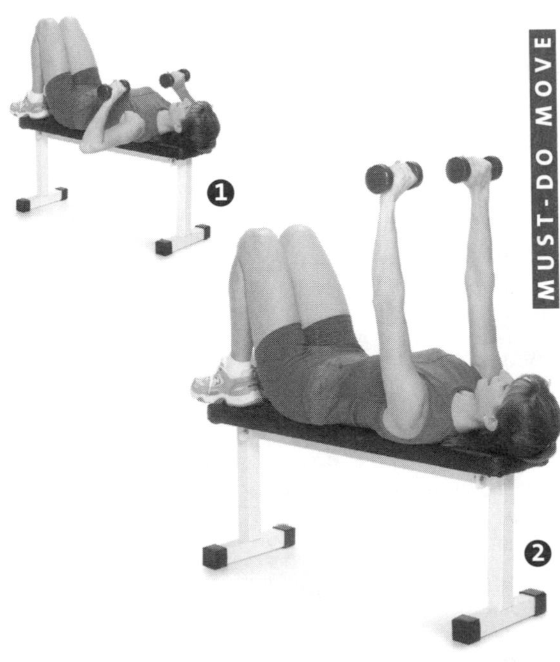

MUST-DO MOVE

Chest Press

Starting position: Lie on the floor (or on a bench) and hold dumbbells end to end, just above your shoulders. Your elbows should be pointing out to the sides.

Movement: Exhale as you press the dumbbells straight up over your chest, extending your arms. Hold for a second and then inhale as you slowly lower them.

Technique: Don't press the dumbbells back toward your head or forward toward your feet: They should go straight up and down. Don't arch your back.

Alternate position: If it's uncomfortable to have your feet on the bench, you can place them on the floor. Make sure your back doesn't arch in that position.

MUST-DO MOVE

Bent-Over Row

Starting position: Stand with your feet shoulder width apart, knees bent slightly. Hold a dumbbell in each hand with your arms at your sides. Keep your back flat and lean forward, bending at the hips so that the dumbbells are hanging at arm's length in front of you, palms facing each other.

Movement: Bending your elbows back and squeezing your shoulder blades, lift the weights toward your ribs as you exhale, until your elbows are higher than your back. Hold for a second and then inhale as you slowly lower them.

Technique: Don't arch your back. Don't pull your shoulders up toward your ears. Don't raise your torso as you lift the dumbbells.

Alternate move: If you have back problems, support yourself with one hand on a chair and do the rows one arm at a time.

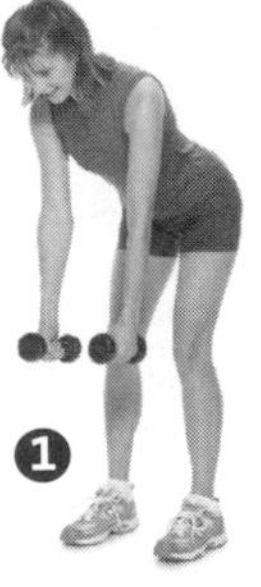

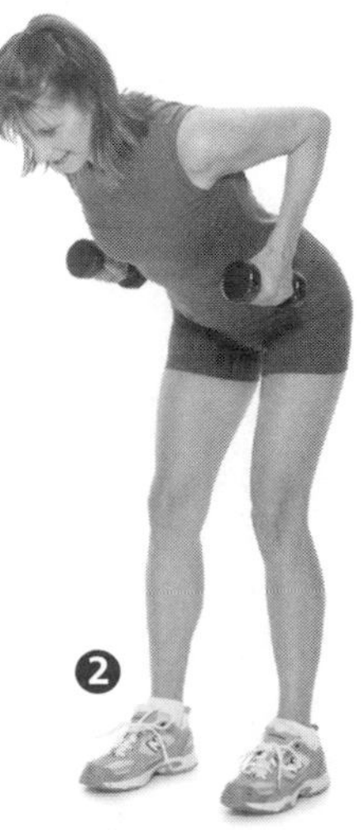

continued

The Workout

Level 2 *continued*

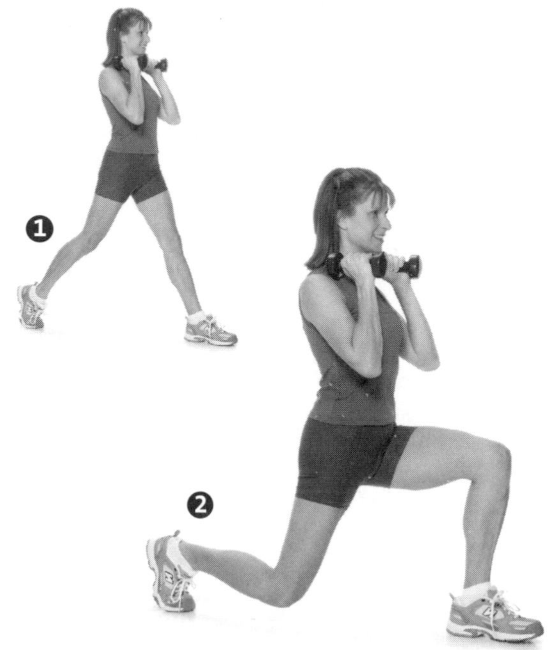

Lunge

Starting position: Stand with your feet 2 to 3 feet apart and your left foot in front of your right. Hold a dumbbell in each hand, either at shoulder height or at your sides.

Movement: Inhale as you bend your left knee and lower your body straight down until your left knee is bent 90 degrees and your right knee nearly touches the floor. Your rear heel will come off the floor. Hold for a second and then exhale as you slowly push yourself back up to the starting position. Finish all of your repetitions, then repeat the exercise with your right foot in front of your left.

Technique: Don't lean forward. Don't let your front knee move forward over your toes.

Biceps Curl

Starting position: Stand with your feet shoulder width apart, knees bent slightly. Hold a dumbbell in each hand with your palms facing forward.

Movement: Bending your elbows, lift the dumbbells toward your shoulders as you exhale. Stop when the dumbbells are at chest height, palms facing your body. Hold for a second and then inhale as you slowly lower them.

Technique: Don't move your upper arms.

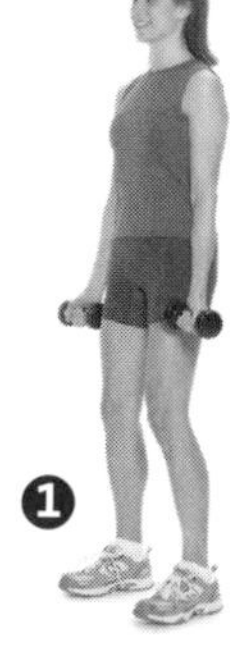

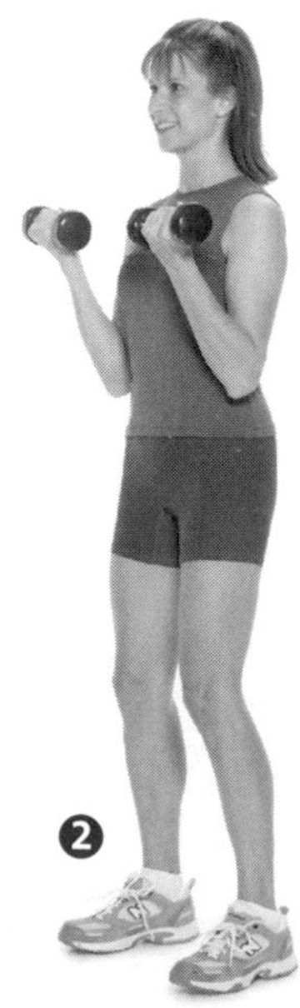

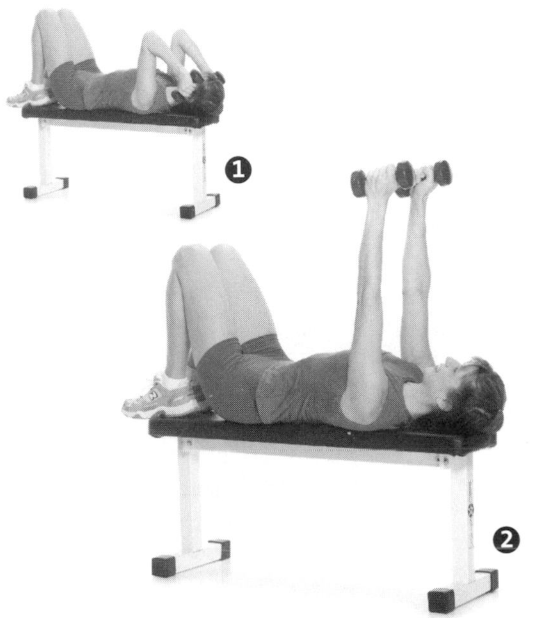

Lying Triceps Extension

Starting position: Lie face up on the floor (or on a bench). Hold a dumbbell in each hand over your chest. Bend your arms so that your elbows are pointing toward the ceiling and the dumbbells are by your ears.

Movement: Without moving your upper arms, press the weights up over your chest as you exhale. Hold for a second and then inhale as you slowly lower them.

Technique: Don't move from your shoulders. Don't arch your back.

Alternate position: If it's uncomfortable to have your feet on the bench, you can place them on the floor. Make sure your back doesn't arch in that position.

Lateral Raise

Starting position: Stand with your feet shoulder width apart, knees bent slightly. Hold a dumbbell in each hand with your arms at your sides, palms facing in, and elbows bent slightly.

Movement: Exhale as you slowly raise the dumbbells out to the sides until they are at about shoulder height. Hold for a second and then inhale as you slowly lower them.

Technique: Don't lift your shoulders. Don't lift higher than shoulder height.

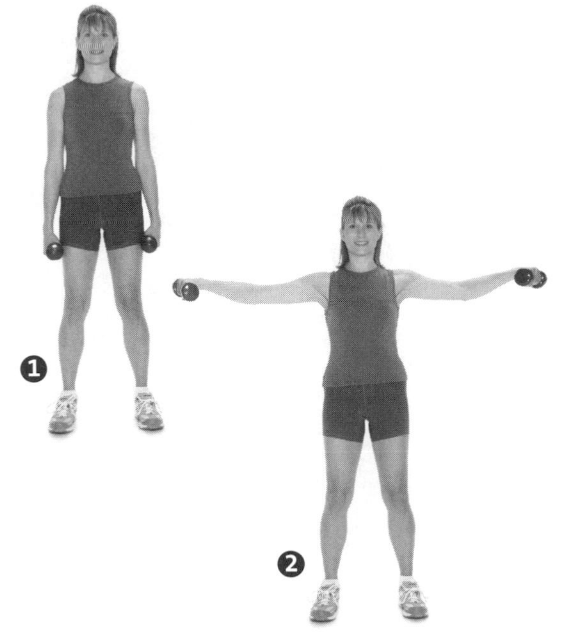

The Workout

Level 3

Easy Walk: 20 Minutes

- 5-minute warmup: Walk 2½ to 3 miles per hour, or 100 to 115 steps per minute.
- 10-minute moderate walk: Increase your speed to 3½ to 4 miles per hour, 125 to 135 steps per minute, or a pace that lets you comfortably carry on a conversation.
- 5-minute cooldown: Slow down to 2½ to 3 miles per hour, or 100 to 115 steps per minute.

Basic Strength Training: 40 Minutes

- Do 10 to 12 reps of each exercise. Repeat the sequence of exercises three times.
- To warm up, use lighter weights, or none at all, the first time through, and for the squat and lunge exercises, only go partway down.

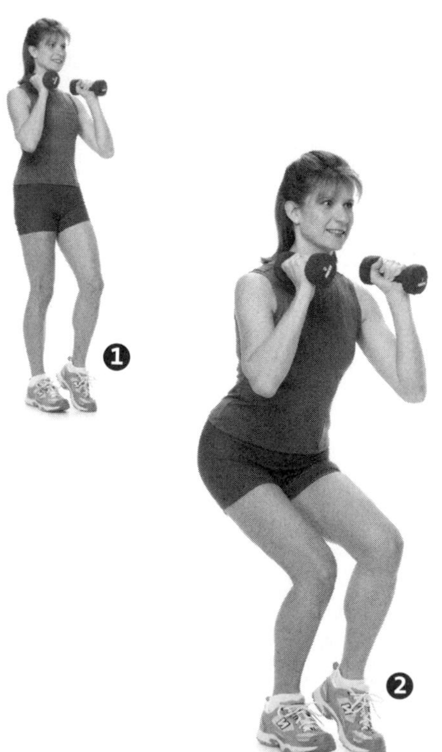

MUST-DO MOVE

One-Leg Squat

Starting position: Hold dumbbells in each hand at shoulder height or down at your sides. Shift your weight to your right foot and lift your left foot off the floor so that only your toes are lightly touching for balance.

Movement: As you inhale, bend your right knee and lean forward slightly from your hips, lowering yourself as if you were sitting in a chair. Go as low as comfortable, but don't go past your right thigh being parallel to the floor. Hold for a second and then exhale as you slowly stand back up. Do the recommended number of reps and then switch legs.

Technique: Don't let your working knee come forward past your toes.

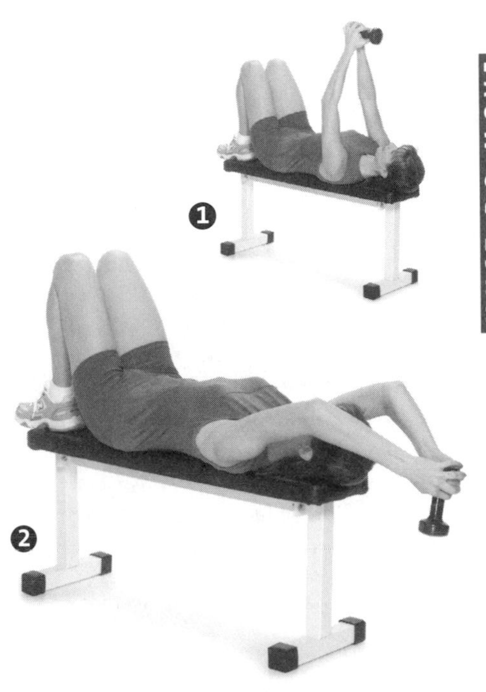

MUST-DO MOVE

Pullover

Starting position: Lie face up on the floor (or on a bench). Grasp a dumbbell with both hands and hold it above your chest with your elbows bent slightly.

Movement: Inhale as you lower the dumbbell backward over your head as far as comfortably possible without bending your elbows any farther than at the start. Hold for a second and then exhale as you slowly raise it to the starting position.

Technique: Don't arch your back. Don't bend your elbows to lower the weight.

Alternate position: If it's uncomfortable to have your feet on the bench, you can place them on the floor. Make sure your back doesn't arch in that position.

MUST-DO MOVE

Wide Bent-Over Row

Starting position: Stand with your feet shoulder width apart, knees bent slightly. Hold a dumbbell in each hand with your arms at your sides. Keep your back flat and lean forward, bending at the hips so that the dumbbells are hanging at arm's length in front of you, palms facing you.

Movement: Bending your elbows out to the sides and squeezing your shoulder blades, lift the dumbbells toward your ribs as you exhale, until your elbows are higher than your back. Hold for a second and then inhale as you slowly lower them.

Technique: Don't arch your back. Don't pull your shoulders up toward your ears. Don't raise your torso as you lift the dumbbells.

Alternate move: If you have back problems, support yourself with one hand on a chair and do the rows one arm at a time.

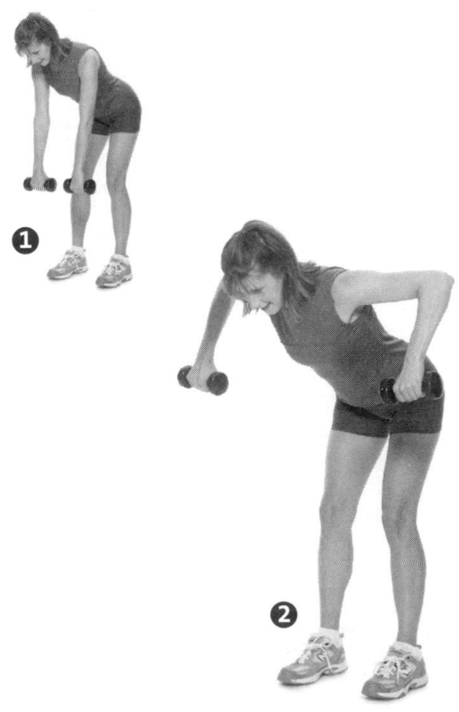

continued

The Workout

Level 3 *continued*

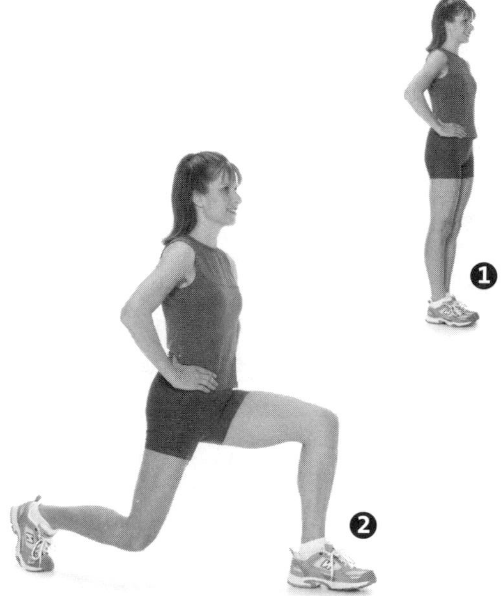

Back Lunge (no weights)

Starting position: Stand with your feet together and place your hands on your hips.

Movement: Step your right foot back 2 to 3 feet. Inhale as you bend your left knee and lower your body straight down until your left knee is bent 90 degrees and your right knee nearly touches the floor. Your rear heel will come off the floor. Hold for a second and then exhale as you push yourself back up, bringing your right foot in. Finish all of your repetitions, then repeat the exercise stepping your left foot back.

Technique: Don't lean forward. Don't let your front knee move forward over your toes.

Biceps Curl

Starting position: Stand with your feet shoulder width apart, knees bent slightly. Hold a dumbbell in each hand with your palms facing forward.

Movement: Bending your elbows, lift the dumbbells toward your shoulders as you exhale. Stop when the dumbbells are at chest height, palms facing your body. Hold for a second and then inhale as you slowly lower them.

Technique: Don't move your upper arms.

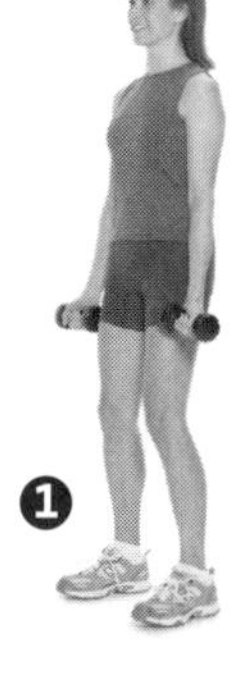

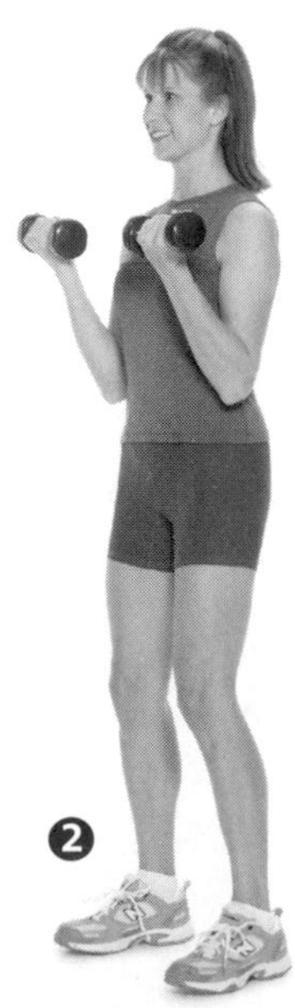

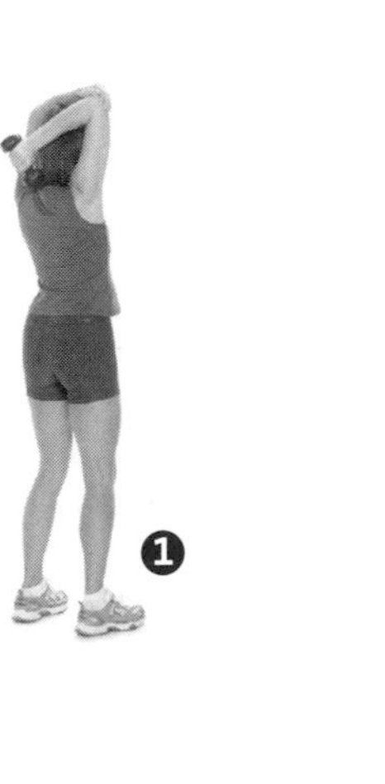

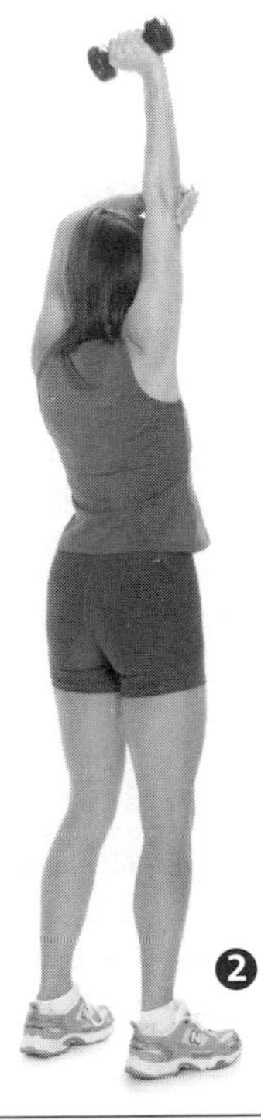

Overhead Triceps Extension

Starting position: Stand with your feet shoulder width apart and knees bent slightly. Hold a dumbbell in your right hand and lift it up over your head. Bend your elbow so that it is pointing toward the ceiling and the dumbbell is behind your head. Place your left hand on your right elbow for support.

Movement: Exhale as you extend your right arm and lift the dumbbell over your head. Hold for a second and then inhale as you slowly lower it. Do the recommended number of reps and then repeat with your left arm.

Technique: Don't lift your shoulders up toward your ears. Don't bend your wrist.

Overhead Press

Starting position: Stand with your feet shoulder width apart and knees bent slightly. Hold a dumbbell in each hand at shoulder height with your palms facing forward and elbows pointing out to the sides.

Movement: Exhale as you slowly press the dumbbells straight up overhead. Hold for a second and then inhale as you slowly lower them.

Technique: Don't arch your back. Don't lift the dumbbells forward or back.

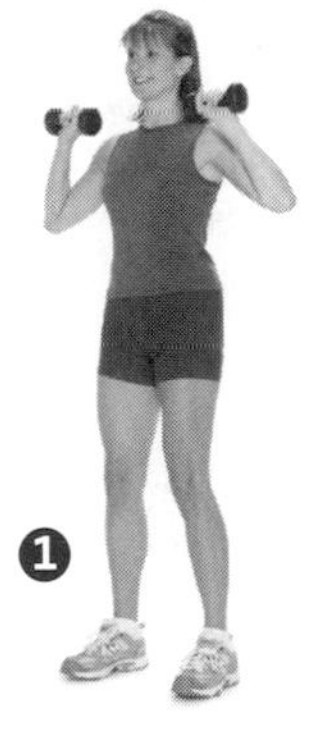

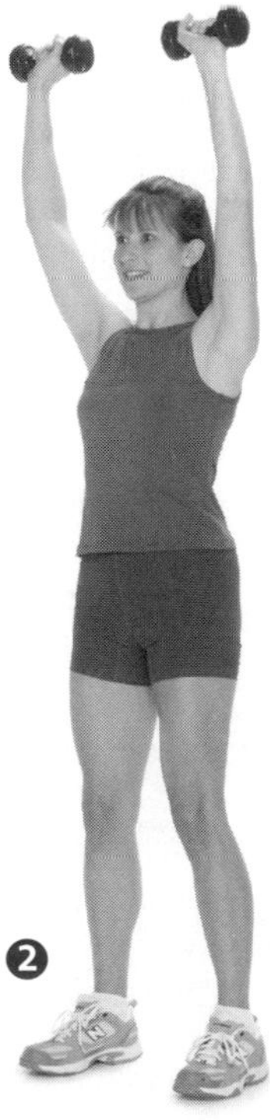

FIRM UP / DAY 4

Real-Life Success Story

In January 2001, Cindy Reinitz, of Henderson, Minnesota, was overweight, and she was in constant pain from headaches and backaches. "I was frustrated with being fat," she says. "I didn't have the energy to keep up with my 6th-grade students." Three years later, she's 40 pounds lighter, running 5-K races and backpacking.

With the typical January resolve to be healthier, Reinitz's transformation began when she started doing *Prevention*'s strength-training program—just 20 minutes, two or three times a week. "At first, I could do only three to five lunges, and I used 1- and 3-pound weights," she says. "Now I use 8- and 10-pound weights, and I can do the advanced moves."

Keeping an exercise calendar was Cindy's secret to working out consistently. "It's so easy to let days slip away without realizing it," she points out. "I keep a calendar by my treadmill, and every day I write down the type of exercise and how many minutes. Then I keep a daily average for the month. At first I used a weekly average, but that made it too easy to skip days. With a daily average, I can correct drops immediately." And she certainly has. Cindy has gone from 20-minute workouts a few times a week to an average of 75 minutes a day: usually 30 minutes in the morning and then 30 to 45 minutes in the evening.

The results are worth it. At age 49, Cindy is a slim 142 pounds. She lowered her cholesterol 87 points, and she feels great. "Exercise used to be a chore, but now I don't feel good if I miss a day," she adds.

FIRM UP TIP

ON YOUR PLATE

Save the best for last. Waiting to eat treats until the end of a meal or party may prevent you from overeating. When overweight people were fed a high-fat meal prior to eating at a buffet, they ate 56 percent more than their lean counterparts. But when offered a low-fat meal ahead of time, neither group overate. It seems to take the body longer to detect that food is being ingested when it's high in fat.

Meal Plan

Most of these recipes are custom designed to make 1 serving–no fuss, no muss; just fix, eat, and go! If a recipe makes more than 1 serving, it's noted below. Save that extra serving for another meal, or share it with your spouse or your walking buddy.

Breakfast

Smoothie to Go: Have 1 Yoplait Nouriche smoothie (any flavor). Serve with 8 peanuts. (This is a healthy smoothie, but it is packed with a hefty dose of refined sugar, so limit yourself to one or two a week.)

Healthy Snack

Fruit and Cheese: Slice a ripe pear or apple; eat with 1 slice (1 ounce) reduced-fat cheese.

Lunch

Meatball and Cheese Sub: Heat 3 (1-ounce) turkey meatballs (from last night's dinner) with ¼ cup spaghetti sauce topped with ⅛ cup reduced-fat shredded cheese. Serve on 1 toasted whole grain hamburger roll with 1½ cups romaine lettuce and ½ chopped paste (Roma-style) tomato, topped with 2 tablespoons light salad dressing.

Indulgent Treat

French Fry Fix: Order a small-size McDonald's french fries (small sizes at other chains have more calories) and a diet soda.

Dinner

Zucchini and Chicken Pasta: Serve ½ cup cooked pasta (any variety) with ¼ cup spaghetti sauce and 2 ounces (¼ cup) cooked chicken strips. Chop ¾ cup zucchini (about 1 small zucchini) and place in a colander. Cook the zucchini by pouring the hot pasta water over it when you drain the cooked pasta into the colander. Mix all the ingredients together and serve.

Healthy Snack

Raisin-Nut Cluster: Have 1 serving from Sunday's recipe.

Nutrient analysis: 1,671 calories, 91 g protein, 223 g carbohydrates, 48 g total fat, 10 g saturated fat, 175 mg cholesterol, 25 g dietary fiber, 1,865 mg sodium, 909 mg calcium

FIRM UP TIPS

FIT FACT

Dehydration can slow your metabolism by 3 percent. So for a woman who weighs 150 pounds, that would be about 45 fewer calories burned a day—which could mean 5 extra pounds a year.

GET FIRM FASTER

Fidget. You can burn up to 700 calories a day! Tap your toes, shift in your seat often, get up and walk around—the more you do, the more calories you can burn.

The Workout

Level 1

Interval Walk: About 30 Minutes

- 5-minute warmup: Walk 2 to 2½ miles per hour, or 95 to 100 steps per minute.
- 4-minute moderate pace: Increase your speed to about 3 miles per hour, or about 115 steps per minute.
- 30-second speedup: Pick up your pace even more to about 3½ miles per hour, or about 125 steps per minute.
- Repeat moderate and speed intervals four times.
- 5-minute cooldown: Slow down to 2 to 2½ miles per hour, or 95 to 100 steps per minute.

Core Training: 10 Minutes

- Do the sequence of exercises one time.

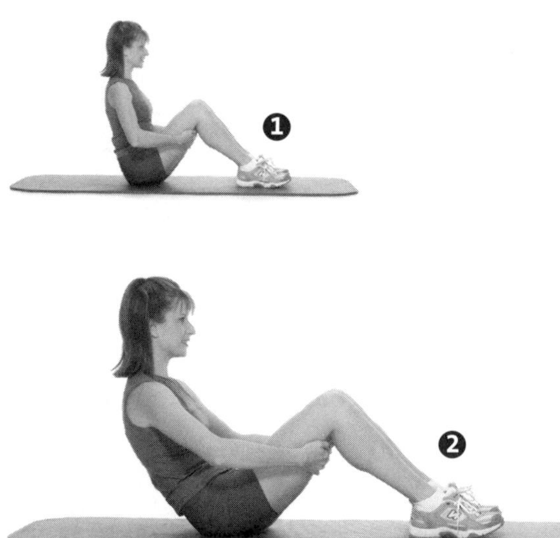

Two-Hand Roll-Down

Starting position: Sit on the floor with your knees bent and your feet flat. Place your hands behind your thighs.

Movement: Using your abs, slowly roll down 2 to 3 inches, one vertebra at a time, as you inhale. Hold for a second and then exhale as you slowly roll back up. Do eight reps.

Technique: Your abs should be powering the move. Don't move quickly.

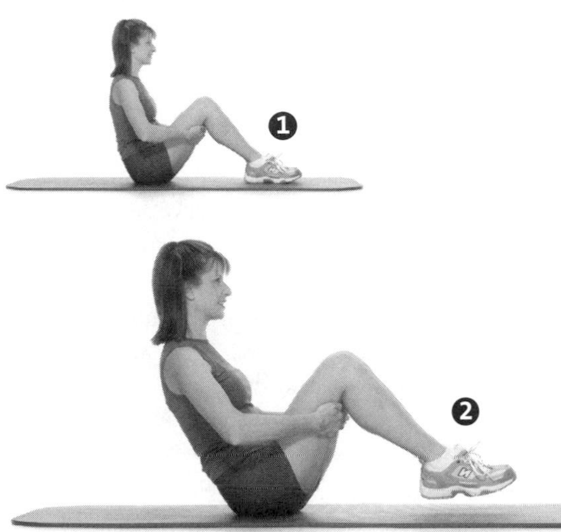

Holding Balance

Starting position: Sit on the floor with your knees bent and your feet flat. Place your hands behind your thighs.

Movement: Lift your feet off the floor slightly and balance on your sitting bones. Hold for three slow breaths and then relax. Do one time only.

Technique: Keep your abs tight and the rest of your body relaxed, especially your shoulders.

MUST-DO MOVE

Easy Ab Crunch

Starting position: Lie on your back with your knees bent, feet flat on the floor, and arms at your sides, palms facing down.

Movement: Using your abs, slowly raise your head, shoulders, and upper back about 45 degrees off the floor as you exhale. Think of shortening the distance between your ribs and pelvis. Hold for a second and then inhale as you slowly lower yourself. Do eight reps.

Technique: Don't pull your chin to your chest. Don't arch your back.

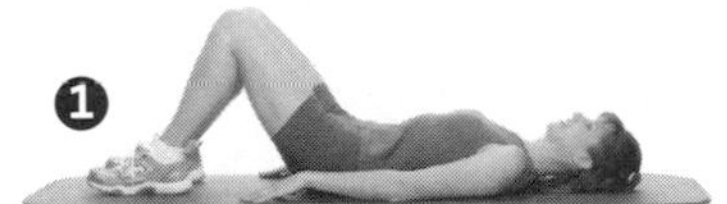

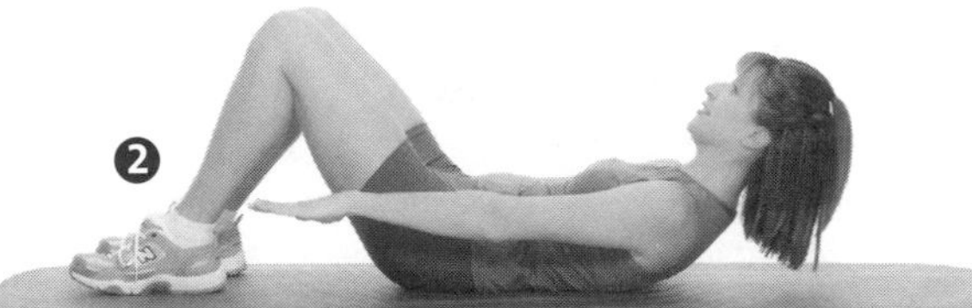

continued

The Workout

Level 1 *continued*

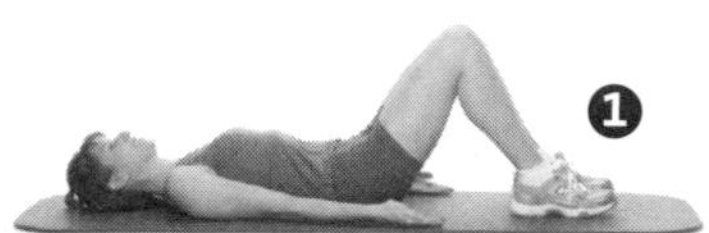

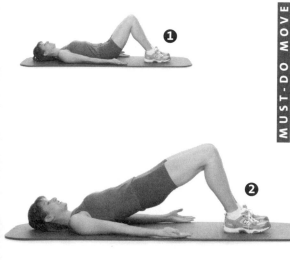

MUST-DO MOVE

Bridge

Starting position: Lie on your back with your knees bent, feet flat on the floor, and arms at your sides, with your palms facing up.

Movement: Contracting your abs, buttocks, and lower back, press into your feet and lift your butt, hips, and back off the floor as you exhale, to form a straight line from your shoulders to your knees. Hold for three slow breaths and then relax. Do one time only.

Technique: Don't lift too high—your upper back and shoulders should remain on the floor. Don't bend at the waist or hips. Don't let your knees fall inward or outward.

MUST-DO MOVE

Knee Plank

Starting position: Lie facedown with your knees bent so that your feet are in the air. Your elbows should be under your shoulders and your forearms and palms on the floor.

Movement: Contracting your abs and back, press into your forearms as you exhale and lift your pelvis off the floor so that your back and thighs form a straight line. Hold for three breaths and then relax. Do one time only.

Technique: Don't lift your head up or let it drop. Don't bend at the waist. Don't arch your back.

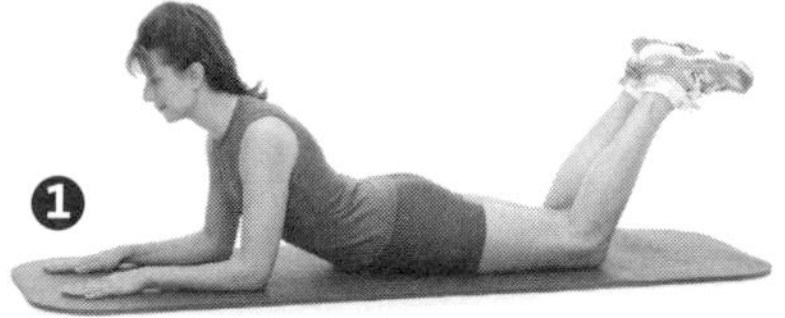

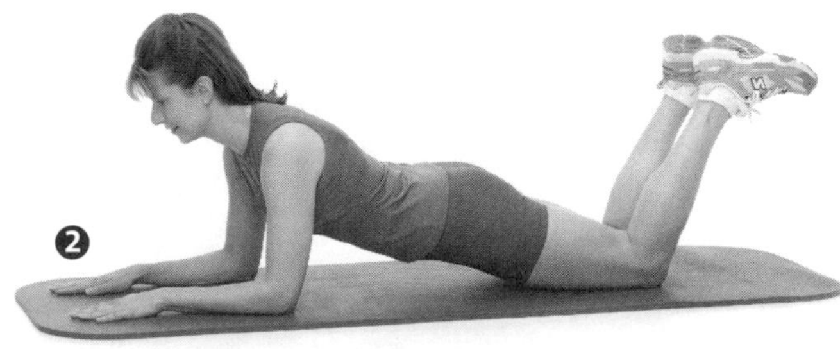

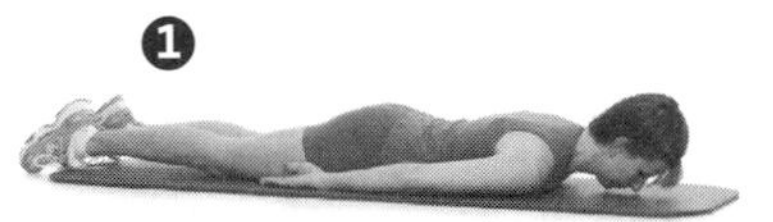

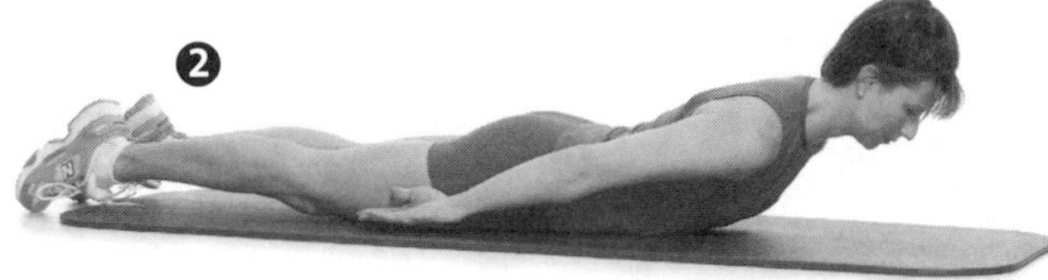

Chest Lift

Starting position: Lie facedown on the floor with your arms at your sides and palms facing up.

Movement: Exhale as you lift your head and chest 5 to 6 inches off the floor. Hold for a second and then inhale as you slowly lower them. Do eight reps.

Technique: Don't look up. Don't lift too high.

FIRM UP TIP

GET FIRM FASTER

Every time you brush your teeth, stand on one foot. The muscles in your abs, back, hips, buttocks, and anchor leg have to spring to action to prevent you from toppling. Try to balance for 1 minute on each leg. Over time, these mini workouts will help firm up your midsection.

The Workout
Level 2

Interval Walk: About 30 Minutes

- 5-minute warmup: Walk 2½ to 3 miles per hour, or 100 to 115 steps per minute.
- 3-minute moderate pace: Increase your speed to about 3½ miles per hour, or about 125 steps per minute.
- 90-second speedup: Pick up your pace even more to about 4 miles per hour, or about 135 steps per minute.
- Repeat moderate and speedup intervals four times.
- 5-minute cooldown: Slow down to 2½ to 3 miles per hour, or 100 to 115 steps per minute.

Core Training: 10 Minutes

- Do the exercise sequence one time.

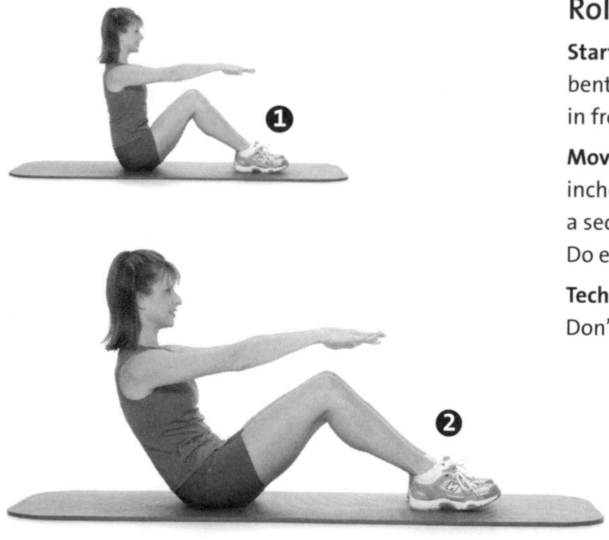

Roll-Down

Starting position: Sit on the floor with your knees bent and your feet flat. Hold your arms straight out in front of you, parallel to the floor.

Movement: Using your abs, slowly roll down 3 to 4 inches, one vertebra at a time, as you inhale. Hold for a second and then exhale as you slowly roll back up. Do eight reps.

Technique: Your abs should be powering the move. Don't move quickly.

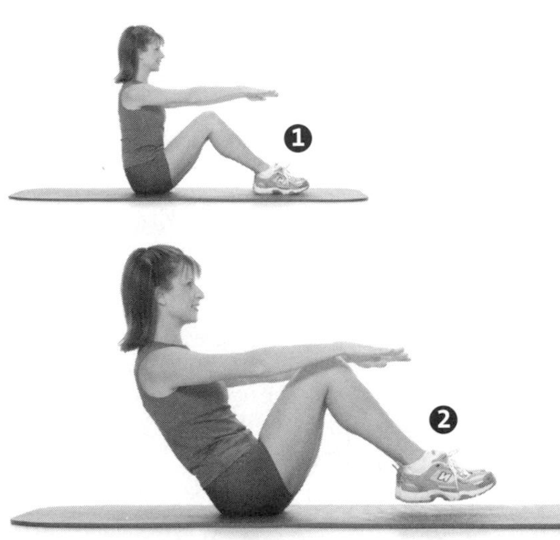

Partial Balance

Starting position: Sit on the floor with your knees bent and your feet flat. Hold your arms straight out in front of you, parallel to the floor.

Movement: Lift your feet off the floor slightly and balance on your sitting bones. Hold for four breaths and then relax. Do one time only.

Technique: Keep your abs tight and the rest of your body relaxed, especially your shoulders.

MUST-DO MOVE

Ab Crunch

Starting position: Lie on your back with your knees bent, feet flat on the floor, and hands behind your head.

Movement: Using your abs, slowly raise your head, shoulders, and upper back about 45 degrees off the floor as you exhale. Think of shortening the distance between your ribs and pelvis. Hold for a second and then inhale as you slowly lower yourself. Do eight reps.

Technique: Don't pull your chin to your chest. Don't arch your back.

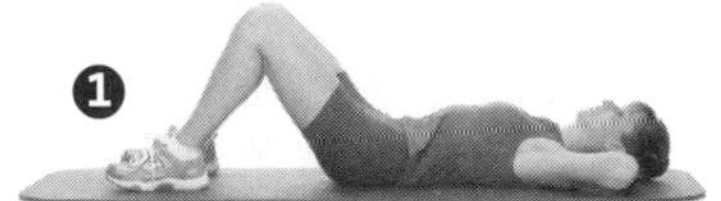

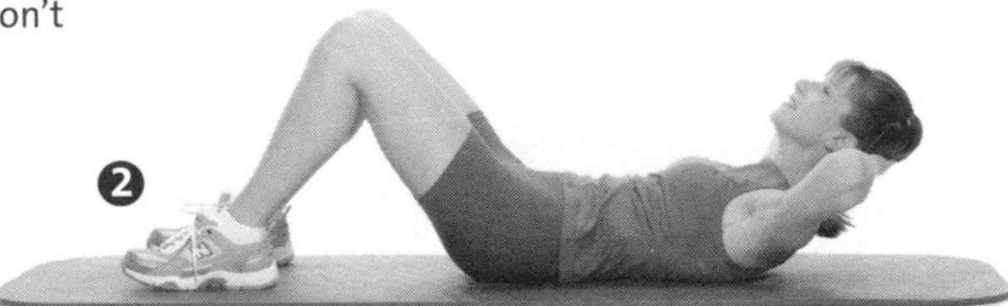

continued

The Workout

Level 2 *continued*

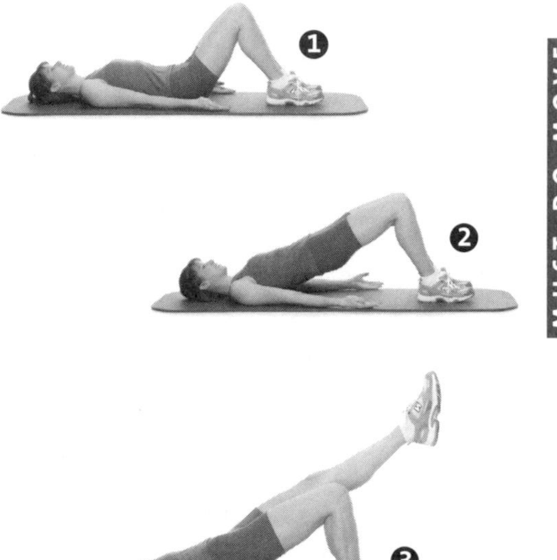

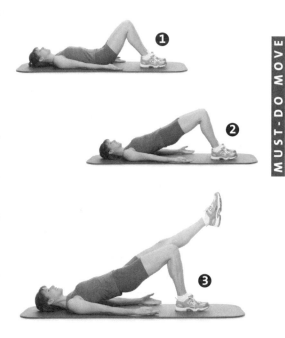

MUST-DO MOVE

Bridge with Leg Lift

Starting position: Lie on your back with your knees bent, feet flat on the floor, and arms at your sides, palms facing up.

Movement: Contracting your abs, buttocks, and lower back, press into your feet and lift your butt, hips, and back off the floor as you exhale, to form a straight line from your shoulders to your knees. Lift one foot off the floor and extend that leg. Hold for two breaths and then lower your foot. Lift the other foot up and hold for two breaths. Lower your foot and return to the starting position. Do one time only.

Technique: Don't lift too high—your upper back and shoulders should remain on the floor. Don't bend at the waist or hips. Don't let your knees fall inward or outward.

MUST-DO MOVE

Plank

Starting position: Lie facedown with your feet flexed and toes tucked. Your elbows should be under your shoulders and your forearms and palms on the floor.

Movement: Contracting your abs and back, press into your forearms as you exhale and lift your pelvis and legs off the floor so that your back and legs form a straight line. Hold for four breaths and then relax. Do one time only.

Technique: Don't lift your head up or let it drop. Don't bend at the waist or hips. Don't let your belly drop toward the floor.

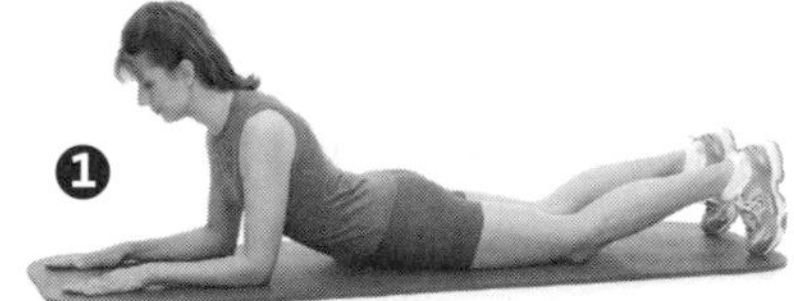

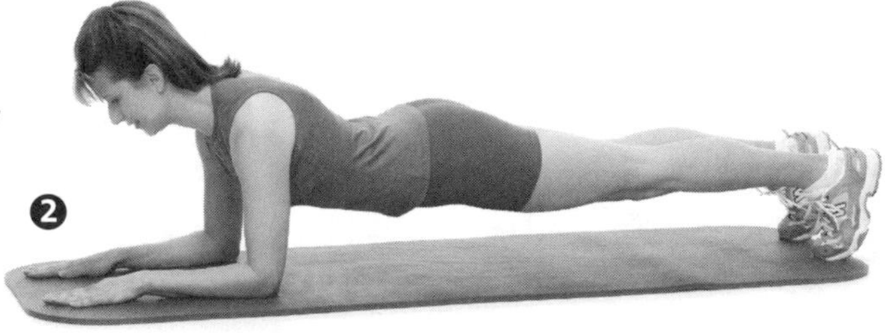

❶

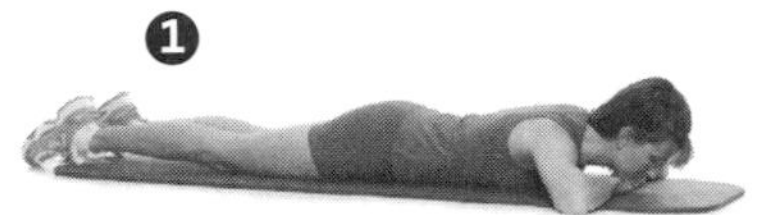

❷

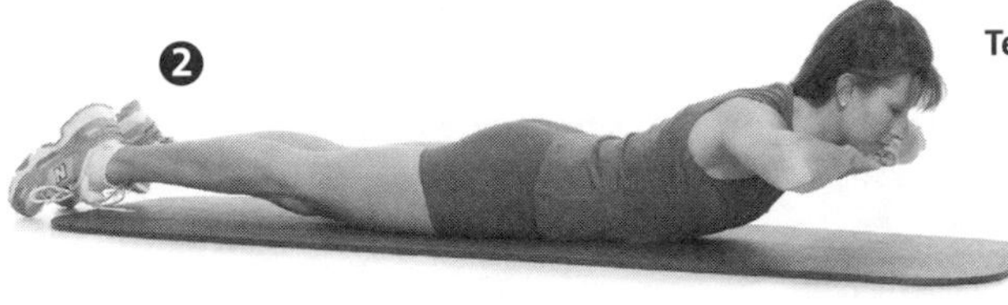

Bent-Arm Chest Lift

Starting position: Lie facedown on the floor with your hands under your chin.

Movement: Exhale as you lift your head and chest 5 to 6 inches off the floor. Hold for a second and then inhale as you slowly lower yourself. Do eight reps.

Technique: Don't lift too high.

FIRM UP TIP

ENERGY BOOSTER

Pick pink workout clothes. There's something about the color pink that's instantly flattering—and when you look good, you feel good. A pink shirt reflects color on your face, making you look—and feel—fresh and relaxed.

The Workout

Level 3

Interval Walk: About 30 Minutes

- 5-minute warmup: Walk 2½ to 3 miles per hour, or 100 to 115 steps per minute.
- 2-minute moderate pace: Increase your speed to about 4 miles per hour, or about 135 steps per minute.
- 2-minute speedup: Pick up your pace even more to about 4½ miles per hour, or about 145 steps per minute.
- Repeat moderate and speedup intervals five times.
- 5-minute cooldown: Slow down to 2½ to 3 miles per hour, or 100 to 115 steps per minute.

Core Training: 10 Minutes

- Do the exercise sequence one time.

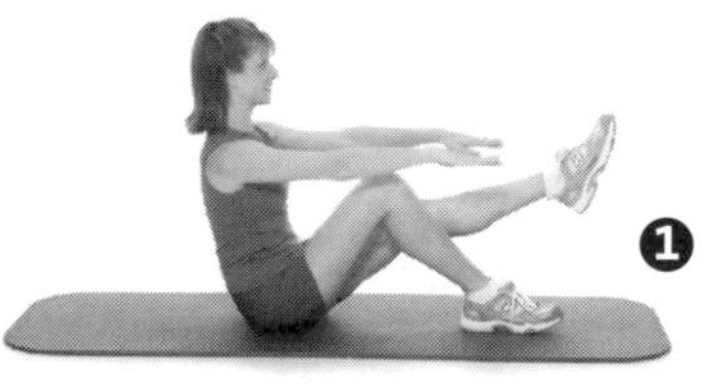

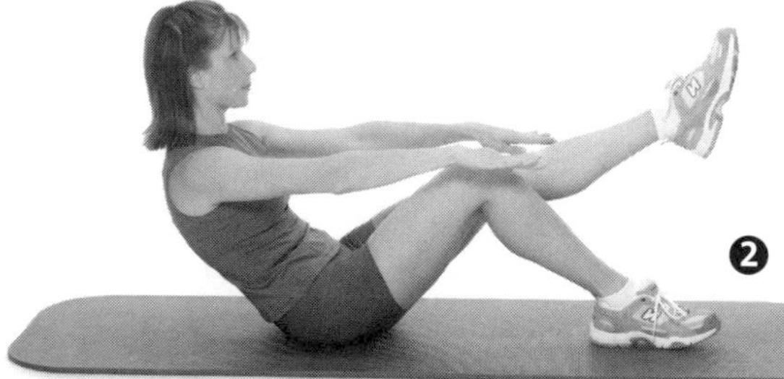

One-Leg Roll-Down

Starting position: Sit on the floor with your knees bent and your feet flat. Lift your left foot off the floor and extend your left leg. Hold your arms straight out in front of you, parallel to the floor.

Movement: Using your abs, slowly roll down 4 to 5 inches, one vertebra at a time, as you inhale. Hold for a second and then exhale as you slowly roll back up. Do four reps, switch legs, and do four more reps.

Technique: Your abs should be powering the move. Don't move quickly.

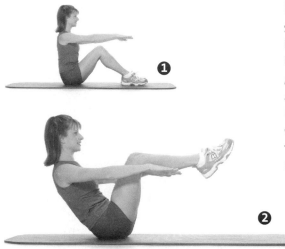

Full Balance

Starting position: Sit on the floor with your knees bent and your feet flat. Hold your arms straight out in front of you, parallel to the floor.

Movement: Lift your feet so that your calves are parallel to the floor, and balance on your sitting bones. Hold for five breaths and then relax. Do one time only.

Technique: Keep your abs tight and the rest of your body relaxed, especially your shoulders.

MUST-DO MOVE

Legs-Up Ab Crunch

Starting position: Lie on your back with your legs in the air and your hands behind your head.

Movement: Using your abs, slowly raise your head, shoulders, and upper back about 45 degrees off the floor as you exhale. Think of shortening the distance between your ribs and pelvis. Hold for a second and then inhale as you slowly lower yourself. Do eight reps.

Technique: Don't pull your chin to your chest.

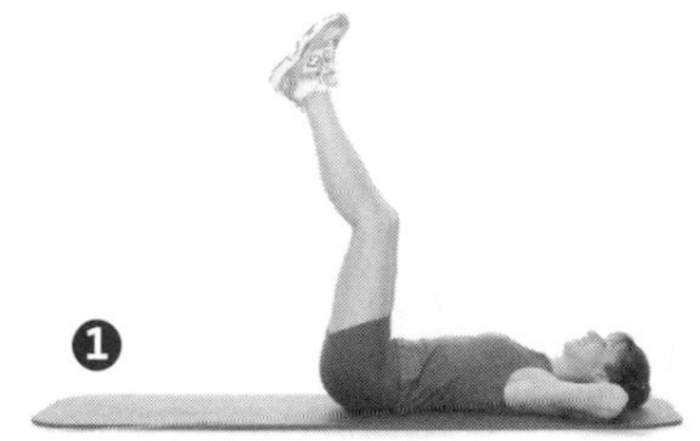

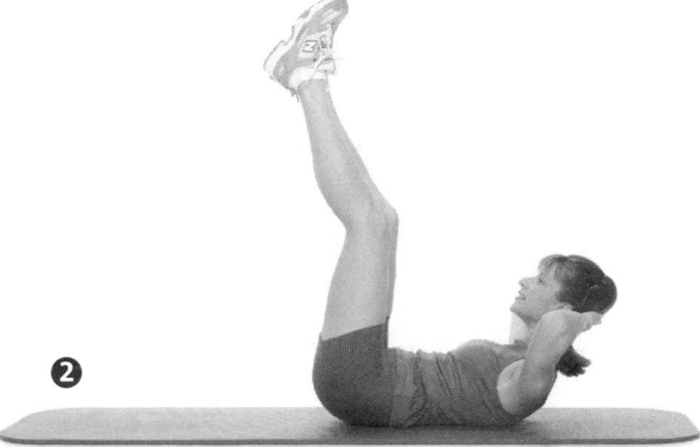

continued

The Workout

Level 3 *continued*

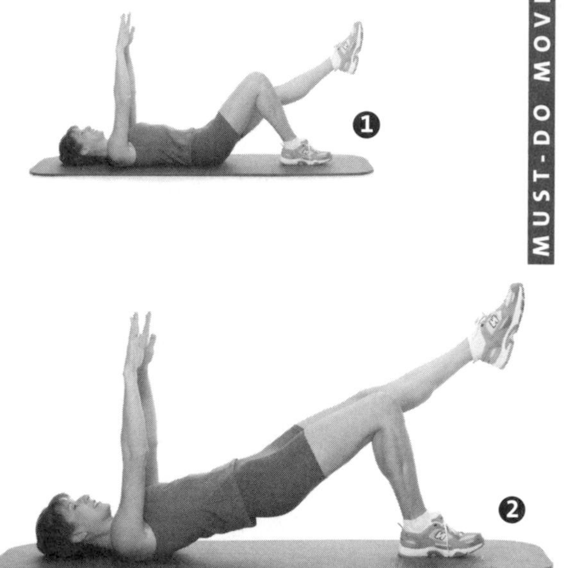

MUST-DO MOVE

One-Leg Bridge with Arms Up

Starting position: Lie on your back with your knees bent, feet flat on the floor, and arms extended over your chest. Lift your left foot off the floor and extend your left leg.

Movement: Contracting your abs, buttocks, and lower back, press into your right foot and lift your butt, hips, and back off the floor as you exhale, to form a straight line from your shoulders to your knees. Hold for three breaths and then lower yourself. Repeat with your right leg extended. Do one time only with each leg.

Technique: Don't lift too high—your upper back and shoulders should remain on the floor. Don't bend at the waist or hips. Don't let your knees fall inward or outward.

MUST-DO MOVE

Plank with Leg Lift

Starting position: Lie facedown with your feet flexed and toes tucked. Your elbows should be under your shoulders and your forearms and palms on the floor.

Movement: Contracting your abs and back, press into your hands and forearms as you exhale and lift your pelvis and legs off the floor so that your back and legs form a straight line. Lift your left foot off the floor, hold for three breaths, and then relax. Repeat by lifting your right foot off the floor. Do one time only with each leg.

Technique: Don't lift your head up or let it drop. Don't bend at the waist or hips. Don't let your belly drop toward the floor.

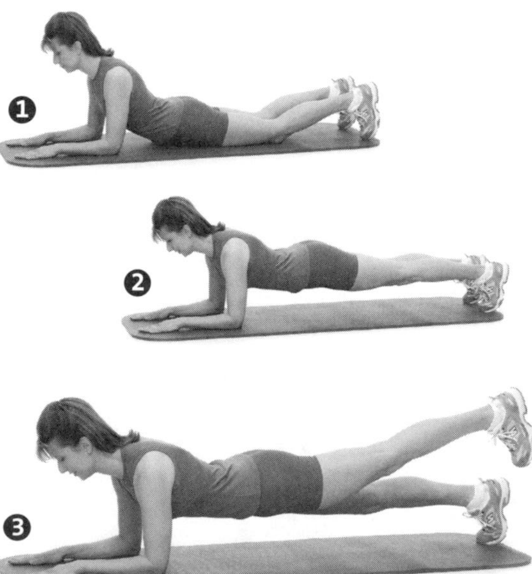

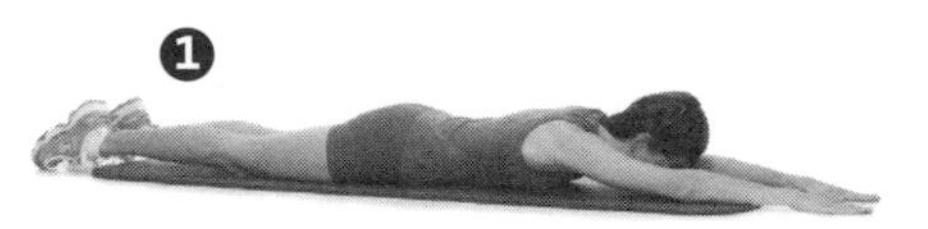

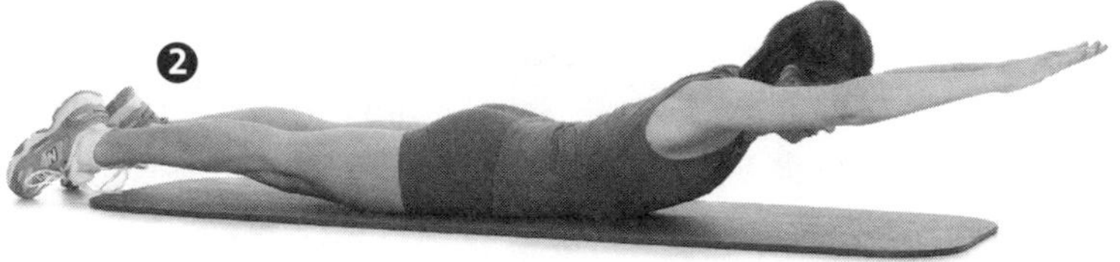

Extended Chest Lift

Starting position: Lie facedown on the floor with your arms extended overhead.

Movement: Exhale as you lift your arms, head, and chest 5 to 6 inches off the floor. Hold for a second and then inhale as you slowly lower yourself. Do eight reps.

Technique: Don't lift too high.

FIRM UP TIP

MYTH BUSTER

Exercising at a slower pace for a longer time will not *burn more fat off your hips. Although you may burn a greater percentage of fat during low-intensity exercise, you'll burn more fat calories and more total calories during high-intensity sessions or intervals. And in the end, it's total calories that determine how many pounds and inches you'll lose. For example, a 150-pound woman who walks 1½ miles for 30 minutes burns 112 total calories. But if she were to run the same distance in 15 minutes, she'd burn 170 total calories. Bonus: Your metabolism will stay elevated five times longer after a vigorous workout than after an easy one.*

FIRM UP / DAY 5

Relax Away Belly Fat

Stress can contribute to headaches, digestive woes, frequent colds, and heart disease. It also can wreck your waistline, because stress even contributes to belly fat.

Uncontrolled stress can boost belly fat in two ways. First, it increases levels of the hormone cortisol, which seems to direct fat to your middle. And it can make you overeat in an effort to reduce tension.

Exercise, sufficient sleep, and stress-reduction techniques, such as the breathing exercise that follows, can lower cortisol levels. Try this quick stress reducer: Find a quiet, comfortable place to sit or lie down, and set a timer for 5 to 10 minutes. Use good posture so that you can fill your lungs with air. Bring your attention to your breath, focusing on the sound and the feel of each inhalation and exhalation. As you inhale, fill your lungs completely, and as you exhale, empty your lungs completely. If other thoughts come into your mind, notice without judgment that your mind is "chattering" and bring your awareness back to your breath.

If you prefer, you can focus on a word—such as "calm" or "peace"—or a meaningful phrase or prayer. Vietnamese Zen master Thich Nhat Hanh suggests mentally reciting this phrase along with your breath: "Breathing in I calm myself, breathing out I smile." Aim to do this once or twice a day, but you can do it anytime, anywhere, to help you calm down and relieve stress.

FIRM UP TIP

ENERGY BOOSTER

Try acupressure. When the midafternoon slump hits, try tapping or massaging three spots: the K27 points, located about an inch below the center of your collarbone in the slight indentations formed below the bone; the thymus point, located in the center of the sternum, or breastbone; and the spleen points, located on the ribs just below each breast. Tap or massage each spot for 15 to 20 seconds, breathing deeply as you do.

Meal Plan

Most of these recipes are custom designed to make 1 serving–no fuss, no muss; just fix, eat, and go! If a recipe makes more than 1 serving, it's noted below. Save that extra serving for another meal, or share it with your spouse or your walking buddy.

Breakfast

Oatmeal: Prepare an instant packet of regular oatmeal, and top with 1 tablespoon chopped nuts. Serve with 1 cup fat-free milk and ½ cup unsweetened applesauce. (Try convenient single-serving peel-top containers, such as Mott's Natural Style or Mott's Healthy Harvest–any flavor.)

Healthy Snack

Raisin-Nut Cluster: Have 1 serving from Sunday's recipe.

Lunch

Vegetarian Chili: Open 1 can vegetarian chili (such as Natural Touch Low-Fat Vegetarian Chili). Warm 1 cup chili topped with ⅓ cup shredded reduced-fat cheese. Serve with ½ apple and ½ cup fat-free milk.

Indulgent Treat

Chocolate-Covered Peanuts or Raisins: Enjoy 16 pieces chocolate-covered peanuts or 40 pieces chocolate-covered raisins.

Dinner

Chinese Meal: Order beef, chicken, or shrimp with broccoli or mixed vegetables. Ask for more vegetables than beef, chicken, or shrimp, and ask to have it stir-fried in very little oil. Have 1¼ cups of the entrée with ¾ cup steamed rice. If the restaurant won't accommodate your requests for less oil and more veggies, then order them steamed with the sauce on the side and use only 4 tablespoons sauce.

Healthy Snack

Apples with Peanut Butter: Have ½ apple topped with 2 teaspoons peanut butter. Serve with 1 cup fat-free milk.

Nutrient analysis: 1,713 calories, 104 g protein, 216 g carbohydrates, 45 g total fat, 12 g saturated fat, 123 mg cholesterol, 29 g dietary fiber, 2,090 mg sodium, 1,104 mg calcium

FIRM UP TIP

ON YOUR PLATE

Start your day with oatmeal. It makes portion control easier at lunch. When 60 people ate high-fiber oatmeal for breakfast instead of low-fiber cornflakes, they ate 30 percent fewer calories at lunch, according to research at the Obesity Research Center, St. Luke's–Roosevelt Hospital in New York City.

The Workout

Level 1

Easy Walk: 20 Minutes

- 5-minute warmup: Walk 2 to 2½ miles per hour, or 95 to 100 steps per minute.
- 10-minute moderate walk: Increase your speed to 2½ to 3 miles per hour, 100 to 115 steps per minute, or a pace that lets you comfortably carry on a conversation.
- 5-minute cooldown: Slow down to 2 to 2½ miles per hour, or 95 to 100 steps per minute.

Basic Strength Training: 20 Minutes

- Do 10 to 12 reps of each exercise. Repeat the sequence of exercises three times.
- To warm up, do not use weights the first time through, and for the squat exercise, only go partway down.

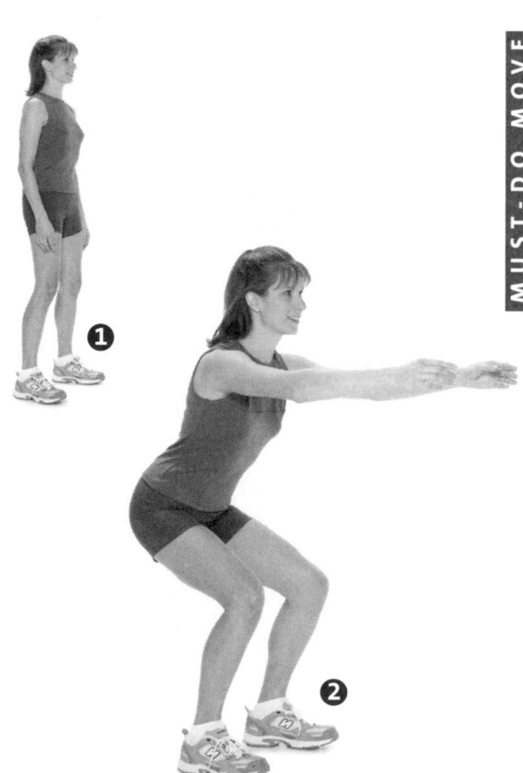

MUST-DO MOVE

Squat

Starting position: Stand with your feet about shoulder width apart, arms at your sides.

Movement: Keeping your back straight, lower yourself, bending from your knees and hips as though you're sitting down, as you inhale. Let your arms come out in front of you to help you balance. Stop just before your thighs are parallel to the floor. Hold for a second and then exhale as you slowly stand back up.

Technique: Don't let your knees move forward over your toes. Don't round your back.

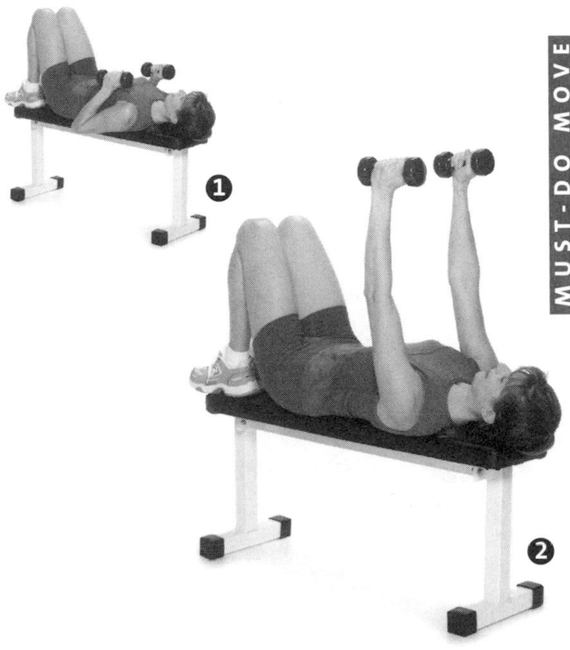

MUST-DO MOVE

Parallel Chest Press

Starting position: Lying on the floor (or on a bench), hold dumbbells parallel and just above your shoulders; your elbows should be pointing toward your feet.

Movement: Exhale as you press the dumbbells straight up over your chest, extending your arms. Hold for a second and then inhale as you slowly lower them.

Technique: Don't press the dumbbells back toward your head or forward toward your feet: They should go straight up and down. Don't arch your back.

Alternate position: If it's uncomfortable to have your feet on the bench, you can place them on the floor. Make sure your back doesn't arch in that position.

MUST-DO MOVE

Seated Bent-Over Row

Starting position: Sit on the edge of a chair with your feet hip width apart and hold a dumbbell in each hand. Keep your back flat and lean forward, bending at the hips so that the dumbbells are hanging at arm's length down by your calves, palms facing each other.

Movement: Bending your elbows back and squeezing your shoulder blades, lift the weights toward your ribs as you exhale. Hold for a second and then inhale as you slowly lower them.

Technique: Don't arch your back. Don't raise your torso as you lift the dumbbells.

Alternate move: If you have back problems, do the rows one arm at a time and place the forearm of your other arm across your thighs for extra support.

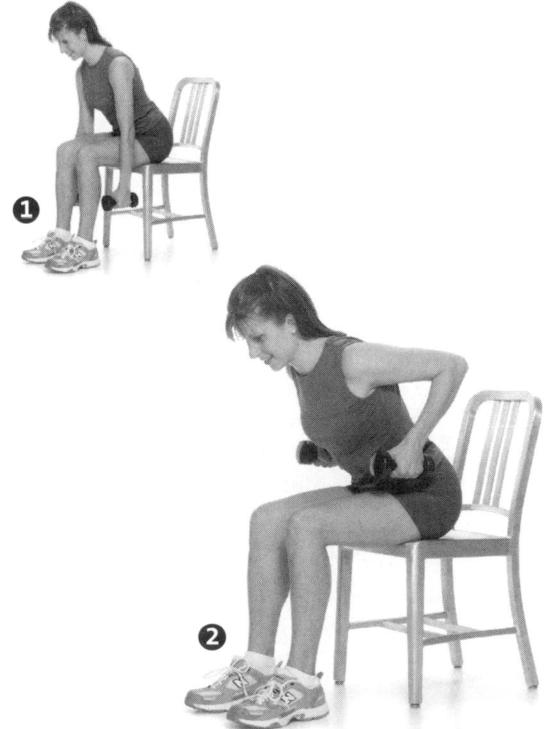

continued

The Workout

Level 1 *continued*

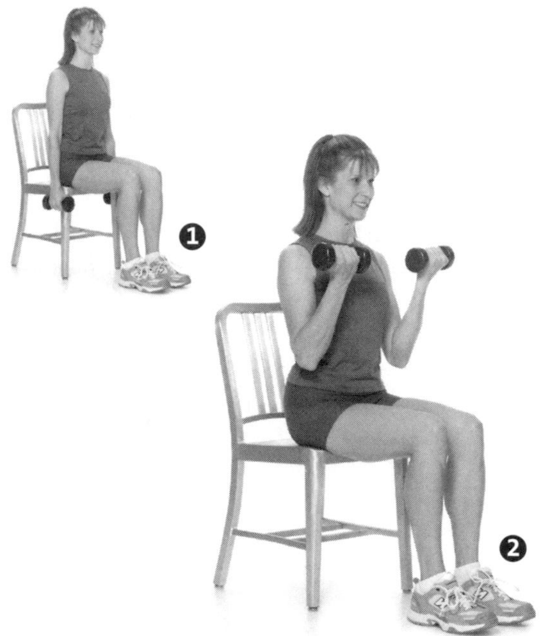

Seated Biceps Curl with a Twist

Starting position: Sit on the edge of a chair with your feet hip width apart and hold dumbbells at your sides, your palms facing in.

Movement: Bending your elbows and turning your wrists upward, lift the dumbbells toward your shoulders as you exhale. Stop when the dumbbells are at chest height, palms facing your body. Hold for a second and then inhale as you slowly lower them.

Technique: Don't move your upper arms.

Seated Triceps Kickback with a Twist

Starting position: Sit on the edge of a chair with your feet hip width apart and hold a dumbbell in each hand. Keep your back flat and lean forward, bending at the hips. Bend your arms at about 90-degree angles with your dumbbells at about hip height.

Movement: Without moving your upper arms, press the dumbbells back as you exhale, extending your arms and turning your wrists so that your palms face the ceiling. Hold for a second and then inhale as you slowly lower them.

Technique: Don't move from your shoulders. Don't raise your torso as you lift the dumbbells.

Alternate move: If you have back problems, do the kickbacks one arm at a time and place the forearm of your other arm across your thighs for extra support.

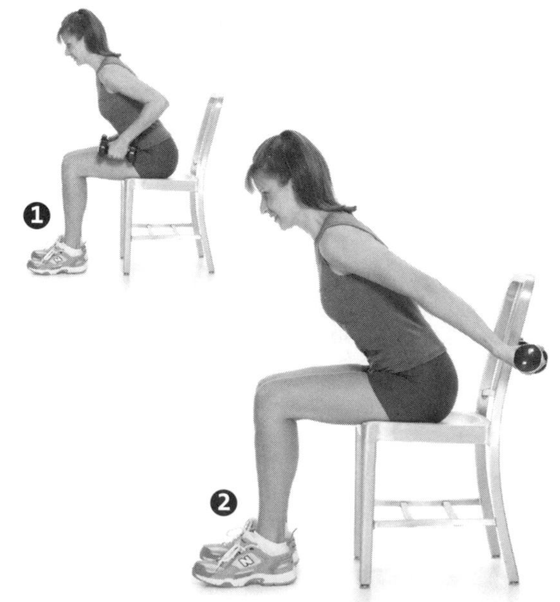

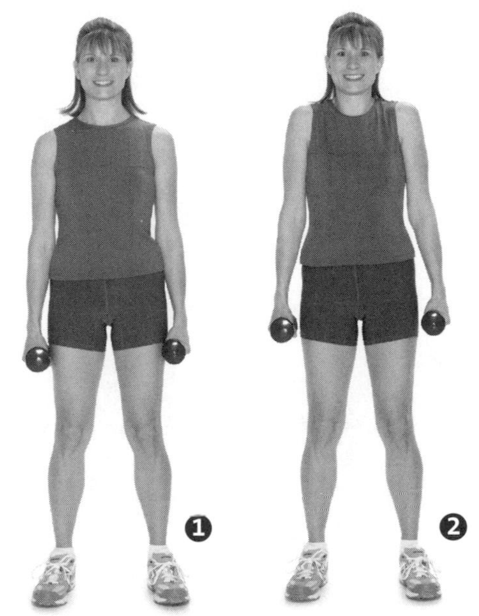

Shoulder Shrug

Starting position: Stand with your feet shoulder width apart, knees bent slightly. Hold a dumbbell in each hand with your arms at your sides, palms facing in.

Movement: Exhale as you slowly lift your shoulders up toward your ears as high as possible. Hold for a second and then inhale as you slowly lower them.

Technique: Don't bend your elbows. Don't use your arms to lift.

FIRM UP TIPS

MIND OVER MATTER	GET FIRM FASTER
Hang out with people who make you laugh. Avoid secondhand pessimism: the kind that rubs off when people complain, criticize, moan, and groan.	*Go slower when you lower dumbbells. Most people drive the weight up and then bring it down too fast. Resist letting gravity take over and lower the weight to a slow count of 1, 2, 3. Your muscles will work harder, so you'll get faster results.*

The Workout

Level 2

Easy Walk: 20 Minutes

- 5-minute warmup: Walk 2½ to 3 miles per hour, or 100 to 115 steps per minute.
- 10-minute moderate walk: Increase your speed to 3 to 3½ miles per hour, 115 to 125 steps per minute, or a pace that lets you comfortably carry on a conversation.
- 5-minute cooldown: Slow down to 2½ to 3 miles per hour, or 100 to 115 steps per minute.

Basic Strength Training: 30 Minutes

- Do 10 to 12 reps of each exercise. Repeat the sequence of exercises three times.
- To warm up, use lighter weights, or none at all, the first time through, and for the squat and lunge exercises, only go partway down.

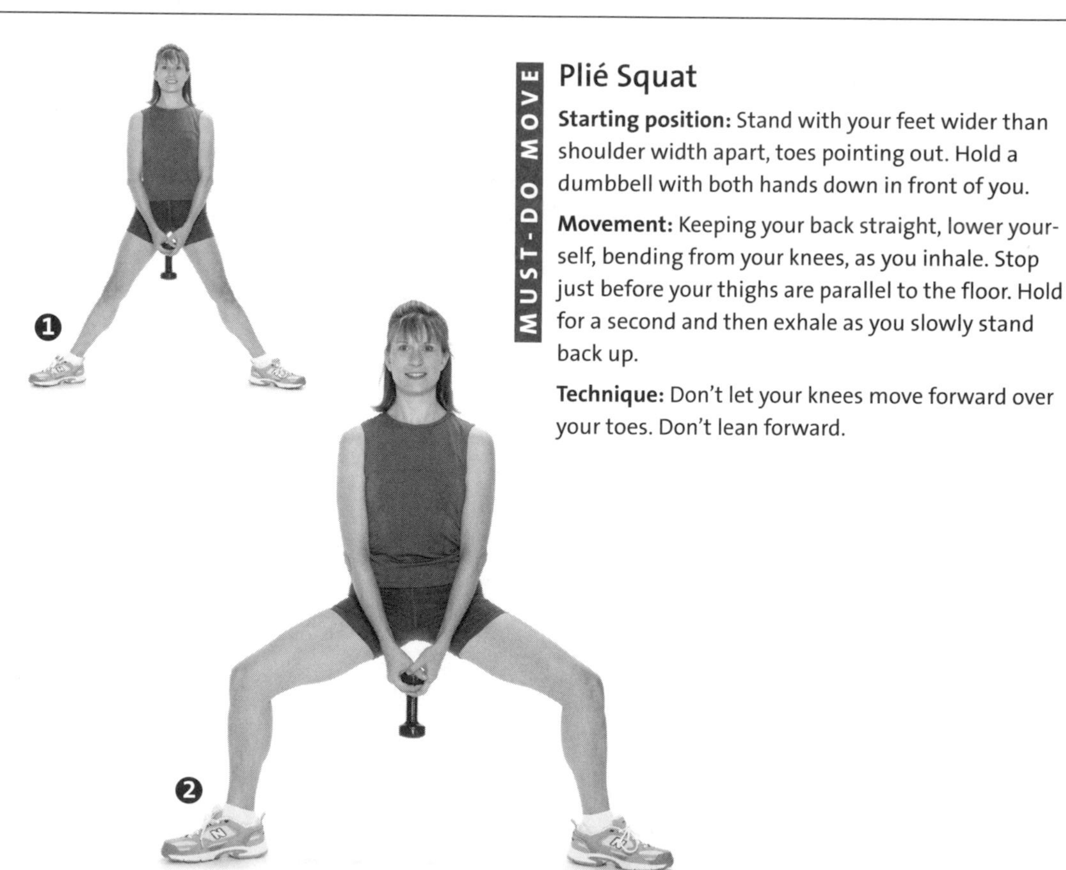

MUST-DO MOVE

Plié Squat

Starting position: Stand with your feet wider than shoulder width apart, toes pointing out. Hold a dumbbell with both hands down in front of you.

Movement: Keeping your back straight, lower yourself, bending from your knees, as you inhale. Stop just before your thighs are parallel to the floor. Hold for a second and then exhale as you slowly stand back up.

Technique: Don't let your knees move forward over your toes. Don't lean forward.

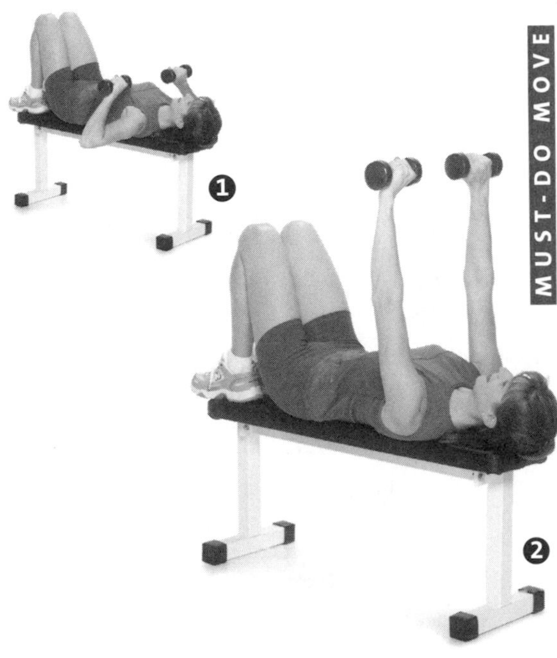

MUST-DO MOVE

Chest Press

Starting position: Lie on the floor (or on a bench) and hold dumbbells end to end, just above your shoulders. Your elbows should be pointing out to the sides.

Movement: Exhale as you press the dumbbells straight up over your chest, extending your arms. Hold for a second and then inhale as you slowly lower them.

Technique: Don't press the dumbbells back toward your head or forward toward your feet: They should go straight up and down. Don't arch your back.

Alternate position: If it's uncomfortable to have your feet on the bench, you can place them on the floor. Make sure your back doesn't arch in that position.

MUST-DO MOVE

Bent-Over Row

Starting position: Stand with your feet shoulder width apart, knees bent slightly. Hold a dumbbell in each hand with your arms at your sides. Keep your back flat and lean forward, bending at the hips so that the dumbbells are hanging at arm's length in front of you, palms facing each other.

Movement: Bending your elbows back and squeezing your shoulder blades, lift the weights toward your ribs as you exhale, until your elbows are higher than your back. Hold for a second and then inhale as you slowly lower them.

Technique: Don't arch your back. Don't pull your shoulders up toward your ears. Don't raise your torso as you lift the dumbbells.

Alternate move: If you have back problems, support yourself with one hand on a chair and do the rows one arm at a time.

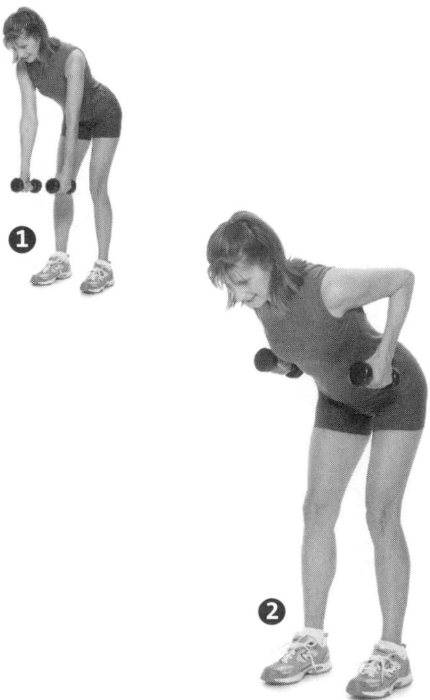

continued

The Workout

Level 2 *continued*

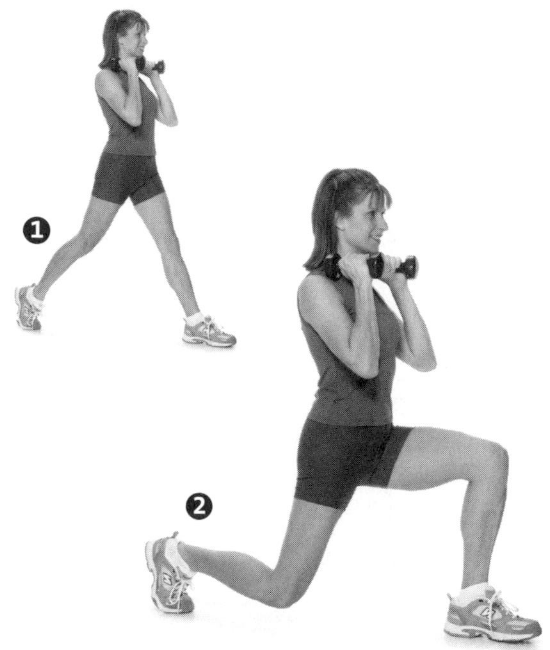

Lunge

Starting position: Stand with your feet 2 to 3 feet apart and your left foot in front of your right. Hold a dumbbell in each hand, either at shoulder height or at your sides.

Movement: Inhale as you bend your left knee and lower your body straight down until your left knee is bent 90 degrees and your right knee nearly touches the floor. Your rear heel will come off the floor. Hold for a second and then exhale as you slowly push yourself back up to the starting position. Finish all of your repetitions, then repeat the exercise with your right foot in front of your left.

Technique: Don't lean forward. Don't let your front knee move forward over your toes.

Biceps Curl

Starting position: Stand with your feet shoulder width apart, knees bent slightly. Hold a dumbbell in each hand with your palms facing forward.

Movement: Bending your elbows, lift the dumbbells toward your shoulders as you exhale. Stop when the dumbbells are at chest height, palms facing your body. Hold for a second, and then inhale as you slowly lower them.

Technique: Don't move your upper arms.

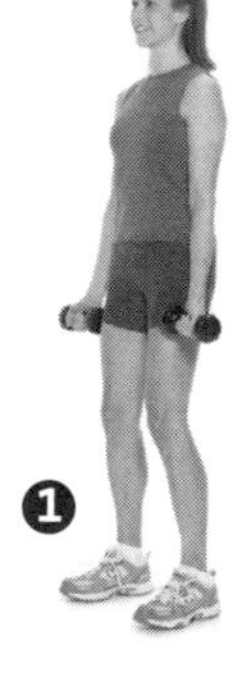

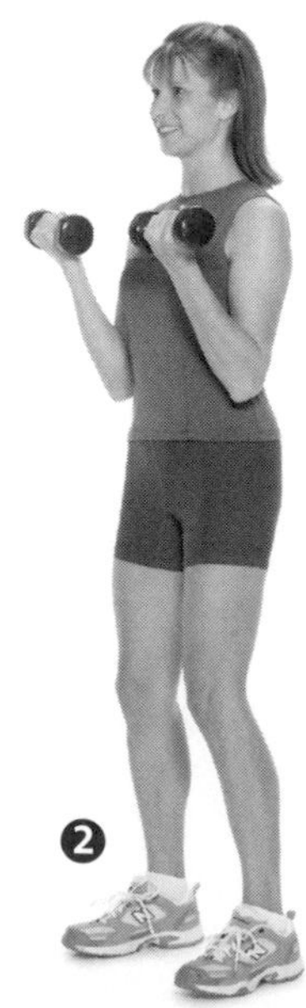

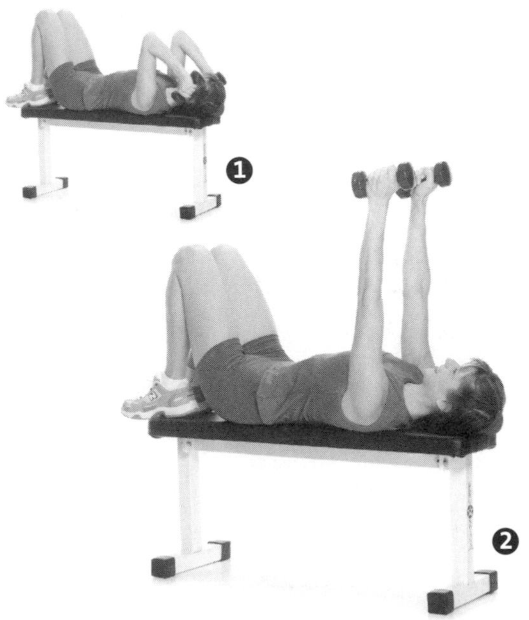

Lying Triceps Extension

Starting position: Lie face up on the floor (or on a bench). Hold a dumbbell in each hand over your chest. Bend your arms so that your elbows are pointing toward the ceiling and the dumbbells are by your ears.

Movement: Without moving your upper arms, press the weights up over your chest as you exhale. Hold for a second and then inhale as you slowly lower them.

Technique: Don't move from your shoulders. Don't arch your back.

Alternate position: If it's uncomfortable to have your feet on the bench, you can place them on the floor. Make sure your back doesn't arch in that position.

Lateral Raise

Starting position: Stand with your feet shoulder width apart, knees bent slightly. Hold a dumbbell in each hand with your arms at your sides, palms facing in, and elbows bent slightly.

Movement: Exhale as you slowly raise the dumbbells out to the sides until they are at about shoulder height. Hold for a second and then inhale as you slowly lower them.

Technique: Don't lift your shoulders. Don't lift higher than shoulder height.

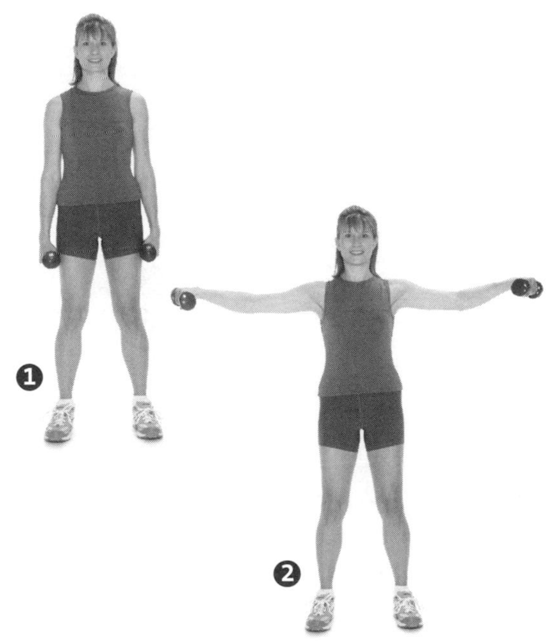

The Workout

Level 3

Easy Walk: 20 Minutes

- 5-minute warmup: Walk 2½ to 3 miles per hour, or 100 to 115 steps per minute.
- 10-minute moderate walk: Increase your speed to 3½ to 4 miles per hour, 125 to 135 steps per minute, or a pace that lets you comfortably carry on a conversation.
- 5-minute cooldown: Slow down to 2½ to 3 miles per hour, or 100 to 115 steps per minute.

Basic Strength Training: 40 Minutes

- Do 10 to 12 reps of each exercise. Repeat the sequence of exercises three times.
- To warm up, use lighter weights, or none at all, the first time through, and for the squat and lunge exercises, only go partway down.

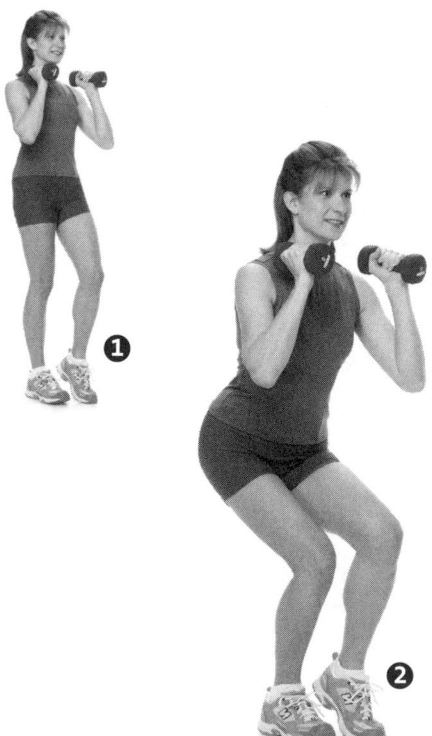

MUST-DO MOVE

One-Leg Squat

Starting position: Hold dumbbells in each hand at shoulder height or down at your sides. Shift your weight to your right foot and lift your left foot off the floor so that only your toes are lightly touching for balance.

Movement: As you inhale, bend your right knee and lean forward slightly from your hips, lowering yourself as if you were sitting in a chair. Go as low as is comfortable, but don't go past your right thigh being parallel to the floor. Hold for a second and then exhale as you slowly stand back up. Do the recommended number of reps and then switch legs.

Technique: Don't let your working knee come forward past your toes.

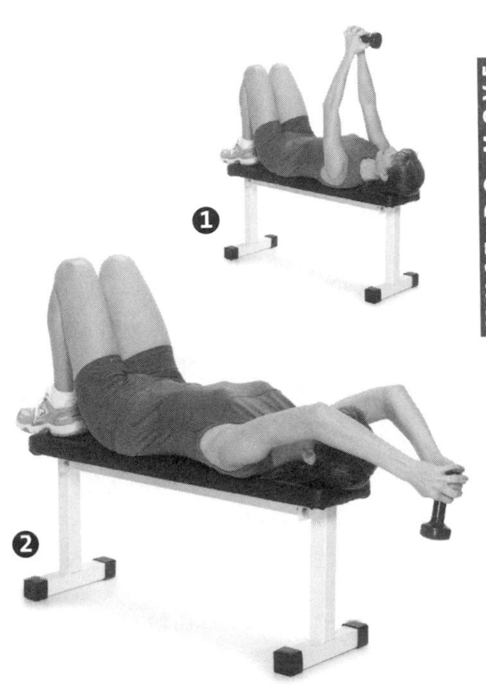

MUST-DO MOVE

Pullover

Starting position: Lie face up on the floor (or on a bench). Grasp a dumbbell with both hands and hold it above your chest with your elbows bent slightly.

Movement: Inhale as you lower the dumbbell backward over your head as far as comfortably possible without bending your elbows any farther than at the start. Hold for a second and then exhale as you slowly raise it to the starting position.

Technique: Don't arch your back. Don't bend your elbows to lower the weight.

Alternate position: If it's uncomfortable to have your feet on the bench, you can place them on the floor. Make sure your back doesn't arch in that position.

MUST-DO MOVE

Wide Bent-Over Row

Starting position: Stand with your feet shoulder width apart, knees bent slightly. Hold a dumbbell in each hand with your arms at your sides. Keep your back flat and lean forward, bending at the hips so that the dumbbells are hanging at arm's length in front of you, palms facing you.

Movement: Bending your elbows out to the sides and squeezing your shoulder blades, lift the dumbbells toward your ribs as you exhale, until your elbows are higher than your back. Hold for a second and then inhale as you slowly lower them.

Technique: Don't arch your back. Don't pull your shoulders up toward your ears. Don't raise your torso as you lift the dumbbells.

Alternate move: If you have back problems, support yourself with one hand on a chair and do the rows one arm at a time.

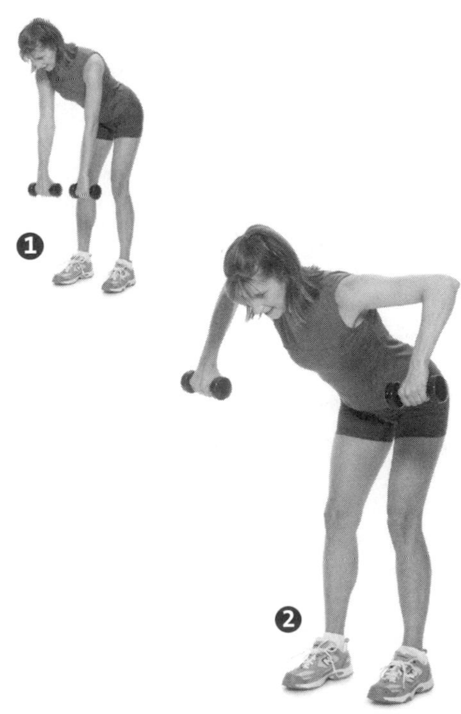

continued

The Workout

Level 3 *continued*

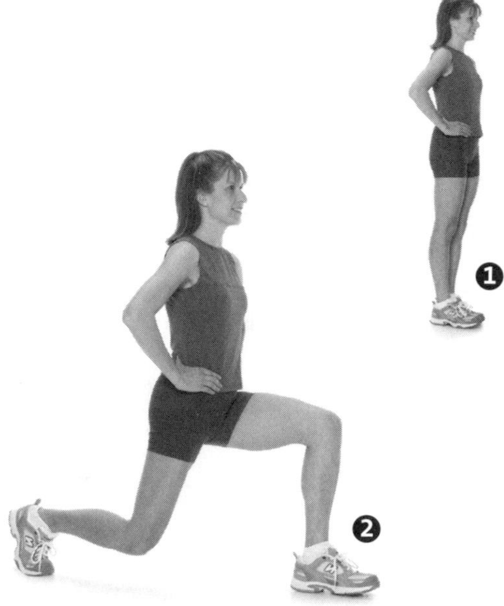

Back Lunge (no weights)

Starting position: Stand with your feet together and place your hands on your hips.

Movement: Step your right foot back 2 to 3 feet. Inhale as you bend your left knee and lower your body straight down until your left knee is bent 90 degrees and your right knee nearly touches the floor. Your rear heel will come off the floor. Hold for a second and then exhale as you push yourself back up, bringing your right foot in. Finish all of your repetitions, then repeat the exercise stepping your left foot back.

Technique: Don't lean forward. Don't let your front knee move forward over your toes.

Biceps Curl

Starting position: Stand with your feet shoulder width apart, knees bent slightly. Hold a dumbbell in each hand with your palms facing forward.

Movement: Bending your elbows, lift the dumbbells toward your shoulders as you exhale. Stop when the dumbbells are at chest height, palms facing your body. Hold for a second and then inhale as you slowly lower them.

Technique: Don't move your upper arms.

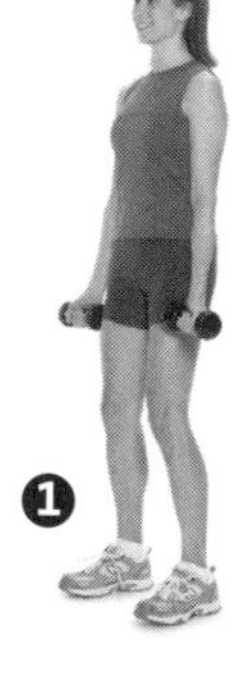

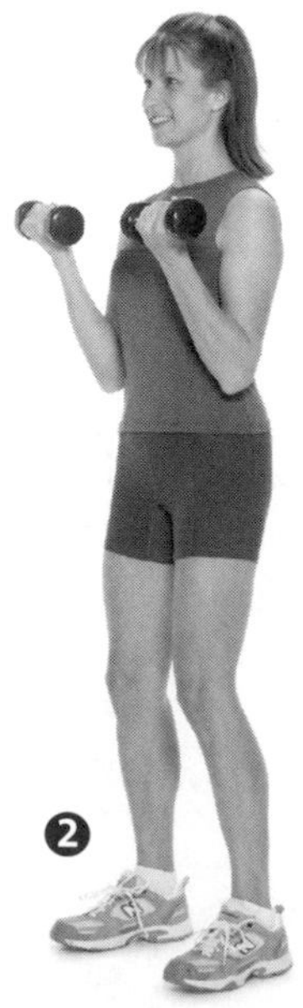

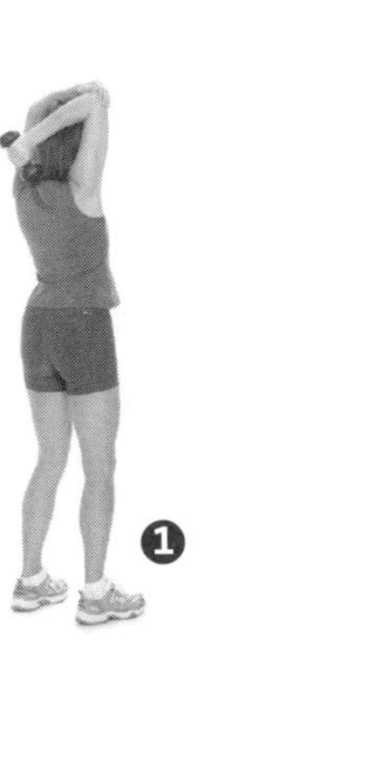

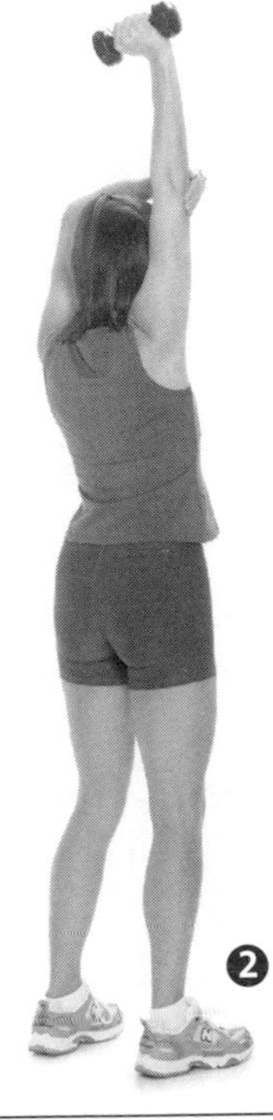

Overhead Triceps Extension

Starting position: Stand with your feet shoulder width apart and knees bent slightly. Hold a dumbbell in your right hand and lift it up over your head. Bend your elbow so that it is pointing toward the ceiling and the dumbbell is behind your head. Place your left hand on your right elbow for support.

Movement: Exhale as you extend your right arm and lift the dumbbell over your head. Hold for a second and then inhale as you slowly lower it. Do the recommended number of reps and then repeat with your left arm.

Technique: Don't lift your shoulders up toward your ears. Don't bend your wrist.

Overhead Press

Starting position: Stand with your feet shoulder width apart and knees bent slightly. Hold a dumbbell in each hand at shoulder height with your palms facing forward and elbows pointing out to the sides.

Movement: Exhale as you slowly press the dumbbells straight up overhead. Hold for a second and then inhale as you slowly lower them.

Technique: Don't arch your back. Don't lift the dumbbells forward or back.

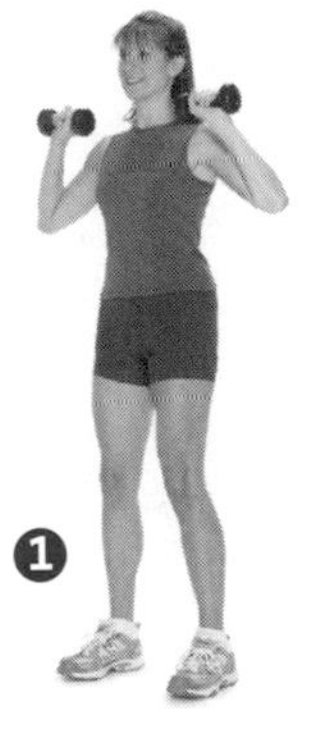

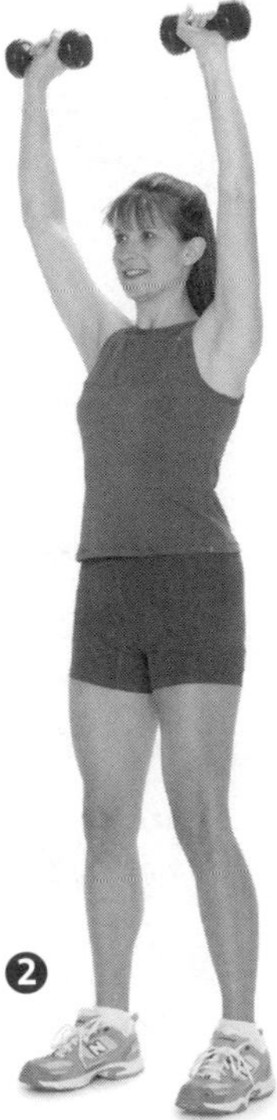

FIRM UP / DAY 6

Don't Drink Your Calories

Some 10 to 14 percent of your daily calories don't come from food at all, according to the USDA. Instead, they sneak through in beverages that wash down those calorie-counted meals. One caffe latte for breakfast, one can of soda at lunch, and a fruit smoothie snack can blow your daily budget by 550 calories!

While they're certainly tasty going down, liquid calories don't register on your appetite meter the way solid food does. In a study in which researchers asked 15 people to drink an extra 450 calories a day (the amount in three cans of soda), they gained weight. When they consumed the same number of additional calories from food, however, their weight didn't change. They made up for the extra food by eating less throughout the day. But they didn't compensate for the drinks, thus adding 450 calories to their normal day's total.

And studies also have found that the more sweetened beverages people drink, the less likely they are to be getting enough essential vitamins and minerals, such as bone-building calcium and heart-protective folate.

That's why the Firm Up Eating Plan limits calorie-filled beverages, except for calcium-rich, low-fat or fat-free dairy or soy milk and antioxidant-rich tomato, orange, or Concord grape juice. Just keep tabs on how much you're drinking, or dilute the juice with sparkling water or diet lemon soda for a refreshing twist. Most of the time, stick to calorie-free beverages such as water, club soda, unsweetened iced tea, or diet soda.

FIRM UP TIP

ENERGY BOOSTER

Didn't get much sleep last night? A 10-minute nap is your best midday recharger. In an Australian study, 12 university students had no nap, a 5-minute nap, a 10-minute nap, or a 30-minute nap following a short night's sleep. Participants whose naps were shorter than 10 minutes didn't get any benefit, while those who slept longer woke up feeling groggy. The 10-minute nap provided immediate improvement in alertness, mood, and performance, because it wasn't long enough to enter deeper sleep, which produces sleep inertia, the researchers explain.

Meal Plan

Most of these recipes are custom designed to make 1 serving—no fuss, no muss; just fix, eat, and go! If a recipe makes more than 1 serving, it's noted below. Save that extra serving for another meal, or share it with your spouse or your walking buddy.

Breakfast

Energy Bar: Have 1 Luna bar, ½ cup fat-free milk, ⅛ cup pistachios, and a 0.9-ounce package Sunsweet dried plums.

Healthy Snack

Applesauce: Try convenient single-serving peel-top containers with ½ cup applesauce (such as Mott's Natural Style or Mott's Healthy Harvest—any flavor). Serve with 20 peanuts.

Lunch

Grilled Cheese and Tomato Sandwich: Between 2 slices whole wheat bread, place 2 slices reduced-fat cheese and 3 slices tomato. Grill in a nonstick skillet coated with cooking spray or in the toaster oven until melted. Serve with 1 cup raw vegetables of your choice (such as cherry tomatoes, sliced green or red peppers, or baby carrots).

Healthy Snack

Fruit and Almond Butter: Slice a ripe pear or apple, and spread with 2 tablespoons almond butter.

Dinner

Ravioli and Garlic Spinach: Heat an entire box (10 ounces) spinach in the microwave. Squeeze out excess water. Mix with ¼ teaspoon salt, ½ teaspoon ground black pepper, and 2 teaspoons minced garlic. Choose refrigerated low-fat ravioli such as Buitoni Light Four-Cheese Ravioli. Prepare the ravioli according to package directions. Serve ¾ cup ravioli topped with ⅓ cup spaghetti sauce. Serve with half of the garlic spinach and 1 small orange, sliced.

Indulgent Treat

Buffalo Wings: Treat yourself to 6 small Buffalo-style chicken wings.

Nutrient analysis: 1,706 calories, 90 g protein, 206 g carbohydrates, 69 g total fat, 18 g saturated fat, 198 mg cholesterol, 28 g dietary fiber, 2,140 mg sodium, 1,343 mg calcium

FIRM UP TIPS

ON YOUR PLATE

Eat it only if it's worth it. Sometimes you pop a high-cal treat into your mouth, only to realize that it's just not worth the extra calories. Don't be embarrassed—just spit it out discreetly into a napkin.

MYTH BUSTER

Eating late at night won't itself cause weight gain. It's how many calories—not when you eat them—that counts.

The Workout

Level 1

Speed Walk: 20 Minutes

- 5-minute warmup: Walk 2 miles per hour, or about 95 steps per minute.
- 10-minute speedup: Increase your speed, walking as quickly as you can. You can do a loop, or you can walk out 5 minutes and then turn around and walk back. If you choose the latter option, note where you turned around, because you'll want to use that same turnaround point for future speed walks.
- 5-minute cooldown: Slow down to 2 miles per hour, or about 95 steps per minute.

Core Training: 10 Minutes

- Do the sequence of exercises one time.

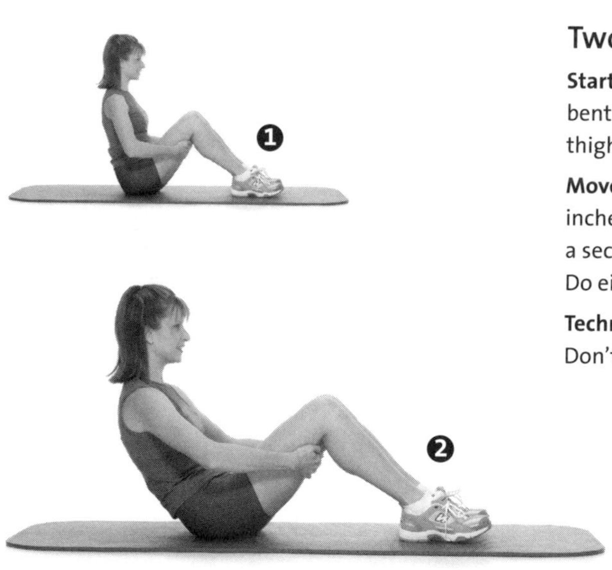

Two-Hand Roll-Down

Starting position: Sit on the floor with your knees bent and your feet flat. Place your hands behind your thighs.

Movement: Using your abs, slowly roll down 2 to 3 inches, one vertebra at a time, as you inhale. Hold for a second and then exhale as you slowly roll back up. Do eight reps.

Technique: Your abs should be powering the move. Don't move quickly.

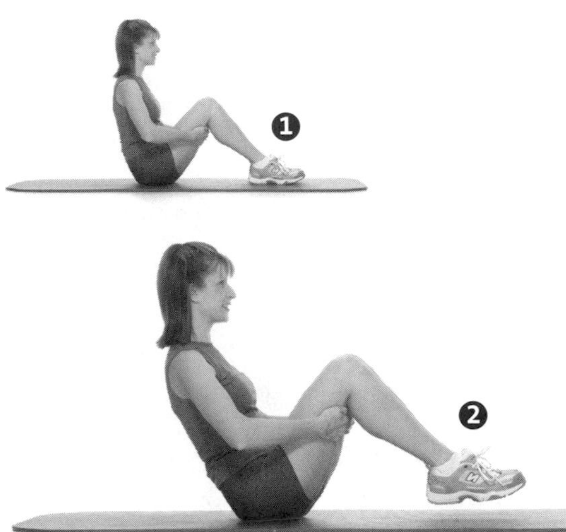

Holding Balance

Starting position: Sit on the floor with your knees bent and your feet flat. Place your hands behind your thighs.

Movement: Lift your feet off the floor slightly and balance on your sitting bones. Hold for three slow breaths and then relax. Do one time only.

Technique: Keep your abs tight and the rest of your body relaxed, especially your shoulders.

MUST-DO MOVE

Easy Ab Crunch

Starting position: Lie on your back with your knees bent, feet flat on the floor, and arms at your sides, palms facing down.

Movement: Using your abs, slowly raise your head, shoulders, and upper back about 45 degrees off the floor as you exhale. Think of shortening the distance between your ribs and pelvis. Hold for a second and then inhale as you slowly lower yourself. Do eight reps.

Technique: Don't pull your chin to your chest. Don't arch your back.

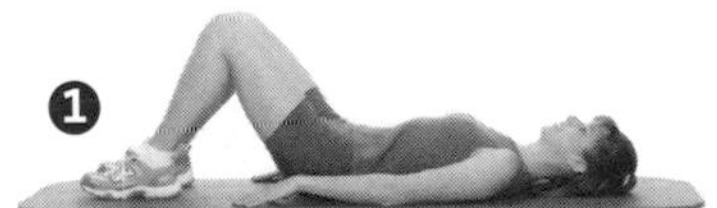

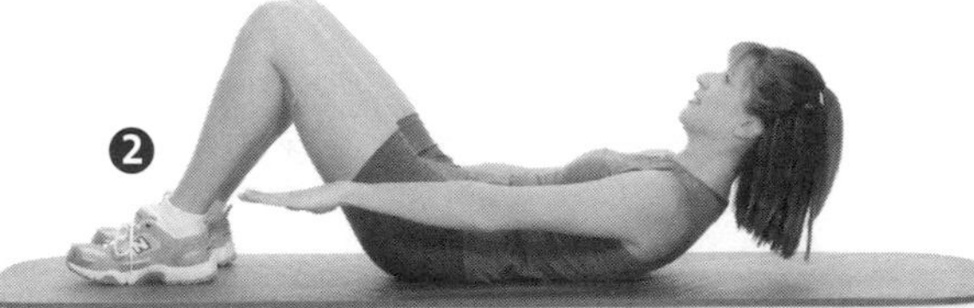

continued

The Workout

Level 1 *continued*

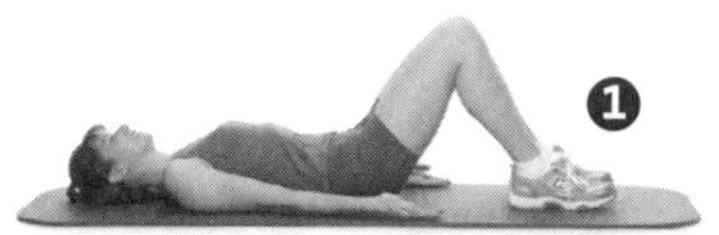

MUST-DO MOVE

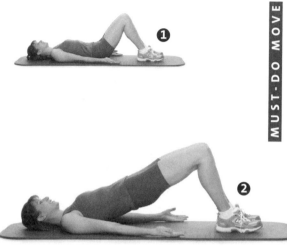

Bridge

Starting position: Lie on your back with your knees bent, feet flat on the floor, and arms at your sides, with palms facing up.

Movement: Contracting your abs, buttocks, and lower back, press into your feet and lift your butt, hips, and back off the floor as you exhale, to form a straight line from your shoulders to your knees. Hold for three slow breaths and then relax. Do one time only.

Technique: Don't lift too high—your upper back and shoulders should remain on the floor. Don't bend at the waist or hips. Don't let your knees fall inward or outward.

MUST-DO MOVE

Knee Plank

Starting position: Lie facedown with your knees bent so that your feet are in the air. Your elbows should be under your shoulders and your forearms and palms on the floor.

Movement: Contracting your abs and back, press into your forearms as you exhale and lift your pelvis off the floor so that your back and thighs form a straight line. Hold for three breaths and then relax. Do one time only.

Technique: Don't lift your head up or let it drop. Don't bend at the waist. Don't arch your back.

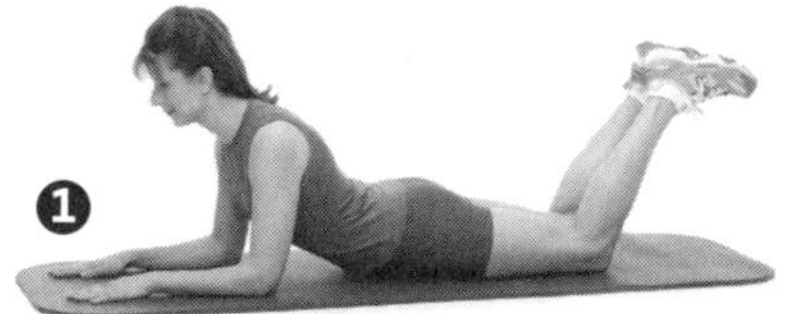

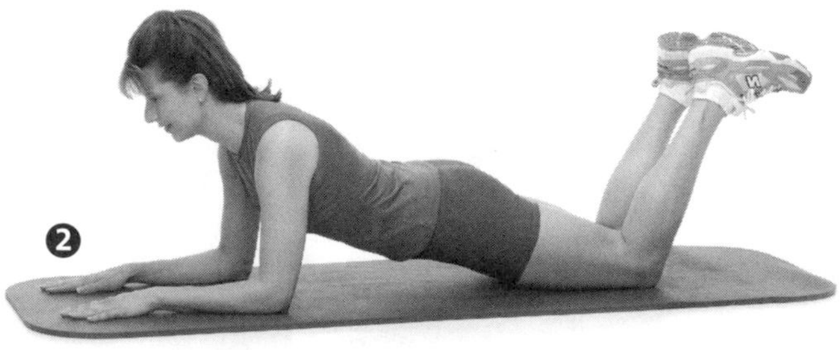

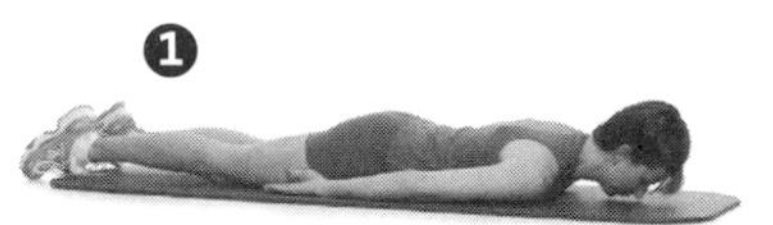

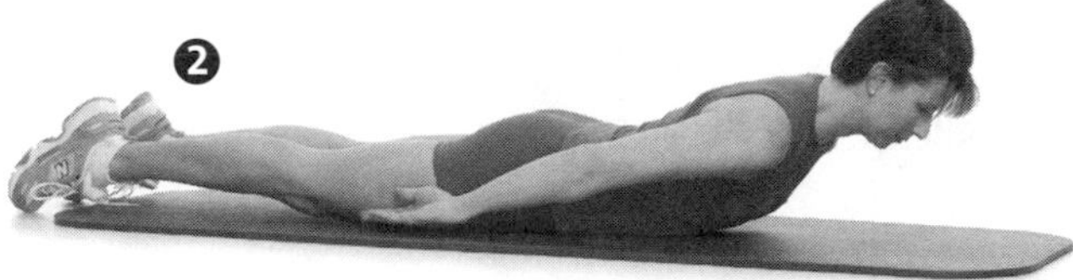

Chest Lift

Starting position: Lie facedown on the floor with your arms at your sides and palms facing up.

Movement: Exhale as you lift your head and chest 5 to 6 inches off the floor. Hold for a second and then inhale as you slowly lower yourself. Do eight reps.

Technique: Don't look up. Don't lift too high.

FIRM UP TIP

GET FIRM FASTER

Remember to cool down. Finishing your workout with 5 minutes of easy activity can make it more enjoyable, according to a study by Britton W. Brewer, Ph.D., of Springfield College in Massachusetts. "People's last impression of exercise is the one that lingers," he says. "With a cooldown, you'll leave feeling the exercise was easier, so you're more likely to do it again."

The Workout

Level 2

Speed Walk: 20 Minutes

- 5-minute warmup: Walk 2 to 2½ miles per hour, or 95 to 100 steps per minute.
- 10-minute speedup: Increase your speed, walking as quickly as you can. You can do a loop, or you can walk out 5 minutes and then turn around and walk back. If you choose the latter option, note where you turned around, because you'll want to use that same turnaround point for future speed walks.
- 5-minute cooldown: Slow down to 2 to 2½ miles per hour, or 95 to 100 steps per minute.

Core Training: 10 Minutes

- Do the sequence of exercises one time.

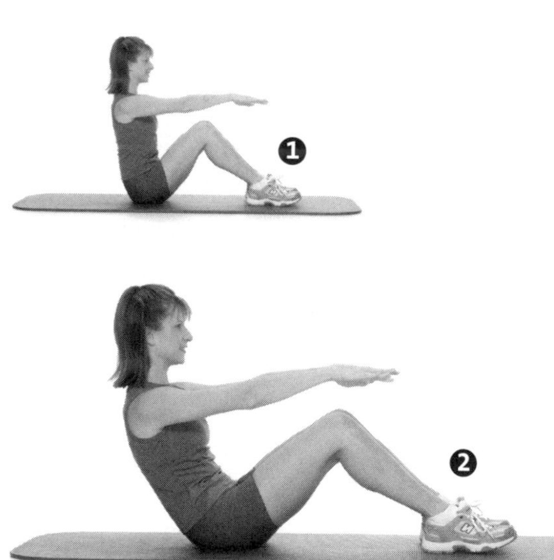

Roll-Down

Starting position: Sit on the floor with your knees bent and your feet flat. Hold your arms straight out in front of you, parallel to the floor.

Movement: Using your abs, slowly roll down 3 to 4 inches, one vertebra at a time, as you inhale. Hold for a second and then exhale as you slowly roll back up. Do eight reps.

Technique: Your abs should be powering the move. Don't move quickly.

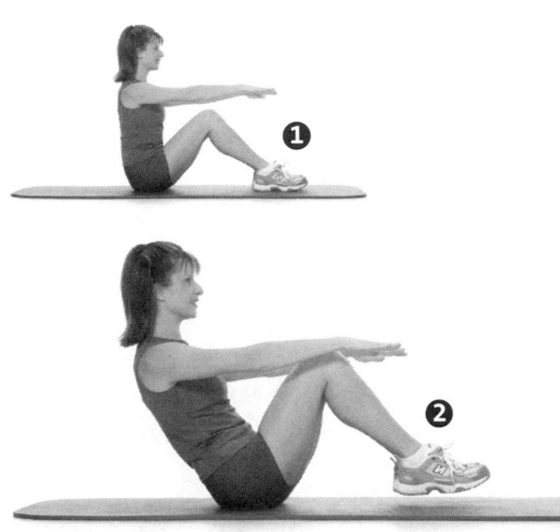

Partial Balance

Starting position: Sit on the floor with your knees bent and your feet flat. Hold your arms straight out in front of you, parallel to the floor.

Movement: Lift your feet slightly off the floor and balance on your sitting bones. Hold for four breaths and then relax. Do one time only.

Technique: Keep your abs tight and the rest of your body relaxed, especially your shoulders.

MUST-DO MOVE

Ab Crunch

Starting position: Lie on your back with your knees bent, feet flat on the floor, and hands behind your head.

Movement: Using your abs, slowly raise your head, shoulders, and upper back about 45 degrees off the floor as you exhale. Think of shortening the distance between your ribs and pelvis. Hold for a second and then inhale as you slowly lower yourself. Do eight reps.

Technique: Don't pull your chin to your chest. Don't arch your back.

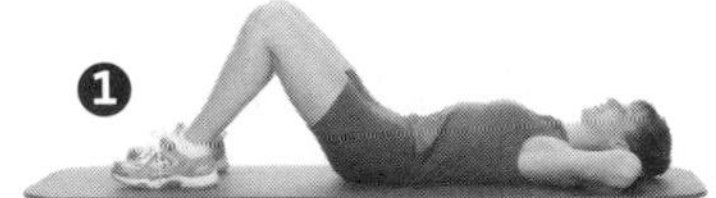

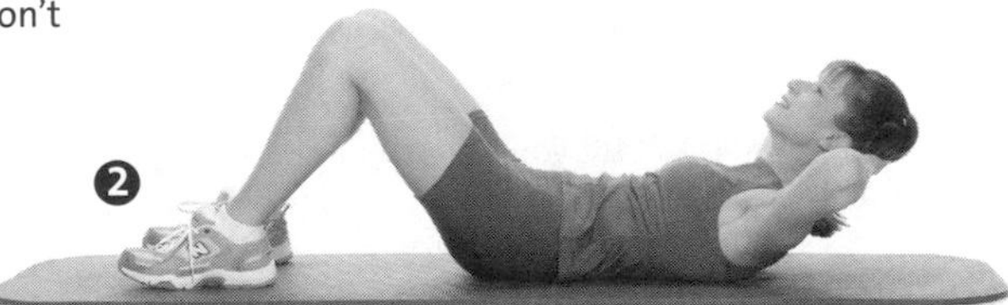

continued

The Workout

Level 2 *continued*

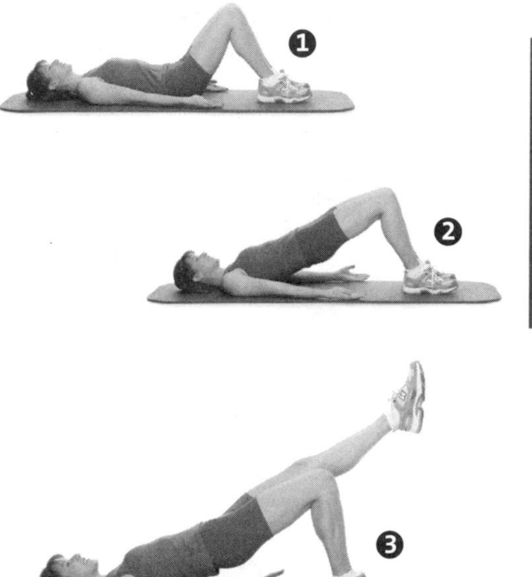

MUST-DO MOVE

Bridge with Leg Lift

Starting position: Lie on your back with your knees bent, feet flat on the floor, and arms at your sides, palms facing up.

Movement: Contracting your abs, buttocks, and lower back, press into your feet and lift your butt, hips, and back off the floor as you exhale, to form a straight line from your shoulders to your knees. Lift one foot off the floor and extend that leg. Hold for two breaths and then lower your foot. Lift the other foot up and hold for two breaths. Lower your foot and return to the starting position. Do one time only.

Technique: Don't lift too high—your upper back and shoulders should remain on the floor. Don't bend at the waist or hips. Don't let your knees fall inward or outward.

MUST-DO MOVE

Plank

Starting position: Lie facedown with your feet flexed and toes tucked. Your elbows should be under your shoulders and your forearms and palms on the floor.

Movement: Contracting your abs and back, press into your forearms as you exhale and lift your pelvis and legs off the floor so that your back and legs form a straight line. Hold for four breaths and then relax. Do one time only.

Technique: Don't lift your head up or let it drop. Don't bend at the waist or hips. Don't let your belly drop toward the floor.

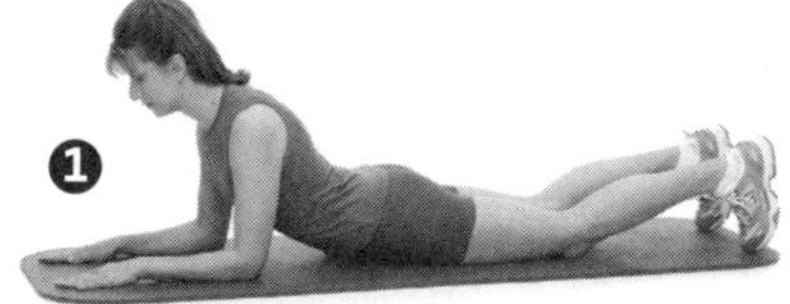

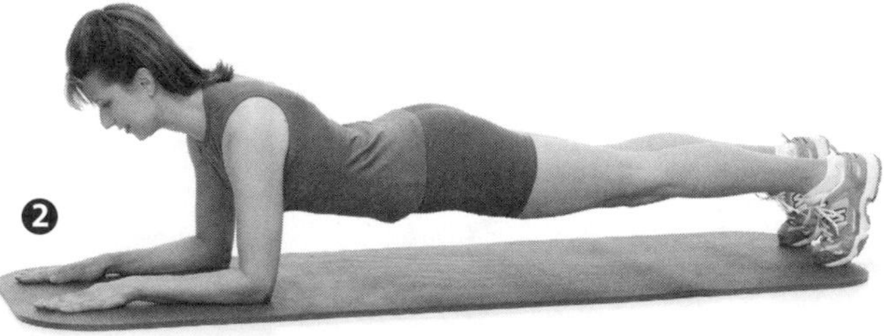

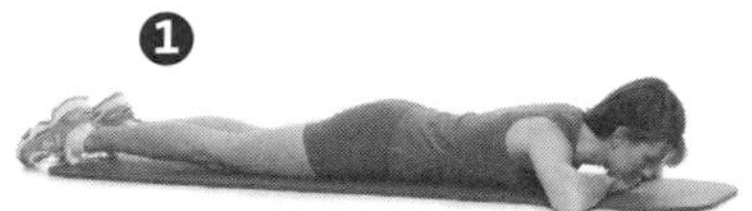

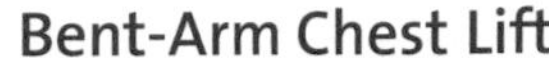

Bent-Arm Chest Lift

Starting position: Lie facedown on the floor with your hands under your chin.

Movement: Exhale as you lift your head and chest 5 to 6 inches off the floor. Hold for a second and then inhale as you slowly lower yourself. Do eight reps.

Technique: Don't lift too high.

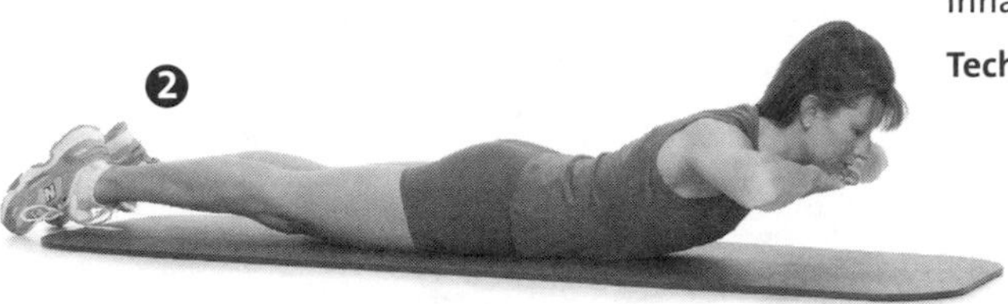

FIRM UP TIP

ENERGY BOOSTER

Do a little dance. When people say they're too tired to exercise, their fatigue is often emotional rather than physical, says Rebecca Gorrell, a movement therapist at Canyon Ranch Health Resort in Tucson, Arizona. "Movement can help people shift their energy, stabilize their emotions, and bring a profound sense of joy." Play your favorite music and just move.

The Workout

Level 3

Speed Walk: 20 Minutes

- 5-minute warmup: Walk 2½ to 3 miles per hour, or 100 to 115 steps per minute.
- 10-minute speedup: Increase your speed, walking as quickly as you can. You can do a loop, or you can walk out 5 minutes and then turn around and walk back. If you choose the latter option, note where you turned around, because you'll want to use that same turnaround point for future speed walks.
- 5-minute cooldown: Slow down to 2½ to 3 miles per hour, or 100 to 115 steps per minute.

Core Training: 10 Minutes

- Do the sequence of exercises one time.

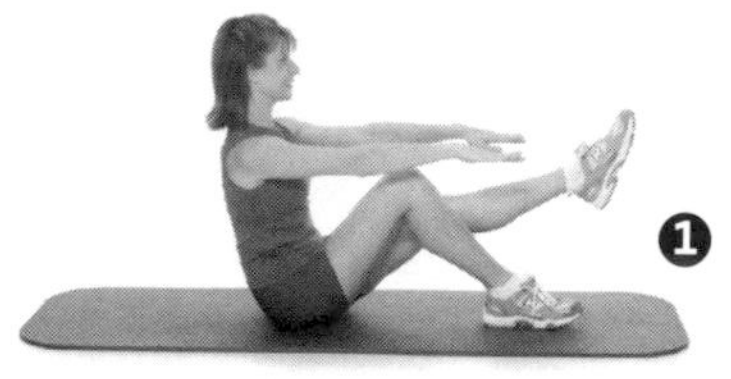

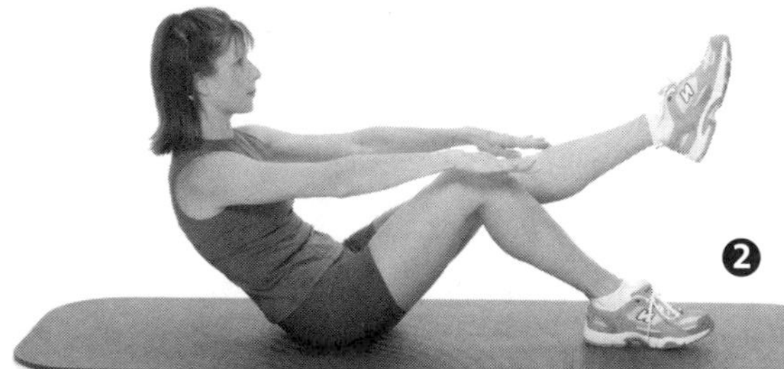

One-Leg Roll-Down

Starting position: Sit on the floor with your knees bent and your feet flat. Lift your left foot off the floor and extend your left leg. Hold your arms straight out in front of you, parallel to the floor.

Movement: Using your abs, slowly roll down 4 to 5 inches, one vertebra at a time, as you inhale. Hold for a second and then exhale as you slowly roll back up. Do four reps, switch legs, and do four more reps.

Technique: Your abs should be powering the move. Don't move quickly.

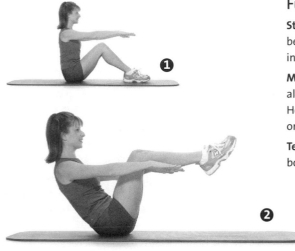

Full Balance

Starting position: Sit on the floor with your knees bent and your feet flat. Hold your arms straight out in front of you, parallel to the floor.

Movement: Lift your feet so that your calves are parallel to the floor, and balance on your sitting bones. Hold for five breaths and then relax. Do one time only.

Technique: Keep your abs tight and the rest of your body relaxed, especially your shoulders.

MUST-DO MOVE

Legs-Up Ab Crunch

Starting position: Lie on your back with your legs in the air and your hands behind your head.

Movement: Using your abs, slowly raise your head, shoulders, and upper back about 45 degrees off the floor as you exhale. Think of shortening the distance between your ribs and pelvis. Hold for a second and then inhale as you slowly lower yourself. Do eight reps.

Technique: Don't pull your chin to your chest.

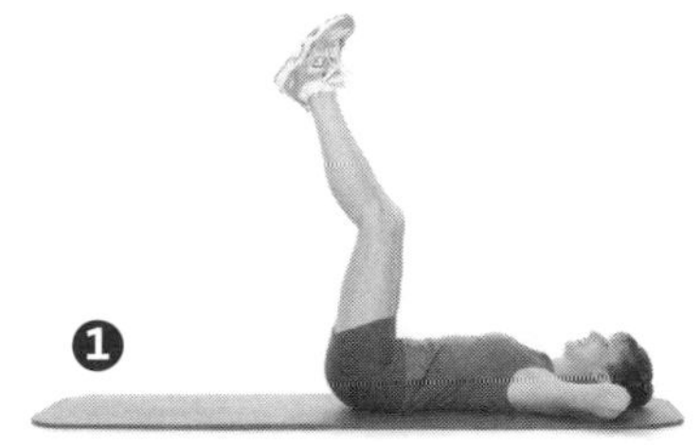

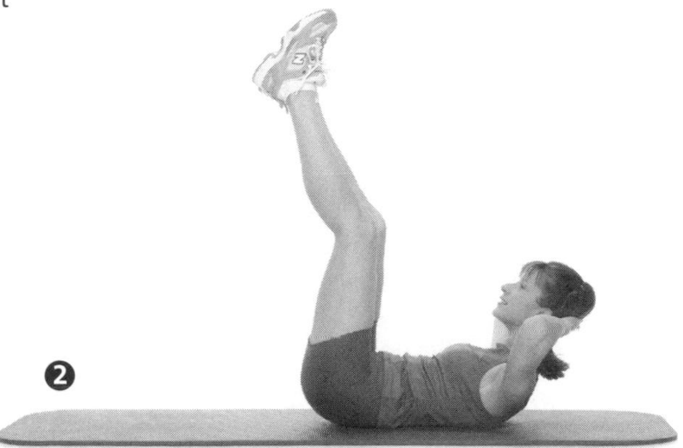

continued

The Workout

Level 3 *continued*

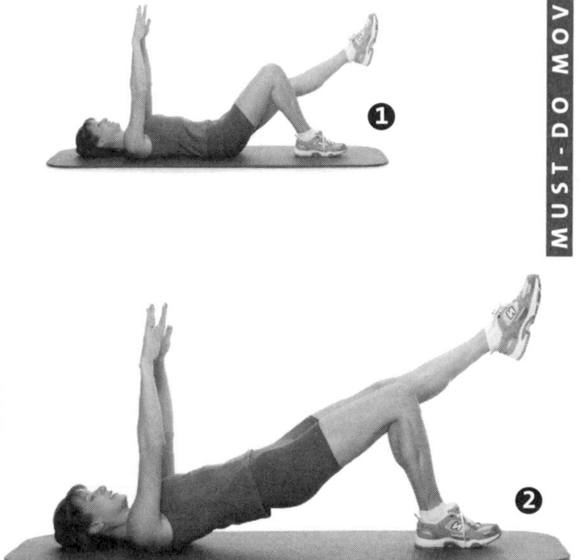

MUST-DO MOVE

One-Leg Bridge with Arms Up

Starting position: Lie on your back with your knees bent, feet flat on the floor, and arms extended over your chest. Lift your left foot off the floor and extend your left leg.

Movement: Contracting your abs, buttocks, lower back, press into your right foot and lift your butt, hips, and back off the floor as you exhale, to form a straight line from your shoulders to your knees. Hold for three breaths and then lower yourself. Repeat with right leg extended. Do one time only with each leg.

Technique: Don't lift too high—your upper back and shoulders should remain on the floor. Don't bend at the waist or hips. Don't let your knees fall inward or outward.

MUST-DO MOVE

Plank with Leg Lift

Starting position: Lie facedown with your feet flexed and toes tucked. Your elbows should be under your shoulders and your forearms and palms on the floor.

Movement: Contracting your abs and back, press into your hands and forearms as you exhale and lift your pelvis and legs off the floor so that your back and legs form a straight line. Lift your left foot off the floor, hold for three breaths, and then relax. Repeat by lifting your right foot off the floor. Do one time only with each leg.

Technique: Don't lift your head up or let it drop. Don't bend at the waist or hips. Don't let your belly drop toward the floor.

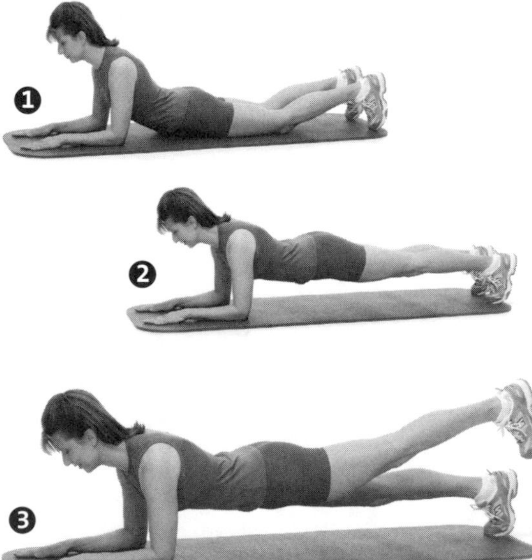

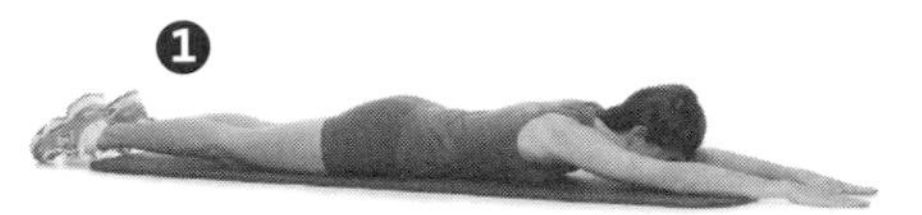

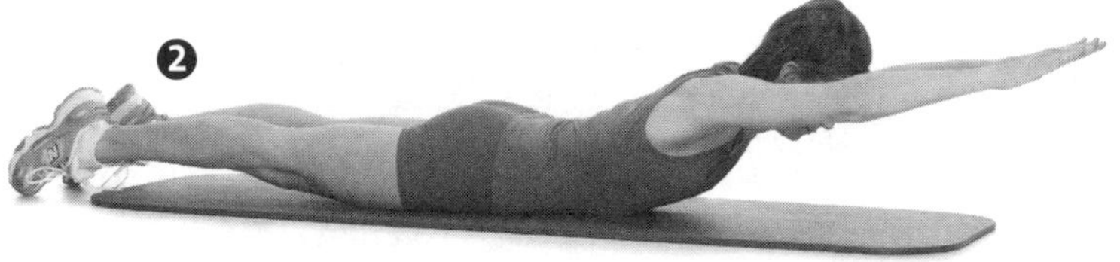

Extended Chest Lift

Starting position: Lie facedown on the floor with your arms extended overhead.

Movement: Exhale as you lift your arms, head, and chest 5 to 6 inches off the floor. Hold for a second and then inhale as you slowly lower yourself. Do eight reps.

Technique: Don't lift too high.

FIRM UP TIP

FIT FACT

In a study of 103 women with type A personalities, researchers found that those with angry temperaments who were unfit had unhealthy cholesterol levels, while their physically fit counterparts had healthy cholesterol levels. Uncontrolled anger appears to elevate cholesterol and triglyceride levels, say researchers, but exercise appears to bring it back down to healthy levels.

FIRM UP / DAY 7

Fun *and* Rewarding

Remember the rewards you wrote down in chapter 2 before you started the Firm Up Program? Well, you've earned the first one, so go out and enjoy it. In fact, why not make today's walk a fun and rewarding experience, too! Here are some ideas to start you off on the right track.

Get off the sidewalk. Check out local hiking trails, Rails-to-Trails paths, or canal towpaths. The uneven terrain will give your body a new kind of workout, and the beautiful surroundings will give your mind a much-needed break. Bring the family along and pack a picnic for an all-day adventure.

Explore new neighborhoods. Drive to a nearby town that you've never walked around. Park your car and start exploring. Window-shop as you walk along the main street. Venture down side streets and check out the architecture, landscaping, and unique decorations–steal a few ideas for your home. After your walk, visit one of the stores that looked interesting and buy yourself something special–you deserve it.

Make it a date. Invite a friend, your spouse, a parent, or one of your children to walk with you. Take advantage of this opportunity for a little one-on-one time to catch up, without all the distractions of home or the calories of meeting for lunch or dinner. You may even be so busy talking that you'll end up walking longer than you had planned!

FIRM UP TIPS

ON YOUR PLATE	FIT FACT
Watch a spooky movie. You're less likely to eat when you're fearful–but more likely when you're angry or happy.	*Watching more than 4 hours of TV a day may double your odds of getting diabetes, compared to watching less than 2 hours weekly. Forty hours a week can triple your risk, according to a study of the viewing habits of nearly 38,000 men.*

Meal Plan

Most of these recipes are custom designed to make 1 serving–no fuss, no muss; just fix, eat, and go! If a recipe makes more than 1 serving, it's noted below. Save that extra serving for another meal, or share it with your spouse or your walking buddy.

Breakfast

Bagel and Cheese: Spread ½ bagel (2½- to 3-ounce size, such as Lender's refrigerated honey wheat bagels, 2.85 ounces) with 2 tablespoons farmer's cheese or reduced-fat cream cheese. Serve with ½ cup fat-free milk and ¾ cup honeydew melon pieces.

Healthy Snack

Café au Lait and Muffin: Mix together 1 cup hot brewed or instant coffee (regular or decaf), 1 cup hot fat-free milk, and 1 teaspoon sugar (if desired). Serve with a mini blueberry muffin (such as a Hostess Blueberry Mini Muffin).

Lunch

Grilled Chicken Caesar Salad: Many restaurants use about 6 ounces chicken; you want to eat 3 ounces, about the size of a deck of cards. (In most cases, that means you'll have chicken to take home for dinner Monday night.) Eat 2 or more cups of salad greens. Ask for dressing on the side; use 2 tablespoons. Top with 3 tablespoons croutons (2 tablespoons if they're the really greasy type). Have ½ cup fruit for dessert.

Healthy Snack

Crackers and Almond Butter: Top 2 Wasa crispbreads with 1 tablespoon almond butter.

Dinner

Homemade Pizza: Top 1 large Neopolitan-style pizza crust with 1¼ cups spaghetti sauce and 1¾ cups (7 ounces) reduced-fat shredded cheese. Top with any vegetables you choose, such as thinly sliced fresh red pepper, thawed frozen (or raw) chopped onion, chopped fresh tomato or a small can stewed tomatoes, and a small can mushrooms (all drained). Remember that the vegetables add only 25 calories per ½ to 1 cup, so be generous. Bake the pizza at 400°F for 12 to 15 minutes. Cut the pizza into 8 equal slices. Serve 1 slice with a salad of 2 cups bagged baby spinach leaves tossed with 2 tablespoons light salad dressing and 2 tablespoons chopped walnuts. Cover the remaining 7 slices with foil and store in the refrigerator for up to 3 days or freeze to use later.

Indulgent Treat

Wine and Cheese: Enjoy 4 ounces wine with 1 Wasa crispbread spread with 1 tablespoon farmer's cheese or reduced-fat cream cheese.

Nutrient analysis: 1,690 calories, 92 g protein, 181 g carbohydrates, 61 g total fat, 16 g saturated fat, 127 mg cholesterol, 23 g dietary fiber, 2,384 mg sodium, 1,170 mg calcium

The Workout

Levels 1 and 2

Long Walk: 40 Minutes

- Drive to a different neighborhood, or find a trail, and walk at a comfortable pace that you can sustain for 40 minutes.

Level 3

Long Walk: 50 Minutes

- Drive to a different neighborhood, or find a trail, and walk at a comfortable pace that you can sustain for 50 minutes.

FIRM UP TIP

GET FIRM FASTER

Don't let rewards outweigh effort. Most people who use food as a reward take in more calories than they've expended. If you're going to use dessert or a nice dinner as your "carrot" to keep going, then reward yourself less frequently. Once a month, if you've exercised consistently, go to your favorite restaurant and get whatever you want. For more frequent rewards, stick to CDs, clothes, and other nonfood items.

Your Reward Diary

Remember to write down your weekly reward here. What are you doing for yourself this week?

____

____

____

____

____

____

____

____

CHAPTER 4

Week 2

Congratulations! You've completed the first week, and you are on your way to firming up and slimming down. Before you move on to week 2 or during this week, take a look at chapter 8, Get a Winning Attitude. Your attitude toward physical activity is an important key to your long-term success.

Grocery List

Photocopy this list and take it with you to the store. You can stock up on everything you need to make the second week's Firm Up meals and snacks, so all the ingredients will be at hand when you need them. The amounts of the fresh ingredients are tailored so that you're buying exactly as much as you need. And you should still have some of the items, such as the spices and condiments, from week 1's shopping list to use this week. For some specific brand recommendations, see page 321 in chapter 7, Mix-and-Match Meals.

Produce Aisle

☐ 1 bunch asparagus (if not in season, choose 1 small package frozen asparagus)

☐ 1 California avocado

☐ 1 banana

☐ 1 head broccoli

☐ 1 head cauliflower

☐ 1 medium cucumber

☐ 1 small bunch grapes

☐ 1 kiwifruit

☐ 1 bag romaine lettuce

☐ 1 small red onion

☐ 1 small sweet yellow or Vidalia onion

☐ 2 oranges

☐ Choose: 2 peaches *or* 2 similar-size fruits

☐ Choose: 2 pears *or* 1 pear and 1 apple

☐ 1 red pepper

☐ 1 large potato

☐ 3 containers raspberries (if unavailable, choose 1 (16-ounce) package frozen unsweetened raspberries)

☐ 1 bag baby spinach leaves

☐ 2 (16-ounce) containers strawberries

☐ 2 tomatoes

Dairy Aisle

☐ 1 package Lender's refrigerated 2½- to 3-ounce honey wheat bagels

☐ 1 (4-ounce) package reduced-fat feta cheese (freeze remainder in sealed plastic bag at end of week)

☐ 1 (8-ounce) package 2% milk reduced-fat shredded mozzarella cheese

☐ 1 (15½-ounce) container low-fat ricotta cheese (or fat-free if low-fat is not available; note: part-skim ricotta cheese is *not* low-fat)

☐ 1 small package 50% reduced-fat string cheese (suggest Healthy Choice or Frigo brands)

☐ 1 (4-ounce) container hummus (any flavor)

☐ 1 gallon plus 1 quart fat-free milk

- [ ] ½ pint orange juice
- [ ] 1 small container reduced-fat sour cream
- [ ] 1 (8-ounce) package low-fat firm tofu (such as Mori-Nu Low-Fat Silken Firm Tofu)
- [ ] 1 package 6½-inch low-fat whole wheat soft tortillas

Canned Fruit/Vegetables/Beans/Soup Aisle

- [ ] 1 (8-ounce) can V8 juice (reduced-sodium is a great choice)

Bread Aisle

- [ ] 1 package whole wheat English muffins

Deli/Meat Aisle

- [ ] 3 ounces 93% lean ground beef
- [ ] 6 ounces sliced lean roast beef (Healthy Choice brand if available)
- [ ] 4 ounces tuna steak

Other/Checkout Aisle

- [ ] 1 Dove miniature dark chocolate bar (or any "fun-size" chocolate bar of your choice)

FIRM UP TIP

ON YOUR PLATE

Curb nighttime eating by going to bed earlier. "People are particularly vulnerable to overeating in the evening because it seems that they don't get the same degree of satisfaction from food that they do earlier in the day," says John De Castro, Ph.D., of Georgia State University in Atlanta, who has looked at how our bodies' natural circadian rhythms affect appetite. It's not that you're actually hungrier, but the same amount of food that satisfied you for breakfast doesn't do the trick at dinner. "The development of artificial lighting has prolonged eating into the time when we're at the low end of our daily satiation cycle."

FIRM UP / DAY 8

Postworkout Stretches

This week, we're going to add some stretches to your workouts. Doing these moves after you exercise will help to increase your flexibility, something that we often lose as we get older and become less active. Perform each move one right after the other and then repeat the sequence using the opposite leg for the final three stretches. It only takes about 5 minutes.

CHEST. Stand with your feet about shoulder width apart and grasp your hands behind your back, fingers intertwined and palms facing in. Keeping your chest lifted and shoulders down, squeeze your shoulder blades and gently lift your arms as high as comfortable. Don't arch your back. Hold while you take three deep breaths and then release.

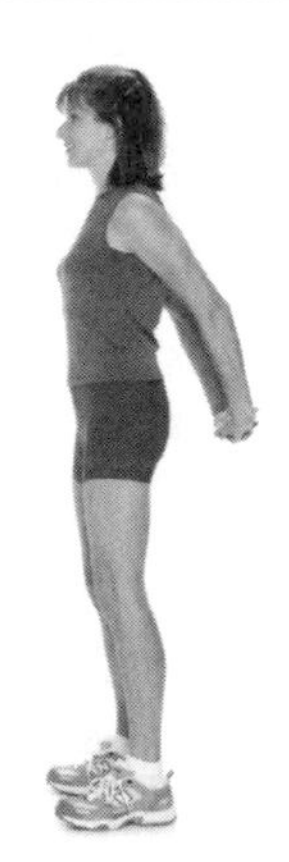

BACK. Stand with your feet about shoulder width apart and your knees bent slightly. Bending at the hips, lean forward and place your hands on your thighs just above your knees. Tuck your hips, round your back, and drop your chin to your chest so that your back forms a C shape. Hold while you take three deep breaths and then release.

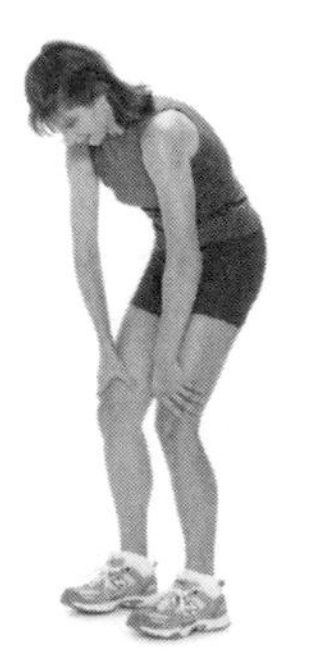

QUADS. Standing with your feet together, bend your left leg behind you, bringing that foot toward your buttocks. Grasp your left foot with your left hand and tuck your hips under so that you feel a stretch in the front of your left thigh and hip. Hold while you take three deep breaths and then release. (You can hold on to a chair or a wall with your right hand for balance if needed.)

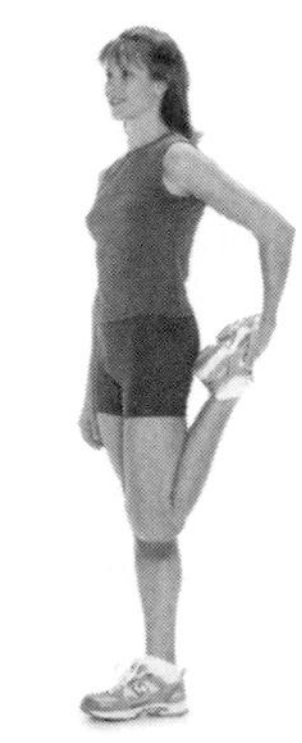

CALF. Bend your right leg and place your left foot about 2 feet behind you, pressing down with your heel. Your left leg should be straight, and you should feel a stretch in your left calf. Hold while you take three deep breaths and then release. Repeat next time with your left leg forward.

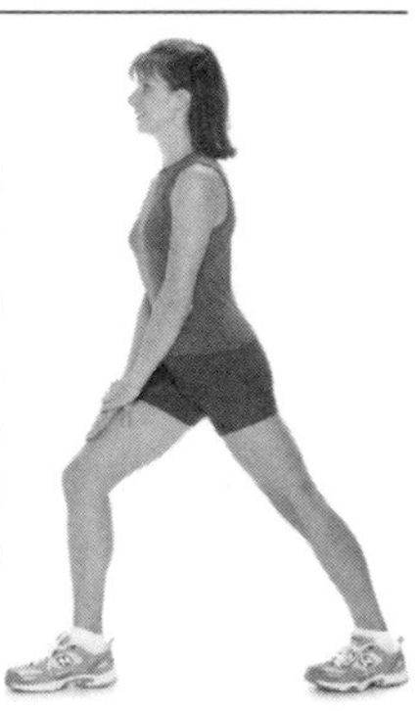

HAMSTRINGS. From the calf stretch position, step your back foot in 6 to 12 inches and bend that leg. Straighten your front leg, bringing your toes off the floor, and sit back, shifting your weight onto your back foot. Don't lock your front knee. Place your hands on your bent leg for support. You should feel a stretch in the back of your straight leg. Hold while you take three deep breaths and then release. Repeat next time with your other leg in front.

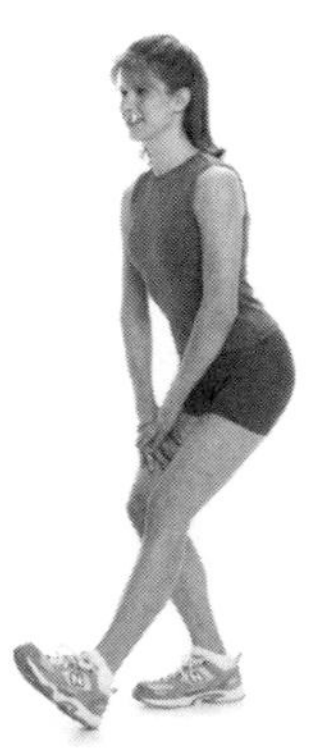

Meal Plan

Most of these recipes are custom designed to make 1 serving–no fuss, no muss; just fix, eat, and go! If a recipe makes more than 1 serving, it's noted below. Save that extra serving for another meal, or share it with your spouse or your walking buddy.

Breakfast

French Toast and Berries: Dip 1 slice whole wheat bread in ¼ cup Egg Beaters or 1 beaten egg white mixed with 2 tablespoons fat-free milk. Grill in a nonstick skillet coated with cooking spray. Top with 1 teaspoon trans-fat-free margarine and ½ tablespoon maple syrup. Serve with 1 cup strawberries and ½ cup fat-free milk.

Healthy Snack

Berry Smoothie: In an electric blender (or with a hand blender), combine 1 cup thawed frozen berries, 1 teaspoon vanilla extract, and 1 cup fat-free milk. Slowly add 1 cup crushed ice.

Lunch

Roast Beef Sandwich: Spread 2 slices whole wheat bread with 1 tablespoon reduced-fat mayo each, plus mustard to taste (horseradish mustard tastes even better). Fill with 3 ounces lean roast beef sliced for sandwiches (usually 3 slices), 4 slices tomato, and romaine lettuce. Serve with an 8-ounce can of reduced-sodium V8.

Healthy Snack

Vegetables and Hummus: Have 8 baby carrots and ½ cup sliced cucumber with 3 tablespoons hummus. Serve with 1 slice (1 ounce) reduced-fat cheese.

Dinner

Grilled Maple-Marinated Tuna: Marinate 4 ounces (uncooked) tuna steak in 1 tablespoon maple syrup, 2 tablespoons orange juice, and freshly ground black pepper (to taste) for 20 minutes. Remove from the marinade and grill or broil approximately 3 minutes on each side. Serve with ½ large baked potato topped with 2 tablespoons low-fat sour cream and 8 large asparagus spears topped with 1 teaspoon trans-fat-free margarine.

Indulgent Treat

Raspberries with Melted Chocolate: Melt 2 tablespoons mini chocolate chips in the microwave (heat in a glass container on 50 percent power for about 50 seconds). Drizzle over 1½ cups fresh raspberries.

Nutrient analysis: 1,681 calories, 100 g protein, 236 g carbohydrates, 45 g total fat, 15 g saturated fat, 106 mg cholesterol, 48 g dietary fiber, 2,378 mg sodium, 1,467 mg calcium

FIRM UP TIP

FIT FACT

In a 15-month study of nearly 50 women, researchers found that those who exercised at home kept off an average of 10 pounds more than those who had to go to a gym.

The Workout

Level 1

Easy Walk: 30 Minutes

- 5-minute warmup: Walk 2 to 2½ miles per hour, or 95 to 100 steps per minute.
- 20-minute moderate walk: Increase your speed to 2½ to 3 miles per hour, 100 to 115 steps per minute, or a pace that lets you comfortably carry on a conversation.
- 5-minute cooldown: Slow down to 2 to 2½ miles per hour, or 95 to 100 steps per minute.

Basic Strength Training: 25 Minutes

- Do 10 to 12 reps of each exercise. Repeat the sequence of exercises three times.
- To warm up, use lighter weights, or none at all, the first time through, and for the lunge exercise, only go partway down.

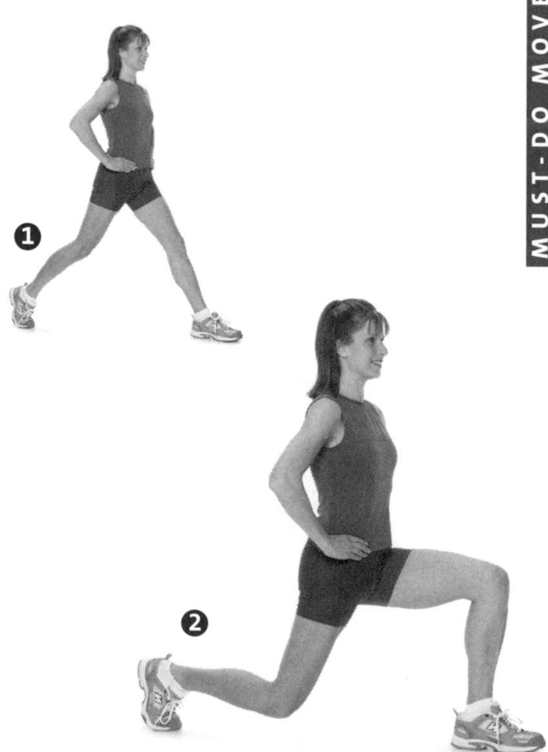

MUST-DO MOVE

Lunge (no weights)

Starting position: Stand with your feet 2 to 3 feet apart, with your left foot in front of your right. Place your hands on your hips.

Movement: Inhale as you bend your left knee and lower your body straight down until your left knee is bent 90 degrees and your right knee nearly touches the floor. Your rear heel will come off the floor. Hold for a second and then exhale as you slowly push yourself back up to the starting position. Finish all of your repetitions, then repeat the exercise with your right foot in front of your left.

Technique: Don't lean forward. Don't let your front knee move forward over your toes.

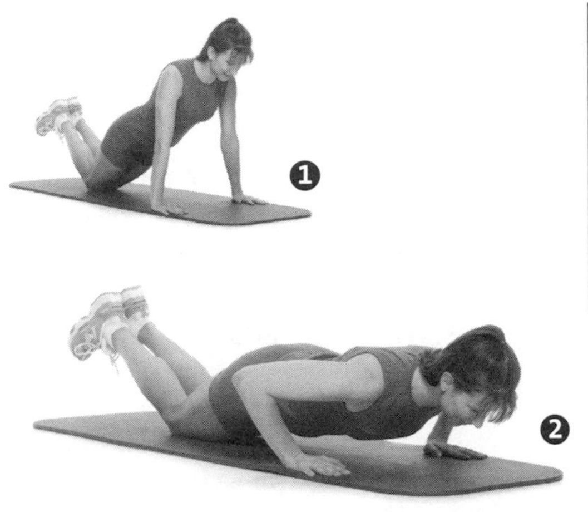

MUST-DO MOVE

Bent-Knee Pushup

Starting position: Lie facedown on the floor. Bend your knees so that your feet are up in the air, and place your palms on the floor near your shoulders so that your elbows are pointing up. Press down with your hands, extend your arms, and lift your body off the floor.

Movement: Keeping your head, back, hips, and knees in a straight line, bend your elbows out to the sides and lower your body as you inhale, until your chest nearly touches the floor. Hold for a second and then exhale as you push back up.

Technique: Don't bend at the hips. Don't arch your back.

MUST-DO MOVE

Seated Back Fly

Starting position: Sit on the edge of a chair with your feet hip width apart and hold a dumbbell in each hand. Keep your back flat and lean forward, bending at the hips so that the dumbbells are hanging at arm's length down by your calves, palms facing each other and elbows bent slightly.

Movement: Keeping your back straight, squeeze your shoulder blades together and lift the dumbbells up and out to the sides as you exhale, pulling your elbows back as far as comfortably possible. Hold for a second and then inhale as you slowly lower them.

Technique: Don't arch your back. Don't raise your torso as you lift the dumbbells.

Alternate move: If you have back problems, do the flies one arm at a time and place the forearm of your other arm across your thighs for extra support.

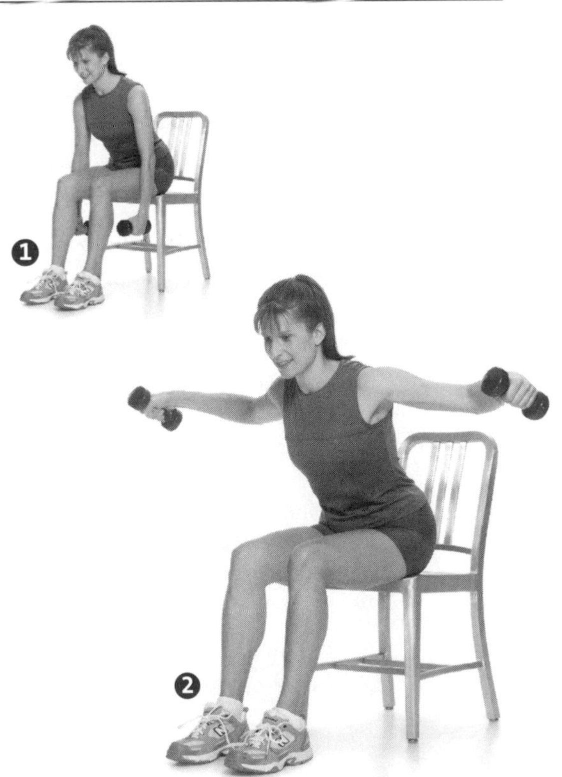

continued

The Workout

Level 1 *continued*

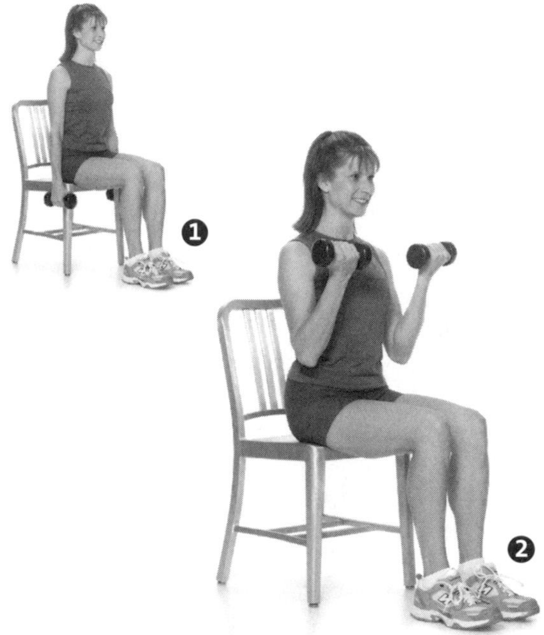

Seated Biceps Curl with a Twist

Starting position: Sit on the edge of a chair with your feet hip width apart. Hold dumbbells at your sides with your palms facing in.

Movement: Bending your elbows and turning your wrists upward, lift the dumbbells toward your shoulders as you exhale. Stop when the dumbbells are at chest height, palms facing your body. Hold for a second and then inhale as you slowly lower them.

Technique: Don't move your upper arms.

Seated Triceps Kickback with a Twist

Starting position: Sit on the edge of a chair with your feet hip width apart and hold a dumbbell in each hand. Keep your back flat and lean forward, bending at the hips. Bend your arms at about 90-degree angles with your dumbbells at about hip height.

Movement: Without moving your upper arms, press the dumbbells back as you exhale, extending your arms and turning your wrists so that your palms face the ceiling. Hold for a second and then inhale as you slowly lower them.

Technique: Don't move from your shoulders. Don't raise your torso as you lift the dumbbells.

Alternate move: If you have back problems, do the kickbacks one arm at a time and place the forearm of your other arm across your thighs for extra support.

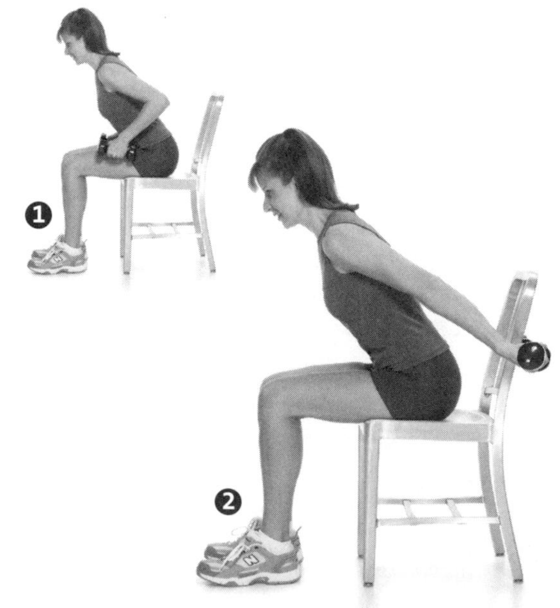

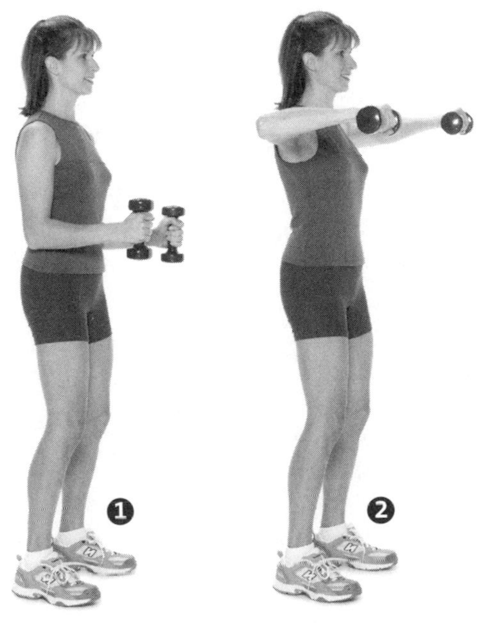

Bent-Arm Lateral Raise

Starting position: Stand with your feet shoulder width apart, knees bent slightly. Hold a dumbbell in each hand with your arms at your sides and bent at 90-degree angles so that your palms are facing in and the dumbbells are in front of you at about waist height.

Movement: Exhale as you slowly raise your elbows out to the sides until they are at about shoulder height. Hold for a second and then inhale as you slowly lower them.

Technique: Don't lift your shoulders. Don't lift higher than shoulder height.

FIRM UP TIPS

GET FIRM FASTER	MIND OVER MATTER
Count backward. Ever notice how your trip back from a great destination seems shorter than your trip there? Apply that principle to exercise by counting reps backward—from 10 to 1, instead of 1 to 10.	*Forgive their trespasses. If you're bitter toward someone who's wronged you, you're just letting them hurt you again. The stress hormones you produce by holding a grudge can increase your chance of a heart attack fivefold. Make an effort to let bygones be bygones. Start by acknowledging that no one can change the past.*

The Workout

Level 2

Easy Walk: 30 Minutes

- 5-minute warmup: Walk 2½ to 3 miles per hour, or 100 to 115 steps per minute.
- 20-minute moderate walk: Increase your speed to 3 to 3½ miles per hour, 115 to 125 steps per minute, or a pace that lets you comfortably carry on a conversation.
- 5-minute cooldown: Slow down to 2½ to 3 miles per hour, or 100 to 115 steps per minute.

Basic Strength Training: 30 Minutes

- Do 10 to 12 reps of each exercise. Repeat the sequence of exercises three times.
- To warm up, use lighter weights, or none at all, the first time through, and for the squat and lunge exercises, only go partway down.

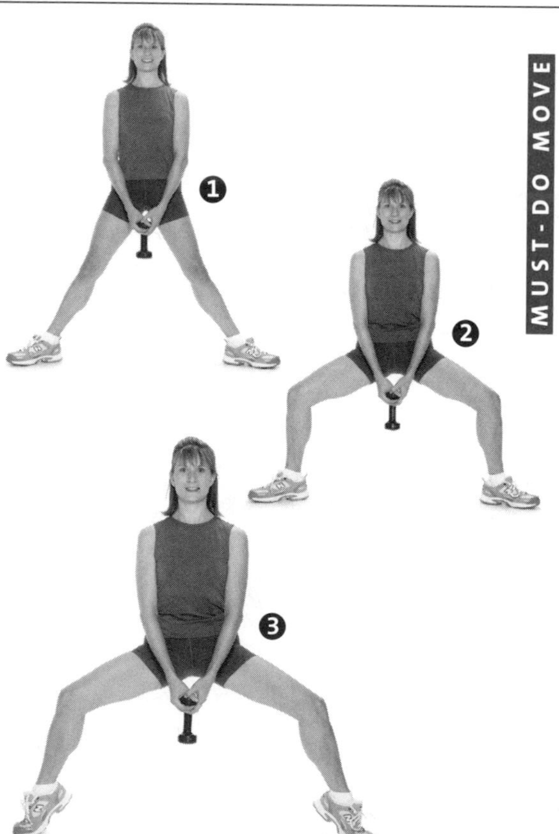

MUST-DO MOVE

Plié Squat with Heel Lift

Starting position: Stand with your feet wider than shoulder width apart, toes pointing out. Hold a dumbbell with both hands down in front of you.

Movement: Keeping your back straight, lower yourself, bending from your knees, as you inhale. Stop just before your thighs are parallel to the floor and then lift your heels off the floor so that you're on your toes. Hold for a second. Exhale as you slowly stand back up and then lower your heels. (You may want to hold on to a chair with one hand for balance, grasping the dumbbell with the other hand.)

Technique: Don't let your knees move forward over your toes. Don't lean forward.

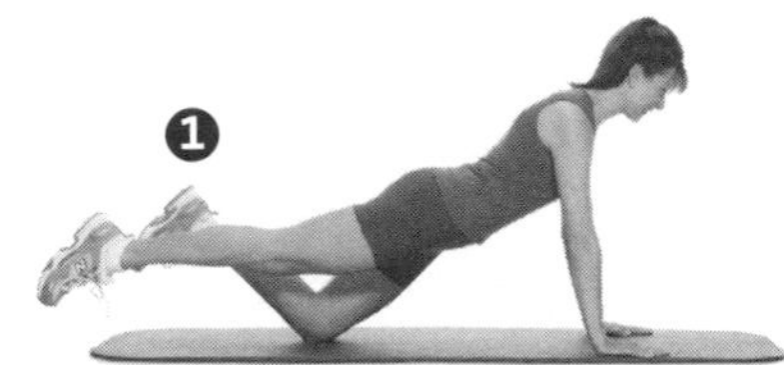

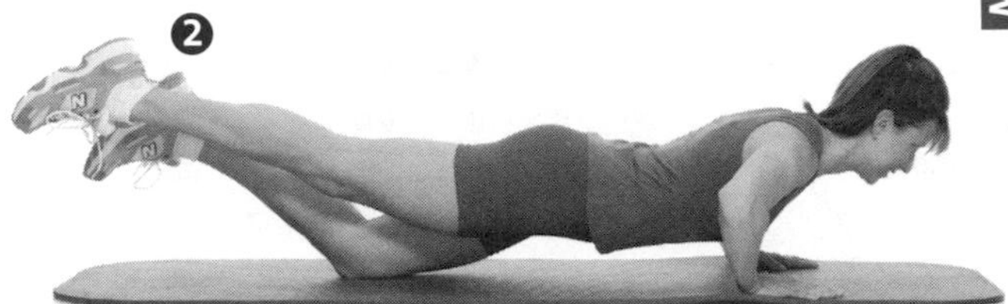

MUST-DO MOVE

One-Knee Pushup

Starting position: Lie facedown on the floor. Bend your knees so that your feet are up in the air, and place your palms on the floor near your shoulders so that your elbows are pointing up. Press down with your hands, extend your arms, lift your body off the floor, and lift one knee off the floor, extending that leg.

Movement: Keeping your head, back, hips, and knees in a straight line, bend your elbows out to the sides and lower your body as you inhale, until your chest nearly touches the floor. Hold for a second and then exhale as you push back up. Do half of the recommended reps and then switch knees.

Technique: Don't bend at the hips. Don't arch your back.

MUST-DO MOVE

Back Fly

Starting position: Stand with your feet shoulder width apart and knees bent slightly. Hold a dumbbell in each hand with your arms at your sides. Keep your back flat and lean forward, bending at the hips so that the dumbbells are hanging at arm's length in front of you, palms facing each other and elbows bent slightly.

Movement: Keeping your back straight, squeeze your shoulder blades together and lift the dumbbells up and out to the sides as you exhale, pulling your elbows back as far as comfortably possible. Hold for a second and then inhale as you slowly lower them.

Technique: Don't arch your back. Don't raise your torso as you lift the dumbbells.

Alternate move: If you have back problems, support yourself with one hand on a chair and do the flies one arm at a time.

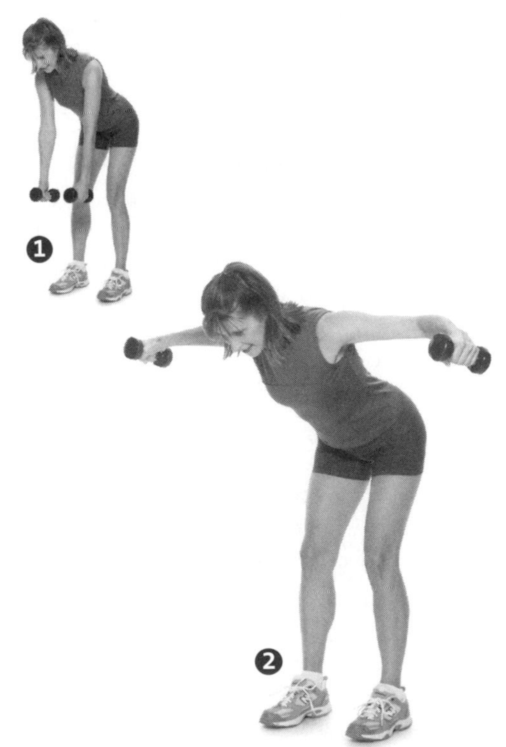

continued

The Workout

Level 2 *continued*

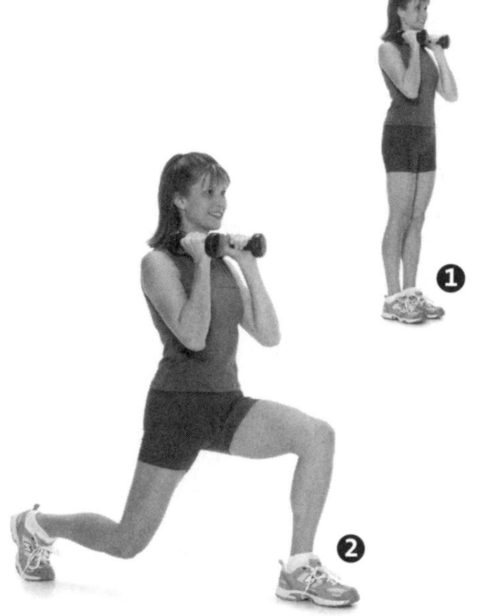

MUST-DO MOVE

Back Lunge

Starting position: Stand with your feet together. Hold a dumbbell in each hand, either at shoulder height or at your sides.

Movement: Step your right foot back 2 to 3 feet. Inhale as you bend your left knee and lower your body straight down until your left knee is bent 90 degrees and your right knee nearly touches the floor. Your rear heel will come off the floor. Hold for a second and then exhale as you push yourself back up, bringing your right foot back in. Finish all of your repetitions, then repeat the exercise stepping back with your left foot.

Technique: Don't lean forward. Don't let your front knee move forward over your toes.

Concentrated Biceps Curl

Starting position: Sit on the edge of a chair with your feet shoulder width apart. Hold a dumbbell in your left hand and lean forward from your hips, resting your left elbow on the inside of your left knee so that your palm is facing your right leg. Place your right hand on your right thigh for support.

Movement: Bending your elbow, lift the dumbbell toward your left shoulder as you exhale. Stop when the dumbbell is at chest height, palm facing your shoulder. Hold for a second and then inhale as you slowly lower it. Do the recommended number of reps and then switch sides.

Technique: Don't move your upper arms.

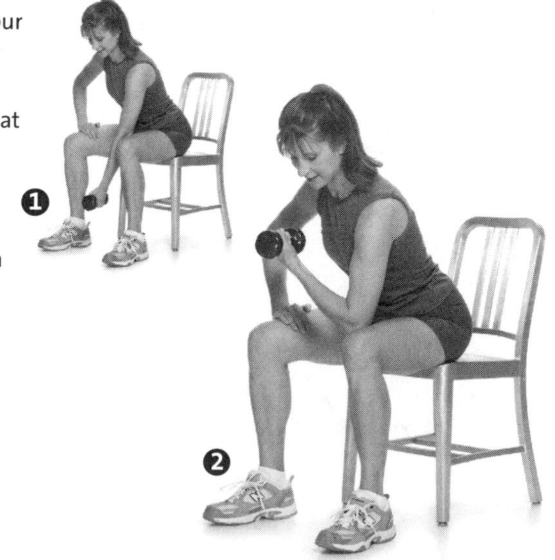

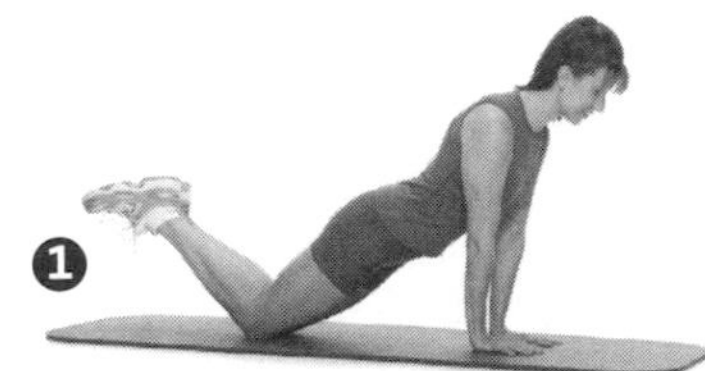

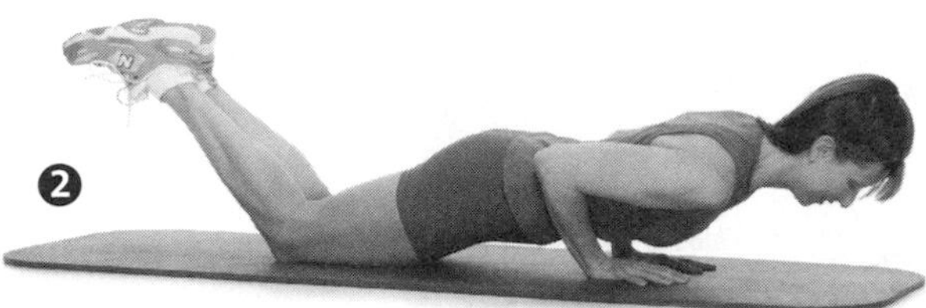

Kneeling Triceps Pushup

Starting position: Lie facedown on the floor. Bend your knees so that your feet are up in the air, and place your palms on the floor close to your ribs so that your elbows are pointing up. Press down with your hands, extend your arms, and lift your body off the floor.

Movement: Keeping your head, back, hips, and knees in a straight line, bend your elbows back, keeping your arms close to your body, as you inhale. Lower your body until your chest nearly touches the floor. Hold for a second and then exhale as you push back up.

Technique: Don't let your elbows point out to the sides. Don't bend at the hips. Don't drop your belly toward the floor.

Parallel Overhead Press

Starting position: Stand with your feet shoulder width apart and knees bent slightly. Hold a dumbbell in each hand at shoulder height, palms facing each other and elbows pointing forward.

Movement: Exhale as you slowly press the dumbbells straight overhead without locking your elbows. Hold for a second and then inhale as you slowly lower them.

Technique: Don't arch your back. Don't lift the dumbbells forward or back.

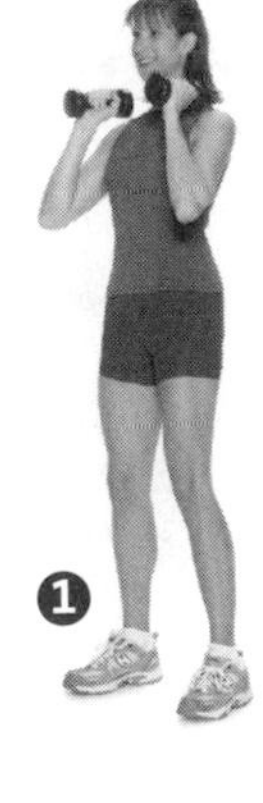

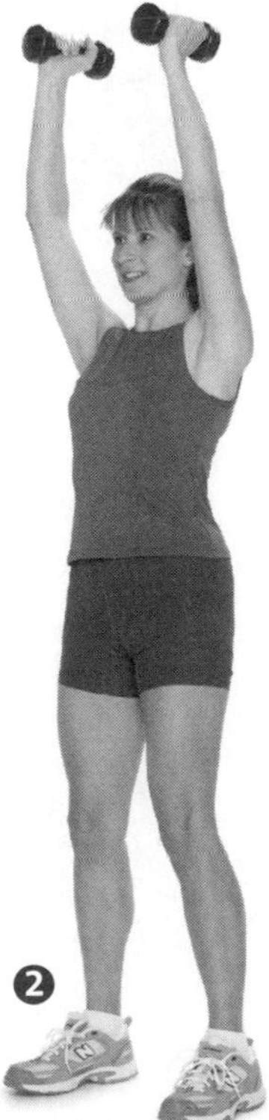

The Workout
Level 3

Easy Walk: 30 Minutes

- 5-minute warmup: Walk 2½ to 3 miles per hour, or 100 to 115 steps per minute.
- 20-minute moderate walk: Increase your speed to 3½ to 4 miles per hour, 125 to 135 steps per minute, or a pace that lets you comfortably carry on a conversation.
- 5-minute cooldown: Slow down to 2½ to 3 miles per hour, or 100 to 115 steps per minute.

Basic Strength Training: 40 Minutes

- Do 10 to 12 reps of each exercise. Repeat the sequence of exercises three times.
- To warm up, use lighter weights, or none at all, the first time through, and for the squat and lunge exercises, only go partway down.

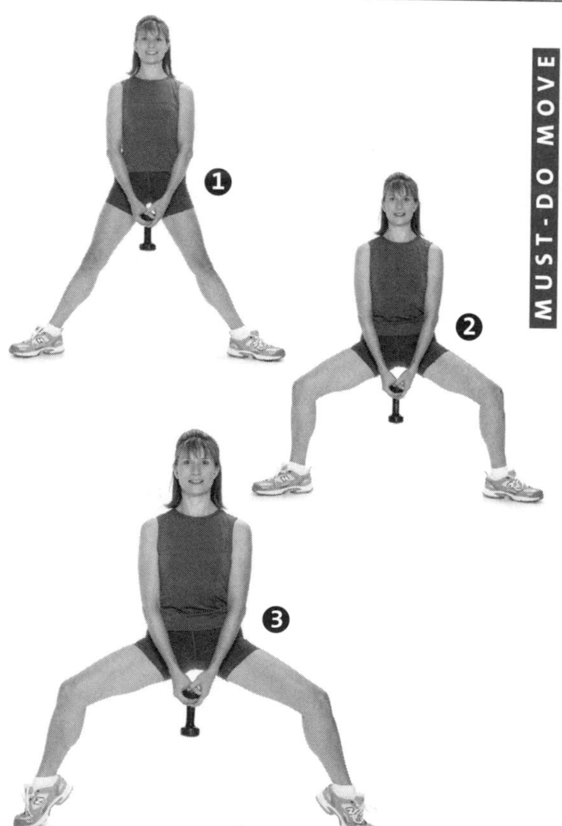

MUST-DO MOVE

Plié Squat with Heel Lift

Starting position: Stand with your feet wider than shoulder width apart, toes pointing out. Hold a dumbbell with both hands down in front of you.

Movement: Keeping your back straight, lower yourself, bending from your knees, as you inhale. Stop just before your thighs are parallel to the floor and then lift your heels off the floor so that you're on your toes. Hold for a second. Exhale as you slowly stand back up and then lower your heels. (You may want to hold on to a chair with one hand for balance, grasping the dumbbell with the other hand.)

Technique: Don't let your knees move forward over your toes. Don't lean forward.

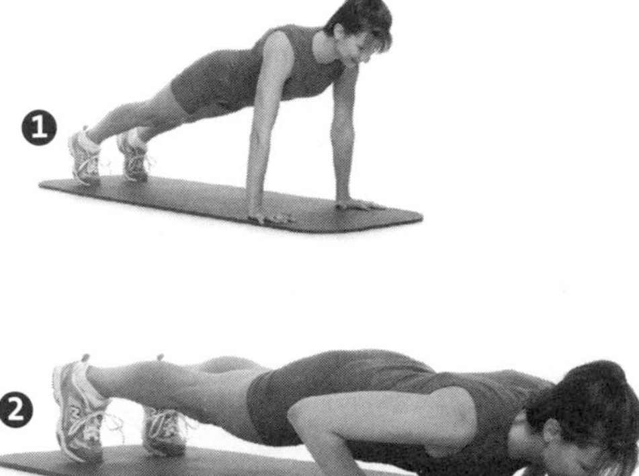

MUST-DO MOVE

Pushup

Starting position: Lie facedown on the floor with your feet flexed and toes tucked. Place your palms on the floor near your shoulders so that your elbows are pointing up. Press down with your hands, extend your arms, and lift your body off the floor so that it forms a straight line from head to toe.

Movement: Keeping your head, back, hips, and legs in a straight line, bend your elbows out to the sides and lower your body as you inhale, until your chest nearly touches the floor. Hold for a second and then exhale as you push back up. If you can't do all the recommended reps in this full pushup position, that's okay. Just drop down onto one or both knees and complete the remaining reps.

Technique: Don't bend at the hips. Don't arch your back.

MUST-DO MOVE

Back Fly

Starting position: Stand with your feet shoulder width apart, knees bent slightly. Hold a dumbbell in each hand with your arms at your sides. Keep your back flat and lean forward, bending at the hips so that the dumbbells are hanging at arm's length in front of you, palms facing each other and elbows bent slightly.

Movement: Keeping your back straight, squeeze your shoulder blades together and lift the dumbbells up and out to the sides as you exhale, pulling your elbows back as far as comfortably possible. Hold for a second and then inhale as you slowly lower them.

Technique: Don't arch your back. Don't raise your torso as you lift the dumbbells.

Alternate move: If you have back problems, support yourself with one hand on a chair and do the flies one arm at a time.

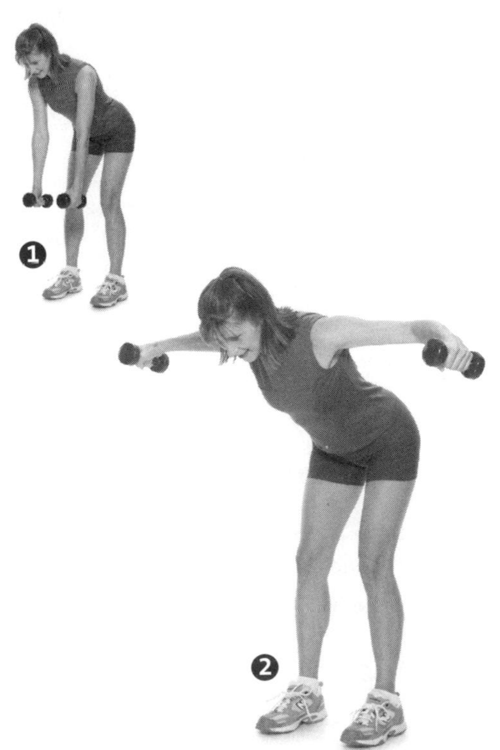

continued

The Workout

Level 3 *continued*

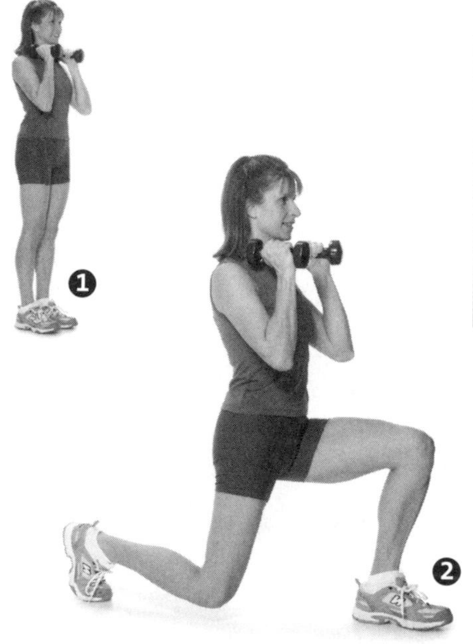

MUST-DO MOVE

Front Lunge

Starting position: Stand with your feet together. Hold a dumbbell in each hand, either at shoulder height or at your sides.

Movement: Step your left foot forward 2 to 3 feet. Inhale as you bend your left knee and lower your body straight down until your left knee is bent 90 degrees and your right knee nearly touches the floor. Your rear heel will come off the floor. Hold for a second and then exhale as you push yourself back up, bringing your left foot back in. Finish all of your repetitions, then repeat the exercise stepping forward with your right foot.

Technique: Don't lean forward. Don't let your front knee move forward over your toes.

Concentrated Biceps Curl

Starting position: Sit on the edge of a chair with your feet shoulder width apart. Hold a dumbbell in your left hand and lean forward from your hips, resting your left elbow on the inside of your left knee so that your palm is facing your right leg. Place your right hand on your right thigh for support.

Movement: Bending your elbow, lift the dumbbell toward your left shoulder as you exhale. Stop when the dumbbell is at chest height, palm facing your shoulder. Hold for a second and then inhale as you slowly lower it. Do the recommended number of reps and then switch sides.

Technique: Don't move your upper arms.

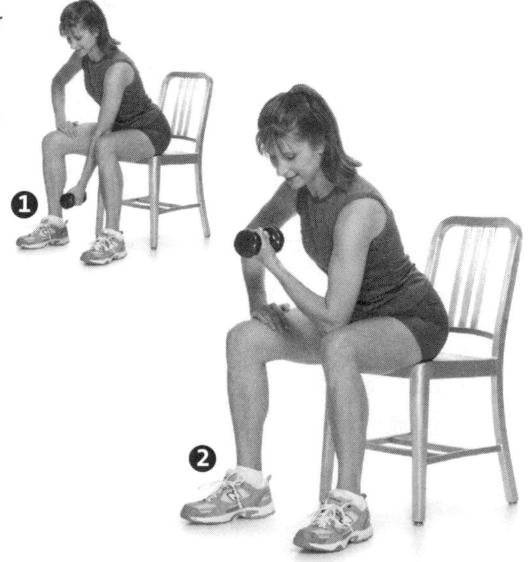

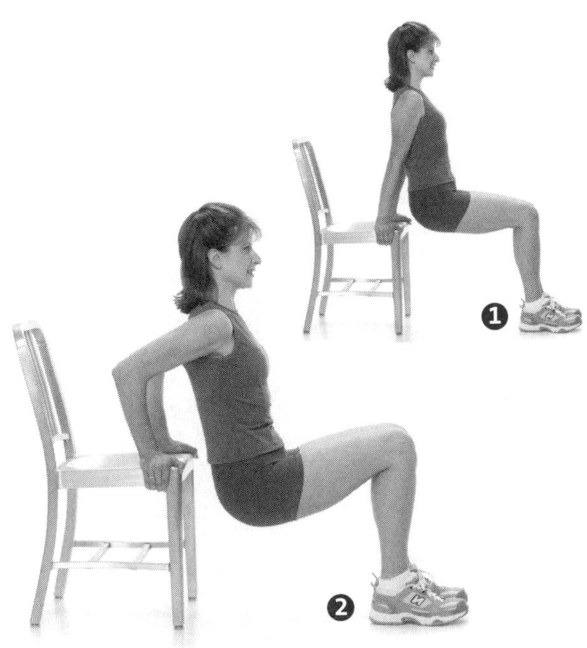

Triceps Dip

Starting position: Sit on the edge of a chair, place your hands on either side of you, and grasp the chair seat. Slide your buttocks off the chair and walk your feet out until your legs are bent at about 90 degrees. You should be balancing on your hands and feet.

Movement: Bending your arms so that your elbows point behind you, slowly lower your body toward the floor as you inhale. Keep your buttocks as close to the chair as possible. Stop when your elbows are bent about 90 degrees. Hold for a second and then exhale as you press back up.

Technique: Don't sink into your arms, allowing your shoulders to come up toward your ears. Don't bend your knees to help lower yourself.

Alternate move: For a more challenging version, lift one leg off the floor.

Lateral Raise

Starting position: Stand with your feet shoulder width apart, knees bent slightly. Hold a dumbbell in each hand with your arms at your sides, palms facing in, and elbows bent slightly.

Movement: Exhale as you slowly raise the dumbbells out to the sides until they are at about shoulder height. Hold for a second and then inhale as you slowly lower them.

Technique: Don't lift your shoulders. Don't lift higher than shoulder height.

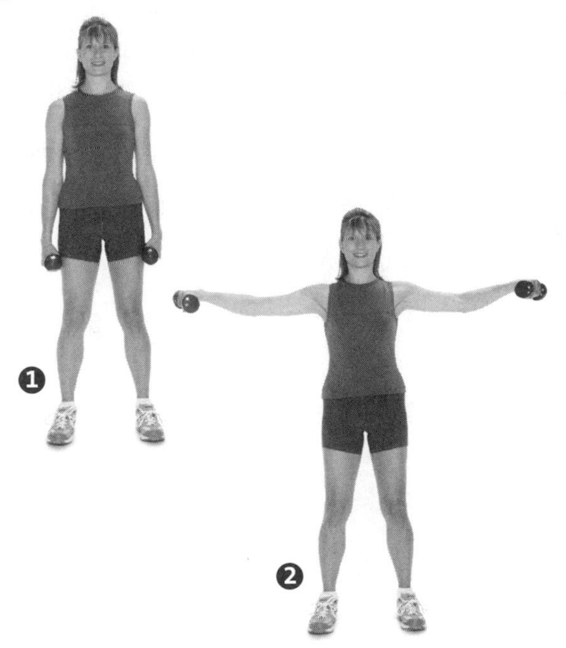

FIRM UP / DAY 9

Real-Life Success Story

Growing up in Jamaica, Yvonne Rubie, of Brooklyn, New York, recalls that "exercise and sweating by women were considered really tacky." But 2 years ago, Yvonne read an article about a woman in her fifties who had walked her first marathon in Honolulu.

"I was turning 50 and looking for something to benchmark this important milestone," she says. "I decided that if she could do it, I could do it."

Yvonne asked three friends to join her. "We walked for an hour each morning before work and would start calling each other around 5:10 A.M.," says Yvonne, who, in addition to working full-time, is earning her master's degree in public health at night. "The social support was key, because the times I didn't want to get out of bed, I knew my friends would be upset with me. Also, with a goal such as a marathon, we knew we had to be in shape to get it done."

On Saturdays, they'd do a long walk, from 1 to 5 hours. The women met their goal of completing the marathon in less than 7 hours—Yvonne's time was 6 hours, 42 minutes—then continued training to complete the Jamaica Marathon in December 2002. They plan to walk the New York City Marathon this year.

"Walking has helped me strengthen my body and control my cholesterol," notes Yvonne, who dropped from 130 to 120 pounds and lowered her cholesterol from an elevated 250 into the normal range, below 200, without using medication.

FIRM UP TIP

FIT FACT

It's not what you did when you were young—it's what you're doing now *that counts. When researchers reviewed the past and recent activity levels of more than 5,000 people, those who were currently active were about 40 percent less likely to die during the 16-year follow-up than the least active group. Sorry, former jocks: Past activity doesn't seem to offer any protection.*

Meal Plan

Most of these recipes are custom designed to make 1 serving—no fuss, no muss; just fix, eat, and go! If a recipe makes more than 1 serving, it's noted below. Save that extra serving for another meal, or share it with your spouse or your walking buddy.

Breakfast

Creamy Ricotta on a Toasted Waffle: Combine a 15½-ounce container low-fat ricotta cheese with 2 tablespoons honey and 3 tablespoons smooth or chunky peanut butter. (This recipe makes six ⅓-cup servings. You'll use another 2 servings later this week. You can keep it in the fridge for up to 7 days or freeze single servings for up to 1 month.) Top a toasted whole grain waffle with ⅓ cup ricotta mixture and serve with 1 cup fat-free milk.

Healthy Snack

Real Raspberry Yogurt: Mix ½ cup fresh or ¼ cup thawed frozen raspberries with 8 ounces (1 cup) fat-free berry-flavored yogurt (make sure it has no more than 120 calories per cup). Serve with 5 almonds or 1 slice reduced-fat cheese.

Lunch

Pizza and Broccoli: Heat 1 slice pizza from Saturday's dinner. Serve with 1 cup cooked broccoli florets topped with 1 tablespoon chopped walnuts.

Healthy Snack

Veggies and Hummus: Serve 8 baby carrots and ½ cup sliced cucumber with 3 tablespoons hummus.

Dinner

Tossed Salad with Roasted Chicken and Feta: Toss 2 cups lettuce (preferably, a dark-green, vitamin-rich variety, such as romaine) with 5 chopped baby carrots; 1 tablespoon sliced black olives; 1 medium tomato, sliced; ¼ avocado; ¼ cup chopped red onion; and 2 tablespoons crumbled feta cheese. Toss with 2 teaspoons olive oil and a generous amount of balsamic vinegar or 2 tablespoons full-fat salad dressing. Top with 3 ounces (½ cup) cold chopped roasted chicken and serve with 7 strawberries.

Indulgent Treat

Popcorn: Have 1 mini bag (about 5 cups popped) Orville Redenbacher Movie Theater Butter Popcorn.

Nutrient analysis: 1,651 calories, 98 g protein, 181 g carbohydrates, 67 g total fat, 16 g saturated fat, 117 mg cholesterol, 29 g dietary fiber, 2,346 mg sodium, 1,884 mg calcium

FIRM UP TIP

ON YOUR PLATE

Don't skip breakfast. A survey of more than 2,000 people who lost an average of 67 pounds and kept the weight off more than 5 years found that 78 percent eat breakfast 7 days a week.

The Workout

Level 1

Interval Walk: About 30 Minutes

- 5-minute warmup: Walk 2 to 2½ miles per hour, 95 to 100 steps per minute.
- 4-minute moderate pace: Increase your speed to about 3 miles per hour, about 115 steps per minute.
- 1-minute speedup: Pick up your pace even more to about 3½ miles per hour, about 125 steps per minute.
- Repeat moderate pace/speedup sequence four times.
- 5-minute cooldown: Slow down to 2 to 2½ miles per hour, 95 to 100 steps per minute.

Core Training: 15 Minutes

- Do the sequence of exercises one time.

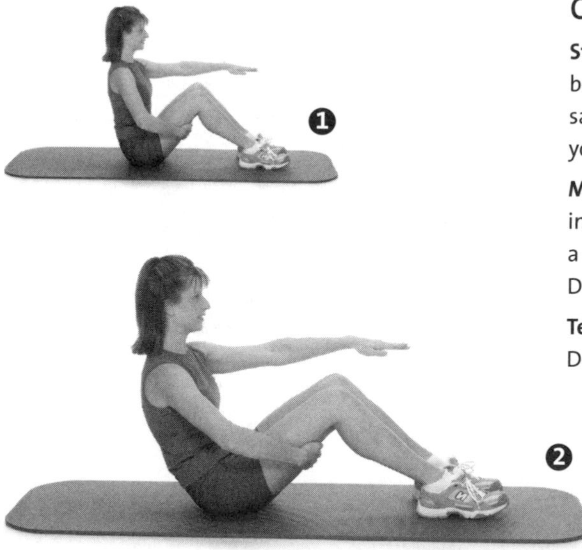

One-Hand Roll-Down

Starting position: Sit on the floor with your knees bent and your feet flat. Place one hand behind the same-side thigh. Keep the other arm out in front of you, parallel to the floor.

Movement: Using your abs, slowly roll down 2 to 3 inches, one vertebra at a time, as you inhale. Hold for a second and then exhale as you slowly roll back up. Do 10 reps.

Technique: Your abs should be powering the move. Don't move quickly.

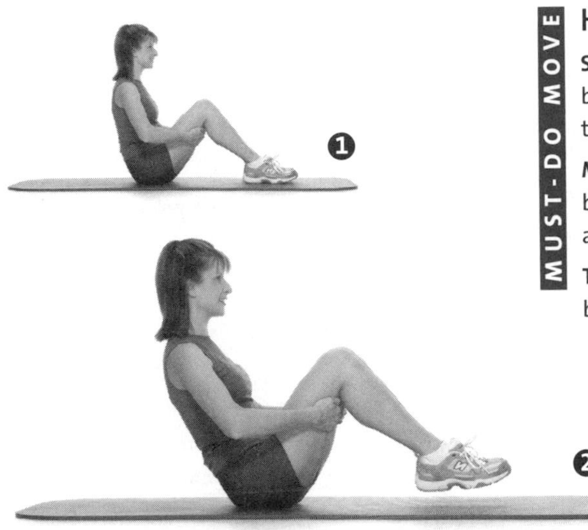

MUST-DO MOVE

Holding Balance

Starting position: Sit on the floor with your knees bent and your feet flat. Place your hands behind your thighs.

Movement: Lift your feet off the floor slightly and balance on your sitting bones. Hold for four breaths and then relax. Do one time only.

Technique: Keep your abs tight and the rest of your body relaxed, especially your shoulders.

Arms-Crossed Ab Crunch

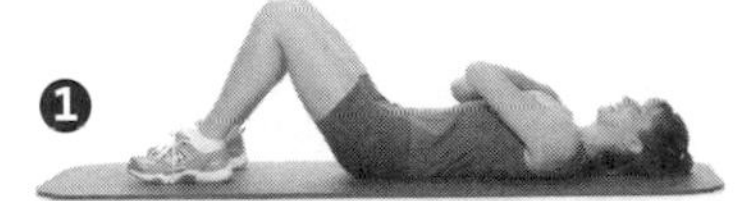

Starting position: Lie on your back with your knees bent, feet flat on the floor, and arms across your chest.

Movement: Using your abs, slowly raise your head, shoulders, and upper back about 45 degrees off the floor as you exhale. Think of shortening the distance between your ribs and pelvis. Hold for a second and then inhale as you slowly lower yourself. Do 10 reps.

Technique: Don't pull your chin to your chest. Don't arch your back.

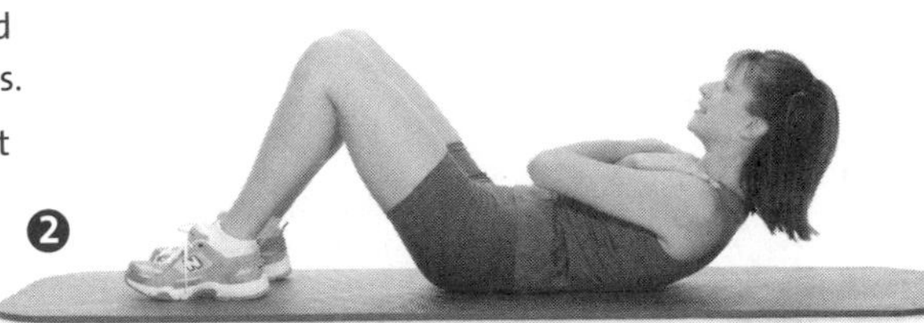

continued

The Workout

Level 1 *continued*

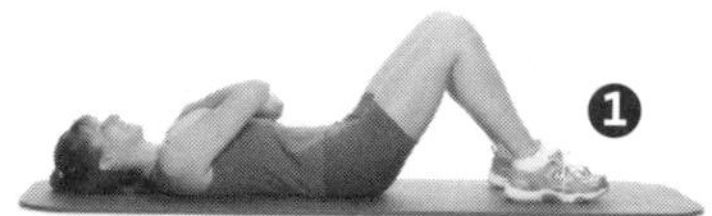

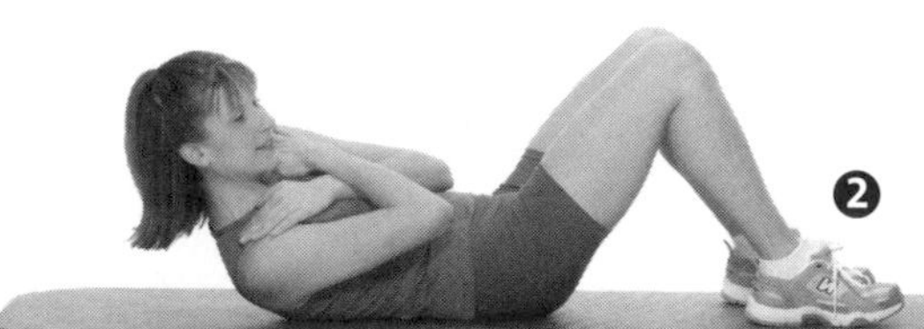

MUST-DO MOVE

Arms-Crossed Twisting Crunch

Starting position: Lie on your back with your knees bent, feet flat on the floor, and arms across your chest.

Movement: Using your abs, slowly lift your head and left shoulder off the floor, twist to the right, and bring your left shoulder toward your right knee as you exhale. Hold for a second and then inhale as you slowly lower yourself. Repeat, alternating sides. Do a total of 10 reps, 5 reps to each side.

Technique: Don't pull your chin to your chest. Don't arch your back.

MUST-DO MOVE

Heel Bridge

Starting position: Lie on your back with your knees bent and arms at your sides, palms facing up. Lift your toes off the floor so that only your heels are touching.

Movement: Contracting your abs, buttocks, and lower back, press into your heels and lift your butt, hips, and back off the floor as you exhale, to form a straight line from your shoulders to your knees. Hold for four breaths and then relax. Do one time only.

Technique: Don't lift too high—your upper back and shoulders should remain on the floor. Don't bend at the waist or hips. Don't let your knees fall inward or outward.

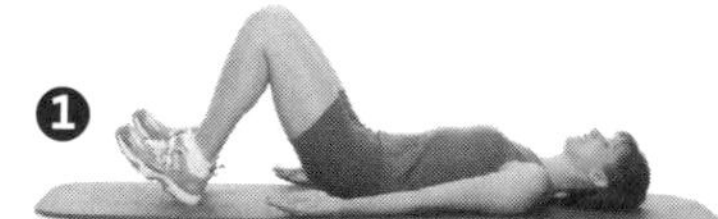

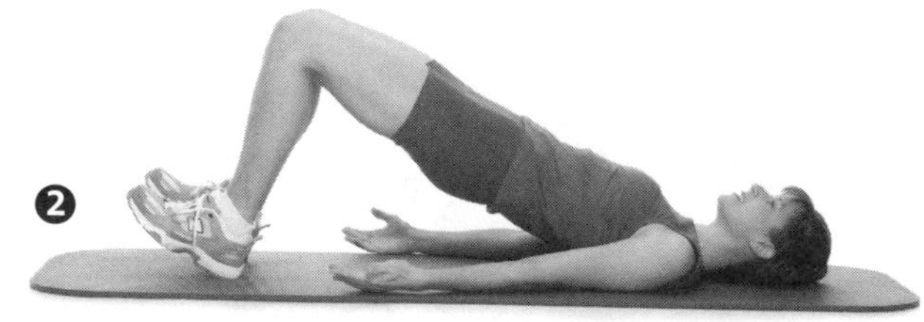

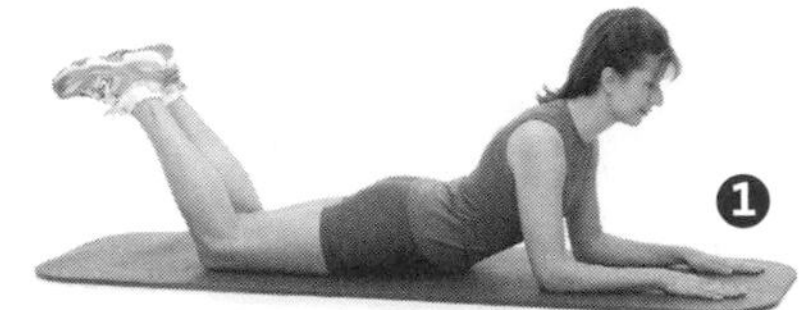

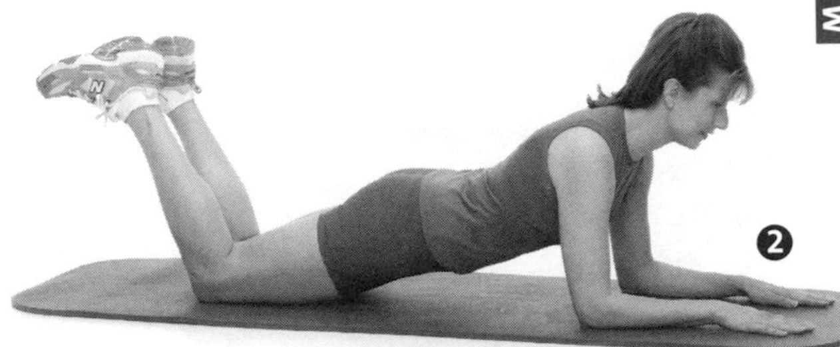

MUST-DO MOVE

Knee Plank

Starting position: Lie facedown with your knees bent so that your feet are in the air. Your elbows should be under your shoulders and your forearms and palms on the floor.

Movement: Contracting your abs and back, press into your forearms as you exhale and lift your pelvis off the floor so that your back and thighs form a straight line. Hold for four breaths and then relax. Do one time only.

Technique: Don't lift your head up or let it drop. Don't bend at the waist. Don't arch your back.

Kneeling T-Stand

Starting position: Sit on your left hip with your left leg bent, your right leg extended, right hand on hip, and left hand on the floor below your shoulder.

Movement: Using your abs, lift your hips off the floor as you exhale. Hold for four breaths, relax, and then repeat on the other side. Do one time only on each side.

Technique: Don't let your body roll forward: Think of it as being sandwiched between two walls. Keep everything in line.

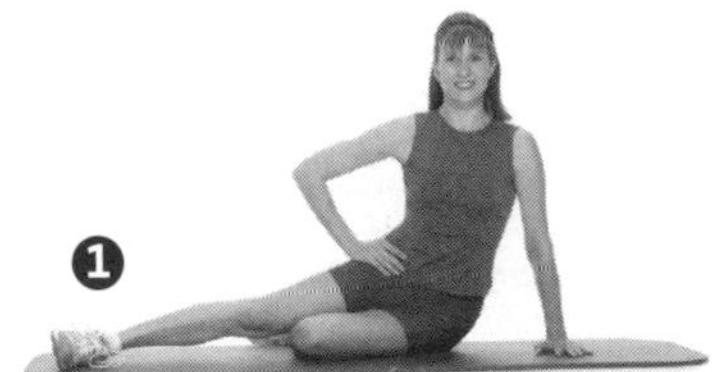

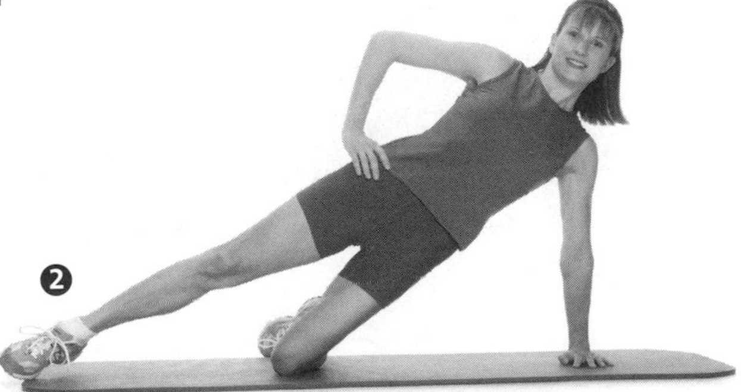

The Workout

Level 2

Interval Walk: About 30 Minutes

- 5-minute warmup: Walk 2½ to 3 miles per hour, 100 to 115 steps per minute.
- 4-minute moderate pace: Increase your speed to about 3½ miles per hour, about 125 steps per minute.
- 2-minute speedup: Pick up your pace even more to about 4 miles per hour, about 135 steps per minute.
- Repeat moderate pace/speedup sequence three times.
- 5-minute cooldown: Slow down to 2½ to 3 miles per hour, 100 to 115 steps per minute.

Core Training: 15 Minutes

- Do the sequence of exercises one time.

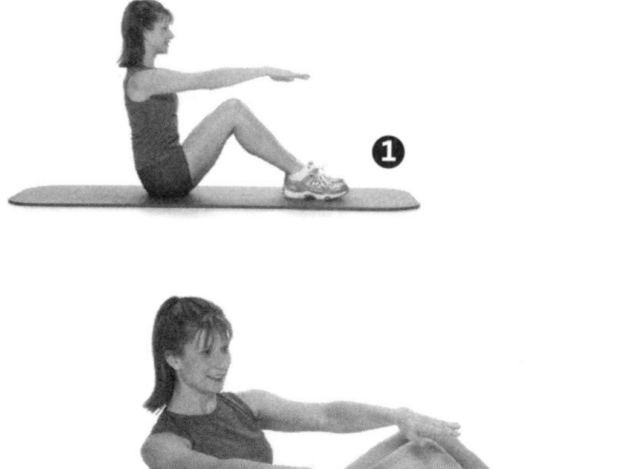

Roll-Down with a Twist

Starting position: Sit on the floor with your knees bent and your feet flat. Hold your arms out in front of you, parallel to the floor.

Movement: Using your abs, slowly roll down 3 to 4 inches, one vertebra at a time, as you inhale and twist to the right. Hold for a second and then exhale as you slowly roll back up. Do 10 reps, alternating the side you twist to each time.

Technique: Your abs should be powering the move. Don't move quickly.

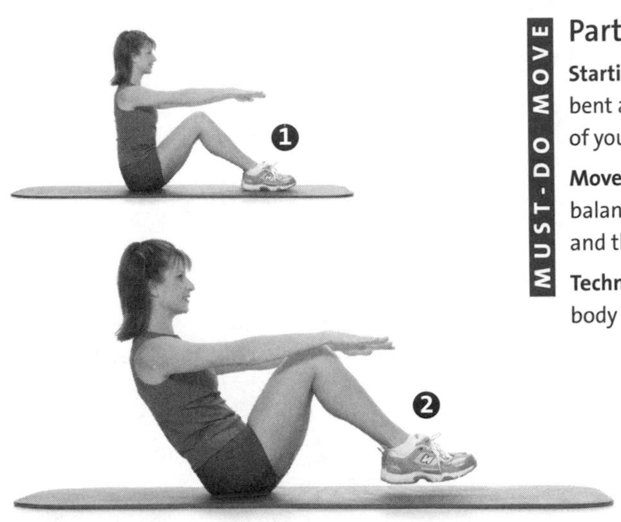

MUST-DO MOVE

Partial Balance

Starting position: Sit on the floor with your knees bent and your feet flat. Hold your arms out in front of you, parallel to the floor.

Movement: Lift your feet off the floor slightly and balance on your sitting bones. Hold for five breaths and then relax. Do one time only.

Technique: Keep your abs tight and the rest of your body relaxed, especially your shoulders.

Ab Crunch

Starting position: Lie on your back with your knees bent, feet flat on the floor, and hands behind your head.

Movement: Using your abs, slowly raise your head, shoulders, and upper back about 45 degrees off the floor as you exhale. Think of shortening the distance between your ribs and pelvis. Hold for a second and then inhale as you slowly lower yourself. Do 10 reps.

Technique: Don't pull your chin to your chest. Don't arch your back.

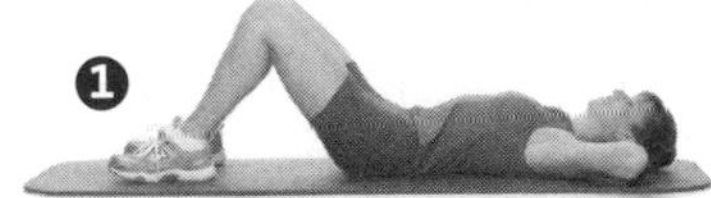

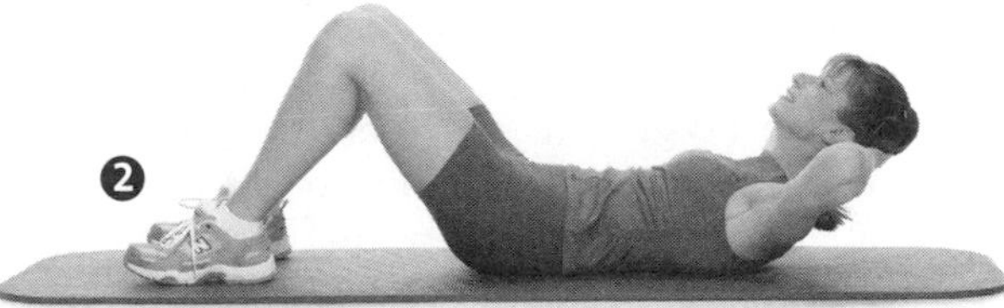

continued

The Workout

Level 2 *continued*

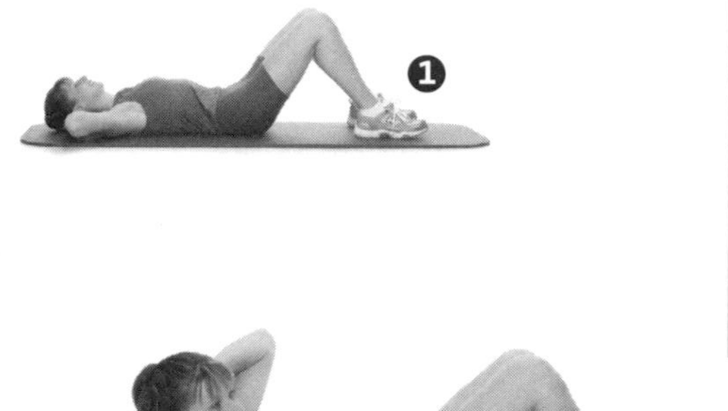

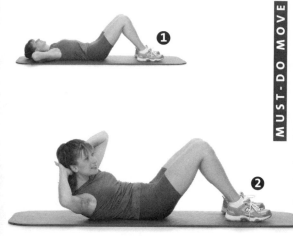

MUST-DO MOVE

Twisting Crunch

Starting position: Lie on your back with your knees bent, feet flat on the floor, and hands behind your head.

Movement: Using your abs, slowly lift your head and left shoulder off the floor, twist to the right, and bring your left shoulder toward your right knee as you exhale. Hold for a second and then inhale as you slowly lower yourself. Repeat, alternating sides. Do a total of 10 reps, 5 reps to each side.

Technique: Don't pull your chin to your chest. Don't arch your back.

MUST-DO MOVE

Bridge with Leg Lift

Starting position: Lie on your back with your knees bent, feet flat on the floor, and arms at your sides, palms facing up.

Movement: Contracting your abs, buttocks, and lower back, press into your feet and lift your butt, hips, and back off the floor as you exhale, to form a straight line from your shoulders to your knees. Lift one foot off the floor and extend that leg. Hold for three breaths and then lower your foot. Lift the other foot up and hold for three breaths. Lower your foot and return to the starting position. Do one time only.

Technique: Don't lift too high—your upper back and shoulders should remain on the floor. Don't bend at the waist or hips. Don't let your knees fall inward or outward.

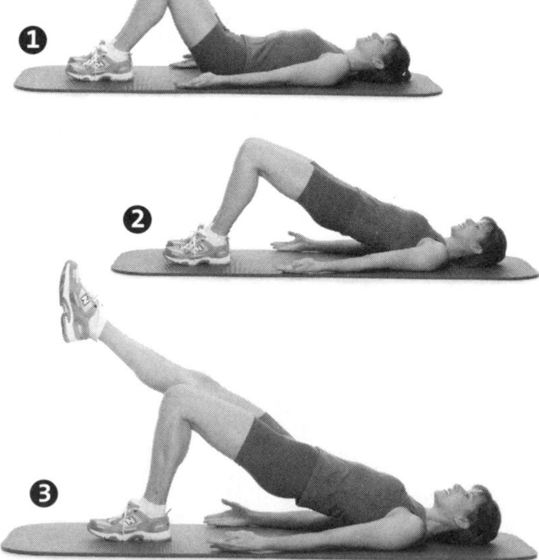

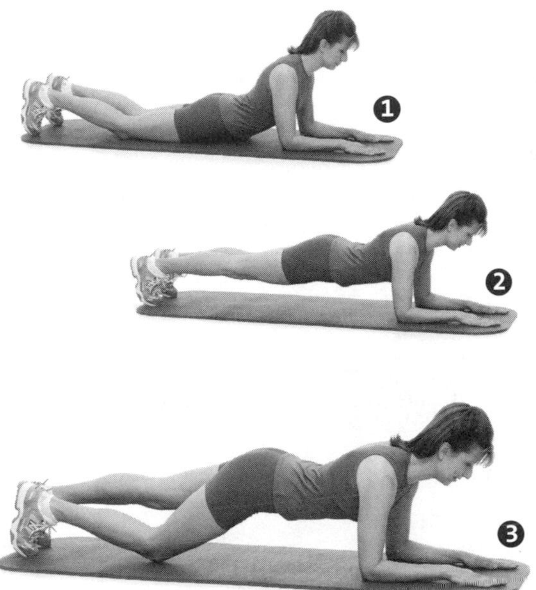

MUST-DO MOVE

Plank with Knee Drop

Starting position: Lie facedown, with your feet flexed and toes tucked. Your elbows should be under your shoulders and your forearms and palms on the floor.

Movement: Contracting your abs and back, press into your forearms as you exhale and lift your pelvis and legs off the floor so that your back and legs form a straight line. Slowly drop your right knee toward the floor and then straighten. Do five knee touches with your right leg, hold for three breaths, do five knee touches with your left leg, hold for three breaths, and then relax. Do one time only.

Technique: Don't lift your head up or let it drop. Don't bend at the waist or hips. Don't let your belly drop toward the floor.

T-Stand

Starting position: Sit on your left hip with your legs extended to the side, your right ankle over the left, right hand on your hip, and left hand on the floor below your shoulder.

Movement: Using your abs, lift your hips, legs, and ankles off the floor as you exhale. Hold for five breaths, relax, and then repeat on the other side. Do one time only on each side.

Technique: Don't let your body roll forward: Think of it as being sandwiched between two walls. Keep everything in line. Don't let your ankles touch the floor.

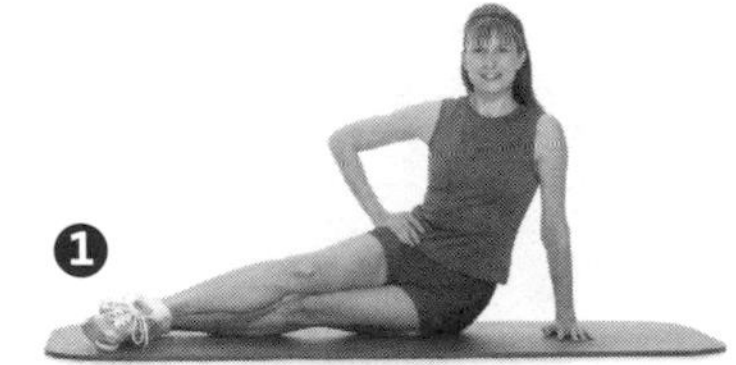

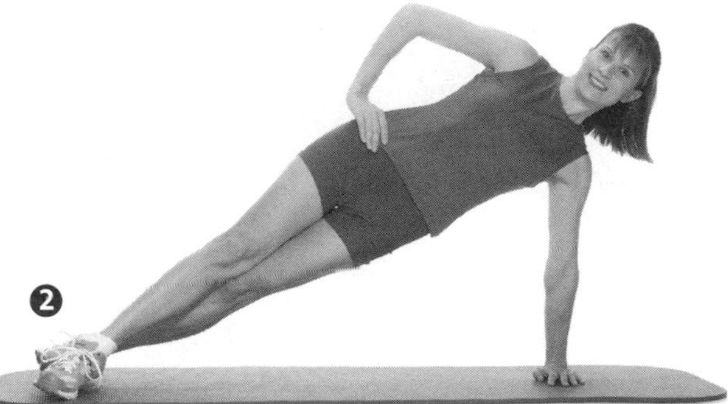

The Workout

Level 3

Interval Walk: About 30 Minutes

- 5-minute warmup: Walk 2½ to 3 miles per hour, 100 to 115 steps per minute.
- 2-minute moderate pace: Increase your speed to about 4 miles per hour, about 135 steps per minute.
- 3-minute speedup: Pick up your pace even more to about 4½ miles per hour, about 145 steps per minute.
- Repeat moderate pace/speedup sequence four times.
- 5-minute cooldown: Slow down to 2½ to 3 miles per hour, 100 to 115 steps per minute.

Core Training: 15 Minutes

- Do the sequence of exercises one time.

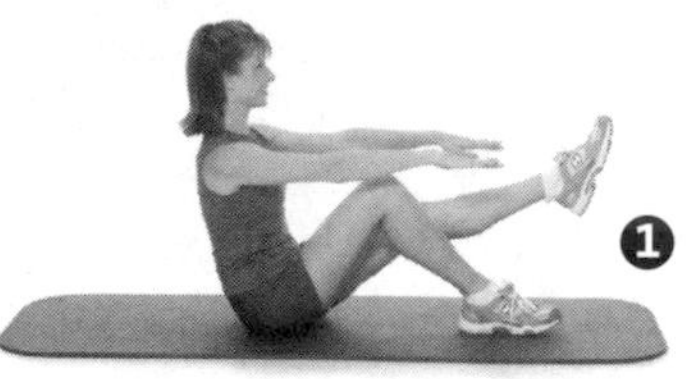

1

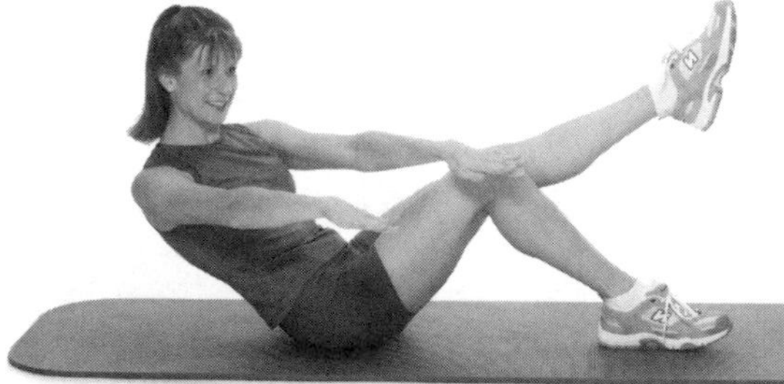

2

One-Leg Roll-Down with a Twist

Starting position: Sit on the floor with your knees bent and your feet flat. Lift your left foot off the floor and extend your left leg. Hold your arms straight out in front of you, parallel to the floor.

Movement: Using your abs, slowly roll down 4 to 5 inches, one vertebra at a time, as you inhale and twist to the right. Hold for a second and then exhale as you slowly roll back up. Do five reps and then switch legs and twist to the left.

Technique: Your abs should be powering the move. Don't move quickly.

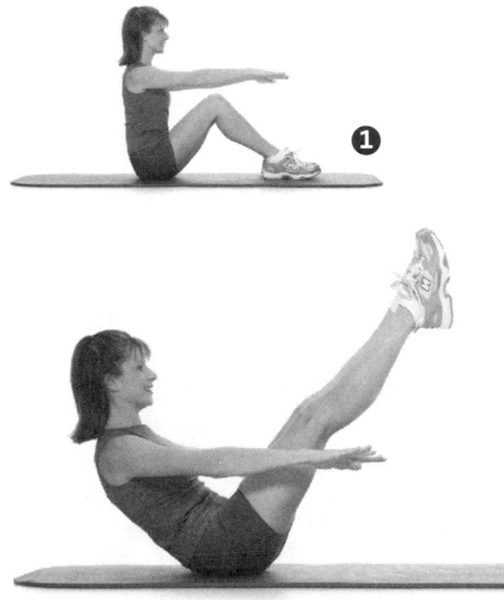

MUST-DO MOVE

Legs-Extended Balance

Starting position: Sit on the floor with your knees bent and your feet flat. Hold your arms out in front of you, parallel to the floor.

Movement: Lift your feet off the floor, extending your legs straight, and balance on your sitting bones. Hold for five breaths and then relax. Do one time only.

Technique: Keep your abs tight and the rest of your body relaxed, especially your shoulders.

Reverse Crunch

Starting position: Lie on your back with your legs up in the air and your hands behind your head. Cross your legs at the shins.

Movement: Slowly contract your abs as you exhale and press your back into the floor, tilting your pelvis and lifting your hips 2 to 4 inches off the floor. Keep your upper body relaxed. Hold for a second and then inhale as you slowly lower. Do 10 reps.

Technique: Don't swing your legs.

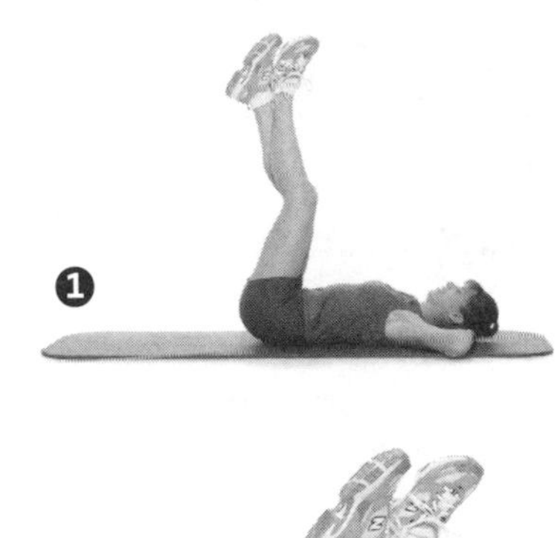

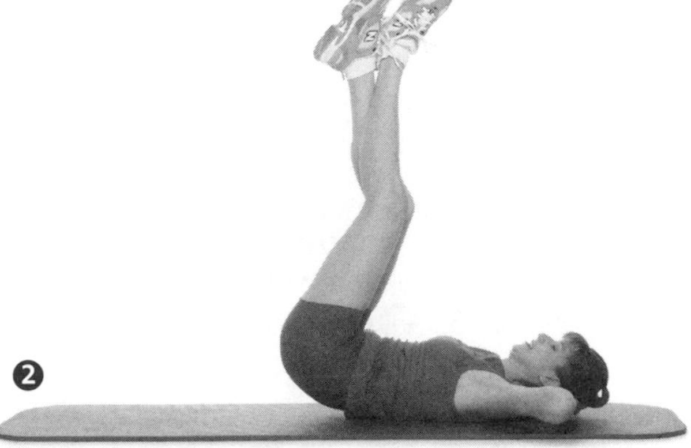

continued

The Workout

Level 3 *continued*

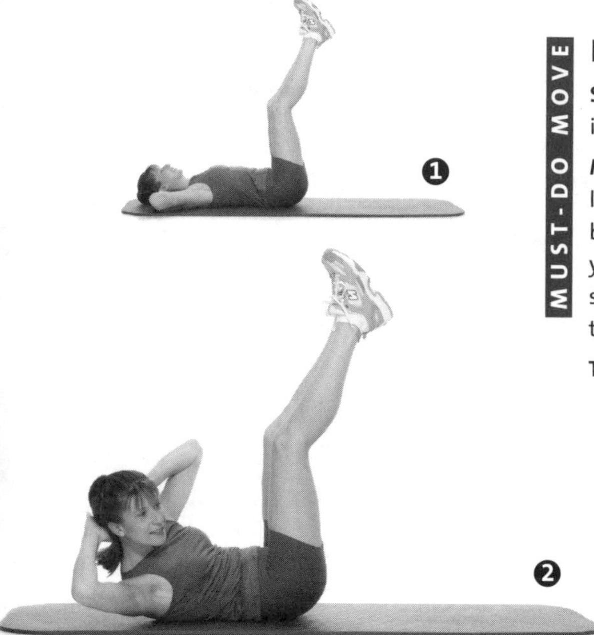

MUST-DO MOVE

Legs-Up Twisting Crunch

Starting position: Lie on your back with your legs up in the air and your hands behind your head.

Movement: Using your abs, slowly lift your head and left shoulder off the floor, twist to the right, and bring your left shoulder toward your right knee as you exhale. Hold for a second and then inhale as you slowly lower yourself. Repeat, alternating sides. Do a total of 10 reps, 5 to each side.

Technique: Don't pull your chin to your chest.

MUST-DO MOVE

Heel Bridge with Leg Lift and Arms Up

Starting position: Lie on your back with your knees bent, feet flat on the floor, and arms extended over your chest. Lift your toes off the floor so that only your heels are touching.

Movement: Contracting your abs, buttocks, and lower back, press into your heels and lift your butt, hips, and back off the floor as you exhale, to form a straight line from your shoulders to your knees. Lift your right foot off the floor and extend that leg. Hold for three breaths and then lower your foot. Lift the other foot up and hold for three breaths. Lower your foot and return to the starting position. Do one time only.

Technique: Don't lift too high—your upper back and shoulders should remain on the floor. Don't bend at the waist or hips. Don't let your knees fall inward or outward.

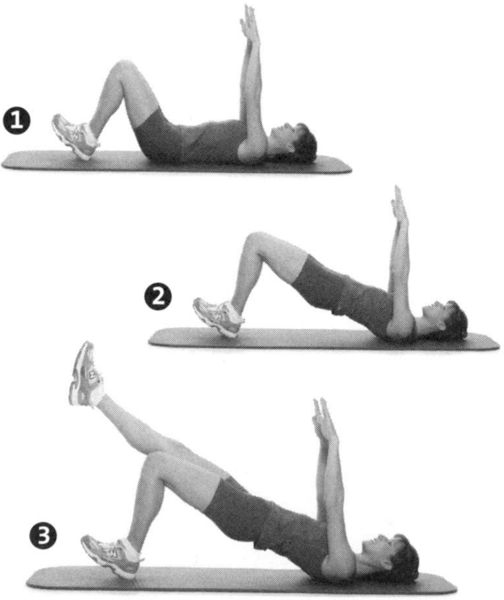

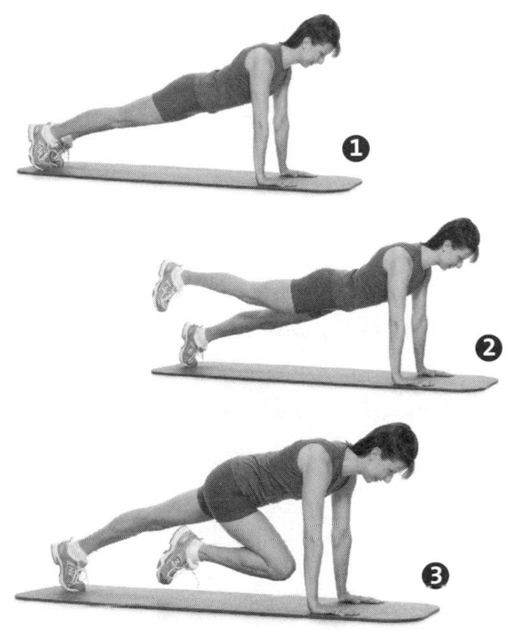

MUST-DO MOVE

Extended Plank with Lift and Bend

Starting position: Lie facedown with your feet flexed and toes tucked. Place your palms on the floor near your shoulders so that your elbows are pointing up. Contracting your abs and back, press into your hands as you exhale, straighten your arms, and lift your torso and legs off the floor so that your head, back, and legs form a straight line.

Movement: Lift your right foot off the floor and hold for three breaths. Next, pull your right knee in toward your chest and press it back out for five reps and then put that foot back on the floor. Lift your left foot off the floor and hold for three breaths. Next, pull your left knee in toward your chest and press it back out for five reps, put that foot back on the floor, and then relax. Do one time only.

Technique: Don't lift your head up or let it drop. Don't bend at the waist or hips. Don't let your belly drop toward the floor.

T-Stand with Arm Up

Starting position: Sit on your left hip with your legs extended to the side, your right ankle over the left, right arm extended on your leg, and left hand on the floor below your shoulder.

Movement: Using your abs, lift your hips, legs, and ankles off the floor and raise your right arm overhead as you exhale. Look up toward your right hand. Hold for five breaths, relax, and then repeat on the other side. Do one time only on each side.

Technique: Don't let your body roll forward; think of it as being sandwiched between two walls. Keep everything in line. Don't let your ankles touch the floor.

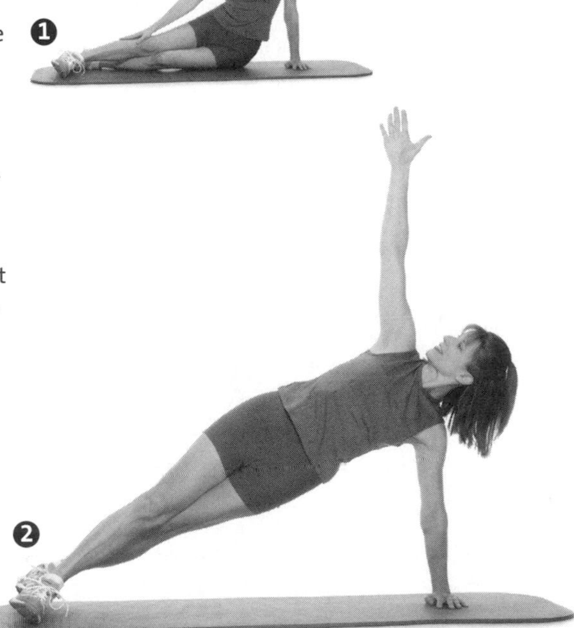

Control Emotional Eating

We've been pairing emotions with food for a long time. (Remember all the cookies you got to cheer you up when you were a kid?) What's more, food works. It can create soothing changes in brain chemistry, and even the simple act of chewing will increase endorphins and ease pain. Unfortunately, the relief lasts only as long as the last bite. To curb emotional eating, you need to figure out what you are really hungering for. Here's how.

Play detective. Every time you eat, write down what you put in your mouth and how you were feeling. Bored? Frustrated? Happy? Before long, you'll see a pattern. Then you can start to break it.

Shop for some stimulants. Do you eat when you're bored? Time to make a new "grocery" list. Buy inexpensive, accessible things such as books, CDs, and tapes or DVDs of favorite films that provide the emotional lift you're seeking from food. Keep them handy and turn to them when you're down.

Make a human connection. Looking for love or companionship? Call your best friend or your sister. Make sure you pick someone who makes you feel good. If you have issues with a parent or friend, calling that person could lead you to finish off an entire row of cookies.

Create new habits. Many people eat every time there's a lull, such as during TV commercials. Be prepared for those times. Keep manicure supplies, stacks of empty photo albums, or a cross-stitch project by the TV for something to do. Even better, find a hobby. When you're engrossed in something you love, you forget all about eating, especially if you're active.

Head toward your dreams. Maybe you're hungering for a big change, such as a more satisfying career. Go for it, one little step at a time. Take a class at a community college, or just start talking to people in that field. Moving toward goals is exhilarating.

Rethink your rewards. Like most people, you probably eat to celebrate happiness. (Don't most happy occasions involve eating?) Find new, affordable rewards, such as earrings or tickets to a play or movie.

FIRM UP TIP

ON YOUR PLATE

Avoid crash dieting; it can make cellulite worse. When you lose weight quickly, you lose muscle tissue—the stuff that makes your legs and butt look toned and smooth.

Meal Plan

Most of these recipes are custom designed to make 1 serving–no fuss, no muss; just fix, eat, and go! If a recipe makes more than 1 serving, it's noted below. Save that extra serving for another meal, or share it with your spouse or your walking buddy.

Breakfast

Shredded Wheat and Strawberries: Top 1 cup shredded wheat (such as Post Bite-Size Shredded Wheat 'n Bran or other cereal containing about 160 calories per 1-cup serving) with 1 cup sliced strawberries and 1 cup fat-free milk. (Drink any leftover milk or add to coffee or tea.) Serve with 10 almonds.

Healthy Snack

Luna Bar and Fruit: Serve 1 Luna bar (any flavor) with ½ orange.

Lunch

Ravioli and Fresh Fruit: Enjoy 1 cup cooked low-fat ravioli (such as Buitoni Light Four-Cheese Ravioli) topped with ⅓ cup spaghetti sauce. Serve with ½ cup fat-free milk and 1 cup raw broccoli with 2 tablespoons balsamic vinegar for dipping.

Indulgent Treat

Chicken McNuggets: Order a 4-piece Chicken McNuggets at McDonald's with your choice of sauce. Have 1 cup raspberries on the side.

Dinner

Cheese Omelet with Tomatoes: Coat a non-stick skillet with olive oil cooking spray and heat over medium heat. Beat 1 whole egg and 2 egg whites (3 total eggs; discard 2 yolks or cook them and feed them to your dog for a special treat) with 2 tablespoons fat-free milk and ½ teaspoon ground black pepper. Mix thoroughly and pour into the skillet. Top with ¼ cup reduced-fat shredded cheese, 1 chopped paste (Roma-style) tomato, and ⅛ cup chopped sweet onion (if desired). Serve with 1 cup fat-free milk and 1 slice whole wheat toast topped with 1 teaspoon trans-fat-free margarine.

Healthy Snack

Crackers and Dip: Dip 2 Wasa crispbreads into ⅓ cup ricotta cheese spread from Monday.

Nutrient analysis: 1,780 calories, 112 g protein, 224 g carbohydrates, 55 g total fat, 16 g saturated fat, 346 mg cholesterol, 29 g dietary fiber, 2,283 mg sodium, 1,921 mg calcium

FIRM UP TIP

MIND OVER MATTER

Smile. There's good evidence that just smiling and looking like you're happy will make you happier. Studies show that muscular changes in your face can elevate your happiness, as can good posture.

The Workout
Level 1

Easy Walk: 30 Minutes

- 5-minute warmup: Walk 2 to 2½ miles per hour, or 95 to 100 steps per minute.
- 20-minute moderate walk: Increase your speed to 2½ to 3 miles per hour, 100 to 115 steps per minute, or a pace that lets you comfortably carry on a conversation.
- 5-minute cooldown: Slow down to 2 to 2½ miles per hour, or 95 to 100 steps per minute.

High-Rep Strength Training: 25 Minutes

- Do three reps of each exercise. Start to do another rep, but stop at the midpoint of the exercise and pulse, moving in a shorter range of motion, three times. Finish by returning to the starting position. Do this three times for each exercise and repeat the sequence of exercises three times. Use a lighter weight, if needed.
- To warm up, use lighter weights, or none at all, the first time through, and for the lunge exercise, only go partway down.

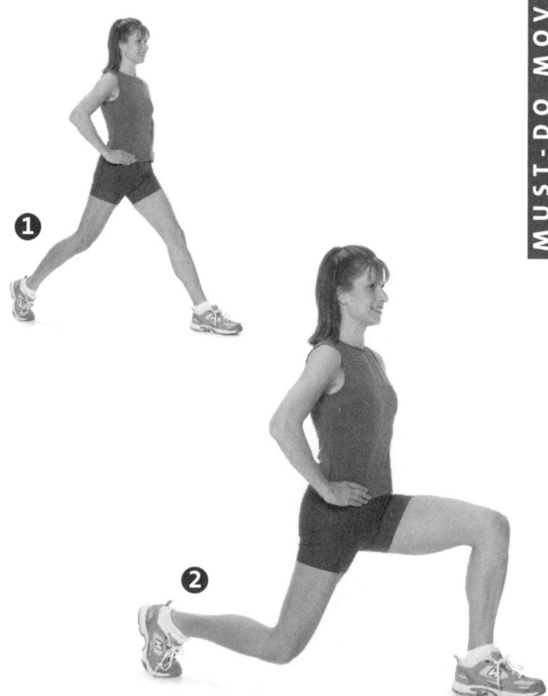

MUST-DO MOVE

Lunge (no weights)

Starting position: Stand with your feet 2 to 3 feet apart, with your left foot in front of your right. Place your hands on your hips.

Movement: Inhale as you bend your left knee and lower your body straight down until your left knee is bent 90 degrees and your right knee nearly touches the floor. Your rear heel will come off the floor. Hold for a second and then exhale as you slowly push yourself back up to the starting position. Finish all of your repetitions, then repeat the exercise with your right foot in front of your left.

Technique: Don't lean forward. Don't let your front knee move forward over your toes.

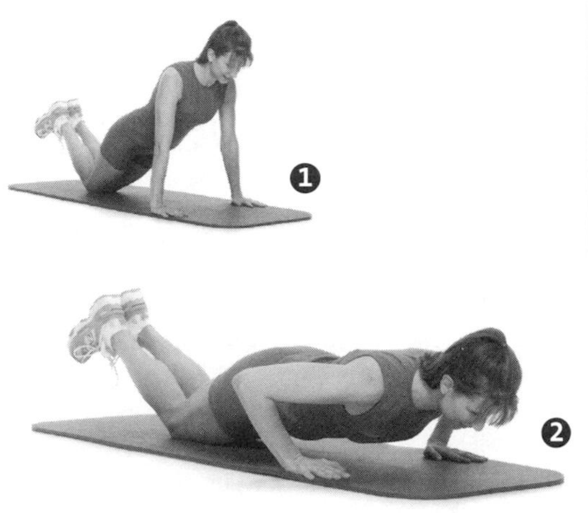

MUST-DO MOVE

Bent-Knee Pushup

Starting position: Lie facedown on the floor. Bend your knees so that your feet are up in the air, and place your palms on the floor near your shoulders so that your elbows are pointing up. Press down with your hands, extend your arms, and lift your body off the floor.

Movement: Keeping your head, back, hips, and knees in a straight line, bend your elbows out to the sides and lower your body as you inhale, until your chest nearly touches the floor. Hold for a second and then exhale as you push back up.

Technique: Don't bend at the hips. Don't arch your back.

MUST-DO MOVE

Seated Back Fly

Starting position: Sit on the edge of a chair with your feet hip width apart and hold a dumbbell in each hand. Keep your back flat and lean forward, bending at the hips so that the dumbbells are hanging at arm's length down by your calves, palms facing each other and elbows bent slightly.

Movement: Keeping your back straight, squeeze your shoulder blades together and lift the dumbbells up and out to the sides as you exhale, pulling your elbows back as far as comfortably possible. Hold for a second and then inhale as you slowly lower them.

Technique: Don't arch your back. Don't raise your torso as you lift the dumbbells.

Alternate move: If you have back problems, do the flies one arm at a time and place the forearm of your other arm across your thighs for extra support.

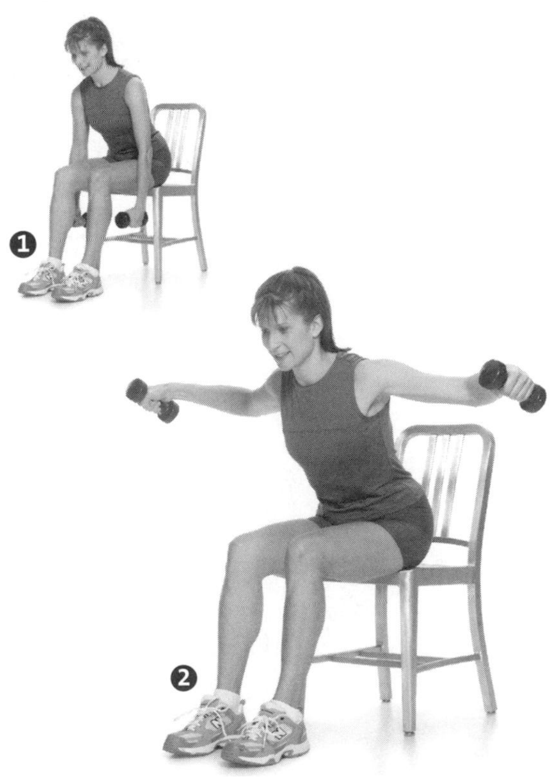

continued

The Workout

Level 1 *continued*

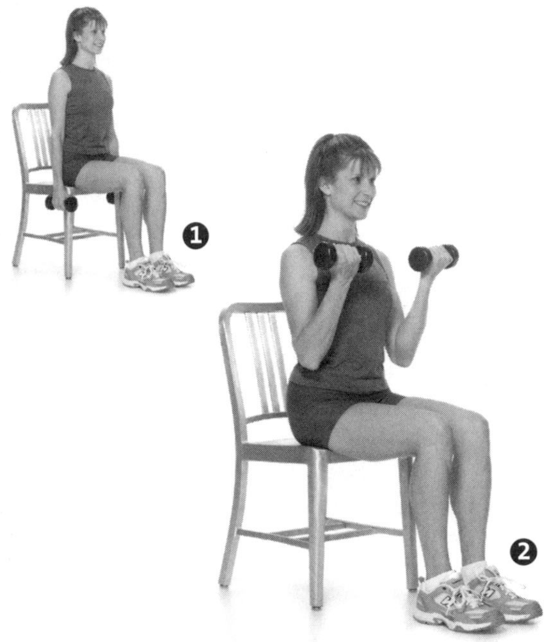

Seated Biceps Curl with a Twist

Starting position: Sit on the edge of a chair with your feet hip width apart. Hold dumbbells at your sides with your palms facing in.

Movement: Bending your elbows and turning your wrists upward, lift the dumbbells toward your shoulders as you exhale. Stop when the dumbbells are at chest height, palms facing your body. Hold for a second and then inhale as you slowly lower them.

Technique: Don't move your upper arms.

Seated Triceps Kickback

Starting position: Sit on the edge of a chair with your feet hip width apart and hold a dumbbell in each hand. Keep your back flat and lean forward, bending at the hips. Bend your arms at about 90-degree angles with your dumbbells at about hip height.

Movement: Without moving your upper arms, press the dumbbells back as you exhale, extending your arms until they are straight. Hold for a second and then inhale as you slowly lower them.

Technique: Don't move from your shoulders. Don't raise your torso as you lift the dumbbells.

Alternate move: If you have back problems, do the kickbacks one arm at a time and place the forearm of your other arm across your thighs for extra support.

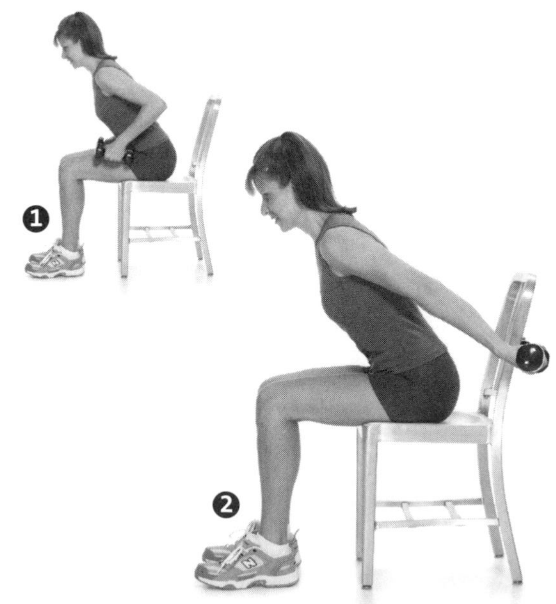

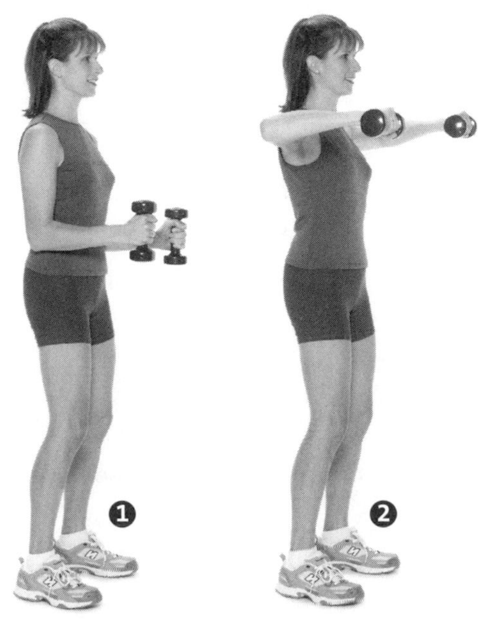

Bent-Arm Lateral Raise

Starting position: Stand with your feet shoulder width apart, knees bent slightly. Hold a dumbbell in each hand with your arms at your sides and bent at 90-degree angles so that your palms are facing in and the dumbbells are in front of you at about waist height.

Movement: Exhale as you slowly raise your elbows out to the sides until they are at about shoulder height. Hold for a second and then inhale as you slowly lower them.

Technique: Don't lift your shoulders. Don't lift higher than shoulder height.

FIRM UP TIPS

GET FIRM FASTER	ENERGY BOOSTER
Drink tea. In two studies, men who drank 3 to 5 cups of green or oolong tea a day burned 80 more calories over 24 hours. Researchers believe that caffeine and polyphenol compounds in the tea work to promote weight loss in two ways: by speeding up metabolism and by turning on your body's fat burners.	*Get more vitamin C. Researchers at Arizona State University in Tempe say that many of us aren't getting enough of this essential vitamin, which helps your body burn fuel for energy. To keep energy levels high, make sure that you're getting enough C-rich foods. Oranges and orange juice are natural choices, but bell peppers, strawberries, and broccoli are also naturally high in vitamin C.*

The Workout

Level 2

Easy Walk: 30 Minutes

- 5-minute warmup: Walk $2\frac{1}{2}$ to 3 miles per hour, or 100 to 115 steps per minute.
- 20-minute moderate walk: Increase your speed to 3 to $3\frac{1}{2}$ miles per hour, 115 to 125 steps per minute, or a pace that lets you comfortably carry on a conversation.
- 5-minute cooldown: Slow down to $2\frac{1}{2}$ to 3 miles per hour, or 100 to 115 steps per minute.

High-Rep Strength Training: 30 Minutes

- Do three reps of each exercise. Start to do another rep but stop at the midpoint of the exercise and pulse, moving in a shorter range of motion, three times. Finish by returning to the starting position. Do this three times for each exercise and repeat the sequence of exercises three times. Use a lighter weight, if needed.
- To warm up, use lighter weights, or none at all, the first time through, and for the squat and lunge exercises, only go partway down.

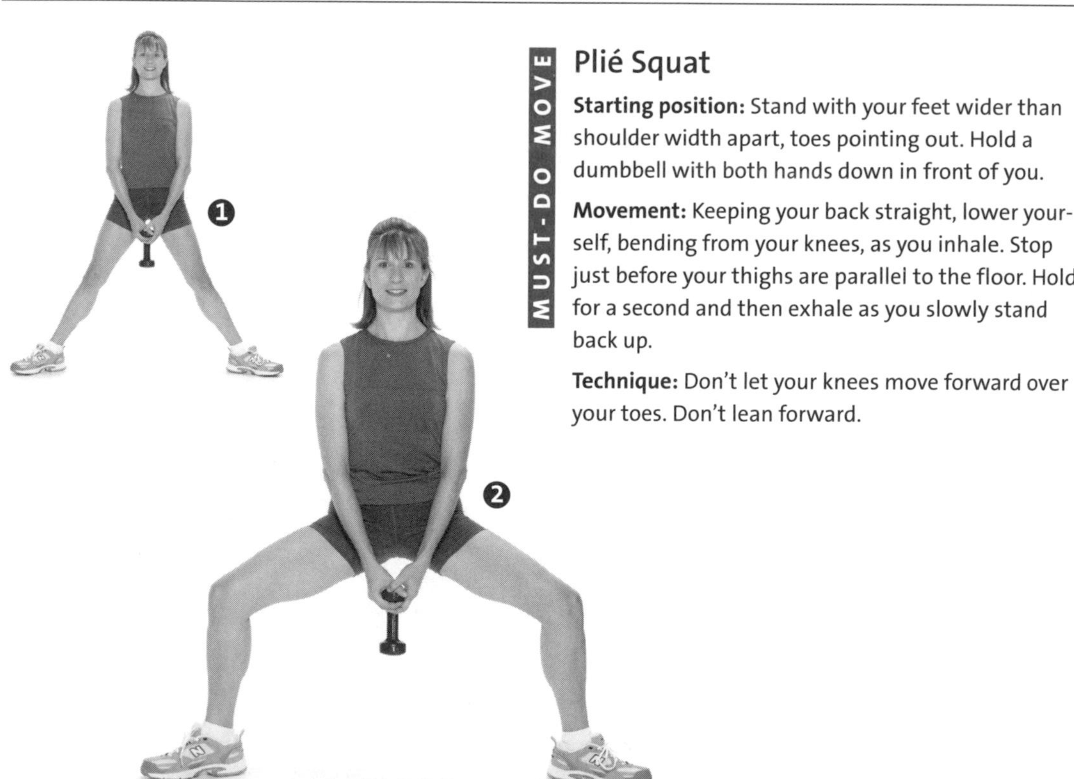

MUST-DO MOVE

Plié Squat

Starting position: Stand with your feet wider than shoulder width apart, toes pointing out. Hold a dumbbell with both hands down in front of you.

Movement: Keeping your back straight, lower yourself, bending from your knees, as you inhale. Stop just before your thighs are parallel to the floor. Hold for a second and then exhale as you slowly stand back up.

Technique: Don't let your knees move forward over your toes. Don't lean forward.

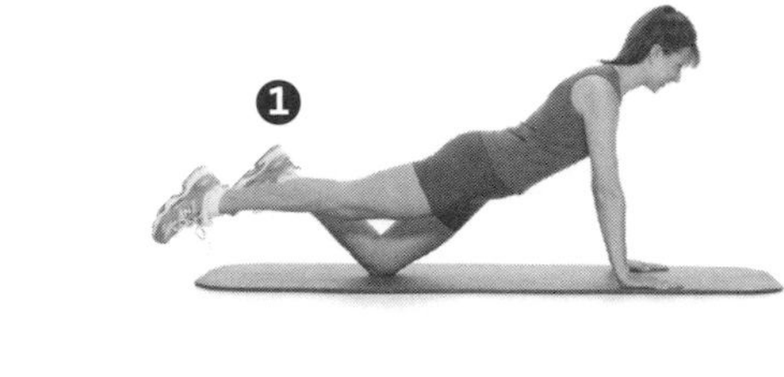

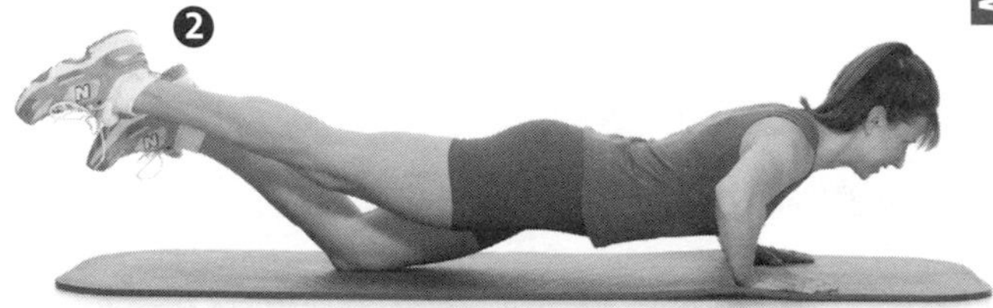

MUST-DO MOVE

One-Knee Pushup

Starting position: Lie facedown on the floor. Bend your knees so that your feet are up in the air, and place your palms on the floor near your shoulders so that your elbows are pointing up. Press down with your hands, extend your arms, lift your body off the floor, and lift one knee off the floor, extending that leg.

Movement: Keeping your head, back, hips, and knees in a straight line, bend your elbows out to the sides and lower your body as you inhale, until your chest nearly touches the floor. Hold for a second and then exhale as you push back up. Do half of the recommended reps and then switch knees.

Technique: Don't bend at the hips. Don't arch your back.

MUST-DO MOVE

Back Fly

Starting position: Stand with your feet shoulder width apart and knees bent slightly. Hold a dumbbell in each hand with your arms at your sides. Keep your back flat and lean forward, bending at the hips so that the dumbbells are hanging at arm's length in front of you, palms facing each other and elbows bent slightly.

Movement: Keeping your back straight, squeeze your shoulder blades together and lift the dumbbells up and out to the sides as you exhale, pulling your elbows back as far as comfortably possible. Hold for a second and then inhale as you slowly lower them.

Technique: Don't arch your back. Don't raise your torso as you lift the dumbbells.

Alternate move: If you have back problems, support yourself with one hand on a chair and do the flies one arm at a time.

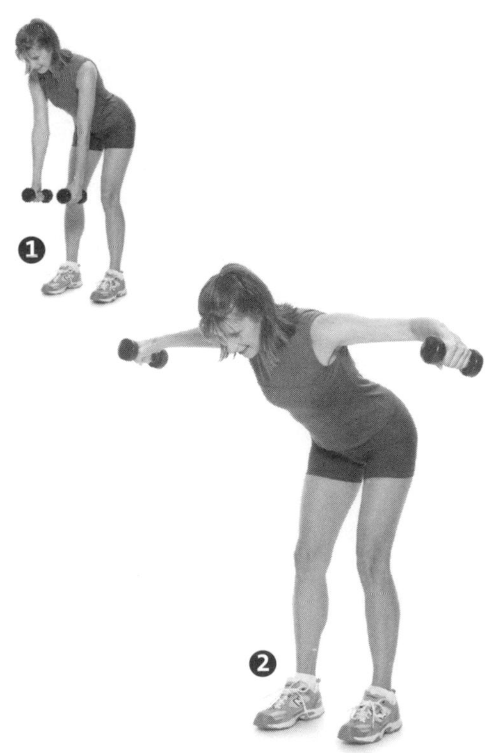

continued

The Workout

Level 2 *continued*

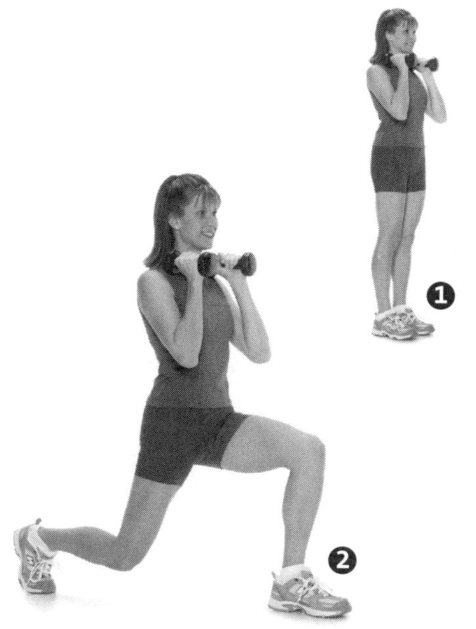

MUST-DO MOVE

Back Lunge

Starting position: Stand with your feet together. Hold a dumbbell in each hand, either at shoulder height or at your sides.

Movement: Step your right foot back 2 to 3 feet. Inhale as you bend your left knee and lower your body straight down until your left knee is bent 90 degrees and your right knee nearly touches the floor. Your rear heel will come off the floor. Hold for a second and then exhale as you push yourself back up, bringing your right foot back in. Finish all of your repetitions, then repeat the exercise, stepping back with your left foot.

Technique: Don't lean forward. Don't let your front knee move forward over your toes.

Concentrated Biceps Curl

Starting position: Sit on the edge of a chair with your feet shoulder width apart. Hold a dumbbell in your left hand and lean forward from your hips, resting your left elbow on the inside of your left knee so that your palm is facing your right leg. Place your right hand on your right thigh for support.

Movement: Bending your elbow, lift the dumbbell toward your left shoulder as you exhale. Stop when the dumbbell is at chest height, palm facing your shoulder. Hold for a second and then inhale as you slowly lower it. Do the recommended number of reps and then switch sides.

Technique: Don't move your upper arms.

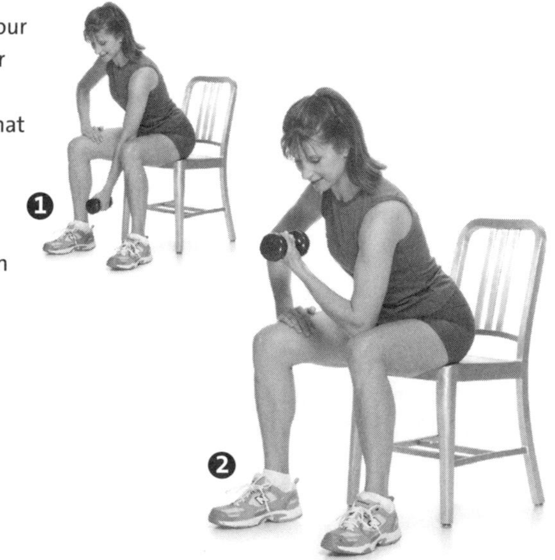

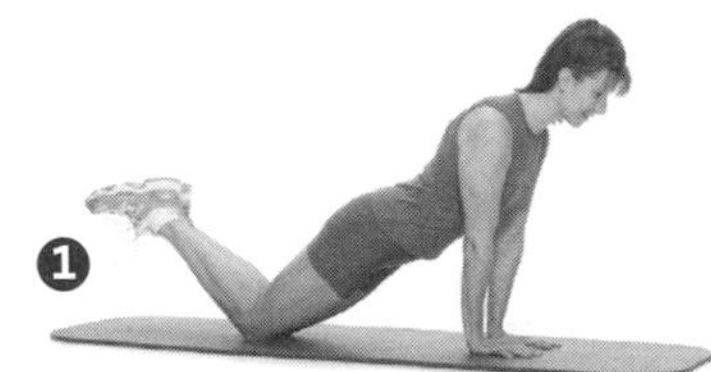

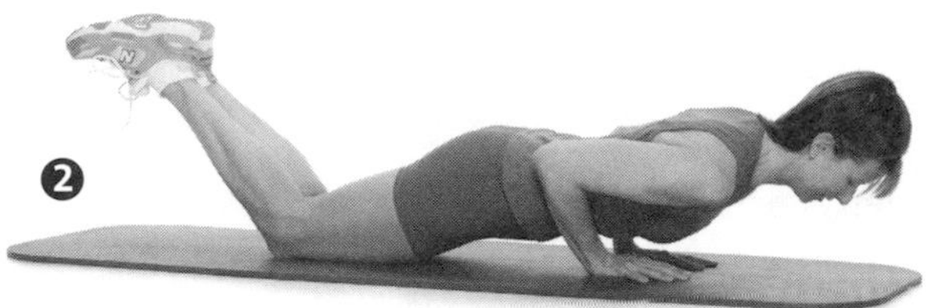

Kneeling Triceps Pushup

Starting position: Lie facedown on the floor. Bend your knees so that your feet are up in the air, and place your palms on the floor close to your ribs so that your elbows are pointing up. Press down with your hands, extend your arms, and lift your body off the floor.

Movement: Keeping your head, back, hips, and knees in a straight line, bend your elbows back, keeping your arms close to your body, as you inhale. Lower your body until your chest nearly touches the floor. Hold for a second and then exhale as you push back up.

Technique: Don't let your elbows point out to the sides. Don't bend at the hips. Don't drop your belly toward the floor.

Parallel Overhead Press

Starting position: Stand with your feet shoulder width apart and knees bent slightly. Hold a dumbbell in each hand at shoulder height, palms facing each other and elbows pointing forward.

Movement: Exhale as you slowly press the dumbbells straight overhead without locking your elbows. Hold for a second and then inhale as you slowly lower them.

Technique: Don't arch your back. Don't lift the dumbbells forward or back.

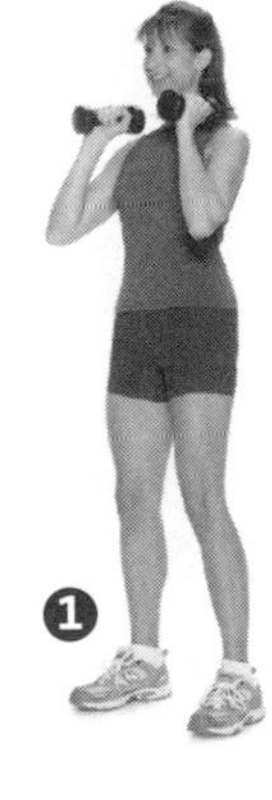

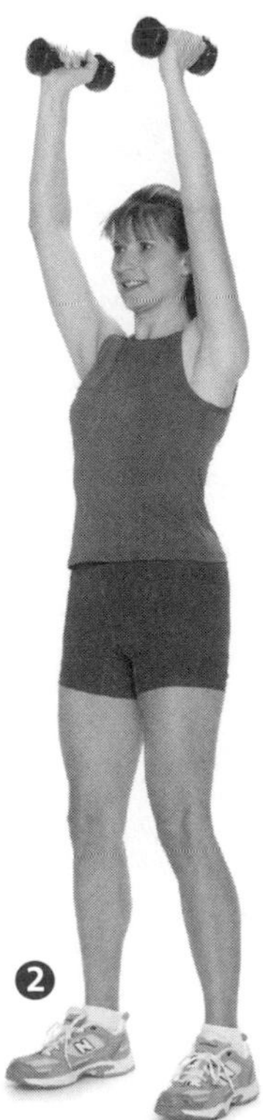

The Workout

Level 3

Easy Walk: 30 Minutes

- 5-minute warmup: Walk 2½ to 3 miles per hour, or 100 to 115 steps per minute.
- 20-minute moderate walk: Increase your speed to 3½ to 4 miles per hour, 125 to 135 steps per minute, or a pace that lets you comfortably carry on a conversation.
- 5-minute cooldown: Slow down to 2½ to 3 miles per hour, or 100 to 115 steps per minute.

High-Rep Strength Training: 30 Minutes

- Do three reps of each exercise. Start to do another rep but stop at the midpoint of the exercise and pulse, moving in a shorter range of motion, three times. Finish by returning to the starting position. Do this three times for each exercise and repeat the sequence of exercises three times. Use a lighter weight, if needed.
- To warm up, use lighter weights, or none at all, the first time through, and for the squat and lunge exercises, only go partway down.

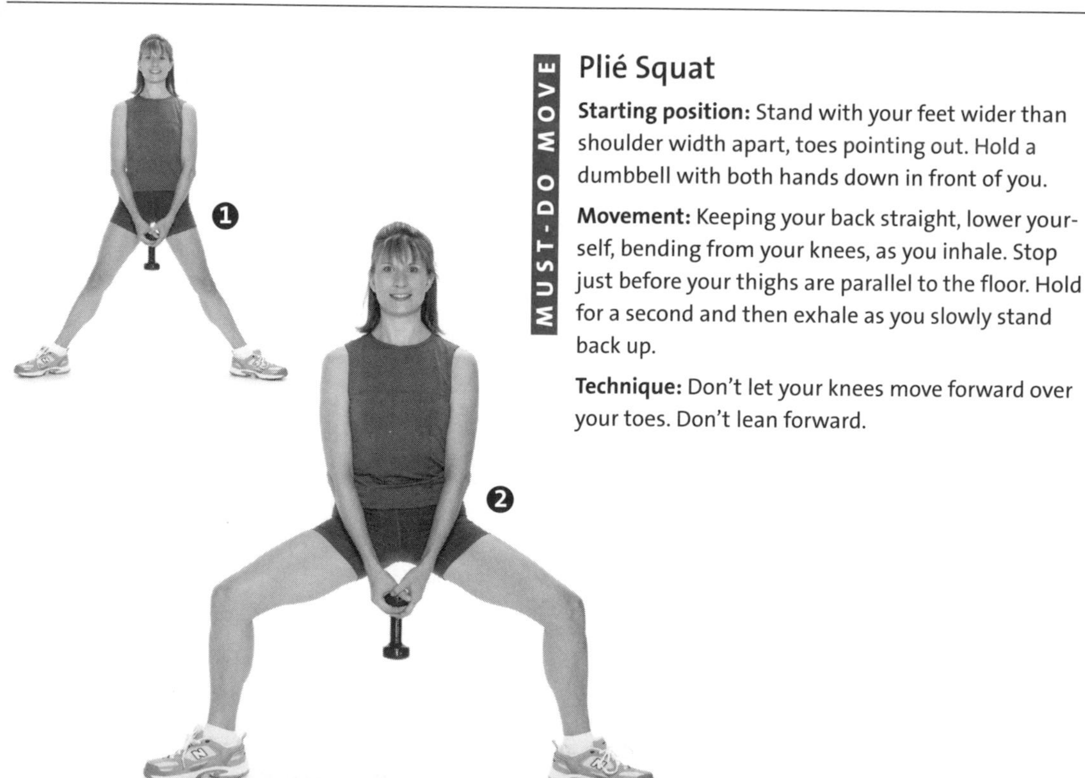

MUST-DO MOVE

Plié Squat

Starting position: Stand with your feet wider than shoulder width apart, toes pointing out. Hold a dumbbell with both hands down in front of you.

Movement: Keeping your back straight, lower yourself, bending from your knees, as you inhale. Stop just before your thighs are parallel to the floor. Hold for a second and then exhale as you slowly stand back up.

Technique: Don't let your knees move forward over your toes. Don't lean forward.

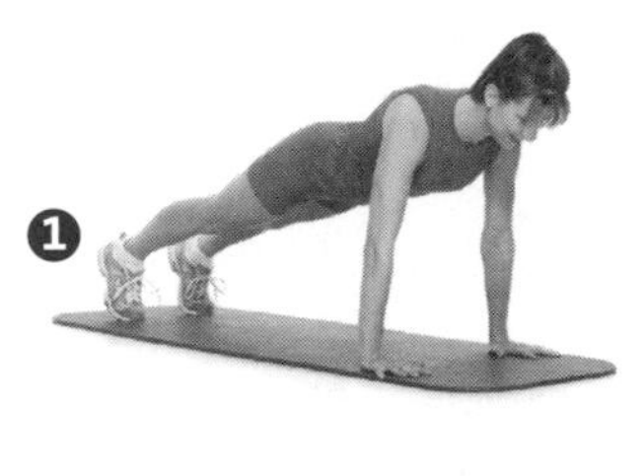

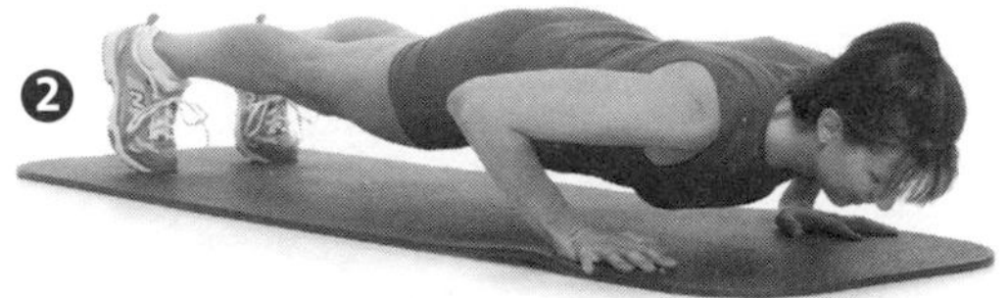

MUST-DO MOVE

Pushup

Starting position: Lie facedown on the floor with your feet flexed and toes tucked. Place your palms on the floor near your shoulders so that your elbows are pointing up. Press down with your hands, extend your arms, and lift your body off the floor so that it forms a straight line from head to toe.

Movement: Keeping your head, back, hips, and legs in a straight line, bend your elbows out to the sides and lower your body as you inhale, until your chest nearly touches the floor. Hold for a second and then exhale as you push back up. If you can't do all the recommended reps in this full pushup position, that's okay. Just drop down onto one or both knees and complete the remaining reps.

Technique: Don't bend at the hips. Don't arch your back.

MUST-DO MOVE

Back Fly

Starting position: Stand with your feet shoulder width apart, knees bent slightly. Hold a dumbbell in each hand with your arms at your sides. Keep your back flat and lean forward, bending at the hips so that the dumbbells are hanging at arm's length in front of you, palms facing each other and elbows bent slightly.

Movement: Keeping your back straight, squeeze your shoulder blades together and lift the dumbbells up and out to the sides as you exhale, pulling your elbows back as far as comfortably possible. Hold for a second and then inhale as you slowly lower them.

Technique: Don't arch your back. Don't raise your torso as you lift the dumbbells.

Alternate move: If you have back problems, support yourself with one hand on a chair and do the flies one arm at a time.

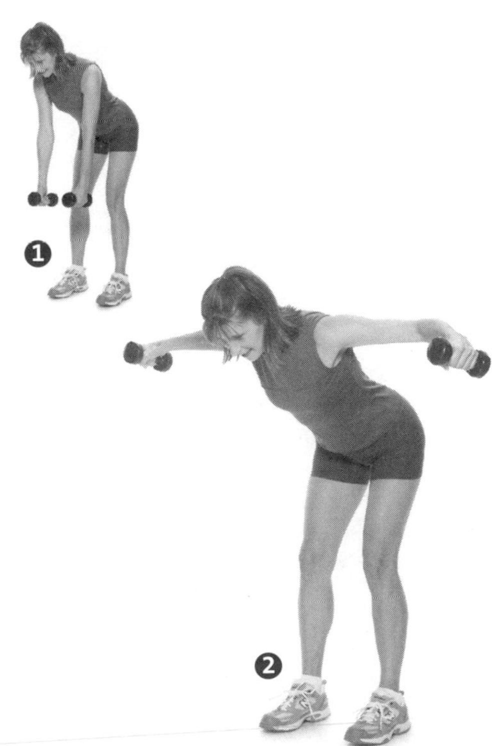

continued

The Workout

Level 3 *continued*

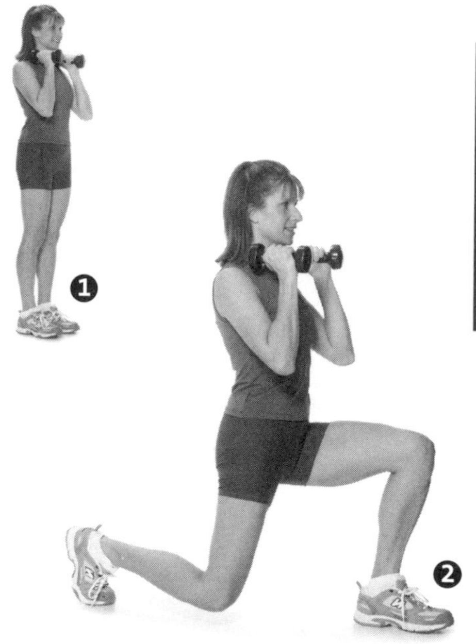

MUST-DO MOVE

Front Lunge

Starting position: Stand with your feet together. Hold a dumbbell in each hand, either at shoulder height or at your sides.

Movement: Step your left foot forward 2 to 3 feet. Inhale as you bend your left knee and lower your body straight down until your left knee is bent 90 degrees and your right knee nearly touches the floor. Your rear heel will come off the floor. Hold for a second and then exhale as you push yourself back up, bringing your left foot back in. Finish all of your repetitions, then repeat the exercise stepping forward with your right foot.

Technique: Don't lean forward. Don't let your front knee move forward over your toes.

Concentrated Biceps Curl

Starting position: Sit on the edge of a chair with your feet shoulder width apart. Hold a dumbbell in your left hand and lean forward from your hips, resting your left elbow on the inside of your left knee so that your palm is facing your right leg. Place your right hand on your right thigh for support.

Movement: Bending your elbow, lift the dumbbell toward your left shoulder as you exhale. Stop when the dumbbell is at chest height, palm facing your shoulder. Hold for a second and then inhale as you slowly lower it. Do the recommended number of reps and then switch sides.

Technique: Don't move your upper arms.

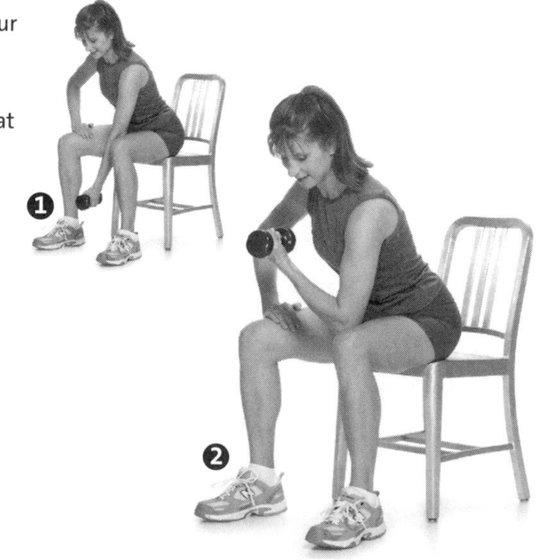

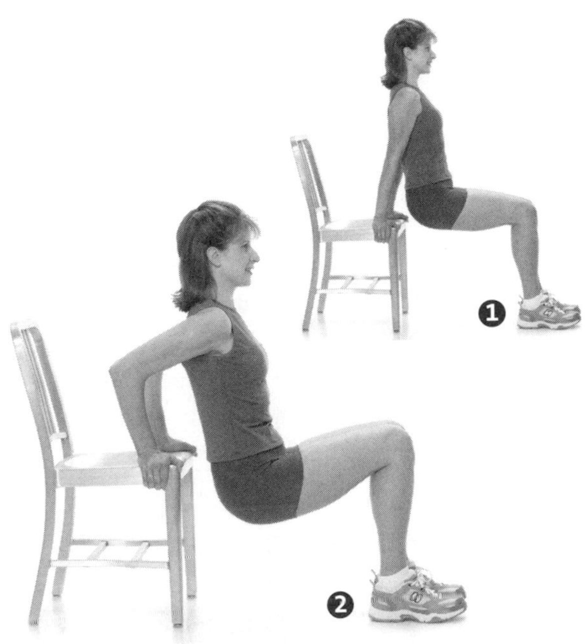

Triceps Dip

Starting position: Sit on the edge of a chair, place your hands on either side of you, and grasp the chair seat. Slide your buttocks off the chair and walk your feet out until your legs are bent at about 90 degrees. You should be balancing on your hands and feet.

Movement: Bending your arms so that your elbows point behind you, slowly lower your body toward the floor as you inhale. Keep your buttocks as close to the chair as possible. Stop when your elbows are bent about 90 degrees. Hold for a second and then exhale as you press back up.

Technique: Don't sink into your arms, allowing your shoulders to come up toward your ears. Don't bend your knees to help lower yourself.

Alternate move: For a more challenging version, lift one leg off the floor.

Lateral Raise

Starting position: Stand with your feet shoulder width apart, knees bent slightly. Hold a dumbbell in each hand with your arms at your sides, palms facing in, and elbows bent slightly.

Movement: Exhale as you slowly raise the dumbbells out to the sides until they are at about shoulder height. Hold for a second and then inhale as you slowly lower them.

Technique: Don't lift your shoulders. Don't lift higher than shoulder height.

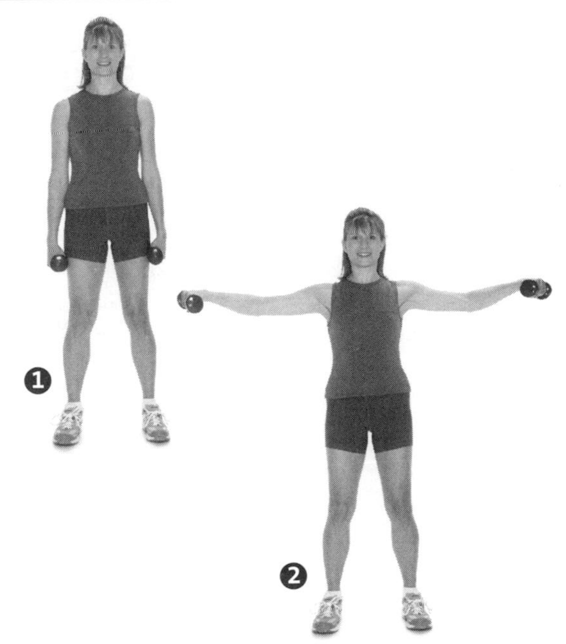

FIRM UP / DAY 11

Look 5 Pounds Slimmer

Virtually everything we do in modern life–from Internet surfing and desk work to driving and eating–rounds our bodies forward. And almost nothing we do reverses this curve, arching us back. As a result, poor posture is common and may contribute to a variety of ailments, from headaches to back spasms. And it can make you look and feel older and heavier than you really are.

Have you ever noticed that people who carry themselves with good alignment appear confident and graceful, while those whose posture reflects a physical slump often seem to be in a mental slump as well? Since our bodies and minds are linked, our posture mirrors our emotional state: When we're depressed, our bodies reflect this collapse. When we're happy, we look–and feel–like we're walking on air.

Stressful emotions can exert a subtle but damaging effect on posture. When we're chronically tense, certain muscles–often in the shoulders, back, and neck–are in a constant state of contraction, pulling the spine out of alignment and creating more stress. Learning to stand and sit with good posture can help muscles relax, which, in turn, can help the mind relax. Learning to lift your head and open your chest can lift your spirits as well. And it makes you look thinner.

Here's a simple posture exercise that you can do anywhere, anytime, standing or sitting, to open up the chest area and prevent rounded shoulders. Try it: Keeping your shoulders down, squeeze your shoulder blades together. Hold for about 10 seconds and repeat as often as possible. It may help you to imagine that you're using your shoulder blades to crack a walnut placed between them. Or pretend that you have a pencil balanced along your spine and squeeze your shoulder blades together to hold the pencil in place.

FIRM UP TIPS

ENERGY BOOSTER	FIT FACT
Up and away. If you have long enough hair, pull it back into a simple ponytail. It'll keep your hair out of your face while you're exercising and help make postworkout grooming simpler. And it's a classic look that doubles as a temporary mini-face-lift.	*In a study of 3,500 men and women, women suffering from moderate depression or anxiety ate an average of 118 extra calories each day. That could translate into a weight gain of 12 pounds over just 1 year.*

Meal Plan

Most of these recipes are custom designed to make 1 serving–no fuss, no muss; just fix, eat, and go! If a recipe makes more than 1 serving, it's noted below. Save that extra serving for another meal, or share it with your spouse or your walking buddy.

Breakfast

Creamy Ricotta English Muffin: Spoon ⅓ cup ricotta mixture from Monday onto ½ whole wheat English muffin and serve with 1 cup fat-free milk.

Healthy Snack

Frozen Grapes: Freeze 1 cup grapes for several hours. Eat them right out of the freezer; they're like candy. Serve with 1 Wasa crispbread topped with 1 tablespoon feta cheese.

Lunch

South of the Border: Microwave according to package directions Lean Cuisine Chicken Enchilada Suiza with Mexican-Style Rice, Smart Ones Chicken Enchilada Suiza, Smart Ones Fajita Chicken Supreme, Amy's Black Bean Enchilada Whole Meal, or a similar frozen meal (check the label for 270 to 280 calories and 6 to 9 grams of fat). Once it's cooked, slice ¼ fresh avocado over the entrée. Serve with 1½ cups cauliflower florets dipped in 1 tablespoon light salad dressing, and ½ cup mandarin oranges.

Indulgent Treat

Chips: Enjoy 1 large snack-size bag (1.25-ounce) potato chips (any variety).

Dinner

Veggie Stir-Fry: Heat a nonstick skillet coated with cooking spray and 2 teaspoons olive oil. Pan-fry 6 ounces low-fat firm tofu in block form for 2 minutes on each side. Break up the tofu into smaller pieces in the skillet and add 2 ounces low-sodium tomato soup and 2 ounces water. Continue cooking for 6 to 8 minutes. Scoop out the tofu; set aside. Using the remaining liquid in the skillet, stir-fry 1 cup fresh or frozen broccoli florets and ½ cup fresh or frozen snow peas with ½ teaspoon each cumin and coriander. Add 2 tablespoons water at a time if needed during cooking. Mix with the tofu and serve in 1 whole wheat tortilla. Have 1 cup chopped fresh fruit (such as 1 peach and 5 strawberries) for dessert.

Healthy Snack

Chocolate Pudding with Peanut Butter: Melt 1 tablespoon peanut butter in the microwave (heat for 30 to 35 seconds on 50 percent power) and immediately mix into 1 ready-to-serve fat-free chocolate pudding cup.

Nutrient analysis: 1,746 calories, 80 g protein, 221 g carbohydrates, 67 g total fat, 18 g saturated fat, 69 mg cholesterol, 23 g dietary fiber, 2,645 mg sodium, 1,411 mg calcium

The Workout

Level 1

Interval Walk: About 30 Minutes

- 5-minute warmup: Walk 2 to 2½ miles per hour, 95 to 100 steps per minute.
- 4-minute moderate pace: Increase your speed to about 3 miles per hour, about 115 steps per minute.
- 1-minute speedup: Pick up your pace even more to about 3½ miles per hour, about 125 steps per minute.
- Repeat moderate pace/speedup sequence four times.
- 5-minute cooldown: Slow down to 2 to 2½ miles per hour, 95 to 100 steps per minute.

Core Training: 15 Minutes

- Do the sequence of exercises one time.

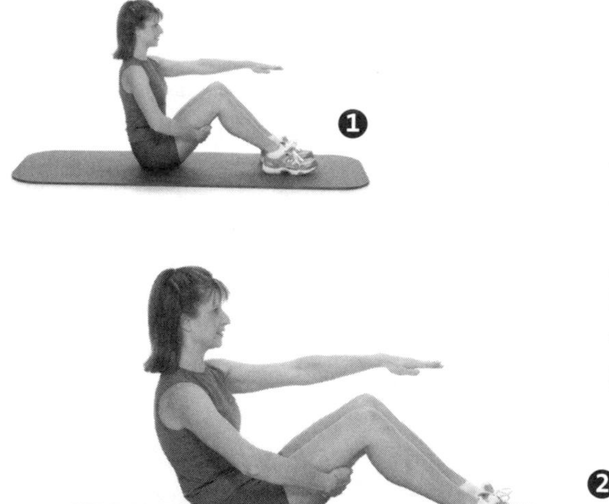

One-Hand Roll-Down

Starting position: Sit on the floor with your knees bent and your feet flat. Place one hand behind the same-side thigh. Keep the other arm out in front of you, parallel to the floor.

Movement: Using your abs, slowly roll down 2 to 3 inches, one vertebra at a time, as you inhale. Hold for a second and then exhale as you slowly roll back up. Do 10 reps.

Technique: Your abs should be powering the move. Don't move quickly.

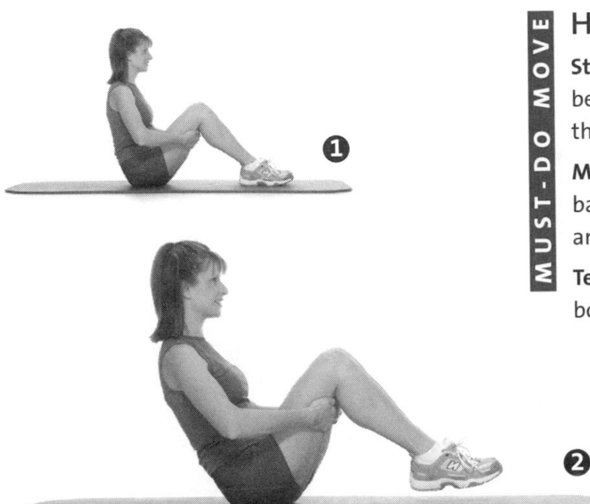

MUST-DO MOVE

Holding Balance

Starting position: Sit on the floor with your knees bent and your feet flat. Place your hands behind your thighs.

Movement: Lift your feet off the floor slightly and balance on your sitting bones. Hold for four breaths and then relax. Do one time only.

Technique: Keep your abs tight and the rest of your body relaxed, especially your shoulders.

Arms-Crossed Ab Crunch

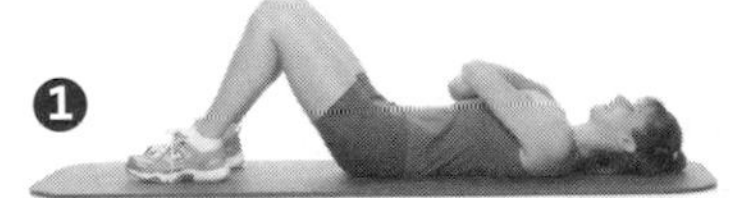

Starting position: Lie on your back with your knees bent, feet flat on the floor, and arms across your chest.

Movement: Using your abs, slowly raise your head, shoulders, and upper back about 45 degrees off the floor as you exhale. Think of shortening the distance between your ribs and pelvis. Hold for a second and then inhale as you slowly lower yourself. Do 10 reps.

Technique: Don't pull your chin to your chest. Don't arch your back.

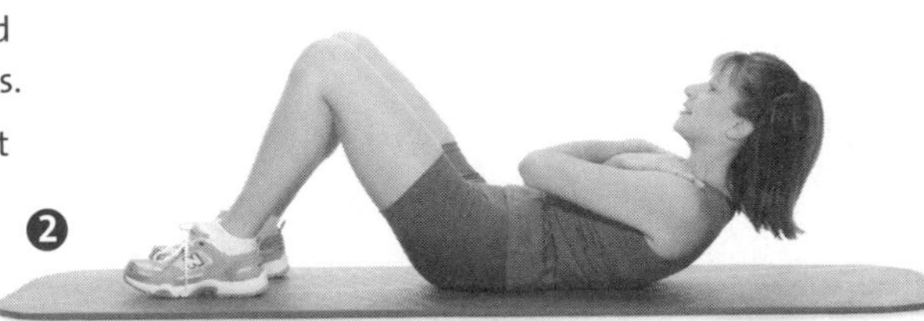

continued

The Workout

Level 1 *continued*

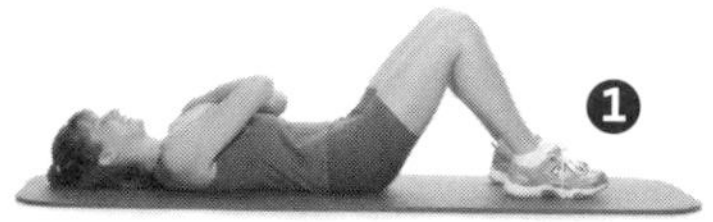

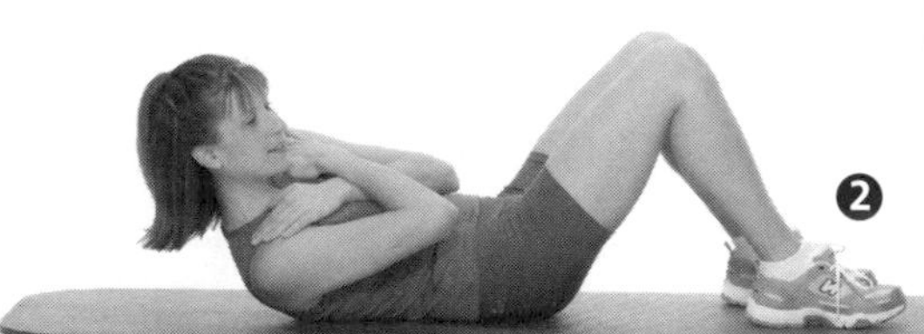

MUST-DO MOVE

Arms-Crossed Twisting Crunch

Starting position: Lie on your back with your knees bent, feet flat on the floor, and arms across your chest.

Movement: Using your abs, slowly lift your head and left shoulder off the floor, twist to the right, and bring your left shoulder toward your right knee as you exhale. Hold for a second and then inhale as you slowly lower yourself. Repeat, alternating sides. Do a total of 10 reps, 5 reps to each side.

Technique: Don't pull your chin to your chest. Don't arch your back.

MUST-DO MOVE

Heel Bridge

Starting position: Lie on your back with your knees bent and arms at your sides, palms facing up. Lift your toes off the floor so that only your heels are touching.

Movement: Contracting your abs, buttocks, and lower back, press into your heels and lift your butt, hips, and back off the floor as you exhale, to form a straight line from your shoulders to your knees. Hold for four breaths and then relax. Do one time only.

Technique: Don't lift too high—your upper back and shoulders should remain on the floor. Don't bend at the waist or hips. Don't let your knees fall inward or outward.

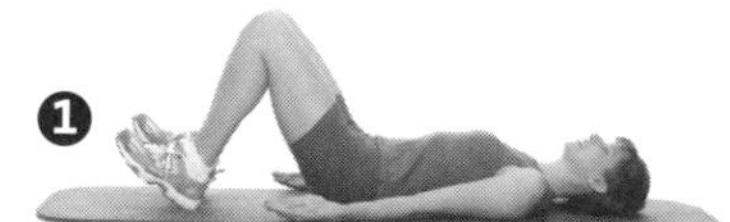

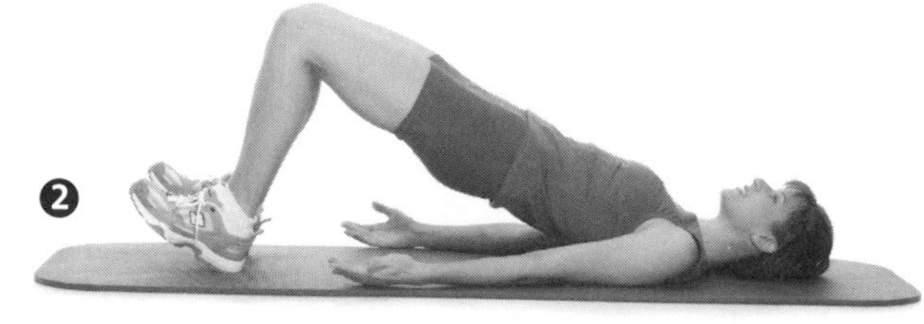

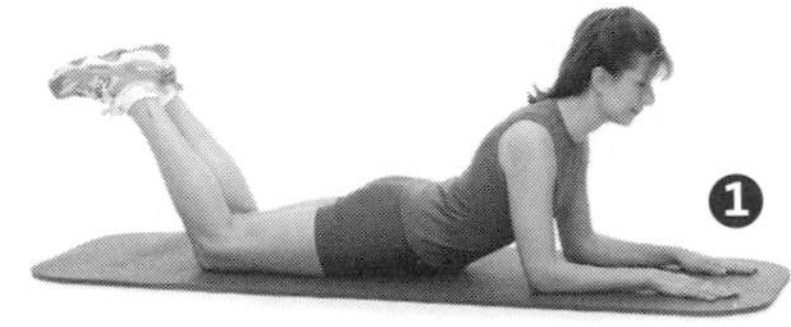

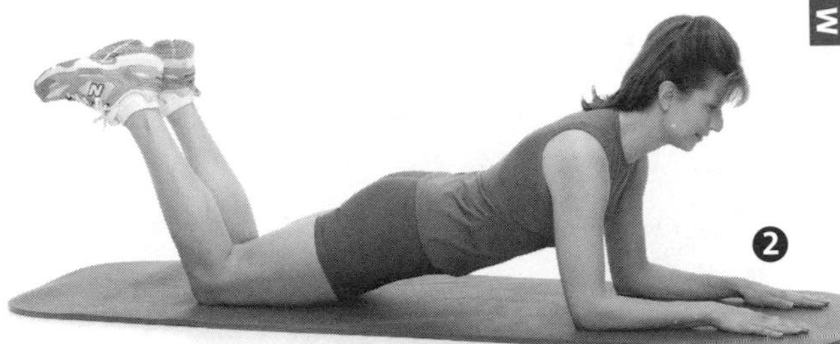

MUST-DO MOVE

Knee Plank

Starting position: Lie facedown with your knees bent so that your feet are in the air. Your elbows should be under your shoulders and your forearms and palms on the floor.

Movement: Contracting your abs and back, press into your forearms as you exhale and lift your pelvis off the floor so that your back and thighs form a straight line. Hold for four breaths and then relax. Do one time only.

Technique: Don't lift your head up or let it drop. Don't bend at the waist. Don't arch your back.

Leg Lift

Starting position: Lie facedown on the floor with your head resting on your hands.

Movement: Exhale as you lift your legs 10 to 12 inches off the floor. Hold for a second and then inhale as you slowly lower them. Do 10 reps.

Technique: Don't lift too high.

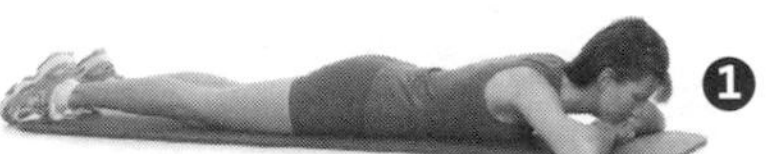

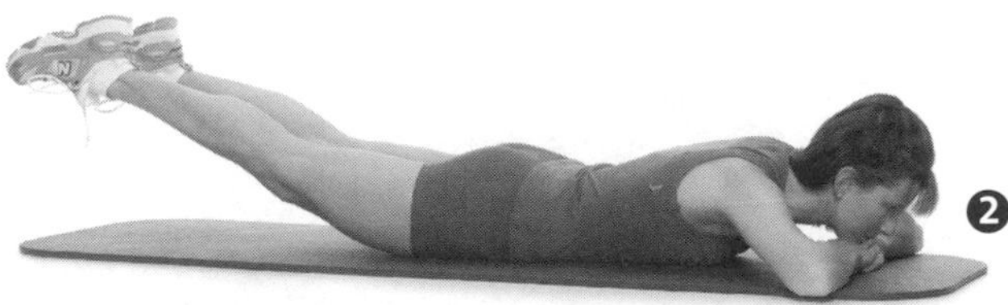

The Workout

Level 2

Interval Walk: About 30 Minutes

- 5-minute warmup: Walk 2½ to 3 miles per hour, 100 to 115 steps per minute.
- 4-minute moderate pace: Increase your speed to about 3½ miles per hour, about 125 steps per minute.
- 2-minute speedup: Pick up your pace even more to about 4 miles per hour, about 135 steps per minute.
- Repeat moderate pace/speedup sequence three times.
- 5-minute cooldown: Slow down to 2½ to 3 miles per hour, 100 to 115 steps per minute.

Core Training: 15 Minutes

- Do the sequence of exercises one time.

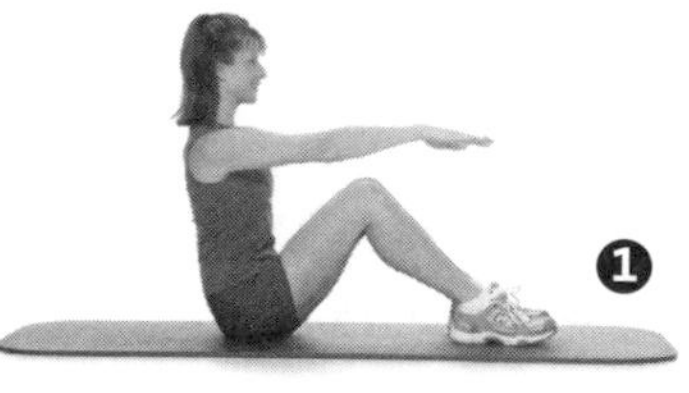

❶

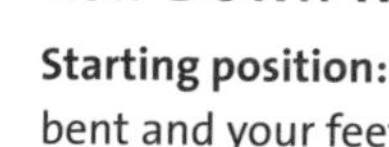

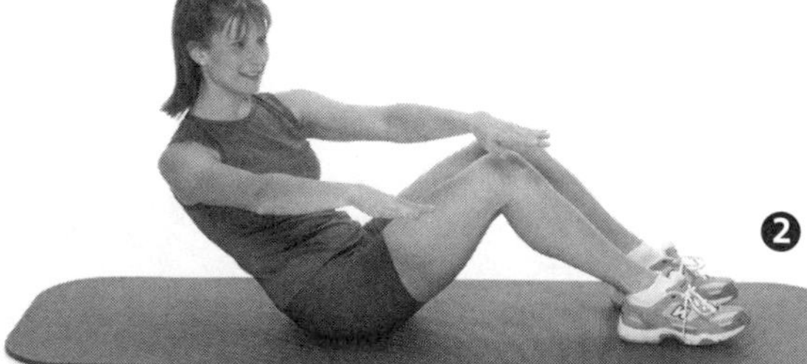

❷

Roll-Down with a Twist

Starting position: Sit on the floor with your knees bent and your feet flat. Hold your arms out in front of you, parallel to the floor.

Movement: Using your abs, slowly roll down 3 to 4 inches, one vertebra at a time, as you inhale and twist to the right. Hold for a second and then exhale as you slowly roll back up. Do 10 reps, alternating the side you twist to each time.

Technique: Your abs should be powering the move. Don't move quickly.

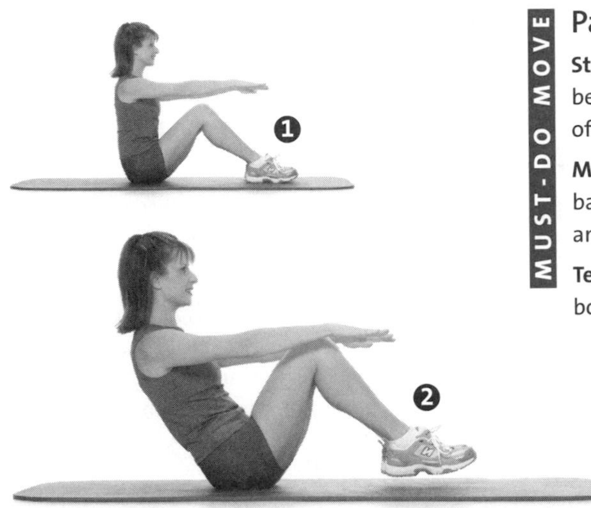

MUST-DO MOVE

Partial Balance

Starting position: Sit on the floor with your knees bent and your feet flat. Hold your arms out in front of you, parallel to the floor.

Movement: Lift your feet off the floor slightly and balance on your sitting bones. Hold for five breaths and then relax. Do one time only.

Technique: Keep your abs tight and the rest of your body relaxed, especially your shoulders.

Ab Crunch

Starting position: Lie on your back with your knees bent, feet flat on the floor, and hands behind your head.

Movement: Using your abs, slowly raise your head, shoulders, and upper back about 45 degrees off the floor as you exhale. Think of shortening the distance between your ribs and pelvis. Hold for a second and then inhale as you slowly lower yourself. Do 10 reps.

Technique: Don't pull your chin to your chest. Don't arch your back.

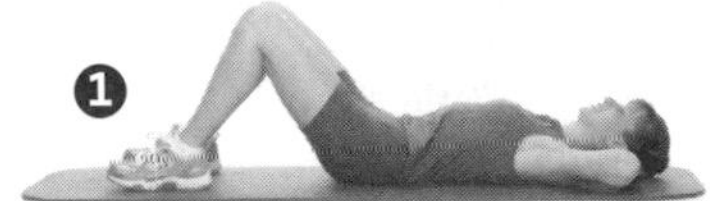

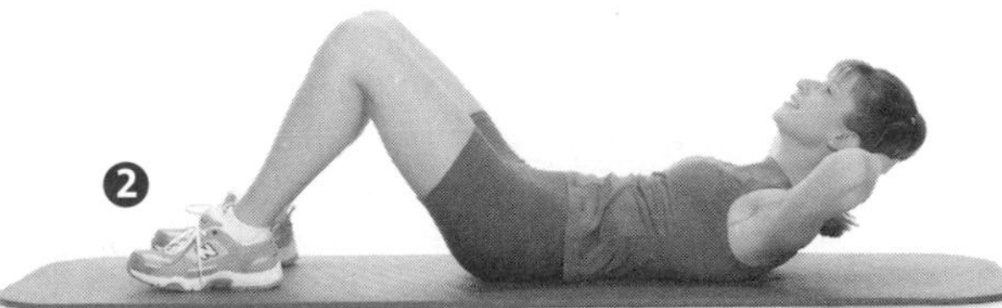

continued

The Workout

Level 2 *continued*

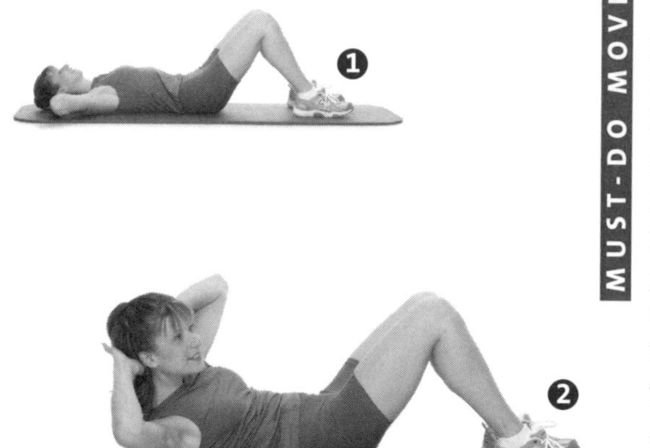

MUST-DO MOVE

Twisting Crunch

Starting position: Lie on your back with your knees bent, feet flat on the floor, and hands behind your head.

Movement: Using your abs, slowly lift your head and left shoulder off the floor, twist to the right, and bring your left shoulder toward your right knee as you exhale. Hold for a second and then inhale as you slowly lower yourself. Repeat, alternating sides. Do a total of 10 reps, 5 reps to each side.

Technique: Don't pull your chin to your chest. Don't arch your back.

MUST-DO MOVE

Bridge with Leg Lift

Starting position: Lie on your back with your knees bent, feet flat on the floor, and arms at your sides, palms facing up.

Movement: Contracting your abs, buttocks, and lower back, press into your feet and lift your butt, hips, and back off the floor as you exhale, to form a straight line from your shoulders to your knees. Lift one foot off the floor and extend that leg. Hold for three breaths and then lower your foot. Lift the other foot up and hold for three breaths. Lower your foot and return to the starting position. Do one time only.

Technique: Don't lift too high—your upper back and shoulders should remain on the floor. Don't bend at the waist or hips. Don't let your knees fall inward or outward.

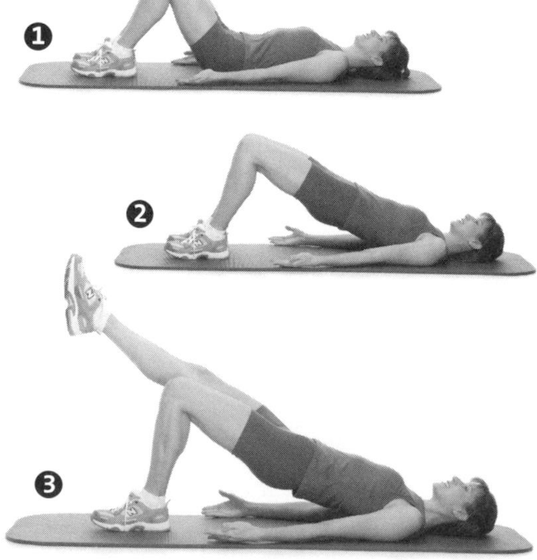

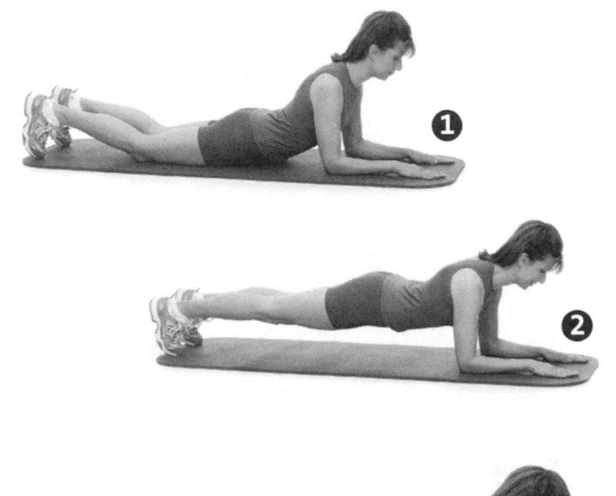

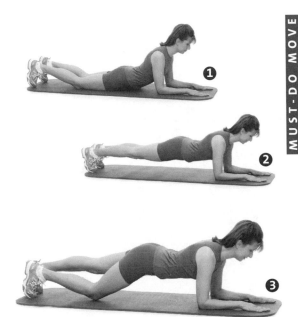

MUST-DO MOVE

Plank with Knee Drop

Starting position: Lie facedown with your feet flexed and toes tucked. Your elbows should be under your shoulders and your forearms and palms on the floor.

Movement: Contracting your abs and back, press into your forearms as you exhale and lift your pelvis and legs off the floor so that your back and legs form a straight line. Slowly drop your right knee toward the floor and then straighten. Do five knee touches with your right leg, hold for three breaths, do five knee touches with your left leg, hold for three breaths, and then relax. Do one time only.

Technique: Don't lift your head up or let it drop. Don't bend at the waist or hips. Don't let your belly drop toward the floor.

Bent-Arm Chest and Leg Lift

Starting position: Lie facedown on the floor with your hands under your chin.

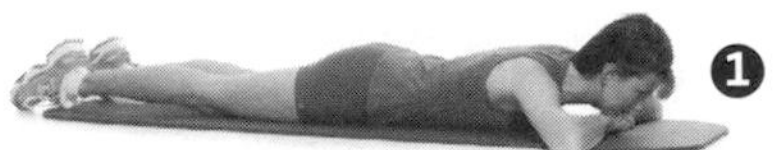

Movement: Exhale as you lift your head, chest, and legs 5 to 10 inches off the floor. Hold for a second and then inhale as you slowly lower yourself. Do 10 reps.

Technique: Don't lift too high.

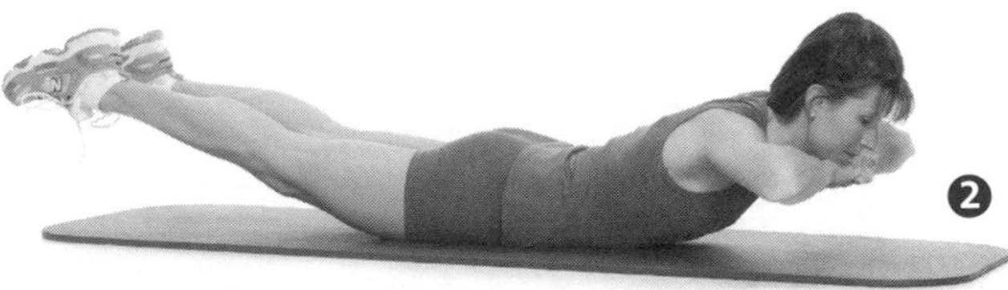

The Workout

Level 3

Interval Walk: About 30 Minutes

- 5-minute warmup: Walk 2½ to 3 miles per hour, 100 to 115 steps per minute.
- 2-minute moderate pace: Increase your speed to about 4 miles per hour, about 135 steps per minute.
- 3-minute speedup: Pick up your pace even more to about 4½ miles per hour, about 145 steps per minute.
- Repeat moderate pace/speedup sequence four times.
- 5-minute cooldown: Slow down to 2½ to 3 miles per hour, 100 to 115 steps per minute.

Core Training: 15 Minutes

- Do the sequence of exercises one time.

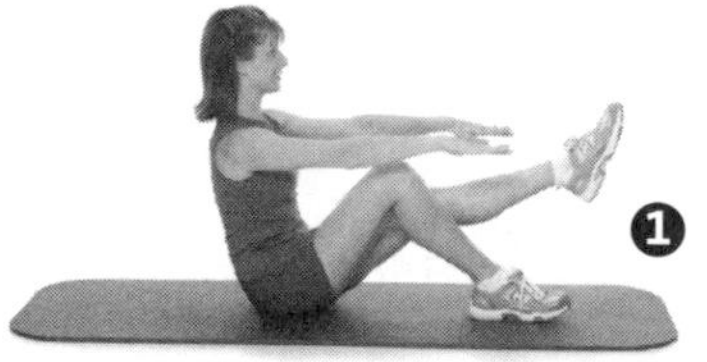

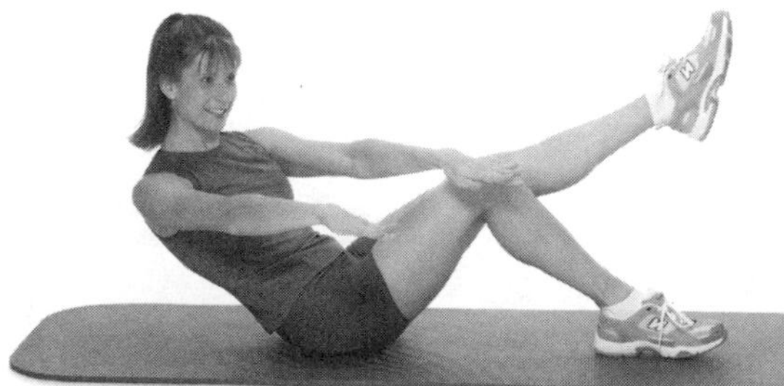

One-Leg Roll-Down with a Twist

Starting position: Sit on the floor with your knees bent and your feet flat. Lift your left foot off the floor and extend your left leg. Hold your arms straight out in front of you, parallel to the floor.

Movement: Using your abs, slowly roll down 4 to 5 inches, one vertebra at a time, as you inhale and twist to the right. Hold for a second and then exhale as you slowly roll back up. Do five reps and then switch legs and twist to the left.

Technique: Your abs should be powering the move. Don't move quickly.

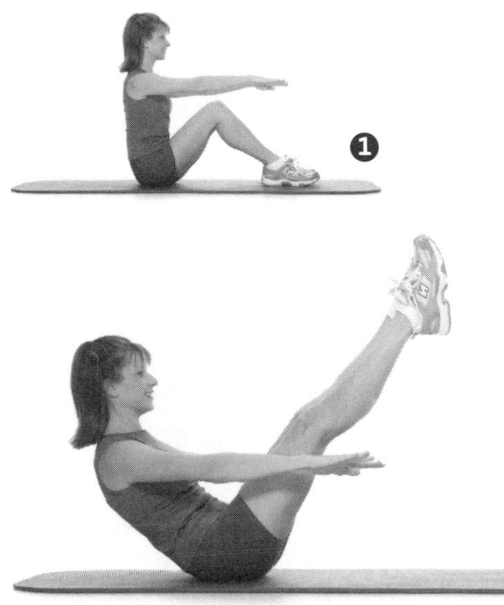

MUST-DO MOVE

Legs-Extended Balance

Starting position: Sit on the floor with your knees bent and your feet flat. Hold your arms out in front of you, parallel to the floor.

Movement: Lift your feet off the floor, extending your legs straight, and balance on your sitting bones. Hold for five breaths and then relax. Do one time only.

Technique: Keep your abs tight and the rest of your body relaxed, especially your shoulders.

Reverse Crunch

Starting position: Lie on your back with your legs up in the air and your hands behind your head. Cross your legs at the shins.

Movement: Slowly contract your abs as you exhale and press your back into the floor, tilting your pelvis and lifting your hips 2 to 4 inches off the floor. Keep your upper body relaxed. Hold for a second and then inhale as you slowly lower. Do 10 reps.

Technique: Don't swing your legs.

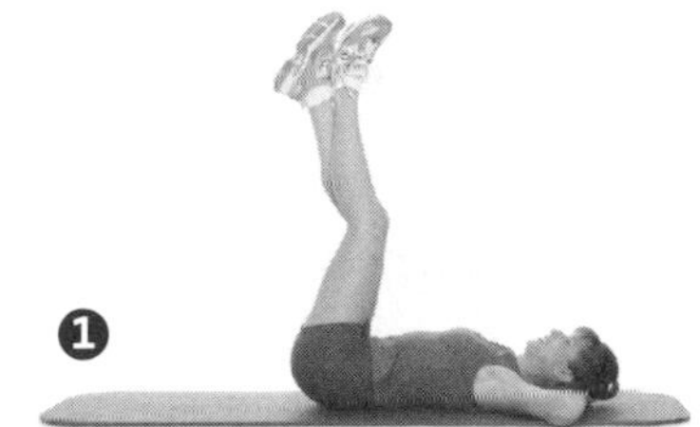

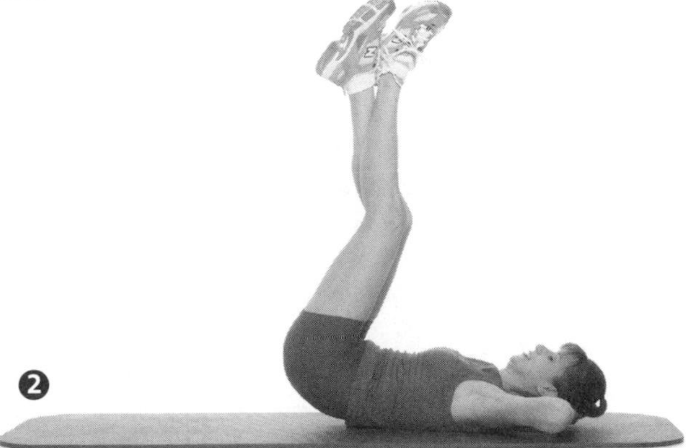

continued

The Workout

Level 3 *continued*

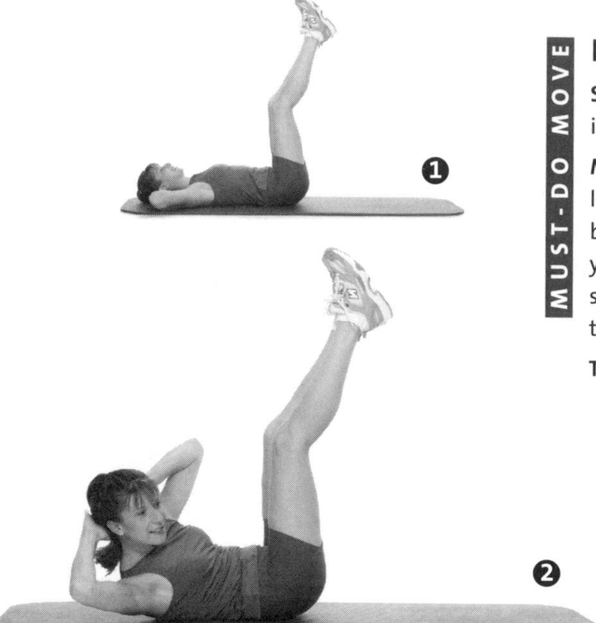

MUST-DO MOVE

Legs-Up Twisting Crunch

Starting position: Lie on your back with your legs up in the air and your hands behind your head.

Movement: Using your abs, slowly lift your head and left shoulder off the floor, twist to the right, and bring your left shoulder toward your right knee as you exhale. Hold for a second and then inhale as you slowly lower yourself. Repeat, alternating sides. Do a total of 10 reps, 5 to each side.

Technique: Don't pull your chin to your chest.

MUST-DO MOVE

Heel Bridge with Leg Lift and Arms Up

Starting position: Lie on your back with your knees bent, feet flat on the floor, and arms extended over your chest. Lift your toes off the floor so that only your heels are touching.

Movement: Contracting your abs, buttocks, and lower back, press into your heels and lift your butt, hips, and back off the floor as you exhale, to form a straight line from your shoulders to your knees. Lift your right foot off the floor and extend that leg. Hold for three breaths and then lower your foot. Lift the other foot up and hold for three breaths. Lower your foot and return to the starting position. Do one time only.

Technique: Don't lift too high—your upper back and shoulders should remain on the floor. Don't bend at the waist or hips. Don't let your knees fall inward or outward.

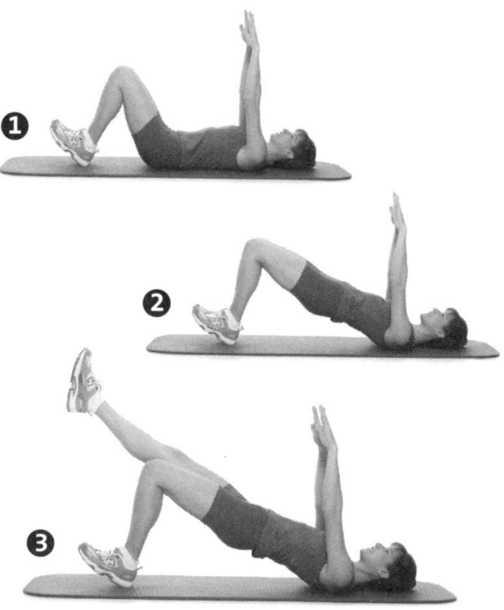

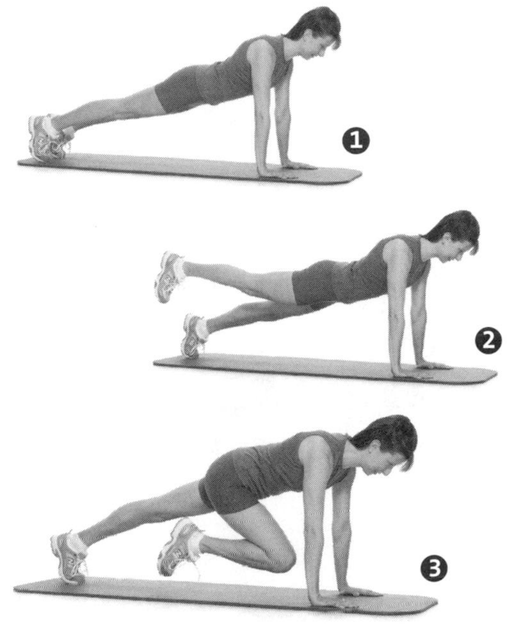

MUST-DO MOVE

Extended Plank with Lift and Bend

Starting position: Lie facedown with your feet flexed and toes tucked. Place your palms on the floor near your shoulders so that your elbows are pointing up. Contracting your abs and back, press into your hands as you exhale, straighten your arms, and lift your torso and legs off the floor so that your head, back, and legs form a straight line.

Movement: Lift your right foot off the floor and hold for three breaths. Next, pull your right knee in toward your chest and press it back out for five reps and then put that foot back on the floor. Lift your left foot off the floor and hold for three breaths. Next, pull your left knee in toward your chest and press it back out for five reps, put that foot back on the floor, and then relax. Do one time only.

Technique: Don't lift your head up or let it drop. Don't bend at the waist or hips. Don't let your belly drop toward the floor.

Swimming Chest Lift

Starting position: Lie facedown on the floor with your arms extended overhead.

Movement: Lift your arms, head, and chest 5 to 6 inches off the floor. Hold as you swim your arms back to your sides and forward again, as if you were doing the breaststroke, and then slowly lower yourself. Do 10 reps.

Technique: Don't lift too high.

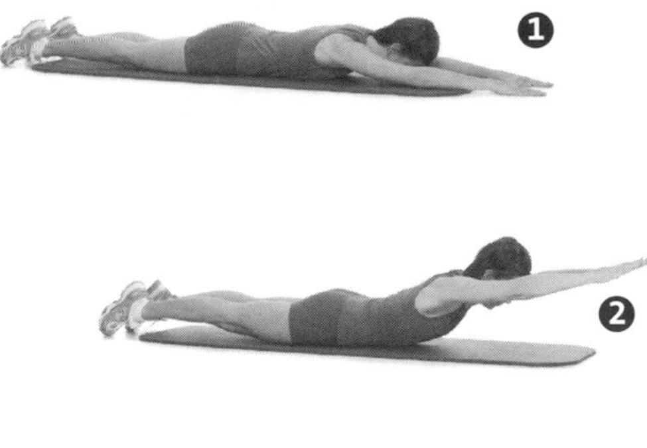

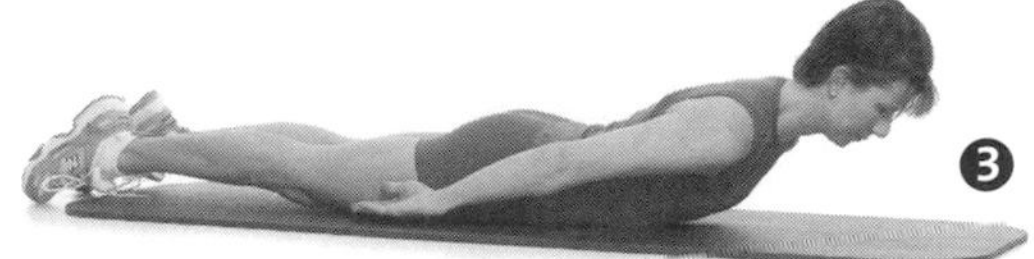

FIRM UP / DAY 12

Find Time to Exercise

"I don't have time." It's the most common excuse for not exercising that I hear (even out of my own mouth). But I've been able to find more time for exercise by controlling distractions in other areas of my life.

My secret: I use my watch for more than telling time. I have a sports watch that can be set to go off every hour. When it beeps, I check to make sure that I'm doing what I'm supposed to be doing. For example, I may come into work knowing that I need to write an article. I sit down at my computer and start writing. Before you know it, I need to find a fact. I start searching the Web, and the next thing I know, I'm reading an interesting article that has nothing to do with what I'm working on. Or I remember that I need to assign an article to a writer, so I call her. By the end of the day, I've done everything except write the article that was my priority for the day. Now when my watch beeps, I realize that I've been distracted and get back to my first priority. If I am sidetracked, it's never for more than an hour, and I get things done more quickly. As a result, I'm working at home and on weekends less often, because I stay focused.

I also have a 10-minute timer that I set (it's just a push of a button) when I know I'm being sidetracked—someone pops into my office to chat or ask a question, or I start to talk with someone at the copier. These breaks are beneficial sometimes, and I'm all for socializing, but it's very easy for these innocent interactions to suck away hours over the course of the day. Now when the timer goes off, I excuse myself, or sometimes the beep is enough to naturally break things up. These strategies work equally well at home.

FIRM UP TIP

ON YOUR PLATE

Add more dairy to your diet. Obese people who ate three servings of fat-free yogurt a day lost 22 percent more weight, 61 percent more body fat, and 81 percent more abdominal fat than those who ate the same number of calories but not the yogurt, according to a study of 34 people. Eating more dairy products may lower levels of cortisol, a hormone that steers fat to the belly, so you lose more fat from your middle.

Meal Plan

Most of these recipes are custom designed to make 1 serving–no fuss, no muss; just fix, eat, and go! If a recipe makes more than 1 serving, it's noted below. Save that extra serving for another meal, or share it with your spouse or your walking buddy.

Breakfast

Waffle and Strawberries: Toast 1 frozen whole grain waffle. Top with 2 tablespoons peanut butter and ¾ cup fresh or ⅓ cup frozen unsweetened strawberries, smashed.

Healthy Snack

Fruit Cocktail Surprise: Drain ¾ cup (6 ounces) fruit cocktail (canned in juice, not syrup). Mix into ⅓ cup ricotta cheese spread from Monday and enjoy.

Lunch

Soup and a Half-Sandwich: Heat ½ cup chicken noodle, chicken rice, beef noodle, chicken gumbo, or 100 calories' worth of any similar soup (such as Campbell's Healthy Request Chicken Noodle soup) with ½ cup water. Spread 1 slice whole wheat bread with mustard to taste and cut in half. Add 2 slices roast beef (2 ounces). Top with ⅛ sliced avocado. Serve with 1 cup fresh cauliflower florets dipped in 2 tablespoons light ranch dressing.

Healthy Snack

Trail Mix: Combine ½ cup dried sweetened cranberries, ½ cup raisins, and ½ cup unsalted peanuts. Divide into 4 equal servings. Have one now and save the others for later.

Dinner

Fettuccini Alfredo: Microwave according to package directions Lean Cuisine Everyday Favorites Chicken Fettuccini or a similar frozen meal (check the label for 270 to 280 calories and 6 to 10 grams of fat). Steam or microwave 1 cup fresh or frozen leaf spinach. Pour the chicken fettuccini over the spinach. Serve with 7 frozen red grapes.

Indulgent Treat

Ice Cream Sundae: Serve ½ cup Healthy Choice ice cream (any variety), Edy's regular chocolate or coffee ice cream, or Baskin-Robbins Cherries Jubilee ice cream with 1½ tablespoons chopped walnuts and 2 tablespoons light whipped topping.

Nutrient analysis: 1,664 calories, 76 g protein, 210 g carbohydrates, 68 g total fat, 19 g saturated fat, 89 mg cholesterol, 29 g dietary fiber, 2,827 mg sodium, 1,393 mg calcium

FIRM UP TIP

MYTH BUSTER

Vigorous exercise won't stimulate you to overeat. It's just the opposite: Exercise at any level helps curb your appetite immediately following the workout.

The Workout

Level 1

Easy Walk: 30 Minutes

- 5-minute warmup: Walk 2 to 2½ miles per hour, or 95 to 100 steps per minute.
- 20-minute moderate walk: Increase your speed to 2½ to 3 miles per hour, 100 to 115 steps per minute, or a pace that lets you comfortably carry on a conversation.
- 5-minute cooldown: Slow down to 2 to 2½ miles per hour, or 95 to 100 steps per minute.

Heavy Strength Training: 25 Minutes

- Do four to six reps of each exercise, using a heavier weight. Repeat the sequence of exercises three times.
- To warm up, use lighter weights, or none at all, the first time through, and for the squat and lunge exercises, only go partway down.

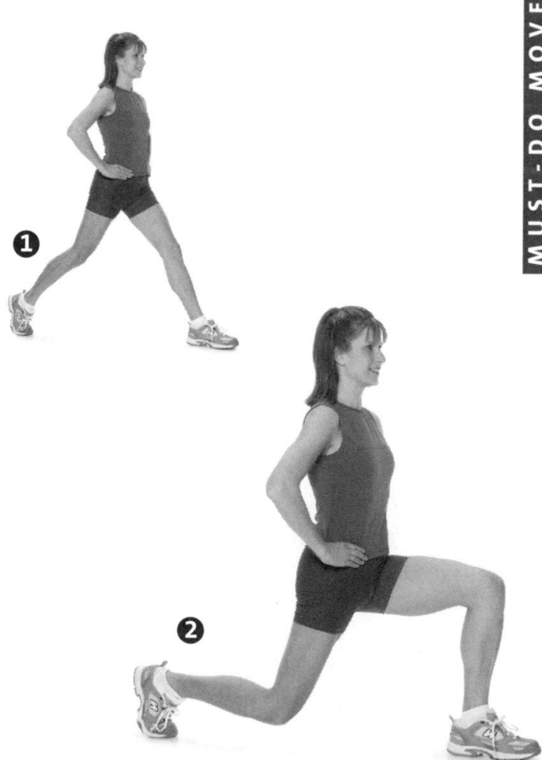

MUST-DO MOVE

Lunge (no weights)

Starting position: Stand with your feet 2 to 3 feet apart, with your left foot in front of your right. Place your hands on your hips.

Movement: Inhale as you bend your left knee and lower your body straight down until your left knee is bent 90 degrees and your right knee nearly touches the floor. Your rear heel will come off the floor. Hold for a second and then exhale as you slowly push yourself back up to the starting position. Finish all of your repetitions, then repeat the exercise with your right foot in front of your left.

Technique: Don't lean forward. Don't let your front knee move forward over your toes.

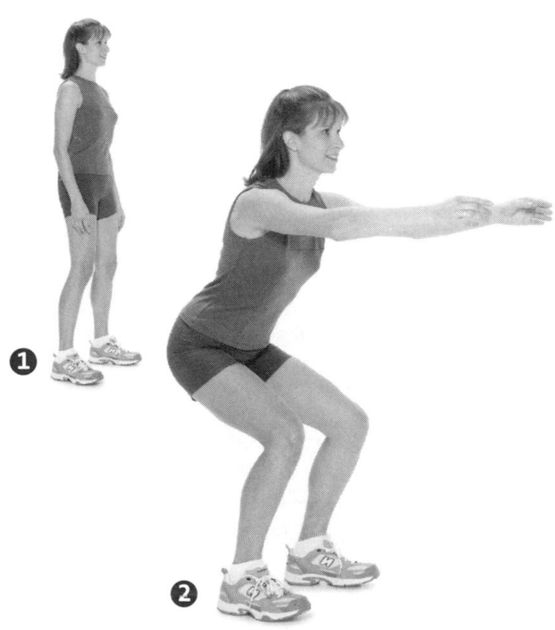

Squat

Starting position: Stand with your feet about shoulder width apart, arms at your sides.

Movement: Keeping your back straight, lower yourself, bending from your knees and hips as though you're sitting down, as you inhale. Let your arms come out in front of you to help you balance. Stop just before your thighs are parallel to the floor. Hold for a second and then exhale as you slowly stand back up.

Technique: Don't let your knees move forward over your toes. Don't round your back.

Parallel Chest Press

Starting position: Lying on the floor (or on a bench), hold dumbbells parallel and just above your shoulders; your elbows should be pointing toward your feet.

Movement: Exhale as you press the dumbbells straight up over your chest, extending your arms. Hold for a second and then inhale as you slowly lower them.

Technique: Don't press the dumbbells back toward your head or forward toward your feet: They should go straight up and down. Don't arch your back.

Alternate position: If it's uncomfortable to have your feet on the bench, you can place them on the floor. Make sure your back doesn't arch in that position.

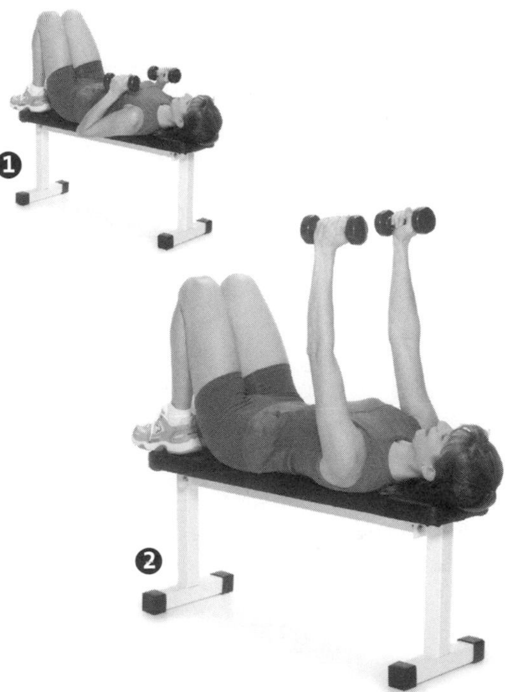

continued

The Workout

Level 1 *continued*

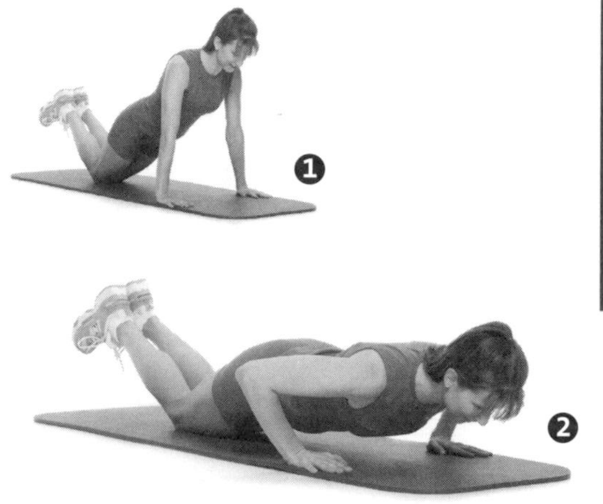

MUST-DO MOVE

Bent-Knee Pushup

Starting position: Lie facedown on the floor. Bend your knees so that your feet are up in the air, and place your palms on the floor near your shoulders so that your elbows are pointing up. Press down with your hands, extend your arms, and lift your body off the floor.

Movement: Keeping your head, back, hips, and knees in a straight line, bend your elbows out to the sides and lower your body as you inhale, until your chest nearly touches the floor. Hold for a second and then exhale as you slowly push back up.

Technique: Don't bend at the hips. Don't arch your back.

Seated Back Fly

Starting position: Sit on the edge of a chair with your feet hip width apart and hold a dumbbell in each hand. Keep your back flat and lean forward, bending at the hips so that the dumbbells are hanging at arm's length down by your calves, palms facing each other and elbows bent slightly.

Movement: Keeping your back straight, squeeze your shoulder blades together and lift the dumbbells up and out to the sides as you exhale, pulling your elbows back as far as comfortably possible. Hold for a second and then inhale as you slowly lower them.

Technique: Don't arch your back. Don't raise your torso as you lift the dumbbells.

Alternate move: If you have back problems, do the flies one arm at a time and place the forearm of your other arm across your thighs for extra support.

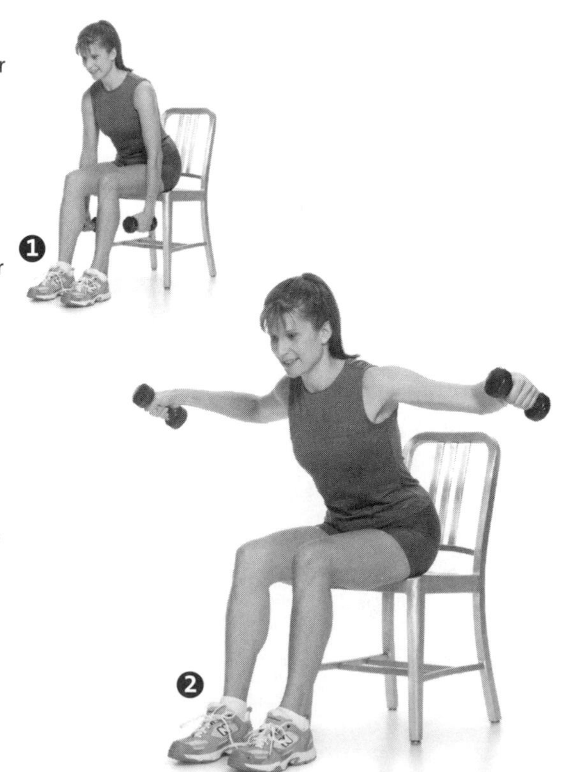

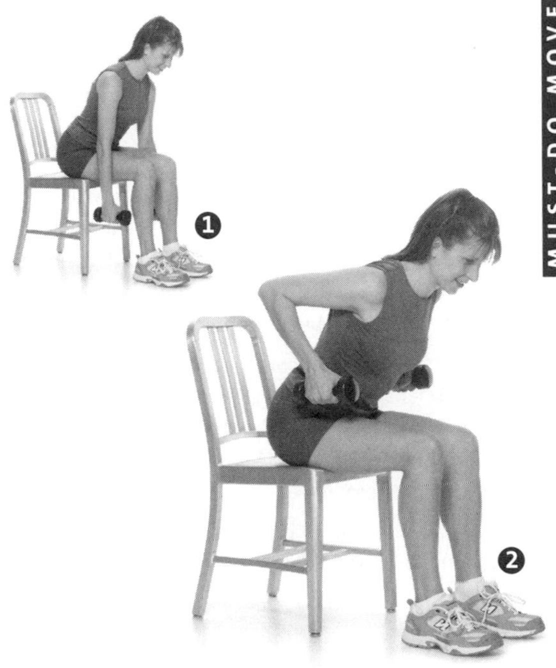

MUST-DO MOVE

Seated Bent-Over Row

Starting position: Sit on the edge of a chair with your feet hip width apart and hold a dumbbell in each hand. Keep your back flat and lean forward, bending at the hips so that the dumbbells are hanging at arm's length down by your calves, palms facing each other.

Movement: Bending your elbows back and squeezing your shoulder blades, lift the weights toward your ribs as you exhale. Hold for a second and then inhale as you slowly lower them.

Technique: Don't arch your back. Don't raise your torso as you lift the dumbbells.

Alternate move: If you have back problems, do the rows one arm at a time and place the forearm of your other arm across your thighs for extra support.

Seated Biceps Curl with a Twist

Starting position: Sit on the edge of a chair with your feet hip width apart. Hold dumbbells at your sides with your palms facing in.

Movement: Bending your elbows and turning your wrists upward, lift the dumbbells toward your shoulders as you exhale. Stop when the dumbbells are at chest height, palms facing your body. Hold for a second and then inhale as you slowly lower them.

Technique: Don't move your upper arms.

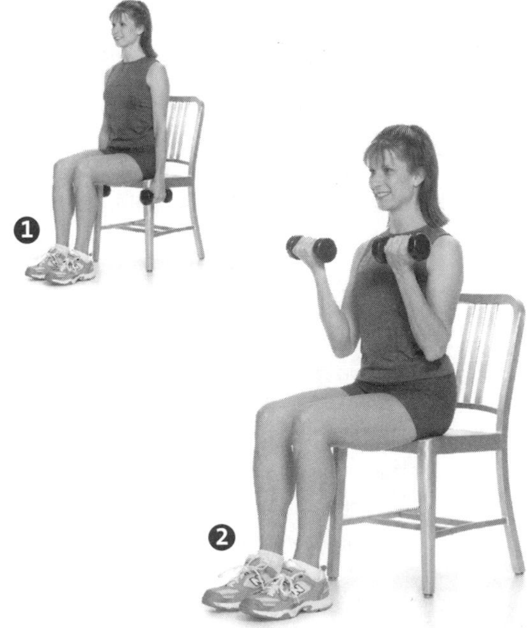

continued

The Workout

Level 1 *continued*

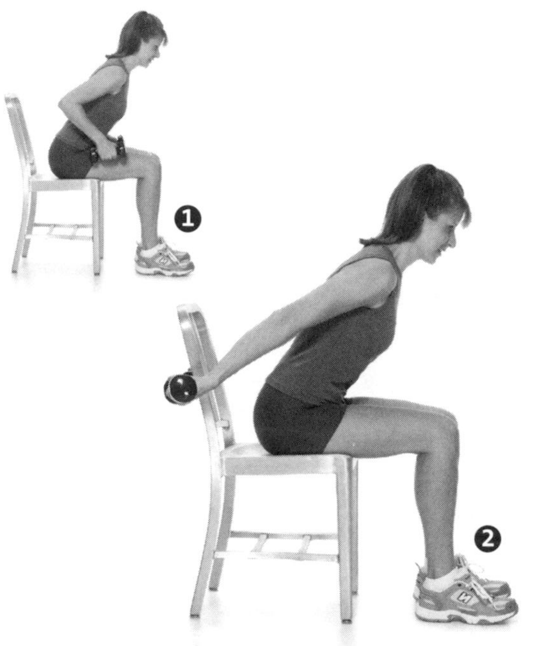

Seated Triceps Kickback with a Twist

Starting position: Sit on the edge of a chair with your feet hip width apart and hold a dumbbell in each hand. Keep your back flat and lean forward, bending at the hips. Bend your arms at about 90-degree angles with your dumbbells at about hip height.

Movement: Without moving your upper arms, press the dumbbells back as you exhale, extending your arms and turning your wrists so that your palms face the ceiling. Hold for a second and then inhale as you slowly lower them.

Technique: Don't move from your shoulders. Don't raise your torso as you lift the dumbbells.

Alternate move: If you have back problems, do the kickbacks one arm at a time and place the forearm of your other arm across your thighs for extra support.

MUST-DO MOVE

Bent-Arm Lateral Raise

Starting position: Stand with your feet shoulder width apart, knees bent slightly. Hold a dumbbell in each hand with your arms at your sides and bent at 90-degree angles so that your palms are facing in and the dumbbells are in front of you at about waist height.

Movement: Exhale as you slowly raise your elbows out to the sides until they are at about shoulder height. Hold for a second and then inhale as you slowly lower them.

Technique: Don't lift your shoulders. Don't lift higher than shoulder height.

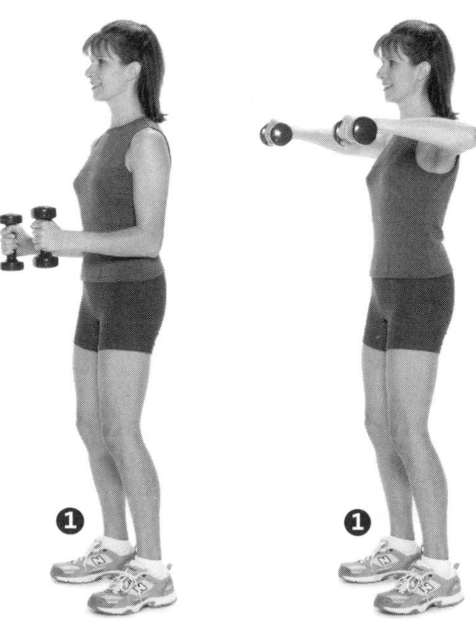

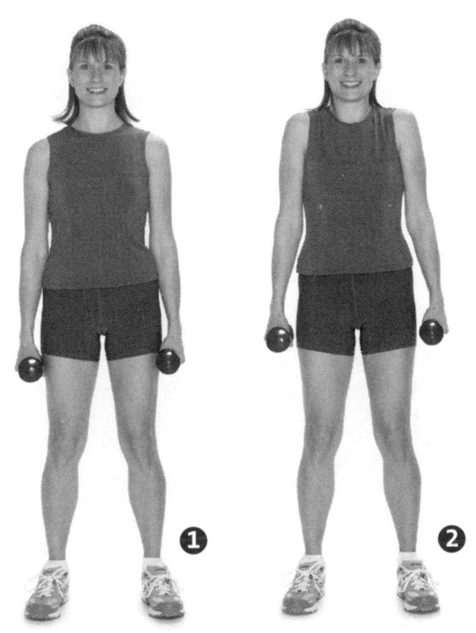

Shoulder Shrug

Starting position: Stand with your feet shoulder width apart, knees bent slightly. Hold a dumbbell in each hand with your arms at your sides, palms facing in.

Movement: Exhale as you slowly lift your shoulders up toward your ears as high as possible. Hold for a second and then inhale as you slowly lower them.

Technique: Don't bend your elbows. Don't use your arms to lift.

FIRM UP TIPS

GET FIRM FASTER	FIT FACT
Hit the bottle. Think you don't need your water bottle for workouts shorter than an hour? Think again. "Research shows that you can get dehydrated in as little as 45 to 50 minutes—and that can drag your energy down," says Nancy Clark, R.D., author of Nancy Clark's Sports Nutrition Guidebook. *"Take a sip of water every 15 to 20 minutes while you work out."*	*German researchers have found a potent germ-killer right below the surface of our skin. This natural antibiotic, called dermcidin, is made in the body's sweat glands. It bubbles to the surface when you exercise and protects you against some bacteria that cause common infections, such as stomach and skin problems.*

The Workout

Level 2

Easy Walk: 30 Minutes

- 5-minute warmup: Walk 2½ to 3 miles per hour, or 100 to 115 steps per minute.
- 20-minute moderate walk: Increase your speed to 3 to 3½ miles per hour, 115 to 125 steps per minute, or a pace that lets you comfortably carry on a conversation.
- 5-minute cooldown: Slow down to 2½ to 3 miles per hour, or 100 to 115 steps per minute.

Heavy Strength Training: 25 Minutes

- Do four to six reps of each exercise, using a heavier weight. Repeat the sequence of exercises three times.
- To warm up, use lighter weights, or none at all, the first time through, and for the squat and lunge exercises, only go partway down.

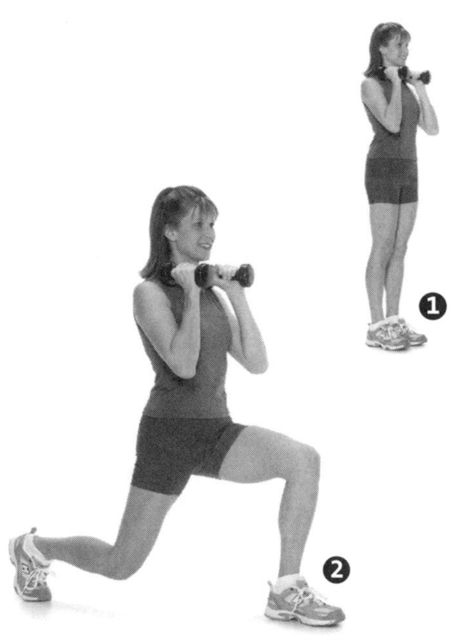

Back Lunge

Starting position: Stand with your feet together. Hold a dumbbell in each hand, either at shoulder height or at your sides.

Movement: Step your right foot back 2 to 3 feet. Inhale as you bend your left knee and lower your body straight down until your left knee is bent 90 degrees and your right knee nearly touches the floor. Your rear heel will come off the floor. Hold for a second and then exhale as you push yourself back up, bringing your right foot back in. Finish all of your repetitions, then repeat the exercise stepping back with your left foot.

Technique: Don't lean forward. Don't let your front knee move forward over your toes.

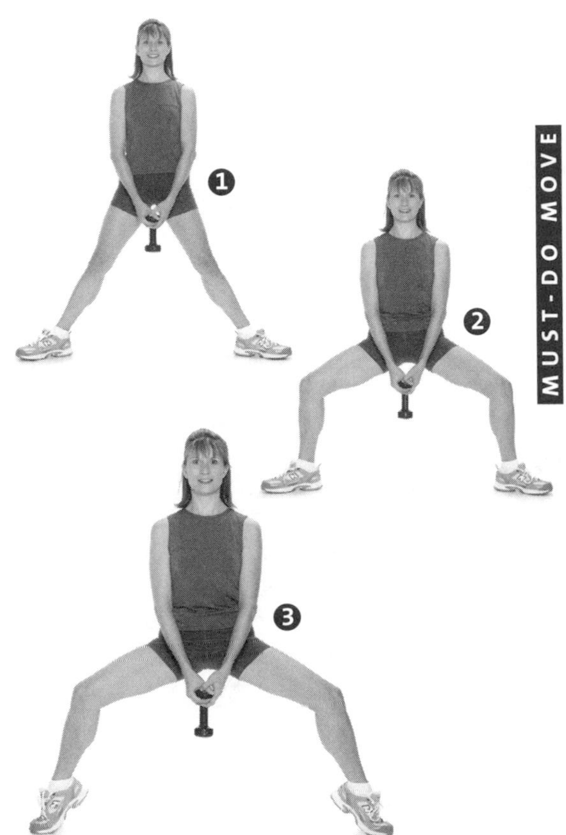

MUST-DO MOVE

Plié Squat with Heel Lift

Starting position: Stand with your feet wider than shoulder width apart, toes pointing out. Hold a dumbbell with both hands down in front of you.

Movement: Keeping your back straight, lower yourself, bending from your knees, as you inhale. Stop just before your thighs are parallel to the floor and then lift your heels off the floor so that you're on your toes. Hold for a second. Exhale as you slowly stand back up and then lower your heels. (You may want to hold on to a chair with one hand for balance, grasping the dumbbell with the other hand.)

Technique: Don't let your knees move forward over your toes. Don't lean forward.

Chest Press

Starting position: Lie on the floor (or on a bench) and hold dumbbells end to end, just above your shoulders. Your elbows should be pointing out to the sides.

Movement: Exhale as you press the dumbbells straight up over your chest, extending your arms. Hold for a second and then inhale as you slowly lower them.

Technique: Don't press the dumbbells back toward your head or forward toward your feet: They should go straight up and down. Don't arch your back.

Alternate position: If it's uncomfortable to have your feet on the bench, you can place them on the floor. Make sure your back doesn't arch in that position.

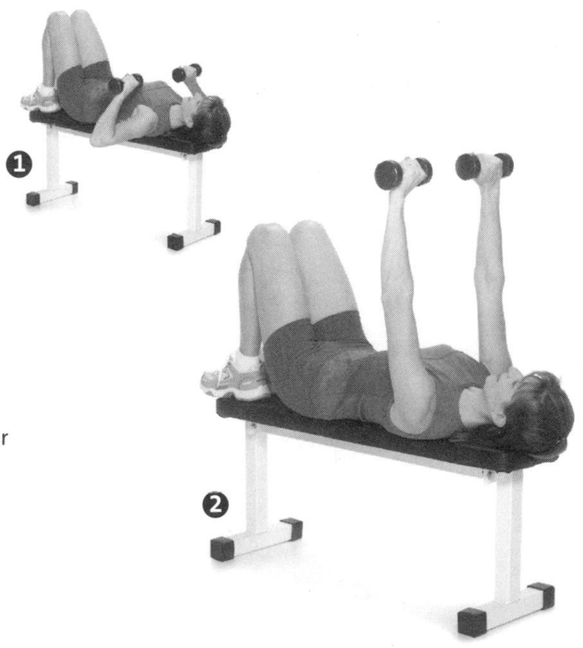

continued

The Workout

Level 2 *continued*

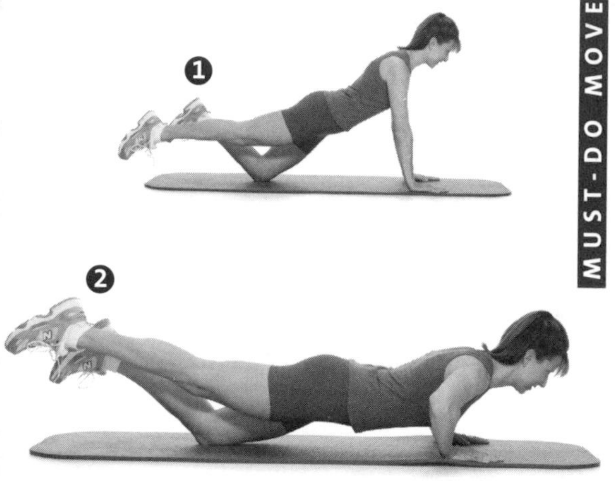

MUST-DO MOVE

One-Knee Pushup

Starting position: Lie facedown on the floor. Bend your knees so that your feet are up in the air, and place your palms on the floor near your shoulders so that your elbows are pointing up. Press down with your hands, extend your arms, lift your body off the floor, and lift one knee off the floor, extending that leg.

Movement: Keeping your head, back, hips, and knees in a straight line, bend your elbows out to the sides and lower your body as you inhale, until your chest nearly touches the floor. Hold for a second and then exhale as you push back up. Do half of the recommended reps and then switch knees.

Technique: Don't bend at the hips. Don't arch your back.

Back Fly

Starting position: Stand with your feet shoulder width apart and knees bent slightly. Hold a dumbbell in each hand with your arms at your sides. Keep your back flat and lean forward, bending at the hips so that the dumbbells are hanging at arm's length in front of you, palms facing each other and elbows bent slightly.

Movement: Keeping your back straight, squeeze your shoulder blades together and lift the dumbbells up and out to the sides as you exhale, pulling your elbows back as far as comfortably possible. Hold for a second and then inhale as you slowly lower them.

Technique: Don't arch your back. Don't raise your torso as you lift the dumbbells.

Alternate move: If you have back problems, support yourself with one hand on a chair and do the flies one arm at a time.

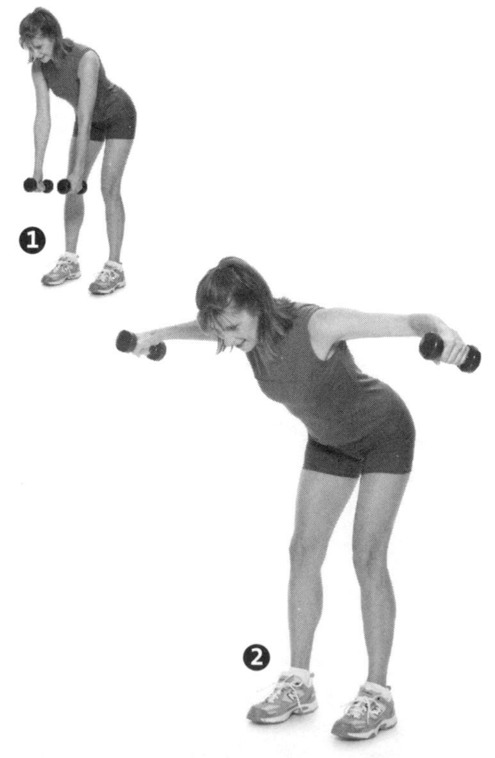

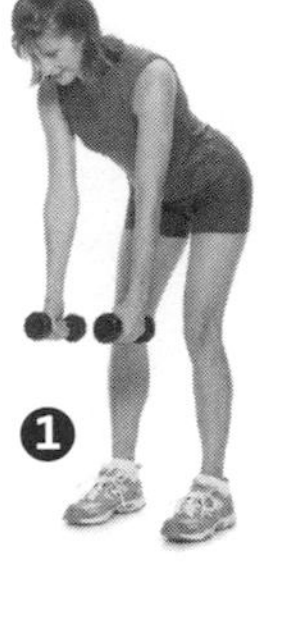

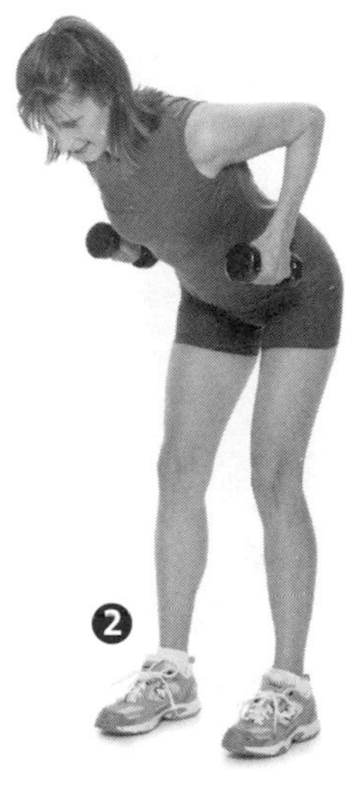

MUST-DO MOVE

Bent-Over Row

Starting position: Stand with your feet shoulder width apart, knees bent slightly. Hold a dumbbell in each hand with your arms at your sides. Keep your back flat and lean forward, bending at the hips so that the dumbbells are hanging at arm's length in front of you, palms facing each other.

Movement: Bending your elbows back and squeezing your shoulder blades, lift the weights toward your ribs as you exhale, until your elbows are higher than your back. Hold for a second and then inhale as you slowly lower them.

Technique: Don't arch your back. Don't pull your shoulders up toward your ears. Don't raise your torso as you lift the dumbbells.

Alternate move: If you have back problems, support yourself with one hand on a chair and do the rows one arm at a time.

Biceps Curl

Starting position: Stand with your feet shoulder width apart, knees bent slightly. Hold a dumbbell in each hand with your palms facing forward.

Movement: Bending your elbows, lift the dumbbells toward your shoulders as you exhale. Stop when the dumbbells are at chest height, palms facing your body. Hold for a second and then inhale as you slowly lower them.

Technique: Don't move your upper arms.

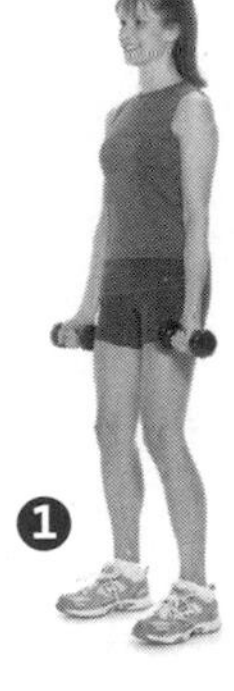

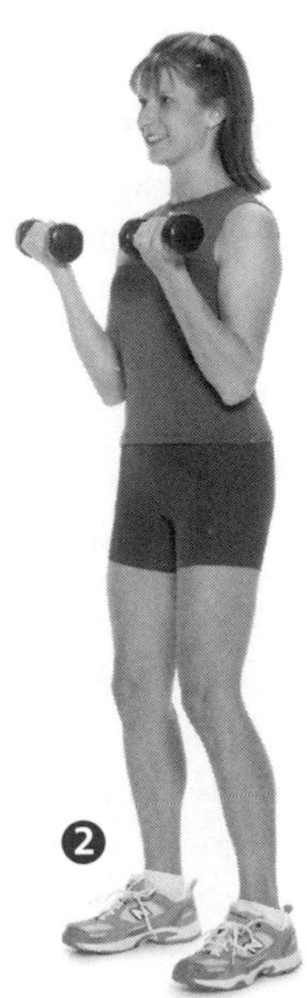

continued

The Workout

Level 2 *continued*

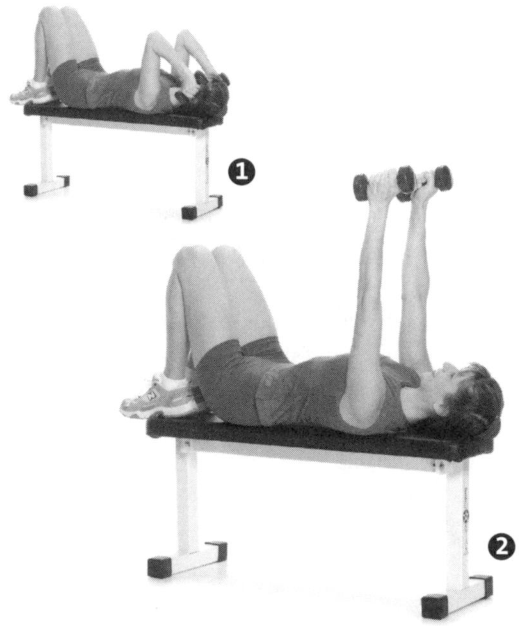

Lying Triceps Extension

Starting position: Lie face up on the floor (or on a bench). Hold a dumbbell in each hand over your chest. Bend your arms so that your elbows are pointing toward the ceiling and the dumbbells are by your ears.

Movement: Without moving your upper arms, press the weights up over your chest as you exhale. Hold for a second and then inhale as you slowly lower them.

Technique: Don't move from your shoulders. Don't arch your back.

Alternate position: If it's uncomfortable to have your feet on the bench, you can place them on the floor. Make sure your back doesn't arch in that position.

Kneeling Triceps Pushup

Starting position: Lie facedown on the floor. Bend your knees so that your feet are up in the air, and place your palms on the floor close to your ribs so that your elbows are pointing up. Press down with your hands, extend your arms, and lift your body off the floor.

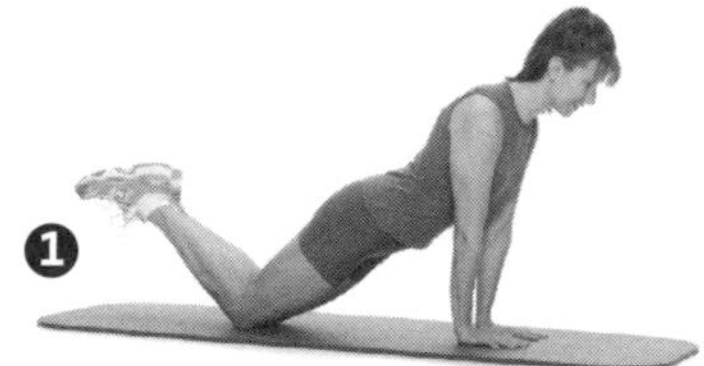

Movement: Keeping your head, back, hips, and knees in a straight line, bend your elbows back, keeping your arms close to your body, as you inhale. Lower your body until your chest nearly touches the floor. Hold for a second and then exhale as you push back up.

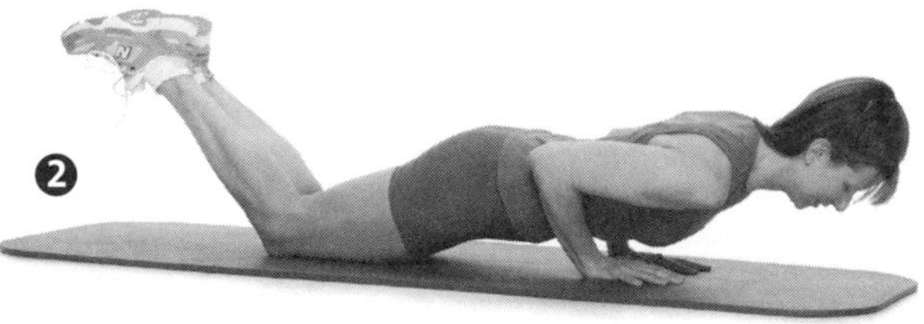

Technique: Don't let your elbows point out to the sides. Don't bend at the hips. Don't drop your belly toward the floor.

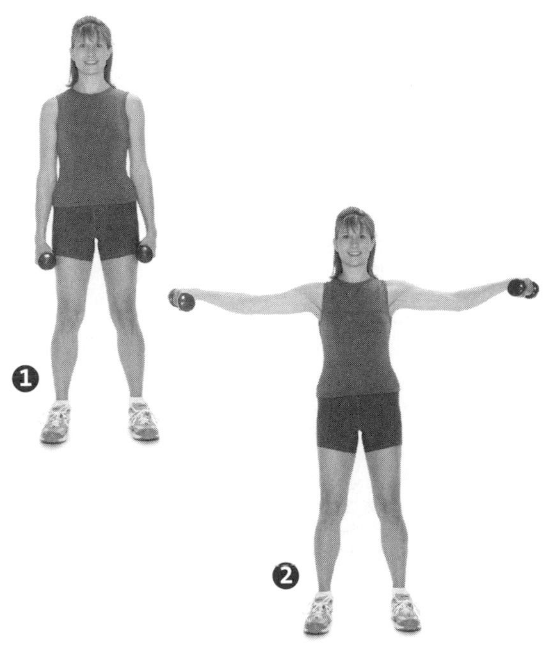

Lateral Raise

Starting position: Stand with your feet shoulder width apart, knees bent slightly. Hold a dumbbell in each hand with your arms at your sides, palms facing in, and elbows bent slightly.

Movement: Exhale as you slowly raise the dumbbells out to the sides until they are at about shoulder height. Hold for a second and then inhale as you slowly lower them.

Technique: Don't lift your shoulders. Don't lift higher than shoulder height.

MUST-DO MOVE

Parallel Overhead Press

Starting position: Stand with your feet shoulder width apart and knees bent slightly. Hold a dumbbell in each hand at shoulder height, palms facing each other and elbows pointing forward.

Movement: Exhale as you slowly press the dumbbells straight overhead without locking your elbows. Hold for a second and then inhale as you slowly lower them.

Technique: Don't arch your back. Don't lift the dumbbells forward or back.

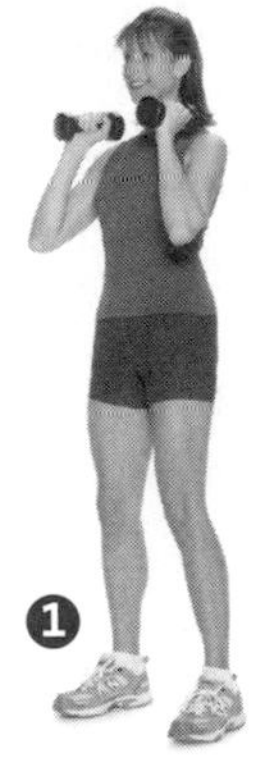

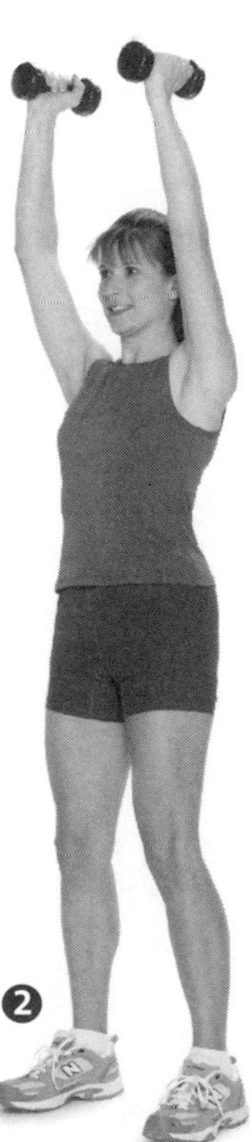

The Workout

Level 3

Easy Walk: 30 Minutes

- 5-minute warmup: Walk 2½ to 3 miles per hour, or 100 to 115 steps per minute.
- 20-minute moderate walk: Increase your speed to 3½ to 4 miles per hour, 125 to 135 steps per minute, or a pace that lets you comfortably carry on a conversation.
- 5-minute cooldown: Slow down to 2½ to 3 miles per hour, or 100 to 115 steps per minute.

Heavy Strength Training: 30 Minutes

- Do four to six reps of each exercise, using a heavier weight. Repeat the sequence of exercises three times.
- To warm up, use lighter weights, or none at all, the first time through, and for the lunge exercise, only go partway down.

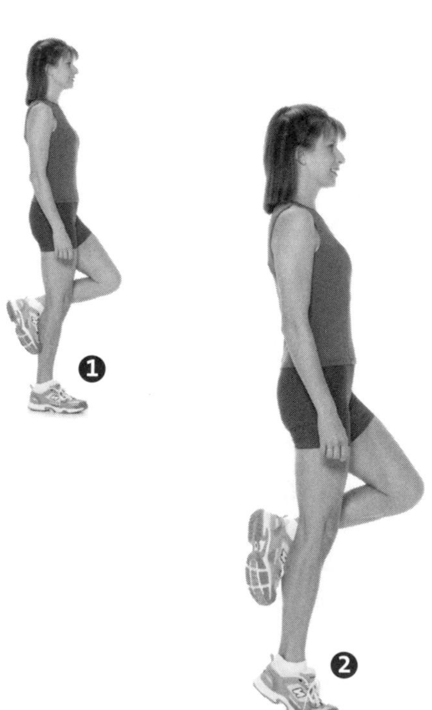

Single-Heel Raise

Starting position: Stand on one foot with the other resting on your calf. Lightly hold on to a chair or wall with one hand if needed for balance.

Movement: Exhale as you slowly lift your heel off the floor, rolling up onto your toes. Hold for a second and then inhale as you slowly lower it. Do the recommended number of reps and then switch feet.

Technique: Don't bend at the waist or lean forward, back, or to the side. Don't bend your supporting leg.

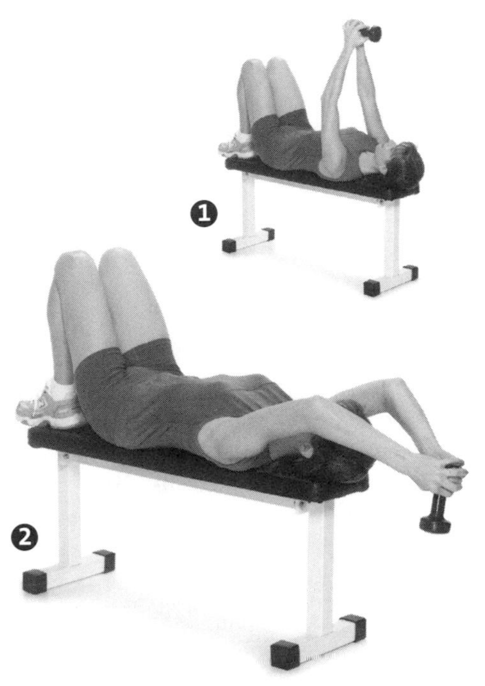

Pullover

Starting position: Lie face up on the floor (or on a bench). Grasp a dumbbell with both hands and hold it above your chest with your elbows bent slightly.

Movement: Inhale as you lower the dumbbell backward over your head as far as comfortably possible without bending your elbows any farther than at the start. Hold for a second and then exhale as you slowly raise it to the starting position.

Technique: Don't arch your back. Don't bend your elbows to lower the weight.

Alternate position: If it's uncomfortable to have your feet on the bench, you can place them on the floor. Make sure your back doesn't arch in that position.

MUST-DO MOVE

Pushup

Starting position: Lie facedown on the floor with your feet flexed and toes tucked. Place your palms on the floor near your shoulders so that your elbows are pointing up. Press down with your hands, extend your arms, and lift your body off the floor so that it forms a straight line from head to toe.

Movement: Keeping your head, back, hips, and legs in a straight line, bend your elbows out to the sides and lower your body as you inhale, until your chest nearly touches the floor. Hold for a second and then exhale as you push back up. If you can't do all the recommended reps in this full pushup position, that's okay. Just drop down onto one or both knees and complete the remaining reps.

Technique: Don't bend at the hips. Don't arch your back.

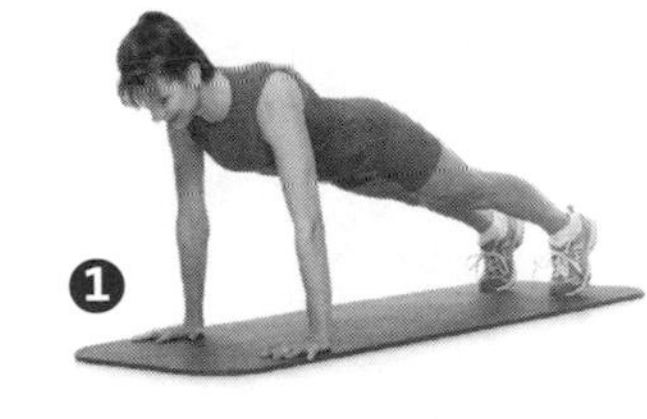

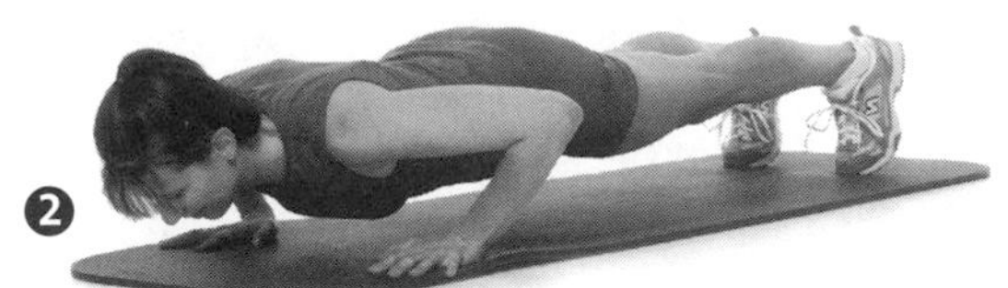

continued

The Workout

Level 3 *continued*

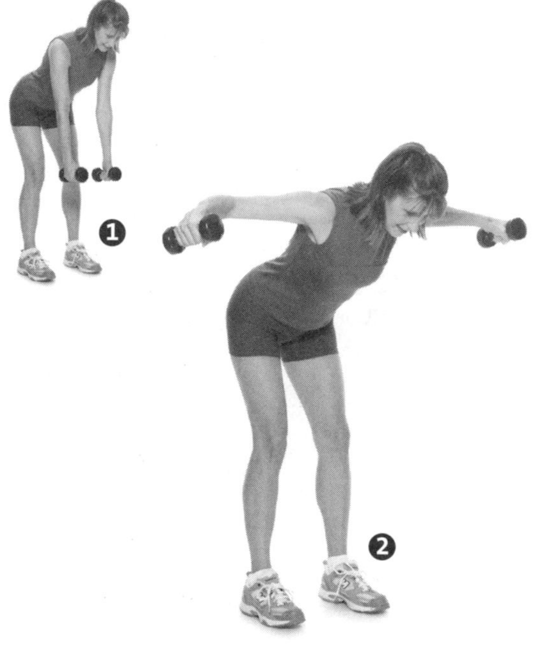

Back Fly

Starting position: Stand with your feet shoulder width apart and knees bent slightly. Hold a dumbbell in each hand with your arms at your sides. Keep your back flat and lean forward, bending at the hips so that the dumbbells are hanging at arm's length in front of you, palms facing each other and elbows bent slightly.

Movement: Keeping your back straight, squeeze your shoulder blades together and lift the dumbbells up and out to the sides as you exhale, pulling your elbows back as far as comfortably possible. Hold for a second and then inhale as you slowly lower them.

Technique: Don't arch your back. Don't raise your torso as you lift the dumbbells.

Alternate move: If you have back problems, support yourself with one hand on a chair and do the flies one arm at a time.

MUST-DO MOVE

Wide Bent-Over Row

Starting position: Stand with your feet shoulder width apart, knees bent slightly. Hold a dumbbell in each hand with your arms at your sides. Keep your back flat and lean forward, bending at the hips so that the dumbbells are hanging at arm's length in front of you, palms facing you.

Movement: Bending your elbows out to the sides and squeezing your shoulder blades, lift the weights toward your ribs as you exhale, until your elbows are higher than your back. Hold for a second and then inhale as you slowly lower them.

Technique: Don't arch your back. Don't pull your shoulders up toward your ears. Don't raise your torso as you lift the dumbbells.

Alternate move: If you have back problems, support yourself with one hand on a chair and do the rows one arm at a time.

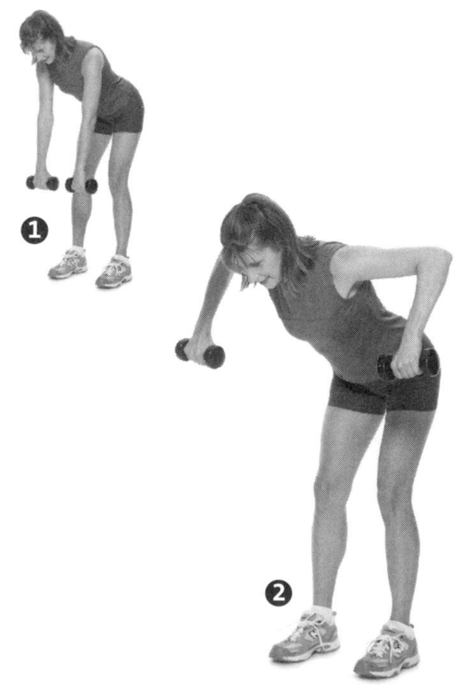

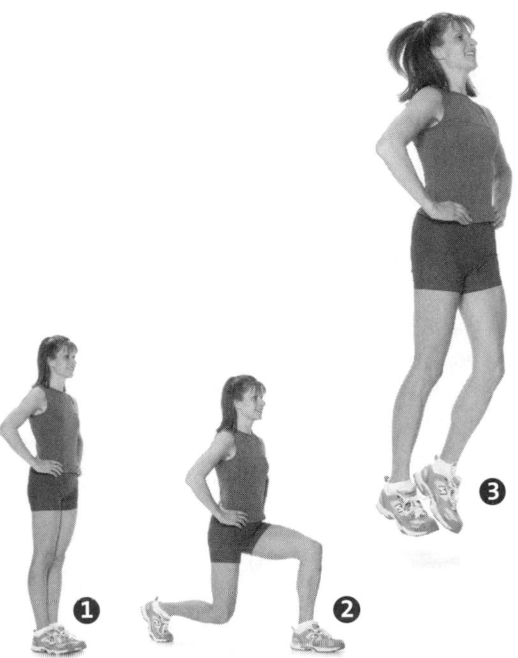

MUST-DO MOVE

Front Lunge with Jump

Starting position: Stand with your feet together and your hands on your hips.

Movement: Step your left foot forward 2 to 3 feet. Inhale as you bend your left knee and lower your body straight down until your left knee is bent 90 degrees and your right knee nearly touches the floor. Your rear heel will come off the floor. Hold for a second and then exhale as you push off with your left foot and jump your feet together. Finish all of your repetitions, then repeat the exercise stepping forward with your right foot.

Technique: Don't lean forward. Don't let your front knee move forward over your toes.

Biceps Curl

Starting position: Stand with your feet shoulder width apart, knees bent slightly. Hold a dumbbell in each hand with your palms facing forward.

Movement: Bending your elbows, lift the dumbbells toward your shoulders as you exhale. Stop when the dumbbells are at chest height, palms facing your body. Hold for a second and then inhale as you slowly lower them.

Technique: Don't move your upper arms.

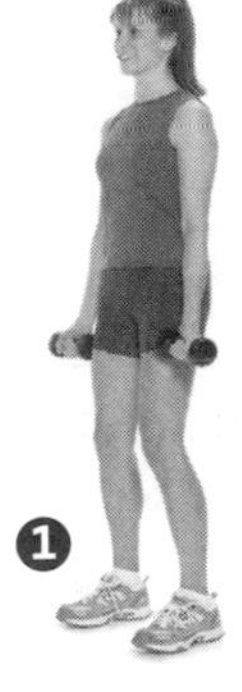

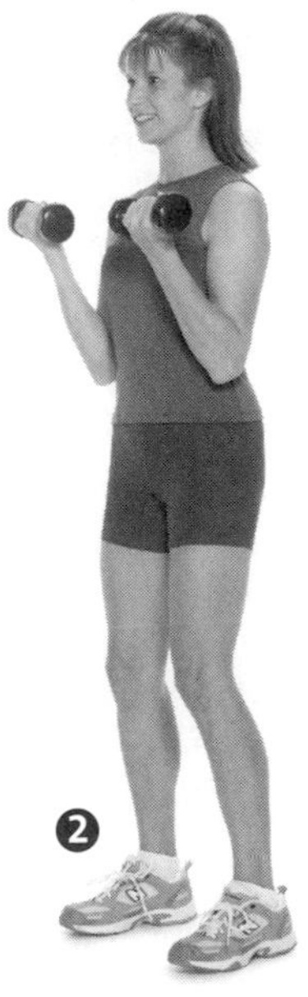

continued

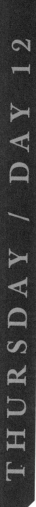

The Workout

Level 3 *continued*

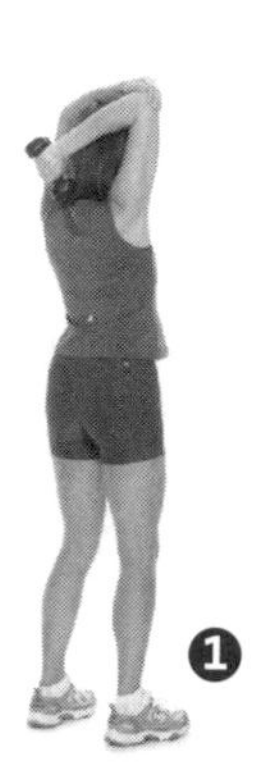

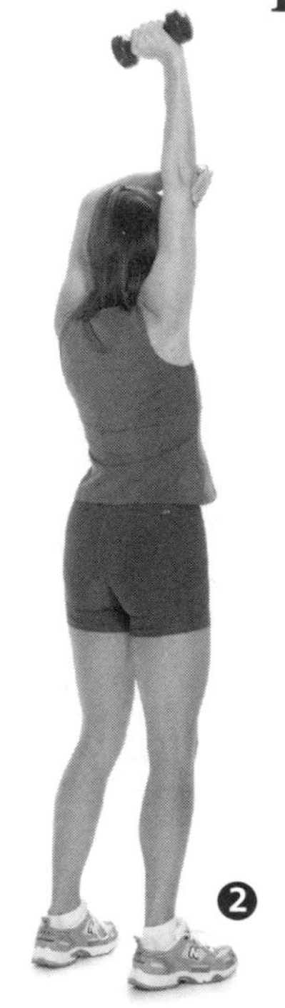

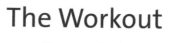

Overhead Triceps Extension

Starting position: Stand with your feet shoulder width apart and knees bent slightly. Hold a dumbbell in your right hand and lift it up over your head. Bend your elbow so that it is pointing toward the ceiling and the dumbbell is behind your head. Place your left hand on your right elbow for support.

Movement: Exhale as you extend your right arm and lift the dumbbell over your head. Hold for a second and then inhale as you slowly lower it. Do the recommended number of reps and then repeat with your left arm.

Technique: Don't lift your shoulders up toward your ears. Don't bend your wrist.

Triceps Dip

Starting position: Sit on the edge of a chair, place your hands on either side of you, and grasp the chair seat. Slide your buttocks off the chair, and walk your feet out until your legs are bent at about 90 degrees. You should be balancing on your hands and feet.

Movement: Bending your arms so that your elbows point behind you, slowly lower your body toward the floor as you inhale. Keep your buttocks as close to the chair as possible. Stop when your elbows are bent about 90 degrees. Hold for a second and then exhale as you press back up.

Technique: Don't sink into your arms, allowing your shoulders to come up toward your ears. Don't bend your knees to help lower yourself.

Alternate move: For a more challenging version, lift one leg off the floor.

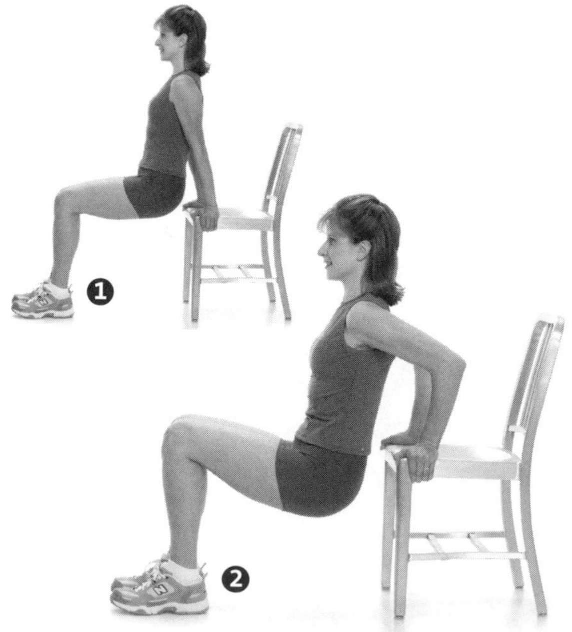

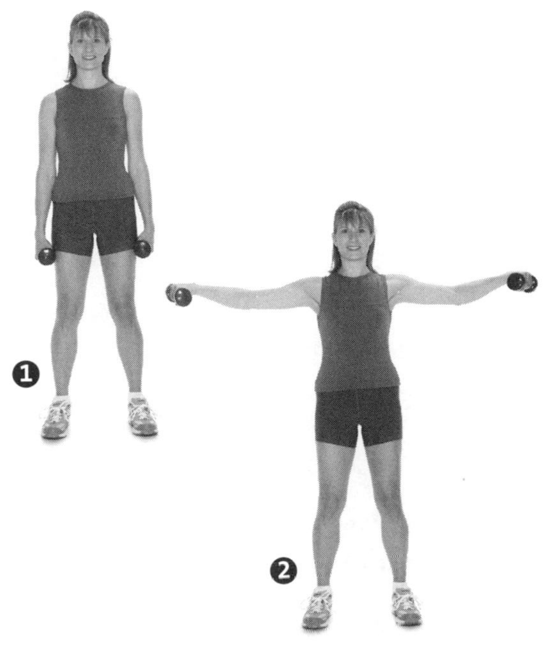

Lateral Raise

Starting position: Stand with your feet shoulder width apart, knees bent slightly. Hold a dumbbell in each hand with your arms at your sides, palms facing in, and elbows bent slightly.

Movement: Exhale as you slowly raise the dumbbells out to the sides until they are at about shoulder height. Hold for a second and then inhale as you slowly lower them.

Technique: Don't lift your shoulders. Don't lift higher than shoulder height.

MUST-DO MOVE

Overhead Press

Starting position: Stand with your feet shoulder width apart and knees bent slightly. Hold a dumbbell in each hand at shoulder height with your palms facing forward and elbows pointing out to the sides.

Movement: Exhale as you slowly press the dumbbells straight up overhead. Hold for a second and then inhale as you slowly lower them.

Technique: Don't arch your back. Don't lift the dumbbells forward or back.

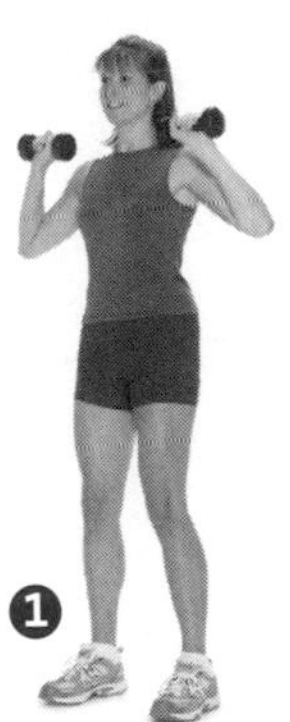

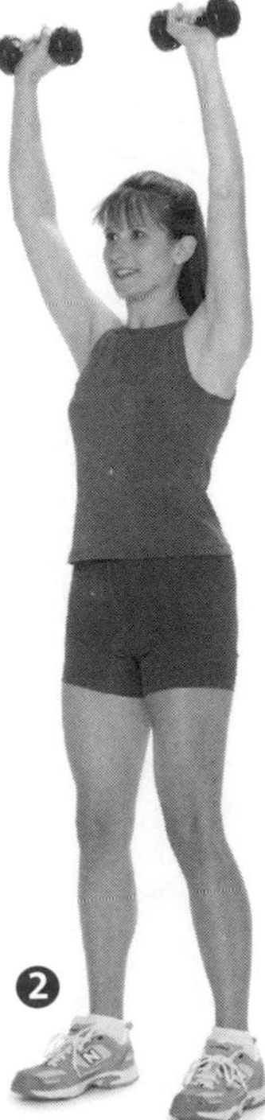

FIRM UP / DAY 13

Real-Life Success Story

"I guess I'll have to give up my pepperoni pizza, huh?" was the first thing Eileen Fehr, 51, of Quakertown, Pennsylvania, said when she joined *Prevention*'s program 5 years ago. Much to her surprise, she didn't! "This program has given me flexibility in eating that I've never had before," raves Eileen, who says her love of fatty foods has always been her weight-loss downfall. "Eating more fiber has saved me. I hate counting calories, servings, and portions. By adding fiber-filled fruits and vegetables to my meals, I don't have to. The fiber fills me up so I don't overeat, and I'm satisfied with less—even when it's a corned beef sandwich or pizza! And when I'm lifting weights regularly, I can still enjoy my favorites without gaining any weight."

Eileen has lost 18 pounds and has kept it off for 5 years. "Weighing myself regularly helps keep me on track," she says. "I don't get upset about the natural fluctuations of a pound or so. But if I see the numbers going up, I know it's time to get serious."

"The biggest benefit for me is that I feel young," Eileen says. "And if you feel young, you *are* young. I do some aerobic exercise, such as walking two or three times a week, but mostly I lift weights. I can run up and down the stairs without feeling winded, and I don't feel sluggish."

FIRM UP TIPS

HAVE FUN!	ON YOUR PLATE
Go swinging. Half an hour pumping your legs and swinging higher burns more than 100 calories and works both the front and back of your thighs. And if you push someone else, you also give your triceps a workout.	*Buy small. The bigger the portion, the more you're likely to eat—up to 44 percent more, according to one study.*

Meal Plan

Most of these recipes are custom designed to make 1 serving–no fuss, no muss; just fix, eat, and go! If a recipe makes more than 1 serving, it's noted below. Save that extra serving for another meal, or share it with your spouse or your walking buddy.

Breakfast

Cheese and Crackers: Take along 3 Wasa crispbreads, 1 stick reduced-fat string cheese, and 1 small peach. Serve with 1 cup fat-free milk.

Healthy Snack

Café au Lait and Muffin: Mix 1 cup hot brewed or instant coffee (regular or decaf), 1 cup hot fat-free milk, and 1 teaspoon sugar (if desired). Serve with a mini blueberry muffin (such as a Hostess Blueberry Mini Muffin).

Lunch

Creamy Tomato Soup: Prepare ½ cup Campbell's Reduced-Sodium Tomato soup with ¾ cup fat-free milk. Heat in a microwave oven to the desired temperature, and stir thoroughly. Top with 1 tablespoon (½ ounce) soy nuts. Serve with ½ small banana and ½ whole wheat English muffin. Place the leftover banana in a zip-top bag and leave it out on the counter for tomorrow.

Healthy Snack

Apricot Indulgence: Have 3 dried apricots (or 6 halves). Serve with 2 graham cracker squares (2½-inch size) spread with 1 tablespoon peanut butter.

Dinner

Greek or Middle Eastern Meal: Order a chicken and vegetable kebab. Have all the skewered vegetables and about 2½ ounces chicken (usually about ⅓ of the serving). Have a side of Greek salad (with 1½ cups of greens and no feta cheese; order dressing on the side and use 1 tablespoon) and 1 cup rice.

Indulgent Treat

Wine and Chocolate: Enjoy 4 ounces wine with 1 Dove miniature dark chocolate bar.

Nutrient analysis: 1,746 calories, 75 g protein, 256 g carbohydrates, 44 g total fat, 13 g saturated fat, 93 mg cholesterol, 23 g dietary fiber, 1,854 mg sodium, 943 mg calcium

FIRM UP TIP

MIND OVER MATTER

Do something new. Do something you've never done before, just for yourself. See the latest blockbuster movie. Paint your toenails orange. Get up and sing in a karaoke bar. It helps fight depression and stimulates your mind, which also boosts your immune system.

The Workout

Level 1

Speed Walk: Less Than 20 Minutes

- Follow the same route as last week. The goal is to complete the distance in less time.
- 5-minute warmup: Walk 2 miles per hour, about 95 steps per minute.
- Under-10-minute speedup: Starting at the same spot as last week, increase your speed, walking as quickly as you can, until you reach the point where you slowed down last week. You should be able to do the same distance and shave off at least a few seconds this week.
- 5-minute cooldown: Slow down to 2 miles per hour, about 95 steps per minute.

Core Training: 15 Minutes

- Do the sequence of exercises one time.

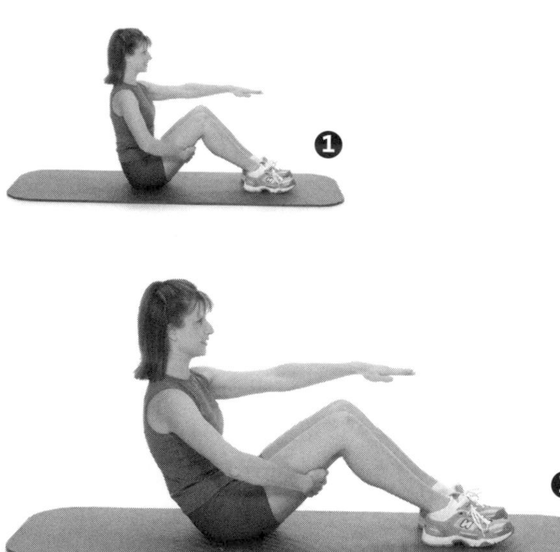

One-Hand Roll-Down

Starting position: Sit on the floor with your knees bent and your feet flat. Place one hand behind the same-side thigh. Keep the other arm out in front of you, parallel to the floor.

Movement: Using your abs, slowly roll down 2 to 3 inches, one vertebra at a time, as you inhale. Hold for a second and then exhale as you slowly roll back up. Do 10 reps.

Technique: Your abs should be powering the move. Don't move quickly.

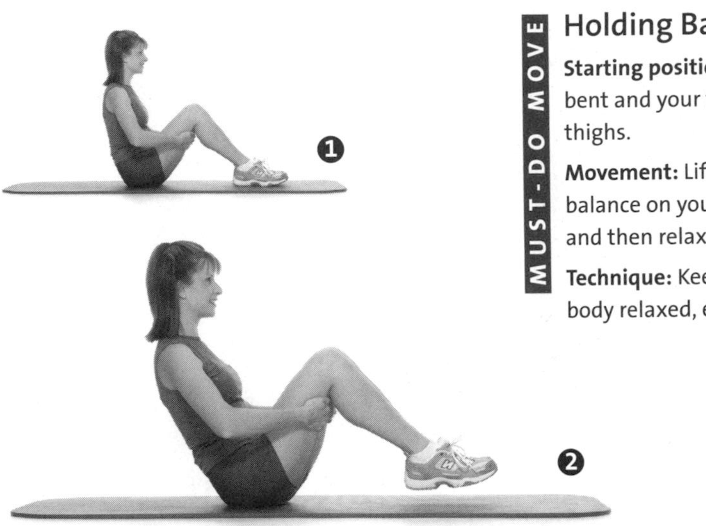

MUST-DO MOVE

Holding Balance

Starting position: Sit on the floor with your knees bent and your feet flat. Place your hands behind your thighs.

Movement: Lift your feet off the floor slightly and balance on your sitting bones. Hold for four breaths and then relax. Do one time only.

Technique: Keep your abs tight and the rest of your body relaxed, especially your shoulders.

Arms-Crossed Ab Crunch

Starting position: Lie on your back with your knees bent, feet flat on the floor, and arms across your chest.

Movement: Using your abs, slowly raise your head, shoulders, and upper back about 45 degrees off the floor as you exhale. Think of shortening the distance between your ribs and pelvis. Hold for a second and then inhale as you slowly lower yourself. Do 10 reps.

Technique: Don't pull your chin to your chest. Don't arch your back.

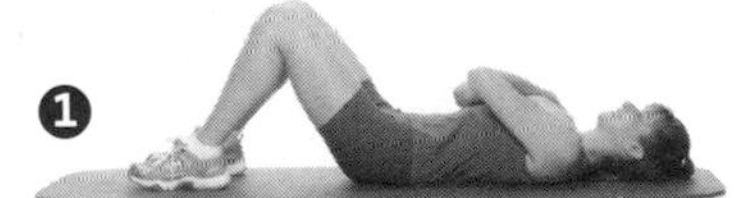

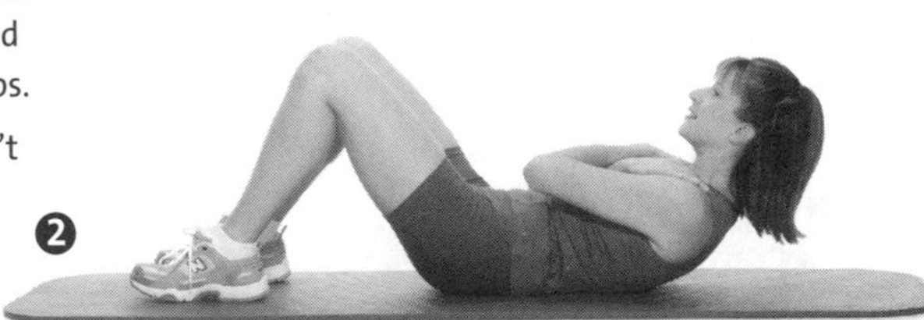

continued

The Workout

Level 1 *continued*

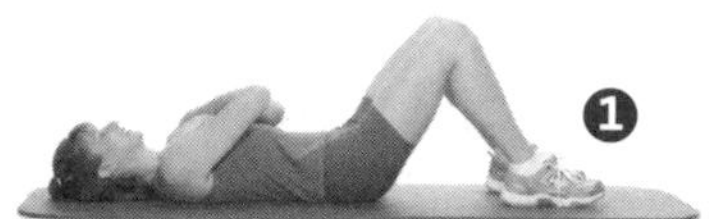

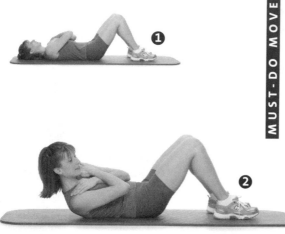

MUST-DO MOVE

Arms-Crossed Twisting Crunch

Starting position: Lie on your back with your knees bent, feet flat on the floor, and arms across your chest.

Movement: Using your abs, slowly lift your head and left shoulder off the floor, twist to the right, and bring your left shoulder toward your right knee as you exhale. Hold for a second and then inhale as you slowly lower yourself. Repeat, alternating sides. Do a total of 10 reps, 5 reps to each side.

Technique: Don't pull your chin to your chest. Don't arch your back.

MUST-DO MOVE

Heel Bridge

Starting position: Lie on your back with your knees bent and your arms at your sides, palms facing up. Lift your toes off the floor so that only your heels are touching.

Movement: Contracting your abs, buttocks, and lower back, press into your heels and lift your butt, hips, and back off the floor as you exhale, to form a straight line from your shoulders to your knees. Hold for four breaths and then relax. Do one time only.

Technique: Don't lift too high—your upper back and shoulders should remain on the floor. Don't bend at the waist or hips. Don't let your knees fall inward or outward.

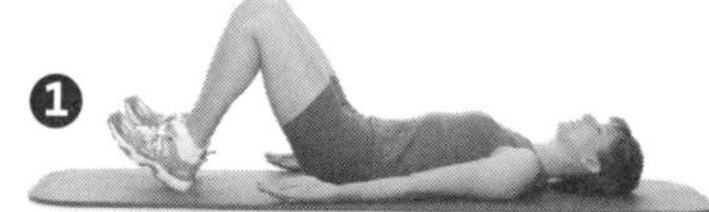

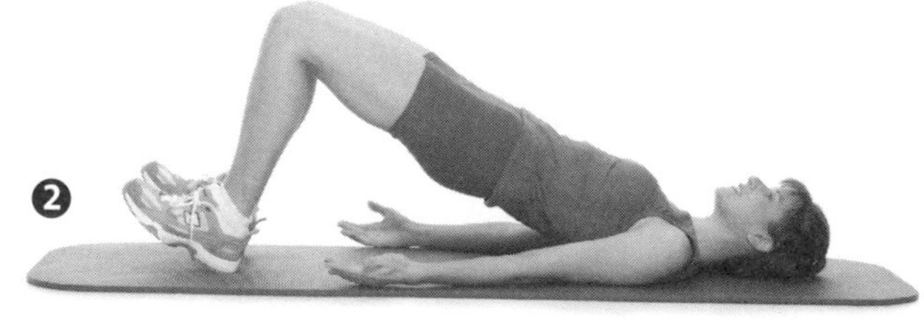

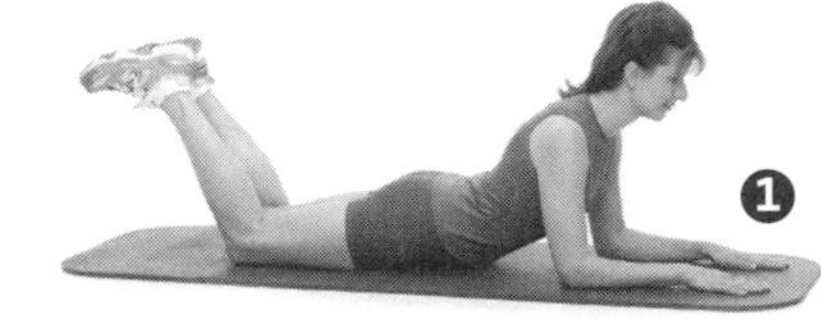

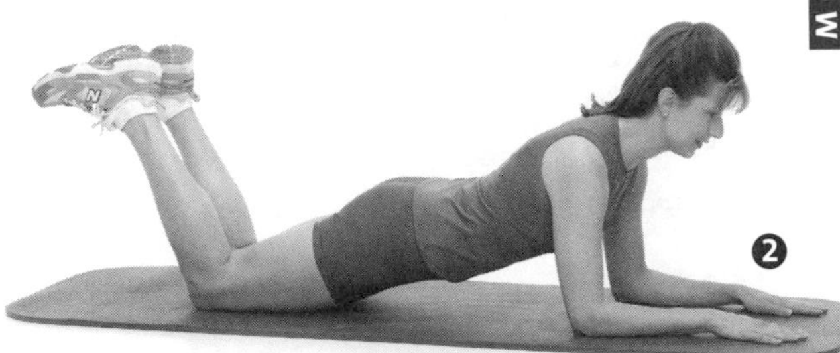

MUST-DO MOVE

Knee Plank

Starting position: Lie facedown with your knees bent so that your feet are in the air. Your elbows should be under your shoulders and your forearms and palms on the floor.

Movement: Contracting your abs and back, press into your forearms as you exhale and lift your pelvis off the floor so that your back and thighs form a straight line. Hold for four breaths and then relax. Do one time only.

Technique: Don't lift your head up or let it drop. Don't bend at the waist. Don't arch your back.

Kneeling T-Stand

Starting position: Sit on your left hip with your left leg bent, your right leg extended, right hand on hip, and left hand on the floor below your shoulder.

Movement: Using your abs, lift your hips off the floor as you exhale. Hold for four breaths, relax, and then repeat on the other side. Do one time only on each side.

Technique: Don't let your body roll forward: Think of it as being sandwiched between two walls. Keep everything in line.

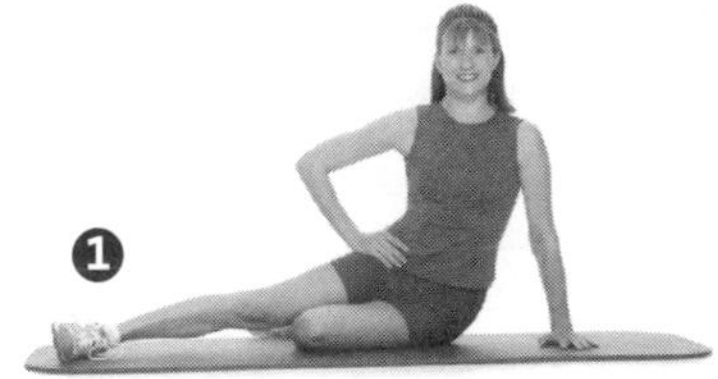

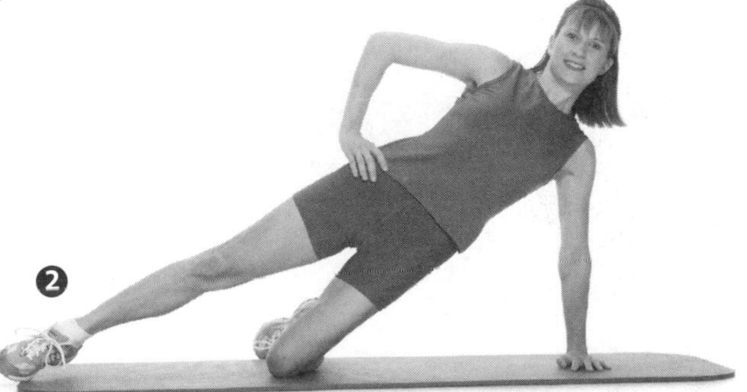

The Workout

Level 2

Speed Walk: Less Than 20 Minutes

- Follow the same route as last week. The goal is to complete the distance in less time.
- 5-minute warmup: Walk 2 to 2½ miles per hour, 95 to 100 steps per minute.
- Under-10-minute speedup: Starting at the same spot as last week, increase your speed, walking as quickly as you can, until you reach the point where you slowed down last week. You should be able to do the same distance and shave off at least a few seconds this week.
- 5-minute cooldown: Slow down to 2 to 2½ miles per hour, 95 to 100 steps per minute.

Core Training: 15 Minutes

- Do the sequence of exercises one time.

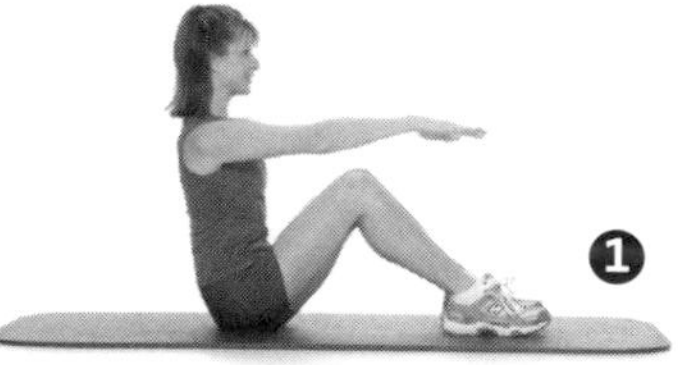

❶

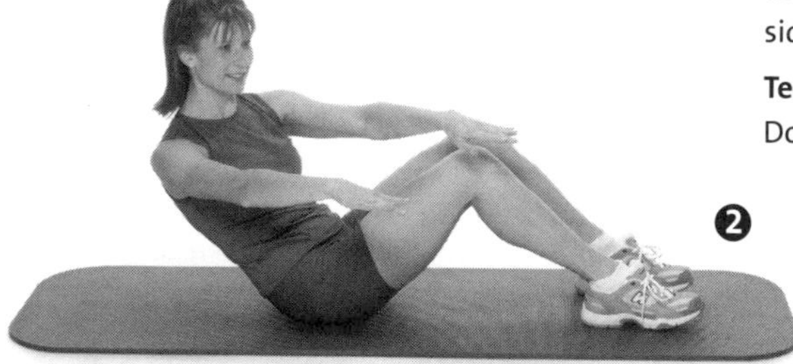

❷

Roll-Down with a Twist

Starting position: Sit on the floor with your knees bent and your feet flat. Hold your arms out in front of you, parallel to the floor.

Movement: Using your abs, slowly roll down 3 to 4 inches, one vertebra at a time, as you inhale and twist to the right. Hold for a second and then exhale as you slowly roll back up. Do 10 reps, alternating the side you twist to each time.

Technique: Your abs should be powering the move. Don't move quickly.

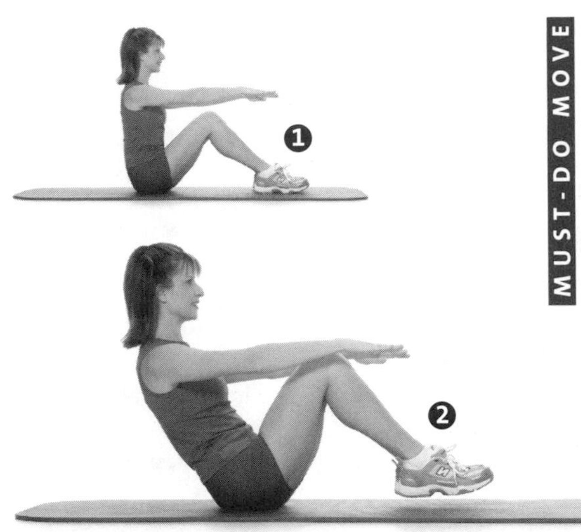

MUST-DO MOVE

Partial Balance

Starting position: Sit on the floor with your knees bent and your feet flat. Hold your arms out in front of you, parallel to the floor.

Movement: Lift your feet slightly off the floor and balance on your sitting bones. Hold for five breaths and then relax. Do one time only.

Technique: Keep your abs tight and the rest of your body relaxed, especially your shoulders.

Ab Crunch

Starting position: Lie on your back with your knees bent, feet flat on the floor, and hands behind your head.

Movement: Using your abs, slowly raise your head, shoulders, and upper back about 45 degrees off the floor as you exhale. Think of shortening the distance between your ribs and pelvis. Hold for a second and then inhale as you slowly lower yourself. Do 10 reps.

Technique: Don't pull your chin to your chest. Don't arch your back.

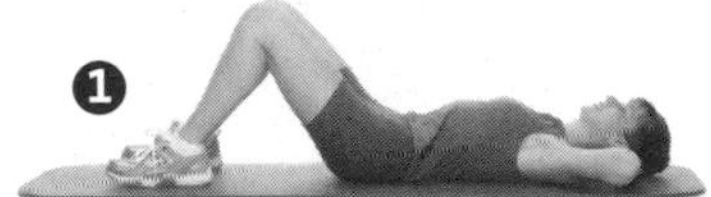

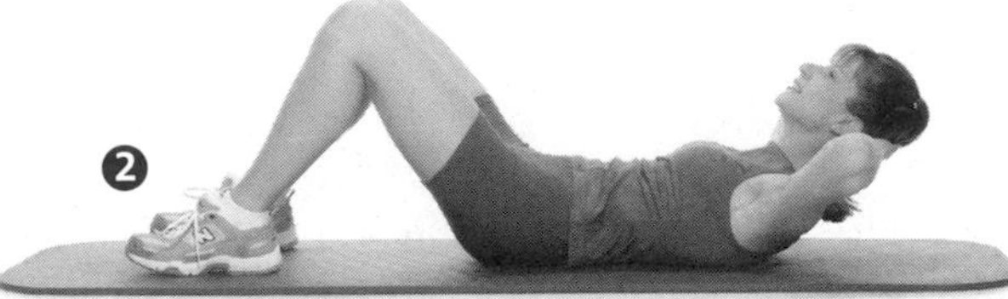

continued

The Workout

Level 2 *continued*

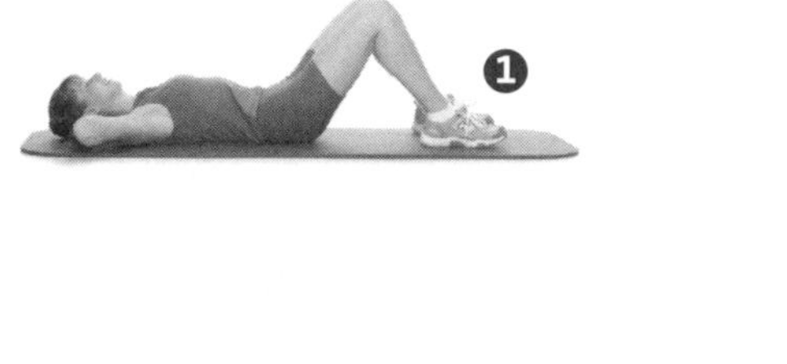

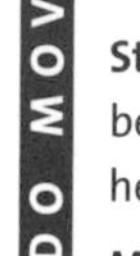

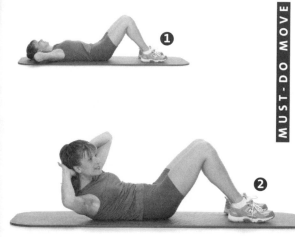

MUST-DO MOVE

Twisting Crunch

Starting position: Lie on your back with your knees bent, feet flat on the floor, and hands behind your head.

Movement: Using your abs, slowly lift your head and left shoulder off the floor, twist to the right, and bring your left shoulder toward your right knee as you exhale. Hold for a second and then inhale as you slowly lower yourself. Repeat, alternating sides. Do a total of 10 reps, 5 reps to each side.

Technique: Don't pull your chin to your chest. Don't arch your back.

MUST-DO MOVE

Bridge with Leg Lift

Starting position: Lie on your back with your knees bent, feet flat on the floor, and arms at your sides, palms facing up.

Movement: Contracting your abs, buttocks, and lower back, press into your feet and lift your butt, hips, and back off the floor as you exhale, to form a straight line from your shoulders to your knees. Lift one foot off the floor and extend that leg. Hold for three breaths and then lower your foot. Lift the other foot up and hold for three breaths. Lower your foot and return to the starting position. Do one time only.

Technique: Don't lift too high—your upper back and shoulders should remain on the floor. Don't bend at the waist or hips. Don't let your knees fall inward or outward.

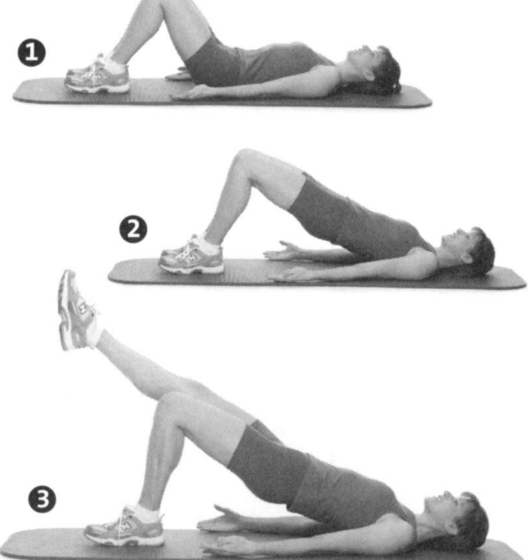

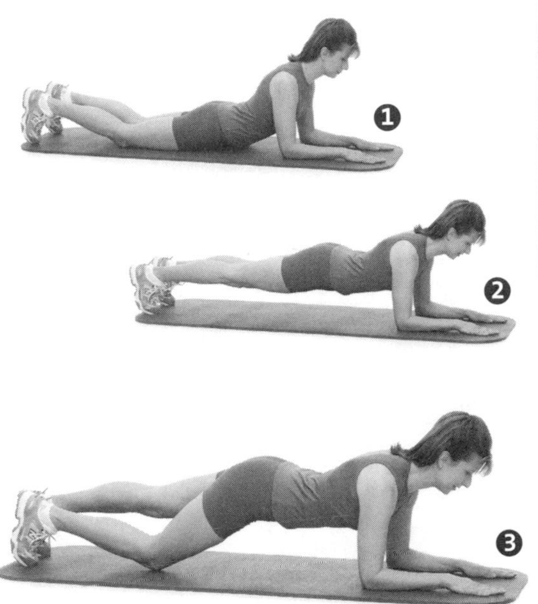

MUST-DO MOVE

Plank with Knee Drop

Starting position: Lie facedown with your feet flexed and toes tucked. Your elbows should be under your shoulders and your forearms and palms on the floor.

Movement: Contracting your abs and back, press into your forearms as you exhale and lift your pelvis and legs off the floor so that your back and legs form a straight line. Slowly drop your right knee toward the floor and then straighten. Do five knee touches with your right leg, hold for three breaths, do five knee touches with your left leg, hold for three breaths, and then relax. Do one time only.

Technique: Don't lift your head up or let it drop. Don't bend at the waist or hips. Don't let your belly drop toward the floor.

T-Stand

Starting position: Sit on your left hip with your legs extended to the side and your right ankle over the left, right hand on your hip, and left hand on the floor below your shoulder.

Movement: Using your abs, lift your hips, legs, and ankles off the floor as you exhale. Hold for five breaths, relax, and then repeat on the other side. Do one time only on each side.

Technique: Don't let your body roll forward: Think of it as being sandwiched between two walls. Keep everything in line. Don't let your ankles touch the floor.

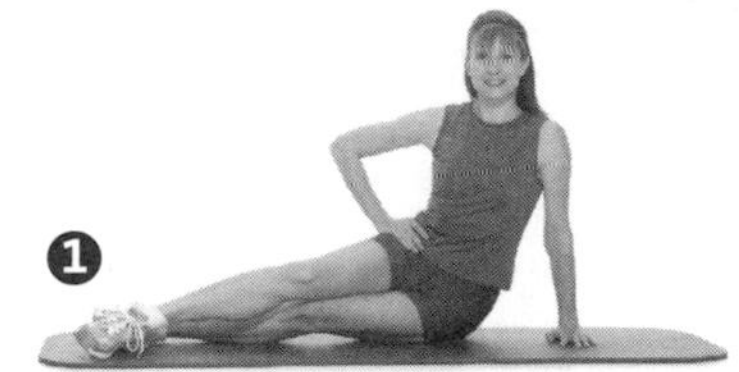

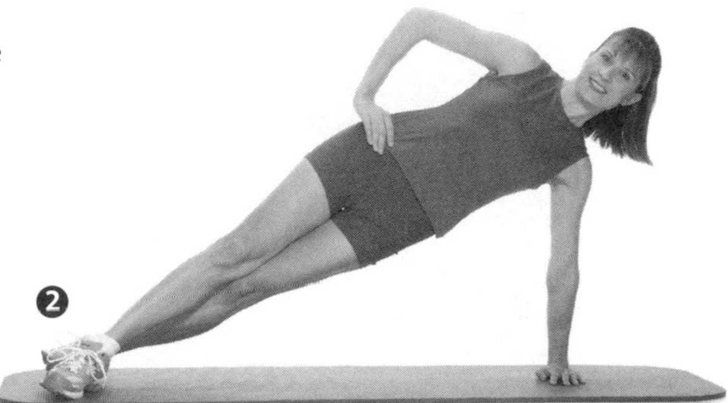

The Workout

Level 3

Speed Walk: Less Than 20 Minutes

- Follow the same route as last week. The goal is to complete the distance in less time.
- 5-minute warmup: Walk 2½ to 3 miles per hour, 100 to 115 steps per minute.
- Under-10-minute speedup: Starting at the same spot as last week, increase your speed, walking as quickly as you can, until you reach the point where you slowed down last week. You should be able to do the same distance and shave off at least a few seconds this week.
- 5-minute cooldown: Slow down to 2½ to 3 miles per hour, 100 to 115 steps per minute.

Core Training: 15 Minutes

- Do the sequence of exercises one time.

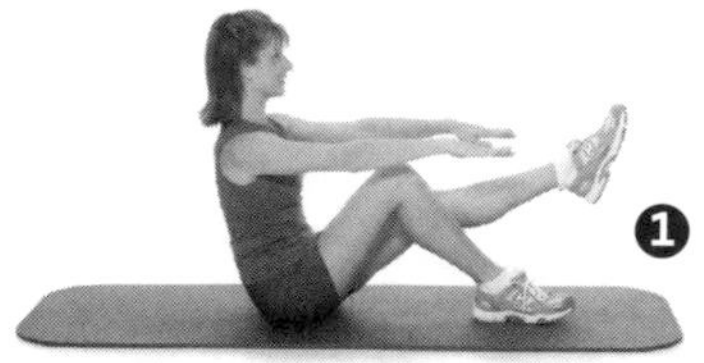

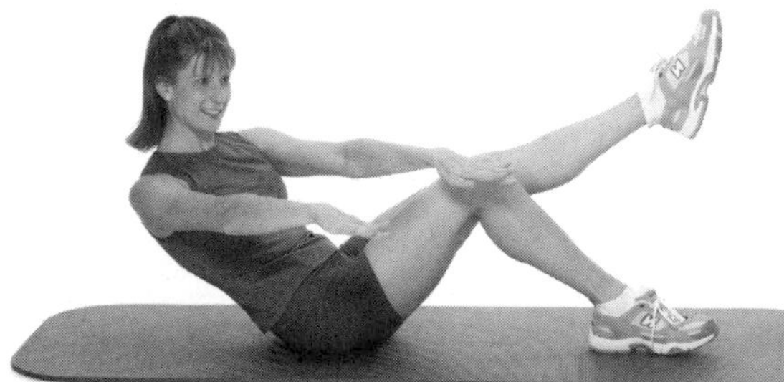

One-Leg Roll-Down with a Twist

Starting position: Sit on the floor with your knees bent and your feet flat. Lift your left foot off the floor and extend your left leg. Hold your arms straight out in front of you, parallel to the floor.

Movement: Using your abs, slowly roll down 4 to 5 inches, one vertebra at a time, as you inhale and twist to the right. Hold for a second and then exhale as you slowly roll back up. Do five reps and then switch legs and twist to the left.

Technique: Your abs should be powering the move. Don't move quickly.

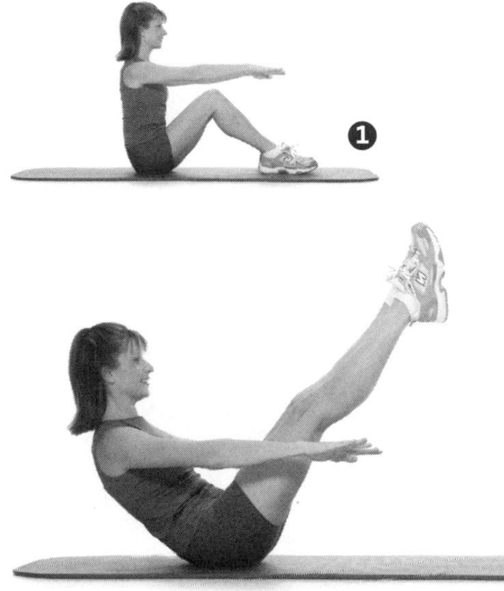

MUST-DO MOVE

Legs-Extended Balance

Starting position: Sit on the floor with your knees bent and your feet flat. Hold your arms out in front of you, parallel to the floor.

Movement: Lift your feet off the floor, extending your legs straight, and balance on your sitting bones. Hold for five breaths and then relax. Do one time only.

Technique: Keep your abs tight and the rest of your body relaxed, especially your shoulders.

Reverse Crunch

Starting position: Lie on your back with your legs up in the air and your hands behind your head. Cross your legs at the shins.

Movement: Slowly contract your abs as you exhale and press your back into the floor, tilting your pelvis and lifting your hips 2 to 4 inches off the floor. Keep your upper body relaxed. Hold for a second and then inhale as you slowly lower yourself. Do 10 reps.

Technique: Don't swing your legs.

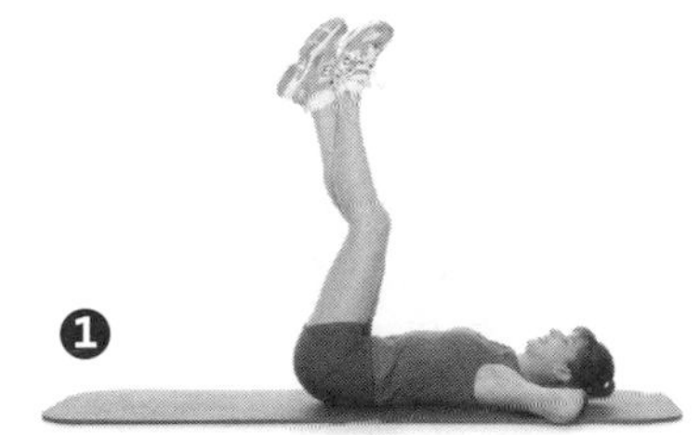

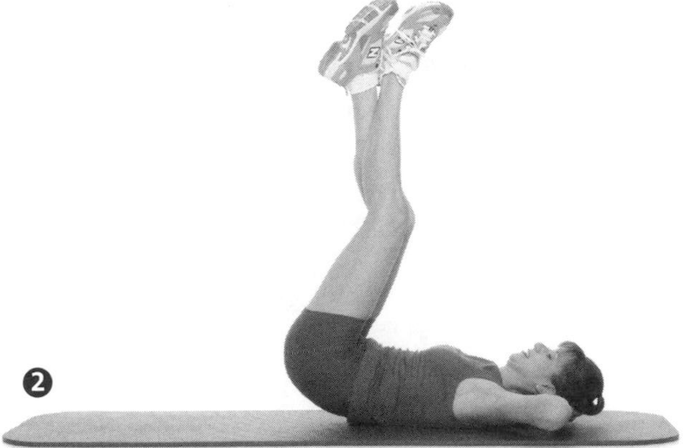

continued

The Workout

Level 3 *continued*

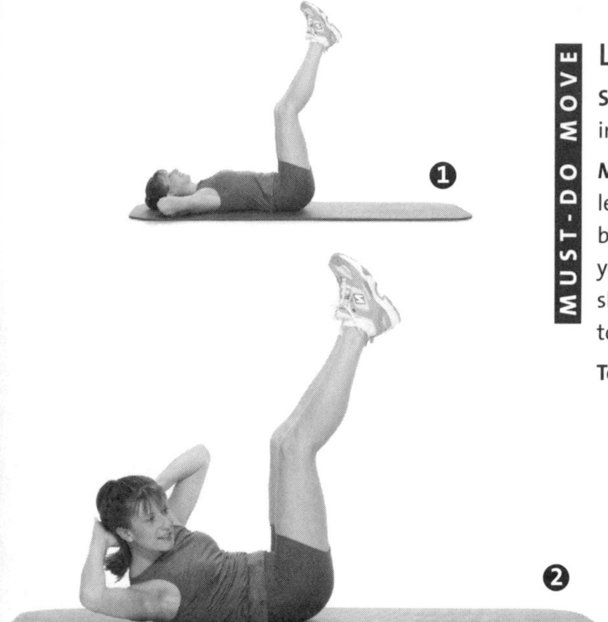

MUST-DO MOVE

Legs-Up Twisting Crunch

Starting position: Lie on your back with your legs up in the air and your hands behind your head.

Movement: Using your abs, slowly lift your head and left shoulder off the floor, twist to the right, and bring your left shoulder toward your right knee as you exhale. Hold for a second and then inhale as you slowly lower yourself. Repeat, alternating sides. Do a total of 10 reps, 5 to each side.

Technique: Don't pull your chin to your chest.

MUST-DO MOVE

Heel Bridge with Leg Lift and Arms Up

Starting position: Lie on your back with your knees bent, feet flat on the floor, and arms extended over your chest. Lift your toes off the floor so that only your heels are touching.

Movement: Contracting your abs, buttocks, and lower back, press into your heels and lift your butt, hips, and back off the floor as you exhale, to form a straight line from your shoulders to your knees. Lift your right foot off the floor and extend that leg. Hold for three breaths and then lower your foot. Lift the other foot up and hold for three breaths. Lower your foot and return to the starting position. Do one time only.

Technique: Don't lift too high—your upper back and shoulders should remain on the floor. Don't bend at the waist or hips. Don't let your knees fall inward or outward.

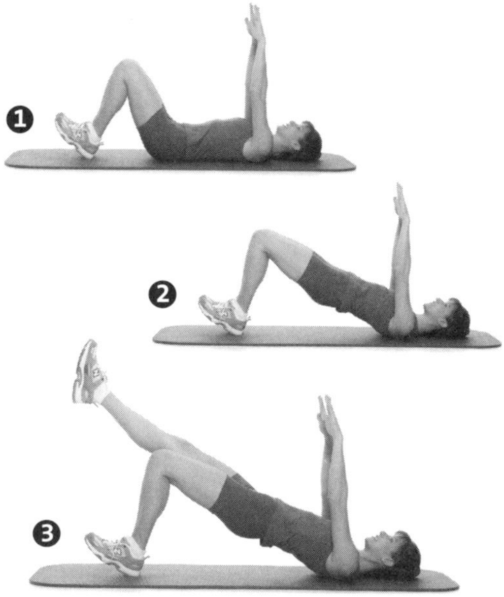

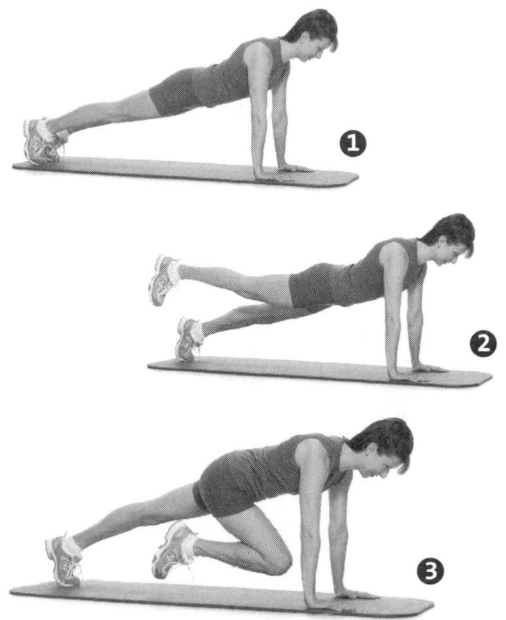

MUST-DO MOVE

Extended Plank with Lift and Bend

Starting position: Lie facedown with your feet flexed and toes tucked. Place your palms on the floor near your shoulders so that your elbows are pointing up. Contracting your abs and back, press into your hands as you exhale, straighten your arms, and lift your torso and legs off the floor so that your head, back, and legs form a straight line.

Movement: Lift your right foot off the floor and hold for three breaths. Next, pull your right knee in toward your chest and press it back out for five reps and then put that foot back on the floor. Lift your left foot off the floor and hold for three breaths. Next, pull your left knee in toward your chest and press it back out for five reps, put that foot back on the floor, and then relax. Do one time only.

Technique: Don't lift your head up or let it drop. Don't bend at the waist or hips. Don't let your belly drop toward the floor.

T-Stand with Arm Up

Starting position: Sit on your left hip with your legs extended to the side, your right ankle over the left, right arm extended on your leg, and left hand on the floor below your shoulder.

Movement: Using your abs, lift your hips, legs, and ankles off the floor and raise your right arm overhead as you exhale. Look up toward your right hand. Hold for five breaths, relax, and then repeat on the other side. Do one time only on each side.

Technique: Don't let your body roll forward; think of it as being sandwiched between two walls. Keep everything in line. Don't let your ankles touch the floor.

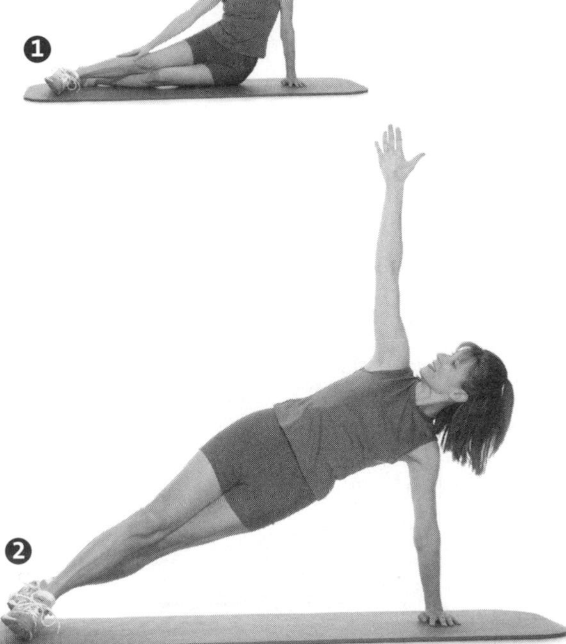

FIRM UP / DAY 14

You Deserve a Pat on the Back

You are awesome! Two weeks, and you're going strong. Time to reward yourself and take a few minutes to bask in all that you've accomplished so far: exercising every day, eating more healthfully, and making any of the other dozens of lifestyle changes that you may have made. You should also be noticing some firmness, especially in your arms and calves, and your clothes may be feeling a little looser. You're on your way to wearing sleeveless tops, tucking in your shirts, and showing off those legs in a pair of shorts. And don't forget how you're feeling. More energized? Stronger? Less stressed? Sleeping better? Exercise can have an enormous impact on so many areas of your life.

Even if you're not following the program to a T, you should still be very proud of yourself. Consistency is the key to getting results and keeping them, so keep up the good work!

FIRM UP TIPS

GET FIRM FASTER	ENERGY BOOSTER
Avoid a side stitch. Instead of gulping one large drink, sip small amounts (4 to 8 ounces) more frequently. If you're still stitch-prone, try these proven remedies. *• Bend forward and tighten your abdominal muscles.* *• Massage the painful area.* *• Breathe without completely exhaling.* *• Wear a wide belt cinched tightly around your waist.* *• Breathe out through pursed lips.*	*Double—or triple—the fun. If you like massage, go for the 90-minute session instead of a 30-minute rubdown. Enjoy a particular friend? Plan a day together: perhaps a hike and dinner, or a morning at a pottery-painting studio, then a long lunch. Need a haircut? Book an appointment with a top stylist and get a manicure or pedicure, too. It will feel like more of a reward, and the more pleasure you get, the less stress you'll have and the stronger your immunity will be.*

Meal Plan

Most of these recipes are custom designed to make 1 serving–no fuss, no muss; just fix, eat, and go! If a recipe makes more than 1 serving, it's noted below. Save that extra serving for another meal, or share it with your spouse or your walking buddy.

Breakfast

Yogurt with Granola and Bananas: Top 4 ounces (½ cup) fat-free fruit-flavored yogurt with ½ cup low-fat granola (without raisins, such as Healthy Choice), 1 tablespoon chopped walnuts, and ½ banana. Serve with 1 cup fat-free milk.

Indulgent Treat

Cookies at the Mall: At Mrs. Fields, have 4 Bite Size Nibbler Chewy Chocolate Fudge Cookies.

Lunch

Grilled Chicken Sandwich: Have Wendy's Grilled Chicken Sandwich or McDonald's Chicken McGrill without the mayo spread. If you must have mayo, ask for just a dab or use ½ tablespoon, max. Bring along a sandwich bag of 2 cups sliced red pepper (or other vegetable) and 1 pear.

Healthy Snack

Trail Mix: Enjoy 1 serving from the batch you made Thursday.

Dinner

Beef and Rice: Prepare ⅓ cup cooked brown rice. In a nonstick skillet over medium heat, cook nearly halfway through 3 ounces crumbled raw 93% lean ground beef. In a bowl, combine ½ cup canned sliced mushrooms (rinse thoroughly and drain), ½ cup raw or frozen chopped onions, ½ cup low-fat/low-sodium cream of mushroom soup, and 1 teaspoon minced garlic. Pour over the ground beef and cook, covered, until the beef is cooked thoroughly. Serve over the brown rice. Have 1 sliced kiwifruit for dessert.

Healthy Snack

Fruit and Cheese: Slice a ripe pear or apple and eat it with 1 slice (1 ounce) reduced-fat cheese.

Nutrient analysis: 1,730 calories, 73 g protein, 245 g carbohydrates, 51 g total fat, 20 g saturated fat, 164 mg cholesterol, 25 g dietary fiber, 1,903 mg sodium, 1,034 mg calcium

FIRM UP TIP

ON YOUR PLATE

Stash chocolate (or other goodies) out of sight. Office workers who stored chocolate kisses in glass jars on their desktops ate three more each day than those who put the candy in their drawers and six more than workers who had to walk 6 feet to their jars.

The Workout

Levels 1, 2, and 3

Long Walk: 50 Minutes

- Drive to a different neighborhood or find a trail and walk at a comfortable pace that you can sustain for 50 minutes.

FIRM UP TIPS

MIND OVER MATTER

Laugh out loud! Humor can actually inoculate you against anxiety: One study found that people who watched an episode of a popular sitcom before tackling a stressful task didn't show the spikes in blood pressure and heart rate that their humor-deprived counterparts did.

FIT FACT

Dining out more than five times a week may make you eat more—nearly 300 calories a day—than if you dine out less frequently.

Your Reward Diary

Remember to write down your weekly reward here. What are you doing for yourself this week?

____

____

____

____

____

____

____

____

CHAPTER 5

Week 3

Two weeks down, and one more to go. You can do it!

If you've noticed a dip in your motivation, take a look right now at chapter 12, Keep Your Motivation Strong. The tips in this chapter can help you get revved up for the final week of the program. Even if your enthusiasm is not waning, the advice in this chapter can help you get over the inevitable dips that occur over the long term.

Grocery List

Photocopy this list and take it with you to the store. You can stock up on everything you need to make the third week's Firm Up meals and snacks, so all the ingredients will be at hand when you need them. The amounts of the fresh ingredients are tailored so that you're buying exactly as much as you need. And you should still have some of the items, such as the spices and condiments, from week 1's shopping list to use this week. For some specific brand recommendations, see page 321 in chapter 7, Mix-and-Match Meals.

Produce Aisle

☐ 1 green apple

☐ 1 bunch asparagus (if not in season, choose 8-ounce box frozen)

☐ 3 bananas

☐ 2 pints blueberries

☐ 1 small bag baby carrots

☐ 3 stalks celery

☐ 1 medium cucumber

☐ 1 bunch (6 ounces) red or green grapes

☐ 2 bags romaine lettuce leaves

☐ 2 peaches

☐ Choose: 3 pears *or* 3 apples (or a combination of both)

☐ 1 bag baby spinach leaves

☐ 1 (16-ounce) container strawberries

☐ 2 tomatoes

Dairy Aisle

☐ 1 (8-ounce) block 50% reduced-fat cheese (any flavor)

☐ 1 (8-ounce) package 2% milk reduced-fat shredded cheese (any flavor; suggest Cheddar)

☐ 1 can Pillsbury Cornbread Twists dough

☐ 1 dozen eggs (option: choose "omega-3" eggs such as Eggland's Best to save 60 milligrams cholesterol and 0.5 gram saturated fat per egg) *or* 2 cartons Egg Beaters (for fat-free eggs)

☐ 1 gallon plus 1 quart fat-free milk

☐ 1 (4-ounce) container reduced-fat sour cream

☐ 3 (8-ounce) containers fat-free yogurt (120 calories or less per cup—choose 1 pineapple or apricot-flavored, if desired)

Canned Fruit/Vegetables/Beans/Soup Aisle

☐ 1 (8-ounce) bottle apple juice

Crackers/Snacks/Cereals/Pasta Aisle

☐ 1 Little Debbie Brownie Lights brownie

☐ 1 small bag tortilla chips

Bread Aisle

☐ 1 (2½-inch-diameter) bran muffin

☐ 1 package honey wheat or oat bran English muffins

☐ 1 package whole grain pita bread (6½-inch size)

Deli/Meat Aisle

☐ 4 (4-ounce) chicken breasts

☐ 6 ounces salmon

Nuts/Baking/Spices Aisle

☐ 1 small spice bottle or tin bay leaves

☐ 1 small spice bottle or tin peppercorns (if desired)

Other/Checkout Aisle

☐ 1 Milky Way Lite candy bar

☐ 1 Pria bar

FIRM UP TIP

MIND OVER MATTER

Reach out. Daily, loving contact with your romantic partner can protect you against the negative effects of stress, such as high blood pressure. Try cuddling for 10 minutes in the morning before you get out of bed.

FIRM UP TIPS

ON YOUR PLATE

Trick your tastebuds. Sucking on a menthol/eucalyptus cough drop can stop cravings instantly.

GET FIRM FASTER

Don't lead with your chin when you walk. The chin-forward position makes your shoulders droop, your stomach sag, and your lower back sway. This slouched posture can make you look older than you are and, down the road, can make it hard to stand tall, so you feel older, too. To straighten up, keep your head level and pull your chin straight back.

FIT FACT

MRI images of unfit people show more evidence of brain shrinkage—a suspected cause of memory loss—compared with those who are fit.

Bedtime Stretches

To help you relax and fall asleep faster, try these stretches to quiet your mind and release tension.

SIDE. Stand with your feet wider than shoulder width apart. Clasp your hands overhead, pressing your palms toward the ceiling. Lift up and then bend slightly to your left. You should feel a stretch down the right side of your torso. Hold for three deep breaths and then release. Repeat to the other side.

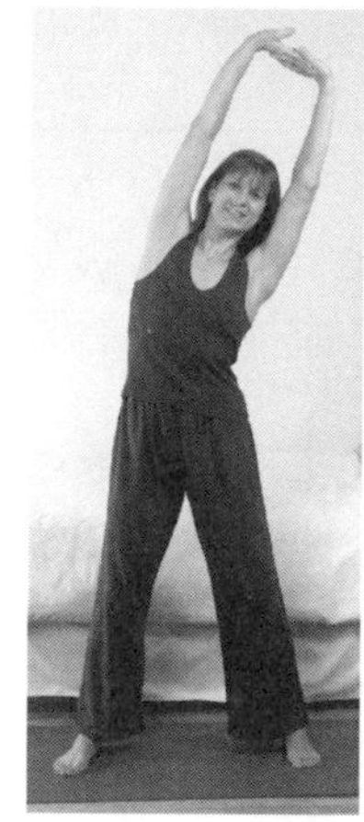

SHIN. Step your right foot back about 6 inches and point your toes back so that the top of your foot rests on the floor. Bending your left knee, press down into your right foot so that you feel a stretch in your right shin. Hold for three deep breaths and then release. Repeat, stretching the left shin. (This is also a great stretch if your shins are aching after a walk. You'll need to remove your shoes, though.)

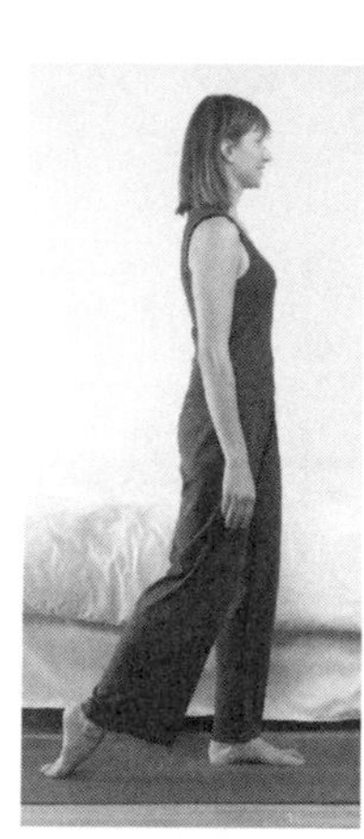

BACK. Sit on the edge of your bed or a chair with your feet flat on the floor. Place your right hand across your body and on top of your left thigh. Gently twist your torso and head to the left. Your hips and lower body should not move. Hold for three deep breaths and then release. Repeat, twisting to the right.

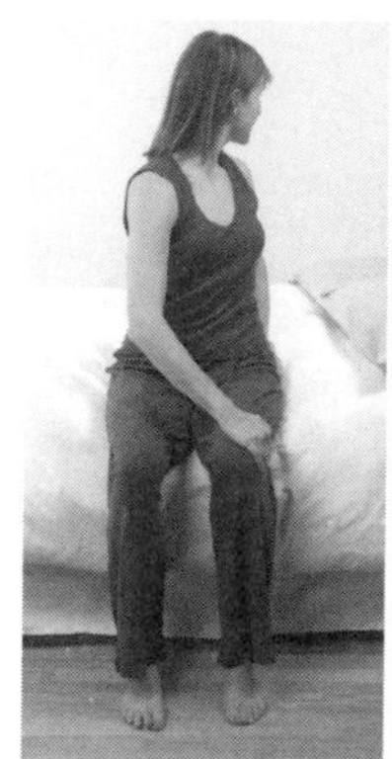

NECK. Sit on the edge of your bed with your feet flat on the floor. Keeping your shoulders back, drop your chin toward your chest. Slowly roll your head toward the right until your right ear is near your right shoulder. Hold for three deep breaths and then roll your head to the left. Hold for three deep breaths and then roll your head down to your chest and then lift it up.

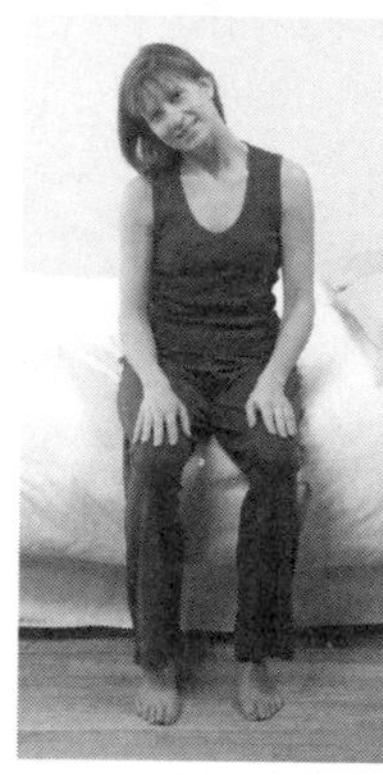

HIP. Sit on the edge of your bed and place your left foot on your right knee. Your right hand should be on top of your left ankle, and your left hand on top of your left knee. Keeping your back straight, bend at the hips and lean forward. You should feel a stretch in your left hip. For a deeper stretch, gently push on your left knee. Hold for three deep breaths and then release. Repeat on the other side.

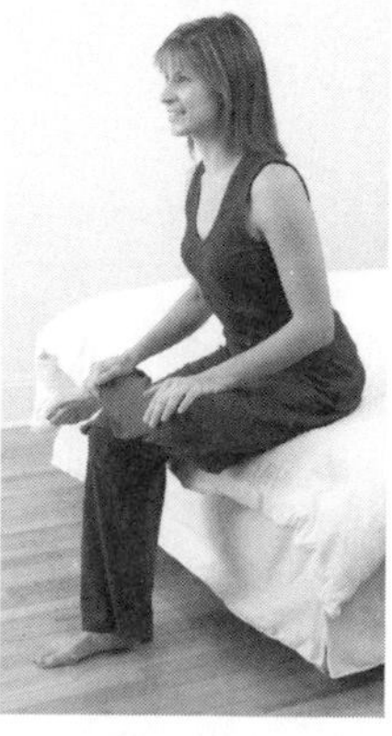

Meal Plan

Most of these recipes are custom designed to make 1 serving–no fuss, no muss; just fix, eat, and go! If a recipe makes more than 1 serving, it's noted below. Save that extra serving for another meal, or share it with your spouse or your walking buddy.

Breakfast

English Muffin with a Scrambled Egg: Scramble 1 egg (or ¼ cup Egg Beaters) in a nonstick skillet with 1 teaspoon trans-fat-free margarine. Gather the scrambled egg onto 1 split and toasted English muffin. Serve with 1 cup fat-free milk.

Healthy Snack

Tropical Yogurt: Stir 2 tablespoons tropical dried-fruit mix into an 8-ounce (1 cup) fat-free pineapple- or apricot-flavored yogurt (check label for no more than 120 calories per cup). Mix in a few drops coconut extract. Top with 1 tablespoon chopped walnuts.

Lunch

Veggie Burger with Baked Fries and Steamed Fresh Baby Spinach: Bake ½ cup Ore-Ida shoestring-style fries in the toaster oven–no oil or spray necessary. While they are baking, heat a nonstick skillet coated with olive oil cooking spray over low to medium heat. When the skillet is hot, toss in 2 cups loose baby spinach leaves and 1 teaspoon minced garlic and gently toss for 2 minutes. The leaves should be a little wilted but not mushy. Top the leaves with 1 to 2 tablespoons balsamic vinegar. Heat a veggie burger in the microwave oven according to package directions and serve with 2 to 3 tablespoons ketchup, if desired. Skip the bun.

Healthy Snack

Vegetables and Dip: Dip 15 baby carrots into 2 tablespoons reduced-fat veggie cream cheese and serve with 1¼ cups fresh strawberries.

Dinner

Salmon, Rice, and Asparagus: Makes 2 servings. Preheat oven to 350°F. In a small (1½-quart) baking dish, pour 1 cup white wine and 1 cup water. Add 5 peppercorns, 2 bay leaves, and 1 peeled clove garlic. Place in the oven. When it comes to a simmer, add 2 pieces (3 ounces each) boneless salmon fillet. Cook skin side down for 8 minutes, or until cooked all the way through. With a slotted spoon, remove the salmon from the liquid. Serve each piece of salmon with 1 cup cooked flavored rice (such as Uncle Ben's Chef Recipe Chicken and Harvest Vegetable Pilaf) and 1 cup steamed or microwaved asparagus with a spritz of lemon.

Indulgent Treat

Banana Split: Slice 1 banana in half lengthwise. Top with ⅓ cup Healthy Choice ice cream (any flavor) and 2 tablespoons light whipped topping.

Nutrient analysis: 1,731 calories, 91 g protein, 249 g carbohydrates, 45 g total fat, 15 g saturated fat, 292 mg cholesterol, 32 g dietary fiber, 1,930 mg sodium, 1,228 mg calcium

The Workout

Level 1

Easy Walk: 40 Minutes

- 5-minute warmup: Walk 2 to 2½ miles per hour, or 95 to 100 steps per minute.
- 30-minute moderate walk: Increase your speed to 2½ to 3 miles per hour, 100 to 115 steps per minute, or a pace that lets you comfortably carry on a conversation.
- 5-minute cooldown: Slow down to 2 to 2½ miles per hour, or 95 to 100 steps per minute.

Basic Strength Training: 30 Minutes

- Do 10 to 12 reps of each exercise. Repeat the sequence of exercises three times.
- To warm up, use lighter weights, or none at all, the first time through, and for the squat and lunge exercises, only go partway down.

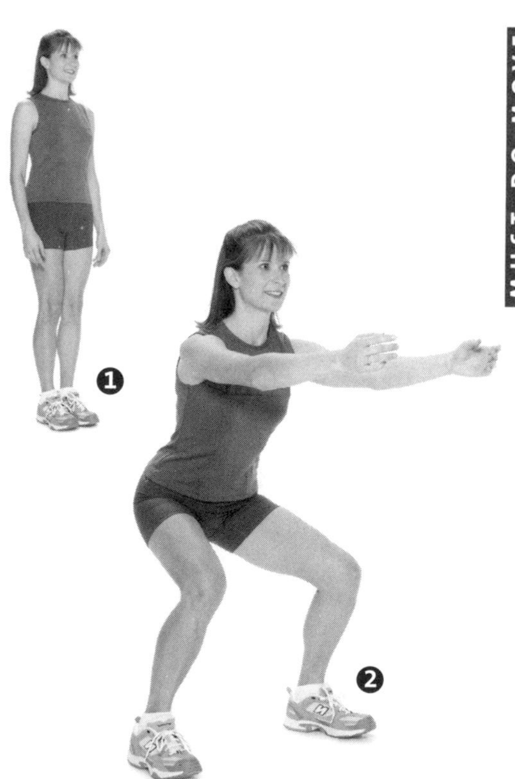

MUST-DO MOVE

Step Squat

Starting position: Stand with your feet together and your hands down at your sides.

Movement: Step your left foot out to the side 2 to 2½ feet. Keeping your back straight, lower yourself, bending from the knees and hips as though you're sitting down, as you inhale. Let your arms come out in front of you to help you balance. Stop just before your thighs are parallel to the floor. Hold for a second and then exhale as you push back up, bringing your left foot back in. Do five or six reps with your left foot and then do five or six reps stepping with your right foot.

Technique: Don't let your knees move forward over your toes. Don't round your back.

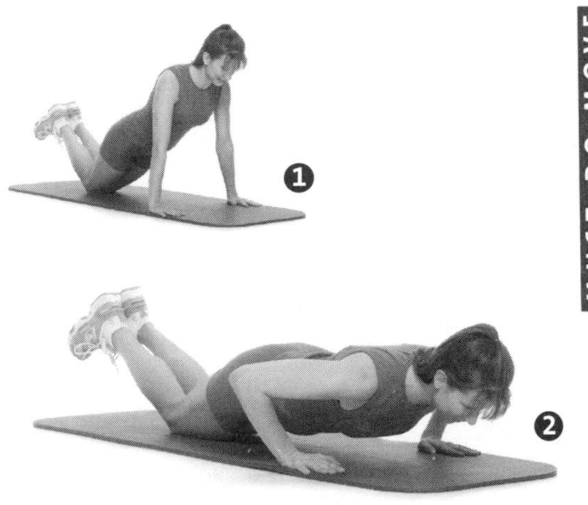

MUST-DO MOVE

Bent-Knee Pushup

Starting position: Lie facedown on the floor. Bend your knees so that your feet are up in the air, and place your palms on the floor near your shoulders so that your elbows are pointing up. Press down with your hands, extend your arms, and lift your body off the floor.

Movement: Keeping your head, back, hips, and knees in a straight line, bend your elbows out to the sides and lower your body as you inhale, until your chest nearly touches the floor. Hold for a second and then exhale as you slowly push back up.

Technique: Don't bend at the hips. Don't arch your back.

MUST-DO MOVE

Back Lunge

Starting position: Stand with your feet together. Hold a dumbbell in each hand, either at shoulder height or at your sides.

Movement: Step your left foot back 2 to 3 feet. Inhale as you bend your right knee and lower your body straight down until your right knee is bent 90 degrees and your left knee nearly touches the floor. Your rear heel will come off the floor. Hold for a second and then exhale as you push yourself back up, bringing your left foot back in. Finish all of your repetitions, then repeat the exercise stepping back with your right foot.

Technique: Don't lean forward. Don't let your front knee move forward over your toes.

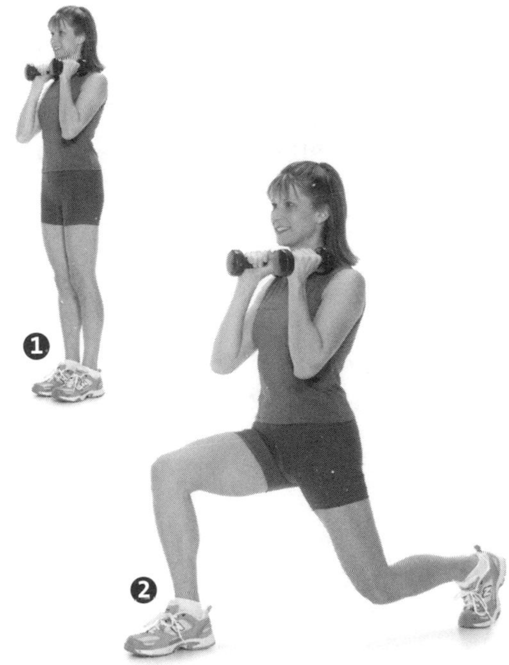

continued

The Workout

Level 1 *continued*

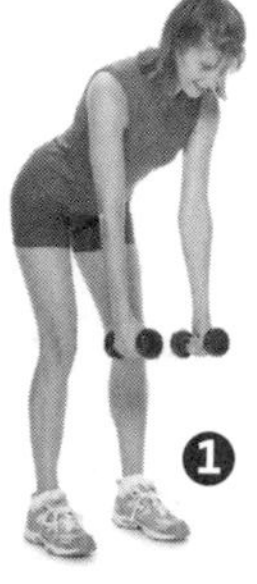

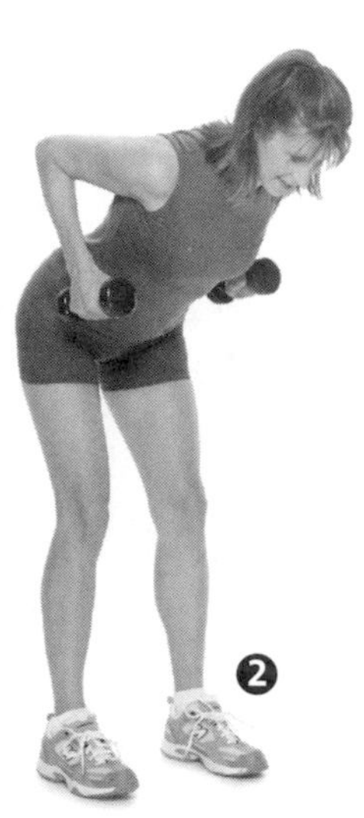

MUST-DO MOVE

Bent-Over Row

Starting position: Stand with your feet shoulder width apart, knees bent slightly. Hold a dumbbell in each hand with your arms at your sides. Keep your back flat and lean forward, bending at the hips so that the dumbbells are hanging at arm's length in front of you, palms facing each other.

Movement: Bending your elbows back and squeezing your shoulder blades, lift the weights toward your ribs as you exhale, until your elbows are higher than your back. Hold for a second and then inhale as you slowly lower them.

Technique: Don't arch your back. Don't pull your shoulders up toward your ears. Don't raise your torso as you lift the dumbbells.

Alternate move: If you have back problems, support yourself with one hand on a chair and do the rows one arm at a time.

Seated Biceps Curl with a Twist

Starting position: Sit on the edge of a chair with your feet hip width apart. Hold dumbbells at your sides with your palms facing in.

Movement: Bending your elbows and turning your wrists upward, lift the dumbbells toward your shoulders as you exhale. Stop when the dumbbells are at chest height, palms facing your body. Hold for a second and then inhale as you slowly lower them.

Technique: Don't move your upper arms.

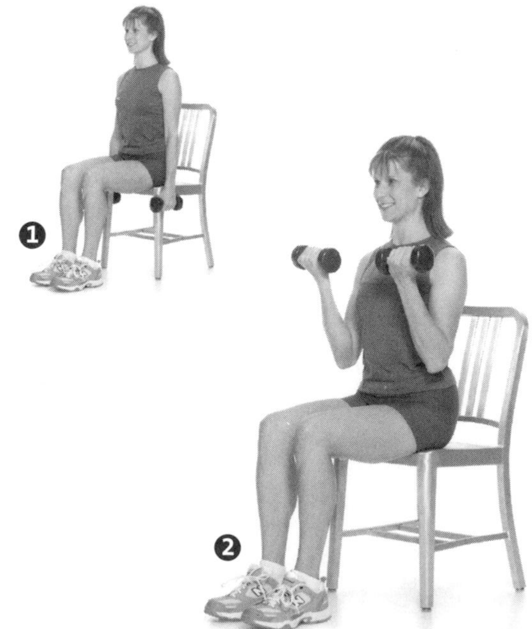

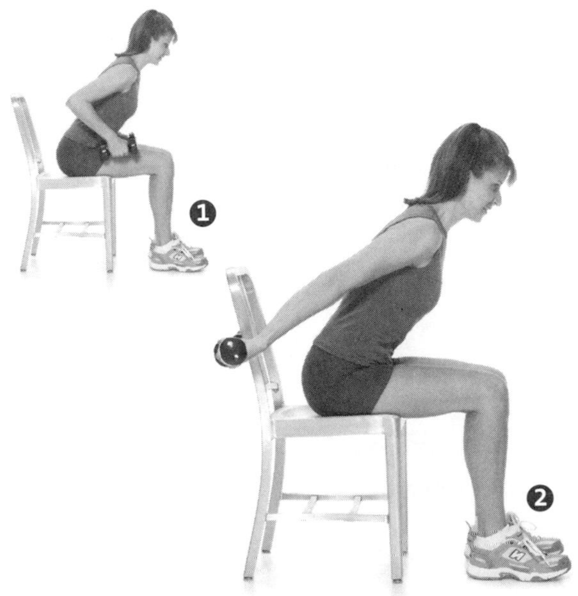

Seated Triceps Kickback with a Twist

Starting position: Sit on the edge of a chair with your feet hip width apart and hold a dumbbell in each hand. Keep your back flat and lean forward, bending at the hips. Bend your arms at about 90-degree angles with your dumbbells at about hip height.

Movement: Without moving your upper arms, press the dumbbells back as you exhale, extending your arms and turning your wrists so that your palms face the ceiling. Hold for a second and then inhale as you slowly lower them.

Technique: Don't move from your shoulders. Don't raise your torso as you lift the dumbbells.

Alternate move: If you have back problems, do the kickbacks one arm at a time and place the forearm of your other arm across your thighs for extra support.

Lateral Raise

Starting position: Stand with your feet shoulder width apart, knees bent slightly. Hold a dumbbell in each hand with your arms at your sides, palms facing in, and elbows bent slightly.

Movement: Exhale as you slowly raise the dumbbells out to the sides until they are at about shoulder height. Hold for a second and then inhale as you slowly lower them.

Technique: Don't lift your shoulders. Don't lift higher than shoulder height.

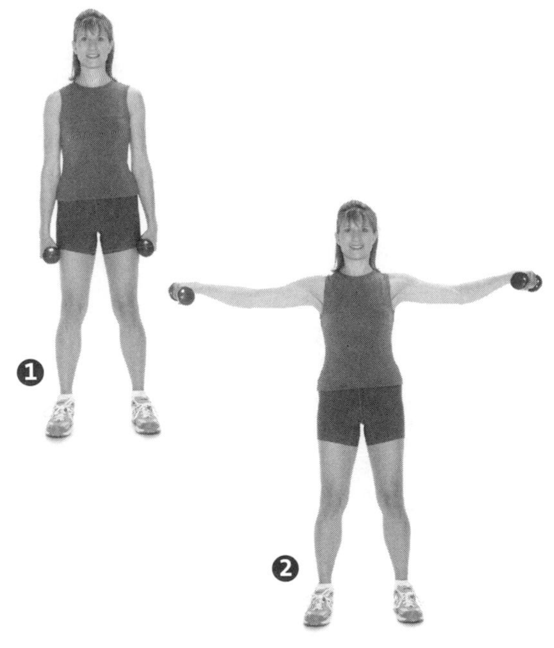

The Workout

Level 2

Easy Walk: 40 Minutes

- 5-minute warmup: Walk 2½ to 3 miles per hour, or 100 to 115 steps per minute.
- 30-minute moderate walk: Increase your speed to 3 to 3½ miles per hour, 115 to 125 steps per minute, or a pace that lets you comfortably carry on a conversation.
- 5-minute cooldown: Slow down to 2½ to 3 miles per hour, or 100 to 115 steps per minute.

Basic Strength Training: 35 Minutes

- Do 10 to 12 reps of each exercise. Repeat the sequence of exercises three times.
- To warm up, through use lighter weights, or none at all, the first time through, and for the squat and lunge exercises, only go partway down.

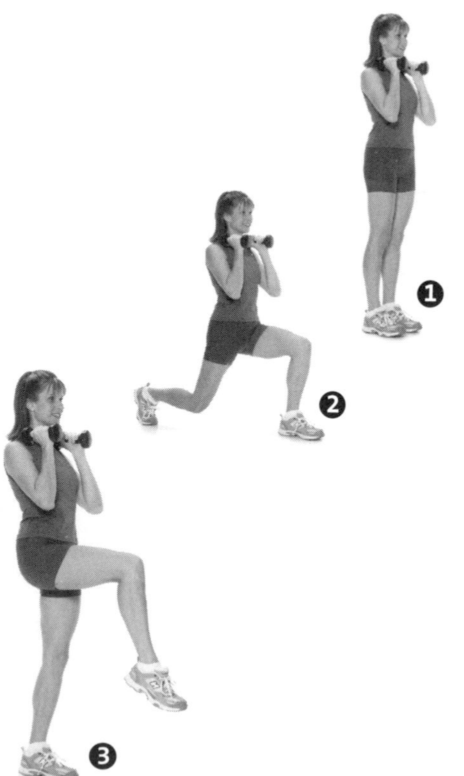

MUST-DO MOVE

Back Lunge with Knee Lift

Starting position: Stand with your feet together. Hold a dumbbell in each hand, either at shoulder height or at your sides.

Movement: Step your right foot back 2 to 3 feet. Inhale as you bend your left knee and lower your body straight down until your left knee is bent 90 degrees and your right knee nearly touches the floor. Your rear heel will come off the floor. Hold for a second and then exhale as you push yourself back up. Lift your right knee up in front of you before bringing it back to the starting position. Finish all of your repetitions, then repeat the exercise stepping back with your left foot.

Technique: Don't lean forward. Don't let your front knee move forward over your toes.

Alternate move: If this move is too challenging, try doing it without dumbbells.

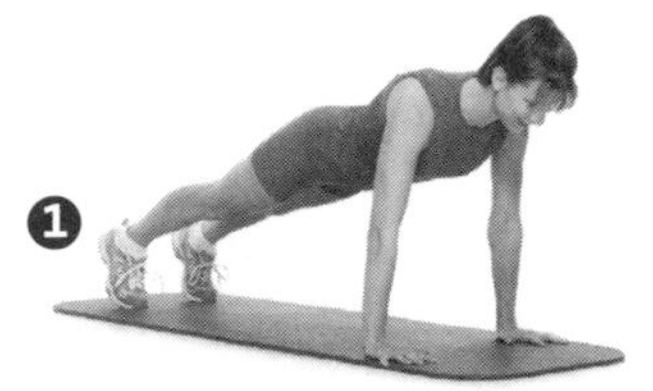

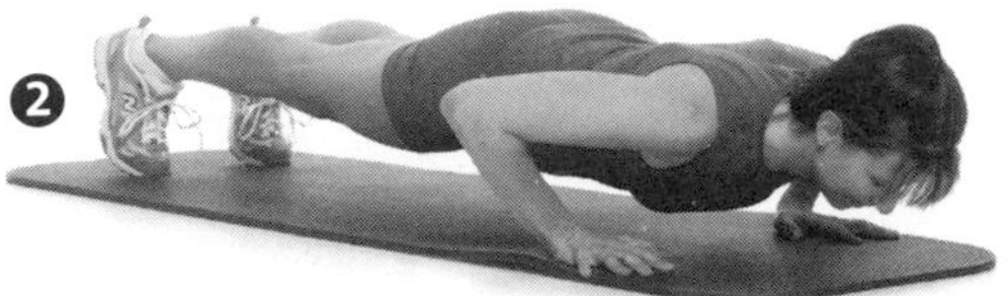

MUST-DO MOVE

Pushup

Starting position: Lie facedown on the floor with your feet flexed and toes tucked. Place your palms on the floor near your shoulders so that your elbows are pointing up. Press down with your hands, extend your arms, and lift your body off the floor so that it forms a straight line from head to toe.

Movement: Keeping your head, back, hips, and legs in a straight line, bend your elbows out to the sides and lower your body as you inhale, until your chest nearly touches the floor. Hold for a second and then exhale as you push back up. If you can't do all the recommended reps in this full pushup position, that's okay. Just drop down onto one or both knees and complete the remaining reps.

Technique: Don't bend at the hips. Don't arch your back.

MUST-DO MOVE

Bent-Over Row

Starting position: Stand with your feet shoulder width apart, knees bent slightly. Hold a dumbbell in each hand with your arms at your sides. Keep your back flat and lean forward, bending at the hips so that the dumbbells are hanging at arm's length in front of you, palms facing each other.

Movement: Bending your elbows back and squeezing your shoulder blades, lift the weights toward your ribs as you exhale, until your elbows are higher than your back. Hold for a second and then inhale as you slowly lower them.

Technique: Don't arch your back. Don't pull your shoulders up toward your ears. Don't raise your torso as you lift the dumbbells.

Alternate move: If you have back problems, support yourself with one hand on a chair and do the rows one arm at a time.

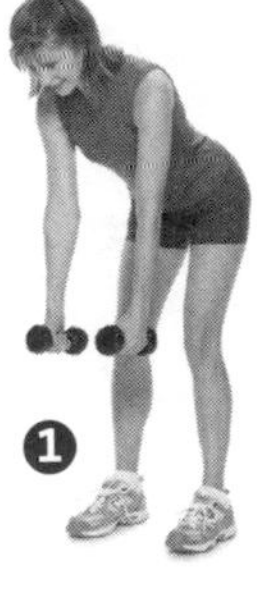

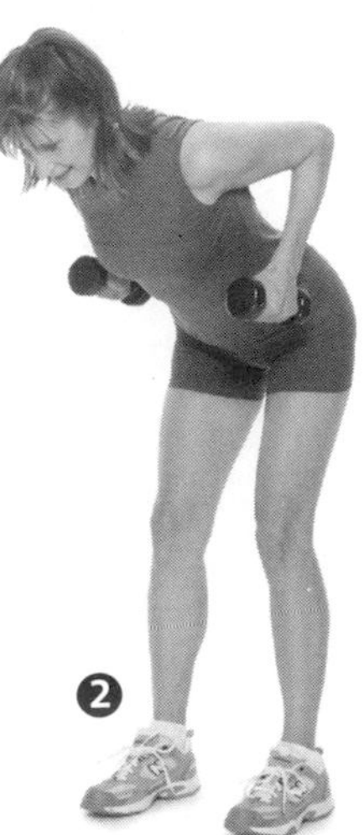

continued

The Workout

Level 2 *continued*

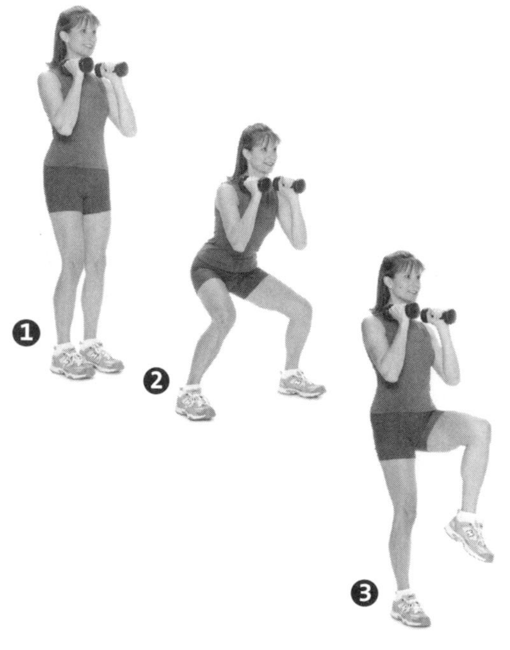

MUST-DO MOVE

Step Squat with Knee Lift

Starting position: Stand with your feet together. Hold a dumbbell in each hand, either at shoulder height or at your sides.

Movement: Step your left foot out to the side 2 to 2½ feet. Keeping your back straight, lower yourself, bending from the knees and hips as though you're sitting down, as you inhale. Stop just before your thighs are parallel to the floor. Hold for a second and then exhale as you push back up, lifting your left knee out in front of you before returning to the starting position. Do five or six reps with your left foot and then do five or six reps stepping with your right foot.

Technique: Don't let your knees move forward over your toes. Don't round your back.

Biceps Curl

Starting position: Stand with your feet shoulder width apart, knees bent slightly. Hold a dumbbell in each hand with your palms facing forward.

Movement: Bending your elbows, lift the dumbbells toward your shoulders as you exhale. Stop when the dumbbells are at chest height, palms facing your body. Hold for a second and then inhale as you slowly lower them.

Technique: Don't move your upper arms.

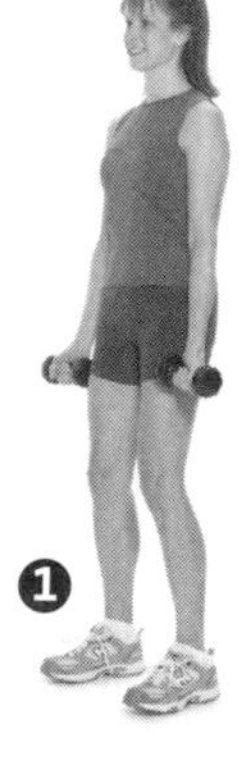

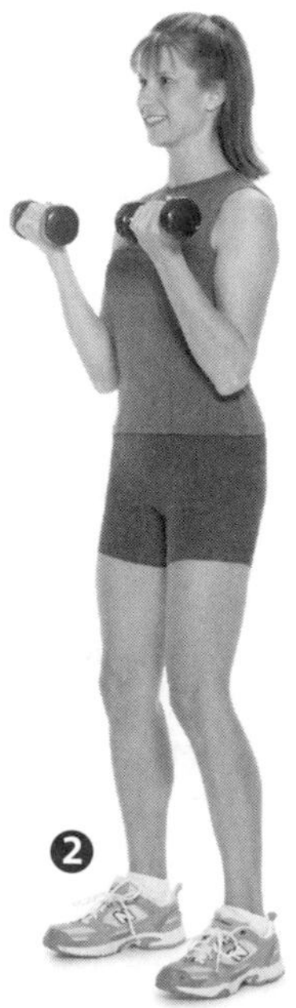

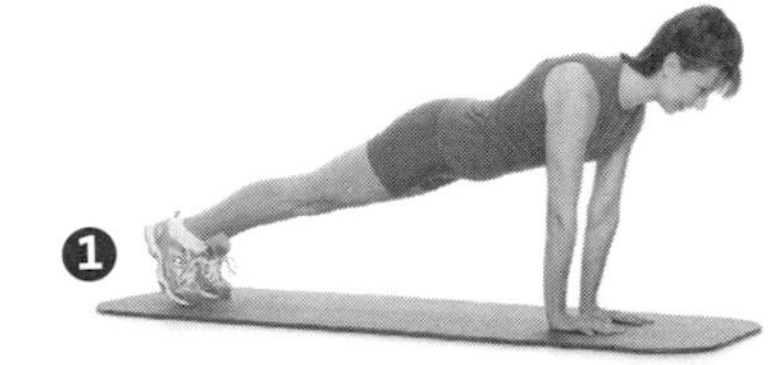

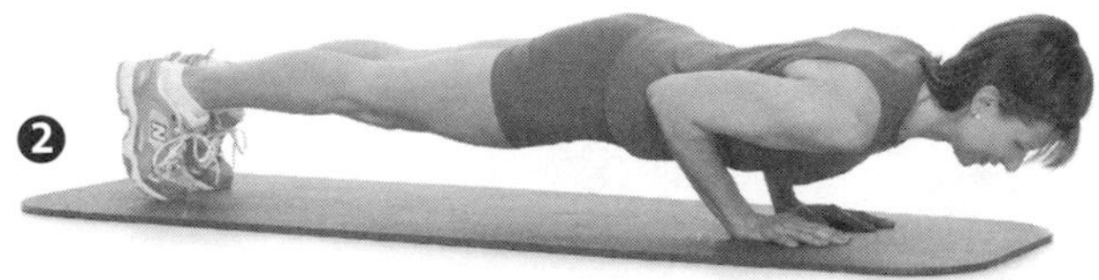

Triceps Pushup

Starting position: Lie facedown on the floor with your feet flexed and toes tucked. Place your palms on the floor close to your ribs so that your elbows are pointing up. Press down with your hands, extend your arms, and lift your body off the floor.

Movement: Keeping your head, back, hips, and legs in a straight line, bend your elbows back, keeping your arms close to your body, as you inhale. Lower your body until your chest nearly touches the floor. Hold for a second and then exhale as you push back up. If you can't do all the recommended reps in this full pushup position, that's okay. Just drop down onto one or both knees and complete the remaining reps.

Technique: Don't let your elbows point out to the sides. Don't bend at the hips. Don't drop your belly toward the floor.

Parallel Overhead Press

Starting position: Stand with your feet shoulder width apart and knees bent slightly. Hold a dumbbell in each hand at shoulder height, palms facing each other and elbows pointing forward.

Movement: Exhale as you slowly press the dumbbells straight overhead without locking your elbows. Hold for a second and then inhale as you slowly lower them.

Technique: Don't arch your back. Don't lift the dumbbells forward or back.

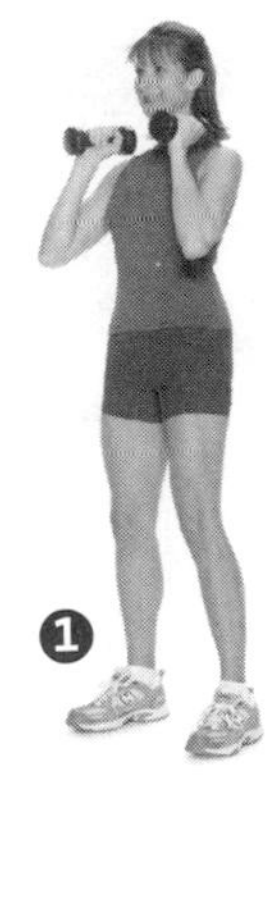

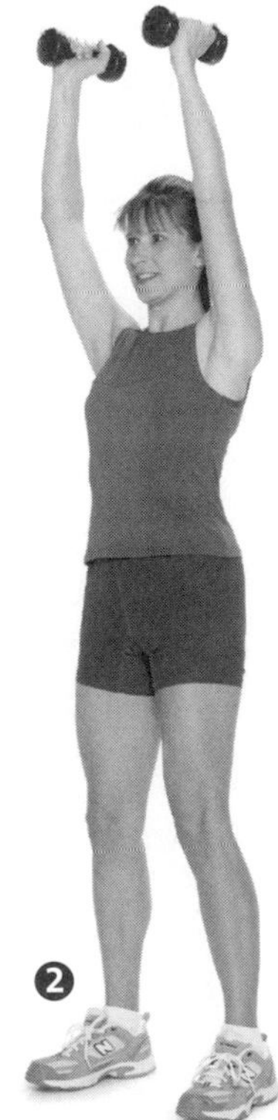

The Workout
Level 3

Easy Walk: 40 Minutes

- 5-minute warmup: Walk 2½ to 3 miles per hour or 100 to 115 steps per minute.
- 30-minute moderate walk: Increase your speed to 3½ to 4 miles per hour, 125 to 135 steps per minute, or a pace that lets you comfortably carry on a conversation.
- 5-minute cooldown: Slow down to 2½ to 3 miles per hour or 100 to 115 steps per minute.

Basic Strength Training: 35 Minutes

- Do 10 to 12 reps of each exercise. Repeat the sequence of exercises three times.
- To warm up, use lighter weights, or none at all, the first time through, and for the squat and lunge exercises, only go partway down.

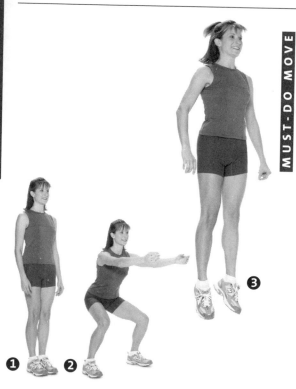

MUST-DO MOVE

Step Squat with Jump

Starting position: Stand with your feet together and your hands down at your sides.

Movement: Step your left foot out to the side 2 to 2½ feet. Keeping your back straight, lowering yourself, bending from the knees and hips as though you're sitting down, as you inhale. Let your arms come out in front of you to help you balance. Stop just before your thighs are parallel to the floor. Hold for a second and then exhale as you jump and bring your left foot back in next to your right foot. Do five or six reps with your left foot and then do five or six reps stepping with your right foot.

Technique: Don't let your knees move forward over your toes. Don't round your back. Don't do this move while holding weights.

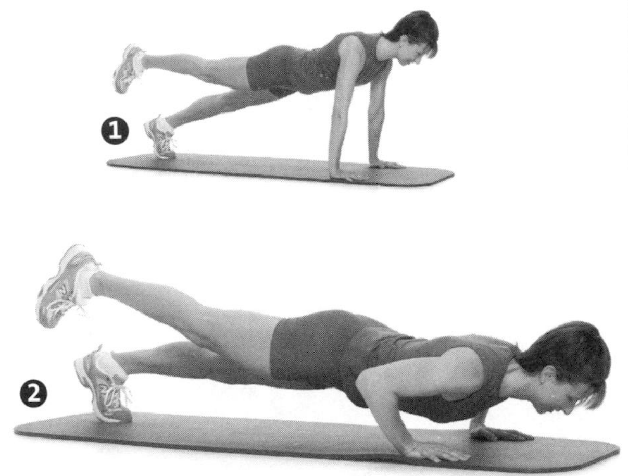

MUST-DO MOVE

One-Leg Pushup

Starting position: Lie facedown on the floor with your feet flexed and toes tucked. Place your palms on the floor near your shoulders so that your elbows are pointing up. Press down with your hands, extend your arms, and lift your body off the floor so that it forms a straight line from head to toe, and lift your right foot off the floor.

Movement: Keeping your head, back, hips, and legs in a straight line, bend your elbows out to the sides and lower your body as you inhale, until your chest nearly touches the floor. Hold for a second and then exhale as you push back up. If you can't do all the recommended reps in this full pushup position, that's okay. Just drop down onto both feet or one or both knees and complete the remaining reps. Do half of the recommended reps with your right leg off the floor and the other half with your left leg off the floor.

Technique: Don't bend at the hips. Don't arch your back.

MUST-DO MOVE

Balancing Bent-Over Row

Starting position: Stand with your right foot in front of your left. Hold a dumbbell in each hand with your arms at your sides. Keep your back flat and lean forward, lifting your back foot off the floor so that your left leg, back, and head are as parallel to the floor as possible. The dumbbells should be hanging at arm's length directly below your shoulders, palms facing each other.

Movement: Bending your elbows back and squeezing your shoulder blades, lift the weights toward your ribs as you exhale, until your elbows are higher than your back. Hold for a second and then inhale as you slowly lower them. Do half of the recommended reps balancing on your right leg and the other half on your left leg.

Technique: Don't arch your back. Don't pull your shoulders up toward your ears. Don't raise your torso as you lift the dumbbells.

Alternate move: If you have back problems, keep both legs down, support yourself with one hand on a chair, and do the rows one arm at a time.

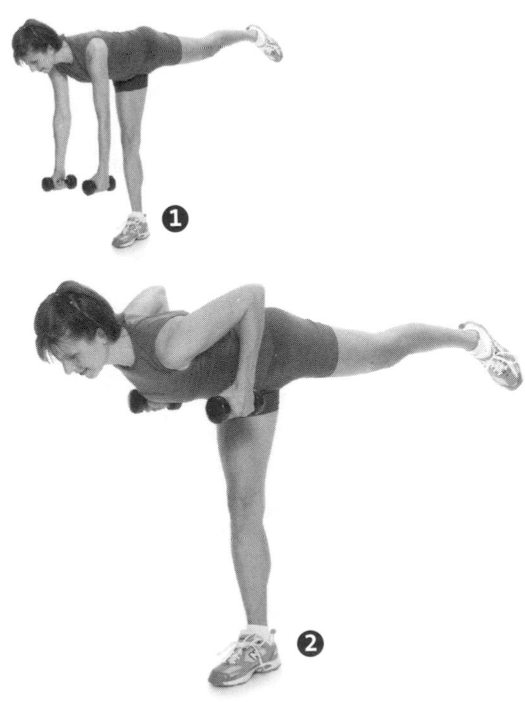

continued

The Workout

Level 3 *continued*

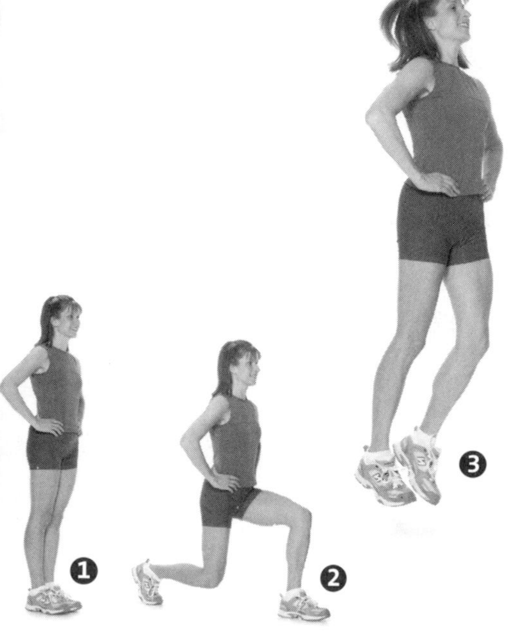

MUST-DO MOVE

Front Lunge with Jump

Starting position: Stand with your feet together and your hands on your hips.

Movement: Step your left foot forward 2 to 3 feet. Inhale as you bend your left knee and lower your body straight down until your left knee is bent 90 degrees and your right knee nearly touches the floor. Your rear heel will come off the floor. Hold for a second and then exhale as you push off with your left foot and jump your feet together. Finish all of your repetitions, then repeat the exercise stepping forward with your right foot.

Technique: Don't lean forward. Don't let your front knee move forward over your toes.

Balancing Biceps Curl

Starting position: Stand with your feet together, knees bent slightly. Hold a dumbbell in each hand with your palms facing forward. Lift your right knee up in front of you so that you're balancing on your left leg.

Movement: Bending your elbows, lift the dumbbells toward your shoulders as you exhale. Stop when the dumbbells are at chest height, palms facing your body. Hold for a second and then inhale as you slowly lower them. Do half of the recommended reps balancing on your left leg and the other half on your right leg.

Technique: Don't move your upper arms.

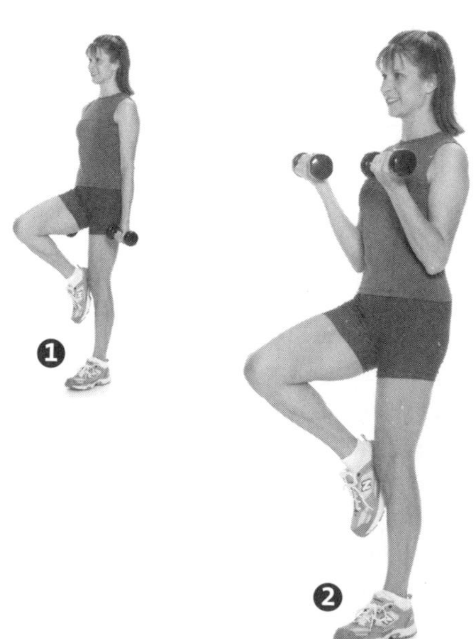

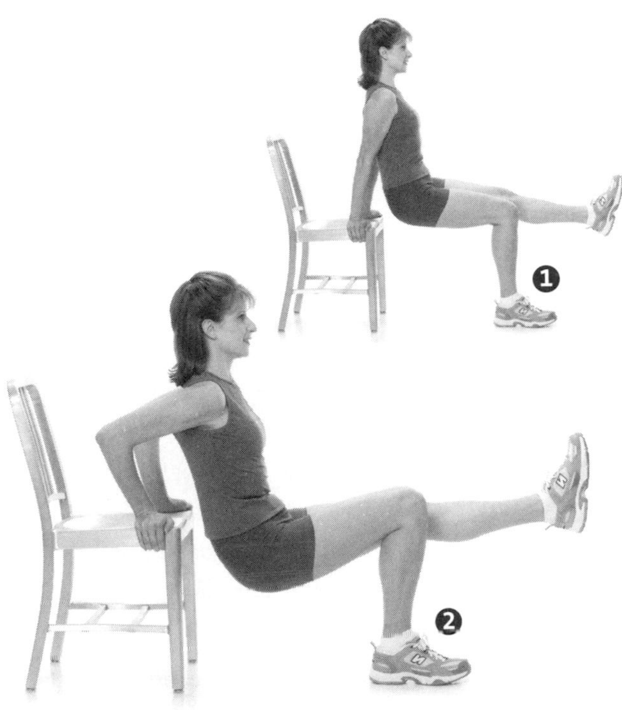

One-Leg Triceps Dip

Starting position: Sit on the edge of a chair, place your hands on either side of you, and grasp the chair seat. Slide your buttocks off the chair, walk your feet out until your legs are bent at about 90 degrees, lift your left foot off the floor, and extend your left leg. You should be balancing on your hands and right foot.

Movement: Bending your arms so that your elbows point behind you, slowly lower your body toward the floor as you inhale. Keep your buttocks as close to the chair as possible. Stop when your elbows are bent about 90 degrees. Hold for a second and then exhale as you press back up. Do half of the recommended reps with your left leg extended and the other half with your right leg extended.

Technique: Don't sink into your arms, allowing your shoulders to come up toward your ears. Don't bend your knees to help lower yourself.

Alternate move: For a more challenging version, extend your legs straight and balance on your heels.

Balancing Overhead Press

Starting position: Stand with your feet together, knees bent slightly. Hold a dumbbell in each hand at shoulder height with your palms facing forward and elbows pointing out to the sides. Lift your right knee up in front of you so that you're balancing on your left leg.

Movement: Exhale as you slowly press the dumbbells straight up overhead. Hold for a second and then inhale as you slowly lower them. Do half of the recommended reps balancing on your left leg and the other half on your right leg.

Technique: Don't arch your back. Don't lift the dumbbells forward or back.

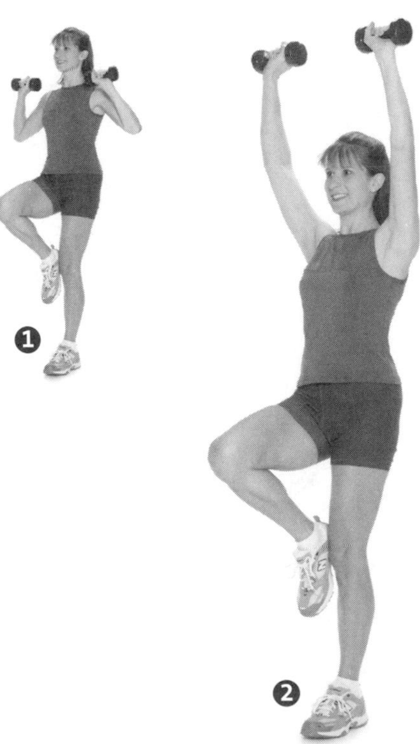

FIRM UP / DAY 16

Take Care of Your Feet

By now, you've been pounding a lot of pavement, and your feet deserve a break. If you're like most people, you probably just walk all over them. But taking them for granted for too long can have painful consequences: 75 percent of Americans get foot pain at some point, and women's feet are four times more likely to hurt. But the good news is that many of these problems are avoidable. Here's how to keep your feet happy.

- Wear appropriate shoes for the activity you are performing: well-cushioned shoes for long periods of standing and activity-specific shoes for exercise. (See chapter 10, Walk Off Pounds and Inches, for specifics on finding the right walking shoe.)
- Stick with heels no higher than ¾ inch. High heels contribute to knee and back problems, falls, and an awkward, unnatural gait. In time, they may cause enough changes in your feet to impair proper function.
- Avoid tight socks or nylons that squeeze your toes or bunch under your feet.
- Massage your feet at least once a week. Put a small, sturdy glass bottle or a golf ball on the floor and roll it under your foot, bearing down with a little pressure. (Chill the bottle or ball for added relief.) Or splurge on a professional foot massage occasionally.
- Give your toes a good stretch at the end of the day by interlacing the fingers of your right hand between the toes of your left foot. Hold for a minute or so, then switch feet.
- Exercise your feet and legs. For specific exercises, see page 401.

FIRM UP TIP

ON YOUR PLATE

Indulge at the right time. It can prevent you from eating the whole box. A recent study found that chocoholics who ate chocolate on a full stomach decreased their desire for chocolate to the level of noncravers. But desire increased in both chocolate cravers and noncravers if they ate candy bars when they were hungry. You learn to crave chocolate if you regularly use it to satisfy your hunger, explains study author Leigh Gibson, Ph.D., of the University College in London. But if you wait until 15 minutes after a meal to indulge, you can retrain your appetite and stay in control of your craving.

Meal Plan

Most of these recipes are custom designed to make 1 serving–no fuss, no muss; just fix, eat, and go! If a recipe makes more than 1 serving, it's noted below. Save that extra serving for another meal, or share it with your spouse or your walking buddy.

Breakfast

Graham Crackers and Yogurt: Spoon 4 ounces (½ cup) fat-free yogurt (any flavor) into a cereal bowl. Crumble 2 graham cracker squares (2½-inch size) over the yogurt, and add 1 tablespoon chopped almonds or walnuts. Serve with ¾ cup blueberries.

Healthy Snack

Ricotta Spread with English Muffin: Top ½ whole wheat English muffin with ⅓ cup ricotta cheese spread from last week.

Lunch

Chili Tortilla: Warm 1 whole wheat tortilla. Top with ¾ cup vegetarian chili (such as Natural Touch Low-Fat Vegetarian Chili), 1 tablespoon light sour cream, and ⅛ cup shredded reduced-fat cheese. Serve with ¾ cup fat-free milk.

Healthy Snack

Apples with Peanut Butter: Cut up 1 small apple and top with 2 teaspoons peanut butter. Serve with 1 cup fat-free milk.

Dinner

Apricot Chicken in the Slow Cooker: Makes 4 servings. Pour ½ cup apple juice and ½ cup water into a slow cooker. Place 4 frozen 4-ounce boneless chicken breasts (one 4-ounce frozen breast is slightly larger than the size of a deck of cards) into the slow cooker. In a small bowl, mix together ¼ cup all-fruit-style apricot jelly with ¼ cup Russian dressing and 1 teaspoon onion powder. Top the chicken breasts with the mixture. Cook on low for 5 to 6 hours. Serve each piece of chicken over ⅔ cup cooked rice or 1 cup cooked pasta.

Indulgent Treat

Little Debbie Snack: Treat yourself to 1 Little Debbie Brownie Lights brownie.

Nutrient analysis: 1,627 calories, 95 g protein, 224 g carbohydrates, 42 g total fat, 12 g saturated fat, 106 mg cholesterol, 45 g dietary fiber, 1,979 mg sodium, 1,977 mg calcium

FIRM UP TIP

FIT FACT

One in four cereal eaters in a recent survey admitted to leaving the milk—and vital nutrients—behind in the bowl. Vitamins added to cereal are sprayed on during processing, so they dissolve in the milk. If you don't drink it all, they go down the drain—along with the milk's calcium and vitamin D.

The Workout

Level 1

Interval Walk: About 30 Minutes

- 5-minute warmup: Walk 2 to 2½ miles per hour, 95 to 100 steps per minute.
- 3-minute moderate pace: Increase your speed to about 3 miles per hour, about 115 steps per minute.
- 1-minute speedup: Pick up your pace even more to about 3½ miles per hour, about 125 steps per minute.
- Repeat moderate pace/speedup sequence five times.
- 5-minute cooldown: Slow down to 2 to 2½ miles per hour, 95 to 100 steps per minute.

Core Training: 20 Minutes

- Do the sequence of exercises one time.

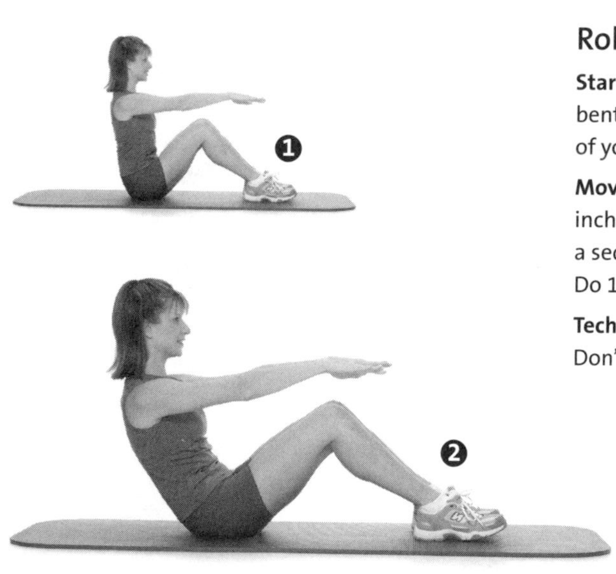

Roll-Down

Starting position: Sit on the floor with your knees bent and your feet flat. Hold your arms out in front of you, parallel to the floor.

Movement: Using your abs, slowly roll down 3 to 4 inches, one vertebra at a time, as you inhale. Hold for a second and then exhale as you slowly roll back up. Do 12 reps.

Technique: Your abs should be powering the move. Don't move quickly.

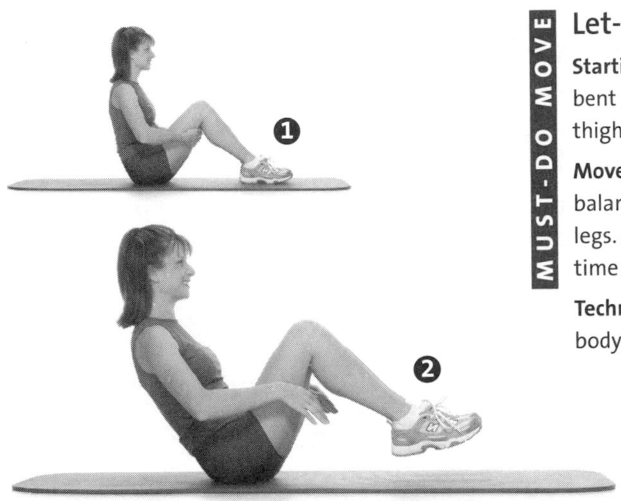

MUST-DO MOVE

Let-Go Balance

Starting position: Sit on the floor with your knees bent and your feet flat. Place your hands behind your thighs.

Movement: Lift your feet off the floor slightly and balance on your sitting bones. Try letting go of your legs. Hold for five breaths and then relax. Do one time only.

Technique: Keep your abs tight and the rest of your body relaxed, especially your shoulders.

Ab Crunch

Starting position: Lie on your back with your knees bent, feet flat on the floor, and hands behind your head.

Movement: Using your abs, slowly raise your head, shoulders, and upper back about 45 degrees off the floor as you exhale. Think of shortening the distance between your ribs and pelvis. Hold for a second and then inhale as you slowly lower yourself. Do 12 reps.

Technique: Don't pull your chin to your chest. Don't arch your back.

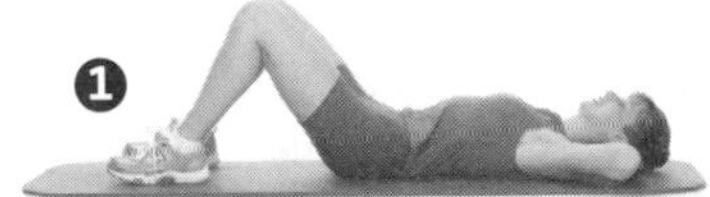

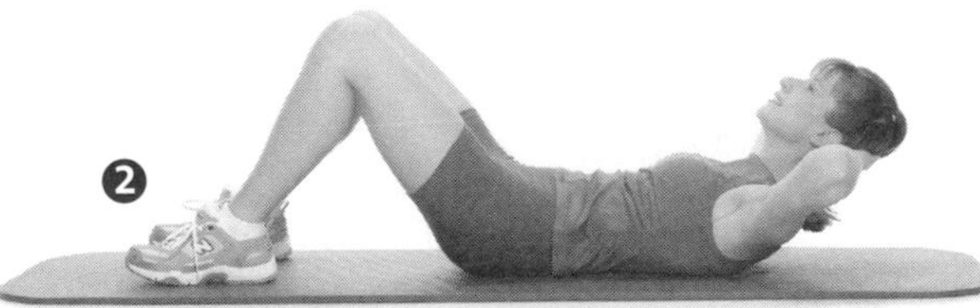

continued

The Workout

Level 1 *continued*

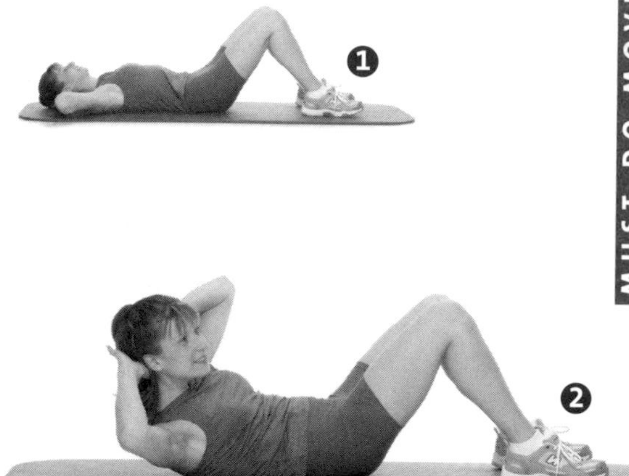

MUST-DO MOVE

Twisting Crunch

Starting position: Lie on your back with your knees bent, feet flat on the floor, and hands behind your head.

Movement: Using your abs, slowly lift your head and left shoulder off the floor, twist to the right, and bring your left shoulder toward your right knee as you exhale. Hold for a second and then inhale as you slowly lower yourself. Repeat, alternating sides. Do a total of 12 reps, 6 reps to each side.

Technique: Don't pull your chin to your chest. Don't arch your back.

MUST-DO MOVE

Bridge with Lift

Starting position: Lie on your back with your knees bent, feet flat on the floor, and arms at your sides, palms facing up.

Movement: Contracting your abs, buttocks, and lower back, press into your feet and lift your butt, hips, and back off the floor as you exhale, to form a straight line from your shoulders to your knees. Lift one foot a few inches off the floor. Hold for three breaths and then lower your foot. Lift the other foot up and hold for three breaths. Lower your foot and then relax. Do one time only.

Technique: Don't lift too high—your upper back and shoulders should remain on the floor. Don't bend at the waist or hips. Don't let your knees fall inward or outward.

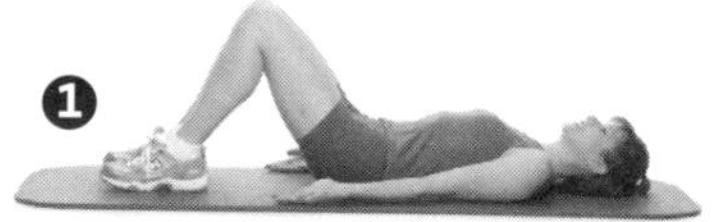

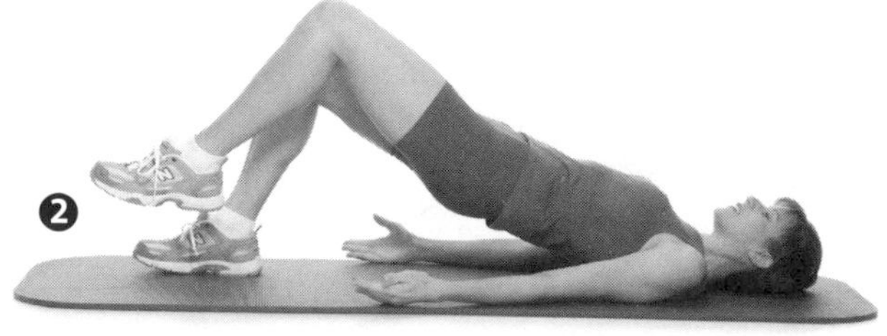

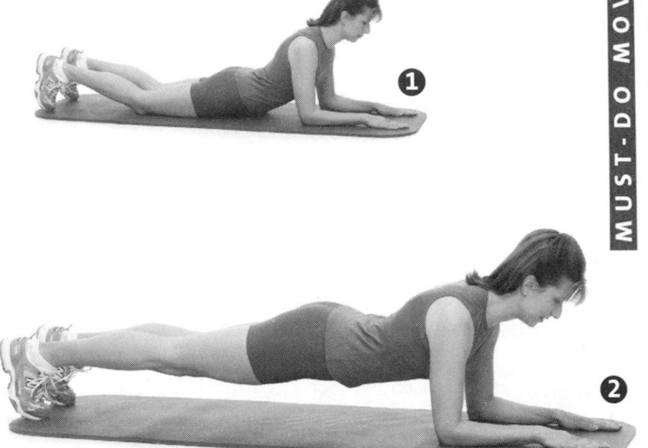

MUST-DO MOVE

Plank

Starting position: Lie facedown with your feet flexed and toes tucked. Your elbows should be under your shoulders and your forearms and palms on the floor.

Movement: Contracting your abs and back, press into your forearms as you exhale and lift your pelvis and legs off the floor so that your back and legs form a straight line. Hold for five breaths and then relax. Do one time only.

Technique: Don't lift your head up or let it drop. Don't bend at the waist or hips. Don't let your belly drop toward the floor.

Chest and Leg Lift

Starting position: Lie facedown on the floor with your arms at your sides.

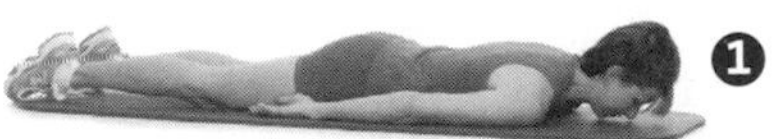

Movement: Exhale as you lift your head, chest, and legs 5 to 10 inches off the floor. Hold for a second and then inhale as you slowly lower yourself. Do 12 reps.

Technique: Don't lift too high.

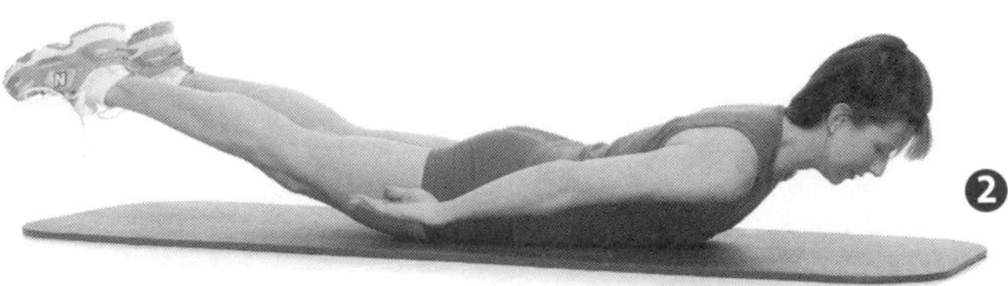

The Workout

Level 2

Interval Walk: About 30 Minutes

- 5-minute warmup: Walk 2½ to 3 miles per hour, 100 to 115 steps per minute.
- 4-minute moderate pace: Increase your speed to about 3½ miles per hour, about 125 steps per minute.
- 3-minute speedup: Pick up your pace even more to about 4 miles per hour, about 135 steps per minute.
- Repeat moderate pace/speedup sequence three times.
- 5-minute cooldown: Slow down to 2½ to 3 miles per hour, 100 to 115 steps per minute.

Core Training: 20 Minutes

- Do the sequence of exercises one time.

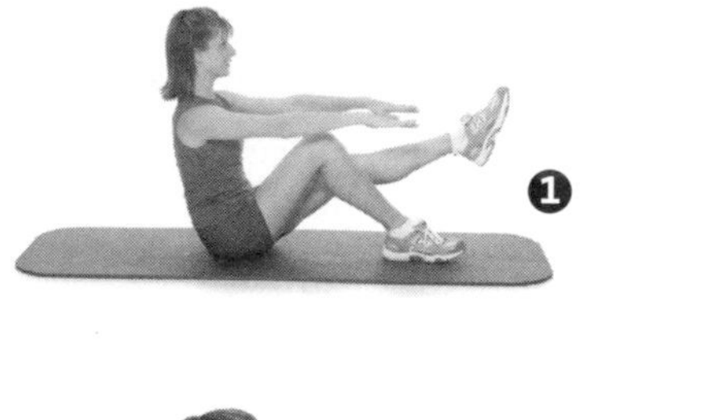

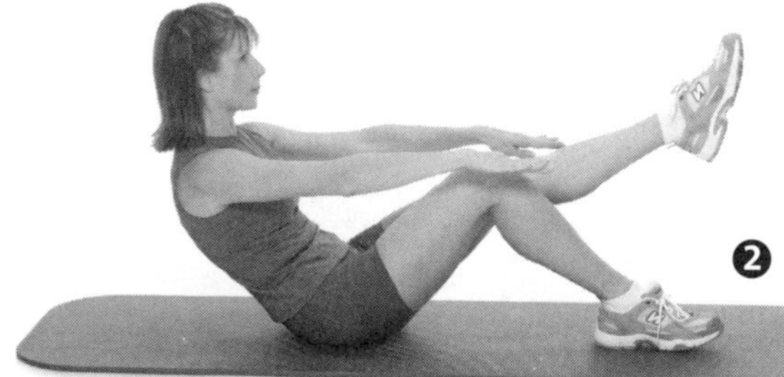

One-Leg Roll-Down

Starting position: Sit on the floor with your knees bent and your feet flat. Lift your left foot off the floor and extend your left leg. Hold your arms out in front of you, parallel to the floor.

Movement: Using your abs, slowly roll down 4 to 5 inches, one vertebra at a time, as you inhale. Hold for a second and then exhale as you slowly roll back up. Do six reps, switch legs, and do six more reps.

Technique: Your abs should be powering the move. Don't move quickly.

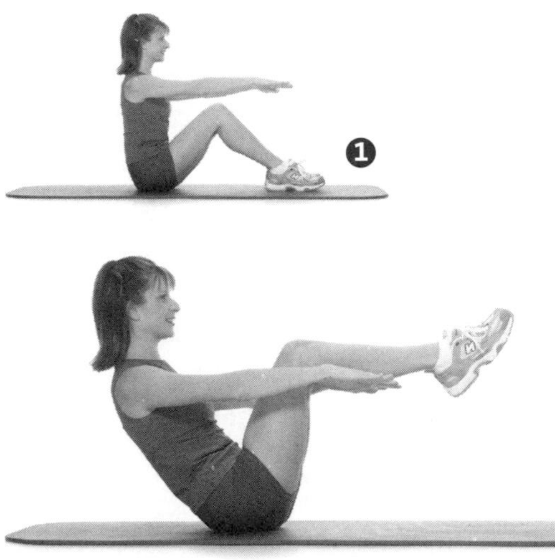

MUST-DO MOVE

Full Balance

Starting position: Sit on the floor with your knees bent and your feet flat. Hold your arms straight out in front of you, parallel to the floor.

Movement: Lift your feet so that your calves are parallel to the floor, and balance on your sitting bones. Hold for five breaths and then relax. Do one time only.

Technique: Keep your abs tight and the rest of your body relaxed, especially your shoulders.

Legs-Up Ab Crunch

Starting position: Lie on your back with your legs in the air and your hands behind your head.

Movement: Using your abs, slowly raise your head, shoulders, and upper back about 45 degrees off the floor as you exhale. Think of shortening the distance between your ribs and pelvis. Hold for a second and then inhale as you slowly lower yourself. Do 12 reps.

Technique: Don't pull your chin to your chest. Don't arch your back.

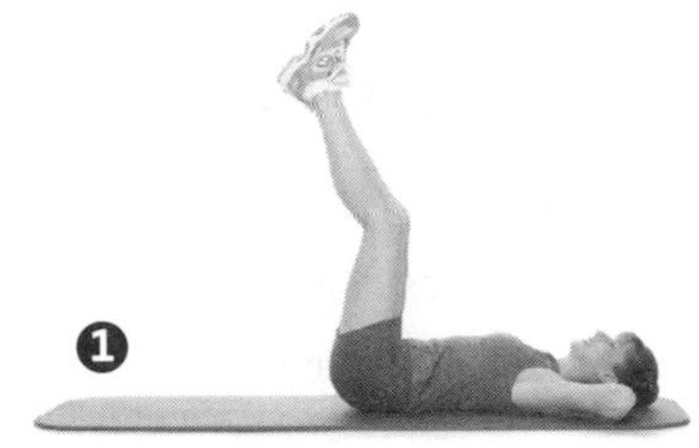

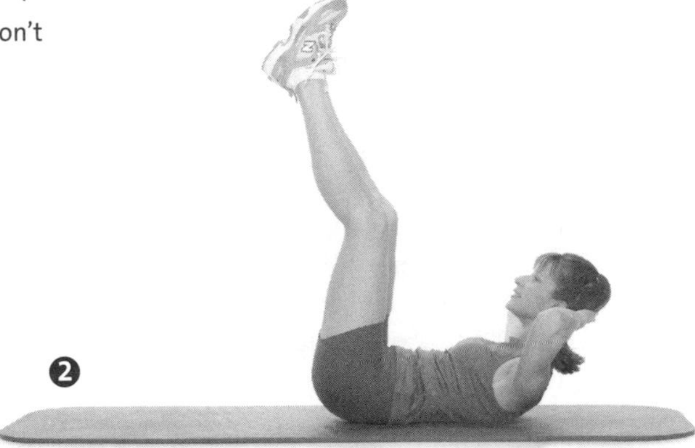

continued

The Workout

Level 2 *continued*

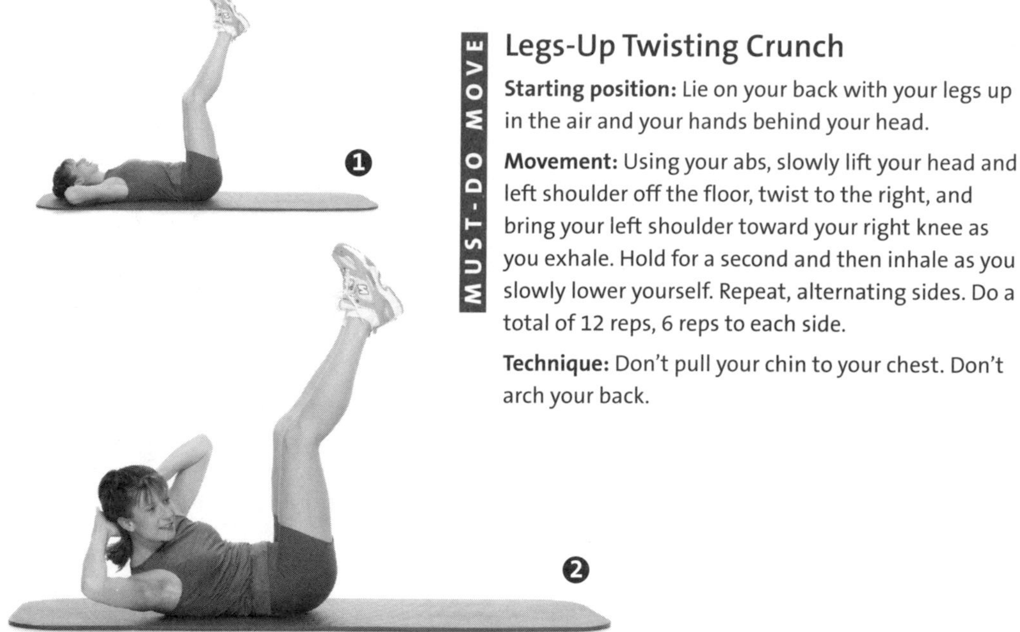

MUST-DO MOVE

Legs-Up Twisting Crunch

Starting position: Lie on your back with your legs up in the air and your hands behind your head.

Movement: Using your abs, slowly lift your head and left shoulder off the floor, twist to the right, and bring your left shoulder toward your right knee as you exhale. Hold for a second and then inhale as you slowly lower yourself. Repeat, alternating sides. Do a total of 12 reps, 6 reps to each side.

Technique: Don't pull your chin to your chest. Don't arch your back.

MUST-DO MOVE

One-Leg Heel Bridge

Starting position: Lie on your back with your knees bent, feet flat on the floor, and arms at your sides, palms facing up. Lift your toes off the floor so that only your heels are touching and then extend your right leg.

Movement: Contracting your abs, buttocks, and lower back, press into your heel and lift your butt, hips, and back off the floor as you exhale, to form a straight line from your shoulders to your knees. Slowly lower your buttocks toward the floor and then lift back up. Do six lifts, hold for three breaths, and then relax. Repeat with the opposite leg extended. Do one time only.

Technique: Don't lift too high—your upper back and shoulders should remain on the floor. Don't bend at the waist or hips. Don't let your knees fall inward or outward.

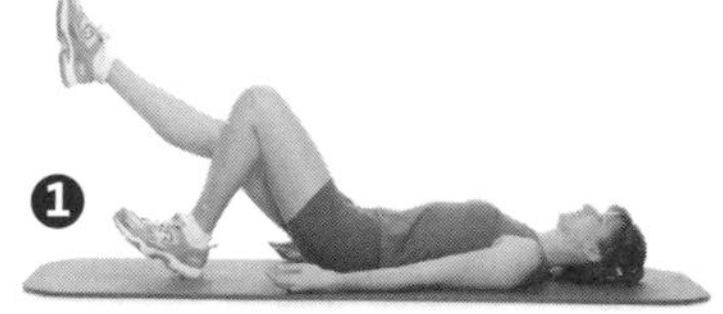

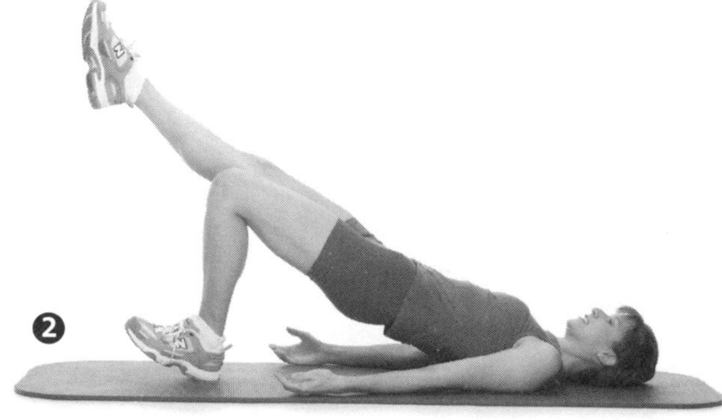

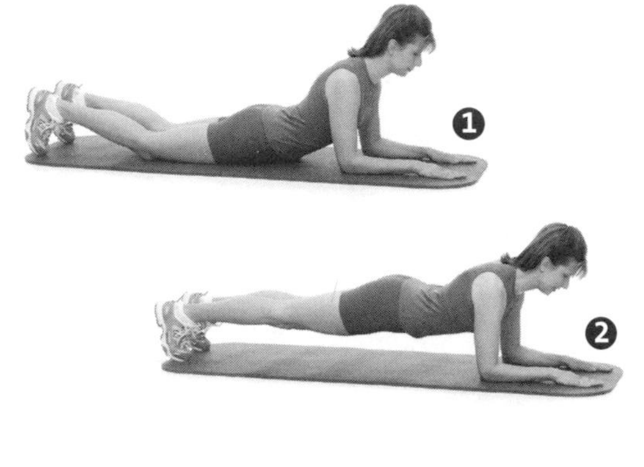

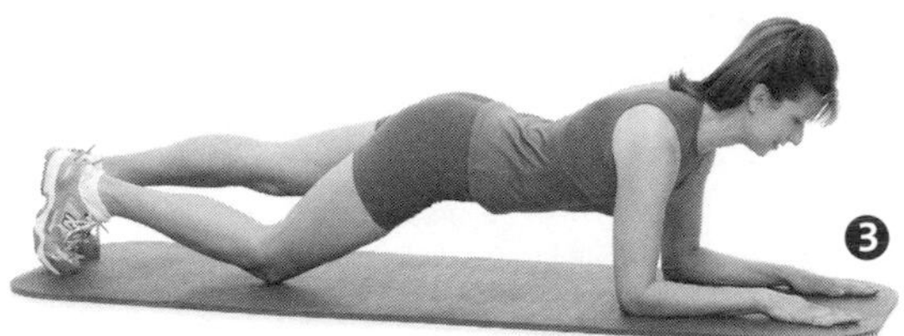

MUST-DO MOVE

Plank with Knee Drop

Starting position: Lie facedown with your feet flexed and toes tucked. Your elbows should be under your shoulders and your forearms and palms on the floor.

Movement: Contracting your abs and back, press into your forearms as you exhale and lift your pelvis and legs off the floor so that your back and legs form a straight line. Slowly drop your right knee toward the floor and then straighten. Do six knee touches with your right leg, hold for three breaths, do six knee touches with your left leg, hold for three breaths, and then relax. Do one time only.

Technique: Don't lift your head up or let it drop. Don't bend at the waist or hips. Don't let your belly drop toward the floor.

Chest Lift with a Twist

Starting position: Lie facedown on the floor with your hands under your chin.

Movement: Exhale as you lift your head and chest 5 to 6 inches off the floor and twist slightly to the right. Hold for a second and then inhale as you slowly lower. Do 12 reps, alternating sides for the twists.

Technique: Don't lift too high.

Alternate move: If this is too challenging or you have back problems, skip the twist and do only the lift.

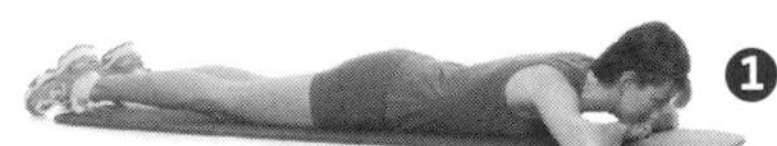

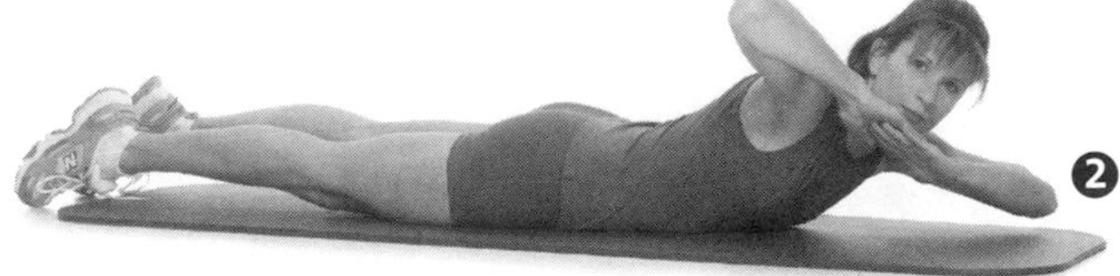

The Workout
Level 3

Interval Walk: About 30 Minutes

- 5-minute warmup: Walk 2½ to 3 miles per hour, 100 to 115 steps per minute.
- 1-minute moderate pace: Increase your speed to about 4 miles per hour, about 135 steps per minute.
- 3-minute speedup: Pick up your pace even more to about 4½ miles per hour, about 145 steps per minute.
- Repeat moderate pace/speedup sequence five times.
- 5-minute cooldown: Slow down to 2½ to 3 miles per hour, 100 to 115 steps per minute.

Core Training: 20 Minutes

- Do the sequence of exercises one time.

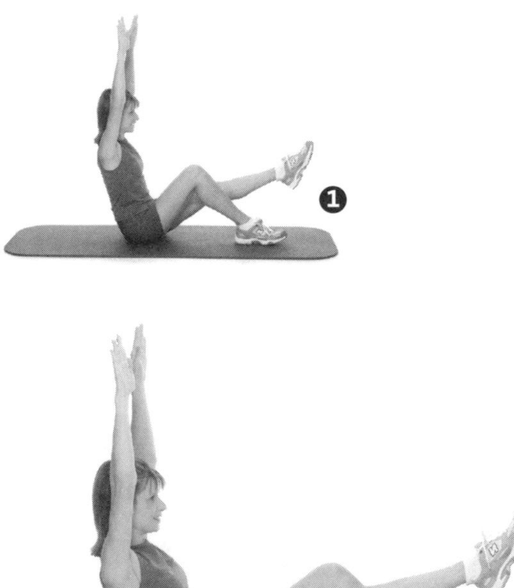

Extended One-Leg Roll-Down

Starting position: Sit on the floor with your knees bent and your feet flat. Lift your left foot off the floor and extend your left leg. Hold your arms up overhead.

Movement: Using your abs, slowly roll down 5 to 6 inches, one vertebra at a time, as you inhale. Hold for a second and then exhale as you slowly roll back up. Do six reps; then switch legs and do six more reps.

Technique: Your abs should be powering the move. Don't move quickly.

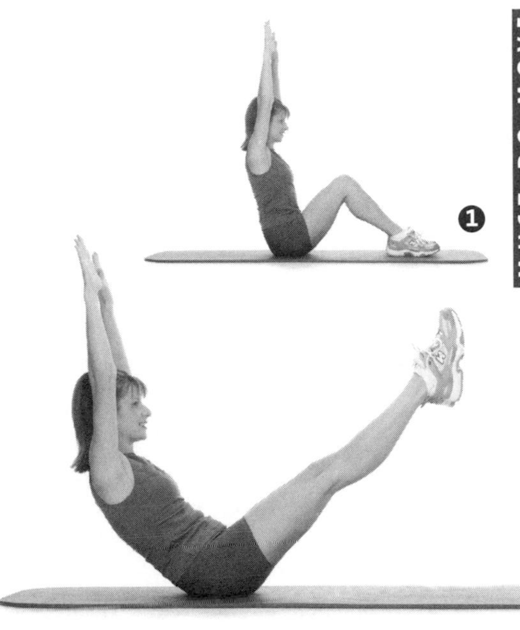

MUST-DO MOVE

Fully Extended Balance

Starting position: Sit on the floor with your knees bent and your feet flat. Hold your arms up overhead.

Movement: Lift your feet off the floor, extending your legs straight, and balance on your sitting bones. Hold for five breaths and then relax. Do one time only.

Technique: Keep your abs tight and the rest of your body relaxed, especially your shoulders.

Reverse Crunch

Starting position: Lie on your back with your legs up in the air and your hands behind your head. Cross your legs at the shins.

Movement: Slowly contract your abs as you exhale, and press your back into the floor, tilting your pelvis and lifting your hips 2 to 4 inches off the floor. Keep your upper body relaxed. Hold for a second and then inhale as you slowly lower. Do 12 reps.

Technique: Don't swing your legs.

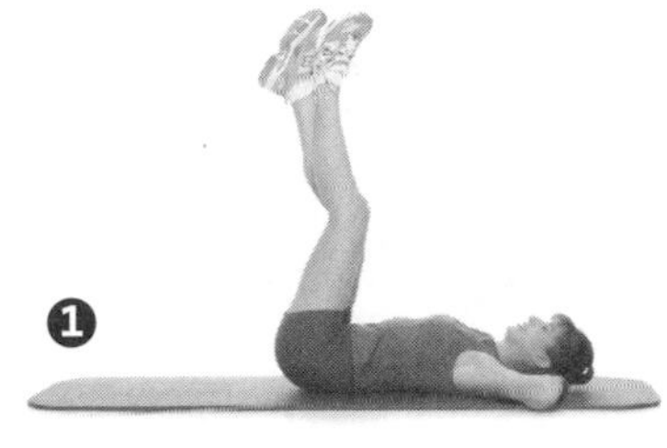

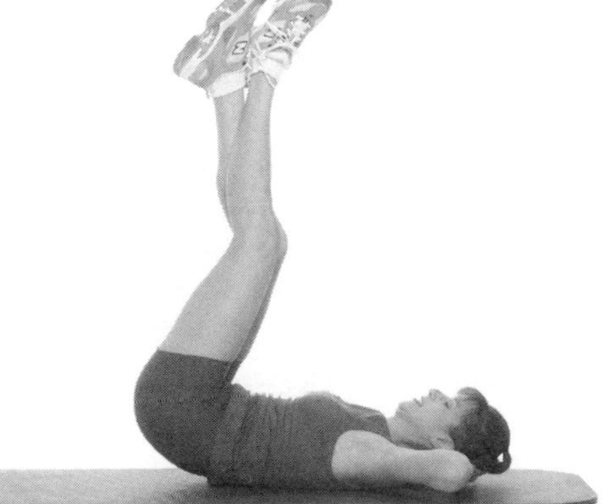

continued

The Workout

Level 3 *continued*

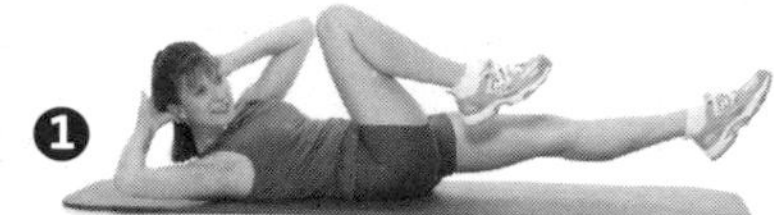

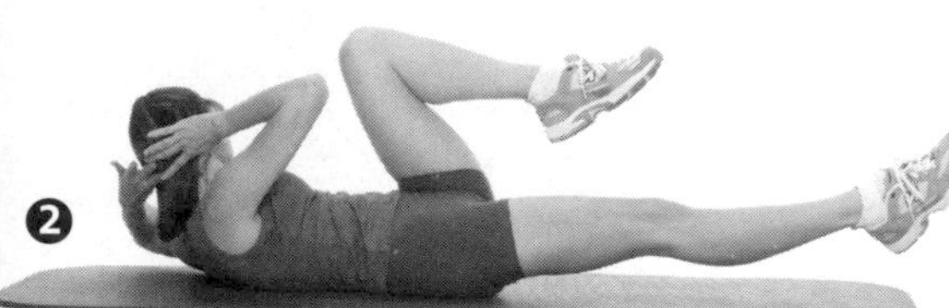

MUST-DO MOVE

Bicycle

Starting position: Lie on your back with your legs bent, feet flat on the floor, and hands behind your head. Lift your head and shoulders off the floor into a crunch position. Lift your feet off the floor, keeping your legs bent about 45 degrees.

Movement: Simultaneously, twist your left shoulder toward your right knee and bend your right knee in toward your chest while straightening your left leg. Then using a bicycle-pedaling motion, straighten your right leg while bringing the left knee in toward your chest and twisting your right shoulder to the left. That's 1 rep; do 12 reps.

Technique: Don't pull your chin to your chest. Don't arch your back.

MUST-DO MOVE

One-Leg Heel Bridge with Arms Up

Starting position: Lie on your back with your knees bent, feet flat on the floor, and arms extended over your chest. Lift your toes off the floor so that only your heels are touching, and then extend your right leg.

Movement: Contracting your abs, buttocks, and lower back, press into your heel and lift your butt, hips, and back off the floor as you exhale, to form a straight line from your shoulders to your knees. Slowly lower your buttocks toward the floor and then lift back up. Do six lifts, hold for three breaths, and then relax. Repeat with the opposite leg extended. Do one time only with each leg.

Technique: Don't lift too high—your upper back and shoulders should remain on the floor. Don't bend at the waist or hips. Don't let your knees fall inward or outward.

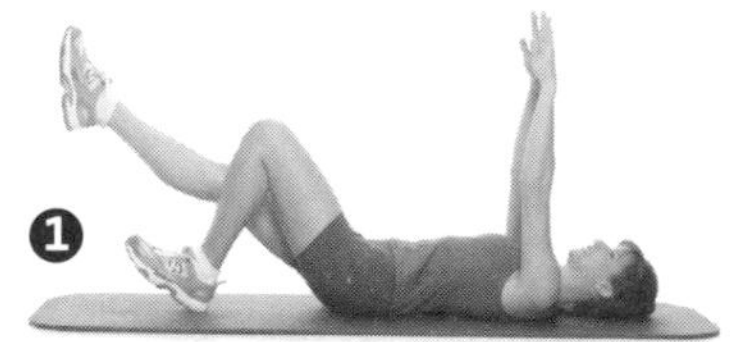

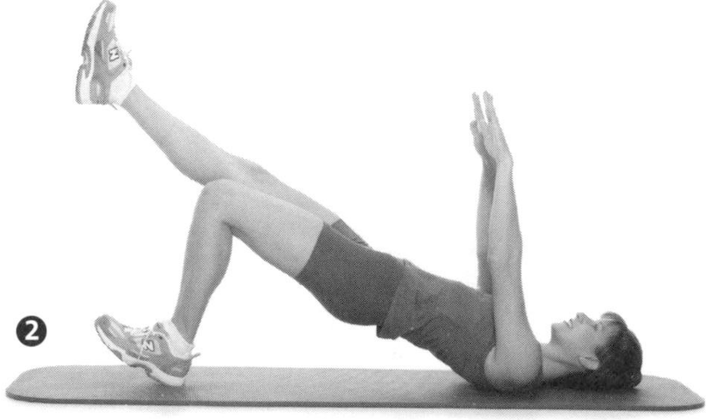

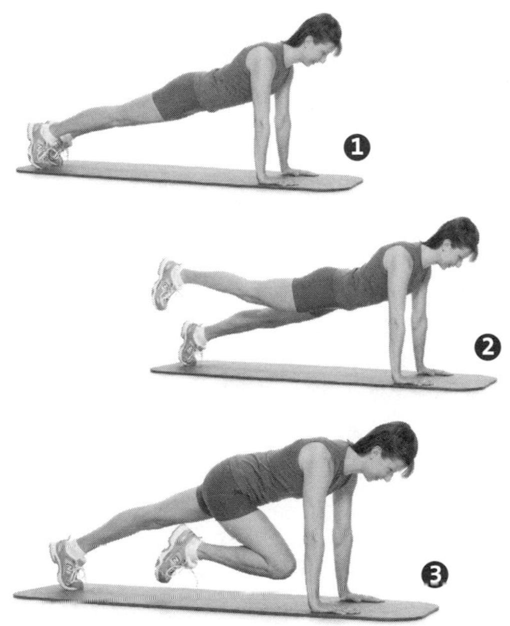

MUST-DO MOVE

Extended Plank with Lift and Bend

Starting position: Lie facedown with your feet flexed and toes tucked. Place your palms on the floor near your shoulders so that your elbows are pointing up. Contracting your abs and back, press into your hands as you exhale, straighten your arms, and lift your torso and legs off the floor so that your head, back, and legs form a straight line.

Movement: Lift your right foot off the floor and hold for three breaths. Next, pull your right knee in toward your chest and press it back out for six reps and then put that foot back on the floor. Lift your left foot off the floor and hold for three breaths. Next, pull your left knee in toward your chest and press it back out for six reps, put that foot back on the floor, and then relax. Do one time only.

Technique: Don't lift your head up or let it drop. Don't bend at the waist or hips. Don't let your belly drop toward the floor.

Swimming Chest and Leg Lift

Starting position: Lie facedown on the floor with your arms extended overhead.

Movement: Lift your arms, head, chest, and legs 5 to 10 inches off the floor. Hold as you swim your arms back to your sides and forward again, as if you were doing the breaststroke, and then slowly lower yourself. Do 12 reps.

Technique: Don't lift too high.

Alternate move: For an easier version, keep your legs down on the floor and lift only your upper body.

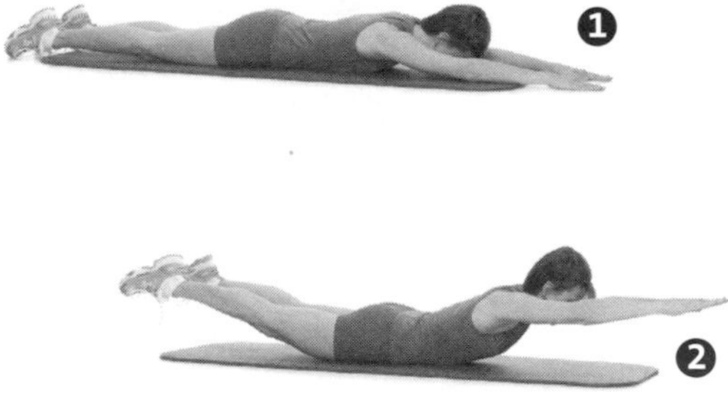

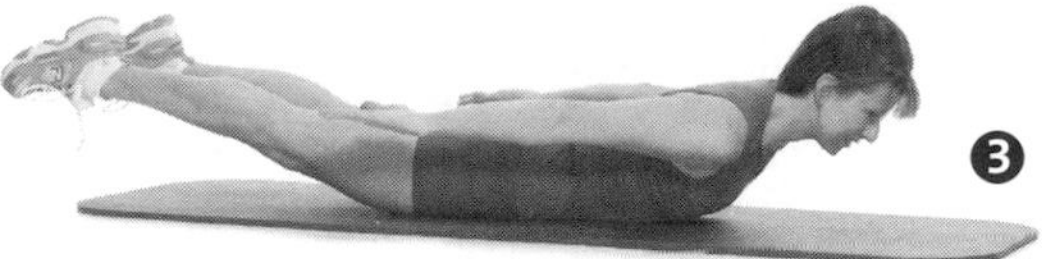

FIRM UP / DAY 17

Real-Life Success Story

For some people, back pain is a reason to stop exercising. But for Fran Mohnke, 48, of St. Johns, Michigan, it was a reason to start.

"I was in a lot of pain, taking medication, and headed for another surgery," she says. For years, she had been sedentary (though she admits that she "made it to the kitchen just fine") and gained 75 pounds.

"I had to lose weight, but as a full-time college student with a night job, I had no time," explains Fran. She began parking farther away and walking 2 to 3 miles from her car to class and back. She lost 30 pounds.

Following her final surgery, Fran had to limit impact exercise, so she started swimming. "It's changed my life," she says. "I lost an additional 35 pounds, and I'm more energetic and healthier than ever. Swimming also keeps me limber. I have much less back pain and need less medication."

FIRM UP TIPS

ON YOUR PLATE	ENERGY BOOSTER
Pick olive oil over butter. When scientists gave 341 diners at Italian restaurants equal amounts of bread and either olive oil or butter, the bread-and-butter eaters ate more slices of bread and 21 percent more calories. So besides protecting your heart, olive oil may keep you from picking the breadbasket clean.	*Eat more oats. This old-fashioned staple is one of the best energy foods around. Certain chemicals in oats are actually similar to the active ingredient in natural stimulants such as ginseng. To get the maximum benefit, try to eat a cup of oats—such as oatmeal or granola—every day.*

Meal Plan

Most of these recipes are custom designed to make 1 serving–no fuss, no muss; just fix, eat, and go! If a recipe makes more than 1 serving, it's noted below. Save that extra serving for another meal, or share it with your spouse or your walking buddy.

Breakfast

Bowl of Berries: Top ½ cup low-fat granola (such as Healthy Choice) with 2 tablespoons toasted walnuts or almonds, ¾ cup blueberries, and ¾ cup fat-free milk (drink it up if you don't use it all with the cereal).

Healthy Snack

Ricotta Spread Surprise and Chocolate Milk: Mix 1 cup cold fat-free milk with ½ tablespoon chocolate syrup. Serve with a 2½-inch graham cracker square crumbled into ⅓ cup ricotta cheese spread from last Monday.

Lunch

No-Mayo Tuna Pasta Salad: Makes 2 servings. Combine 6 ounces water-packed tuna with 4 tablespoons white wine vinegar, 2 teaspoons olive oil, 4 tablespoons finely chopped celery, ¼ cup roasted red peppers from the jar (chopped), and 1 teaspoon ground black pepper. Mix half of the tuna mixture (save the rest for Friday) with 1 cup cooked spiral pasta. Serve with 1 medium tomato, sliced and sprinkled with ground black pepper (if desired) and 1 fresh peach.

Indulgent Treat

Licorice Break: Have 1 vending-machine-size package (50 grams) red or black Twizzler licorice.

Dinner

Vegetarian Chili with Cornbread: Heat 1 cup canned vegetarian chili. Serve with a 2-inch × 3-inch piece of cornbread (about 1½ ounces or 42 grams; check your supermarket bakery department) or 1 serving Pillsbury Cornbread Twists (in refrigerated cans) and 2 cups salad greens topped with either 1 teaspoon olive oil plus ⅛ sliced avocado and 2 tablespoons balsamic vinegar or 2 tablespoons full-fat salad dressing.

Healthy Snack

Banana and Chocolate Dip: Prepare a dip using 2 tablespoons reduced-fat sour cream, ¼ teaspoon vanilla extract, and 1 tablespoon chocolate syrup. Serve with 1 sliced banana. Spear each banana slice with a toothpick for dipping.

Nutrient analysis: 1,710 calories, 60 g protein, 272 g carbohydrates, 54 g total fat, 13 g saturated fat, 46 mg cholesterol, 29 g dietary fiber, 2,148 mg sodium, 1,217 mg calcium

FIRM UP TIP

GET FIRM FASTER

Spread out your exercise. By doing a little bit every day instead of only killer workouts on the weekends, you'll reduce your risk of injury and keep your metabolism revved up.

The Workout

Level 1

Easy Walk: 40 Minutes

- 5-minute warmup: Walk 2 to 2½ miles per hour, or 95 to 100 steps per minute.
- 30-minute moderate walk: Increase your speed to 2½ to 3 miles per hour, 100 to 115 steps per minute, or a pace that lets you comfortably carry on a conversation.
- 5-minute cooldown: Slow down to 2 to 2½ miles per hour, or 95 to 100 steps per minute.

High-Rep Strength Training: 30 Minutes

- Do three reps of each exercise. Start to do another rep, but stop at the midpoint of the exercise and pulse, moving in a shorter range of motion, three times. Finish by returning to the starting position. Do this three times for each exercise and repeat the sequence of exercises three times. Use lighter weight, if needed.
- To warm up, use lighter weights, or none at all, the first time through, and for the squat and lunge exercises, only go partway down.

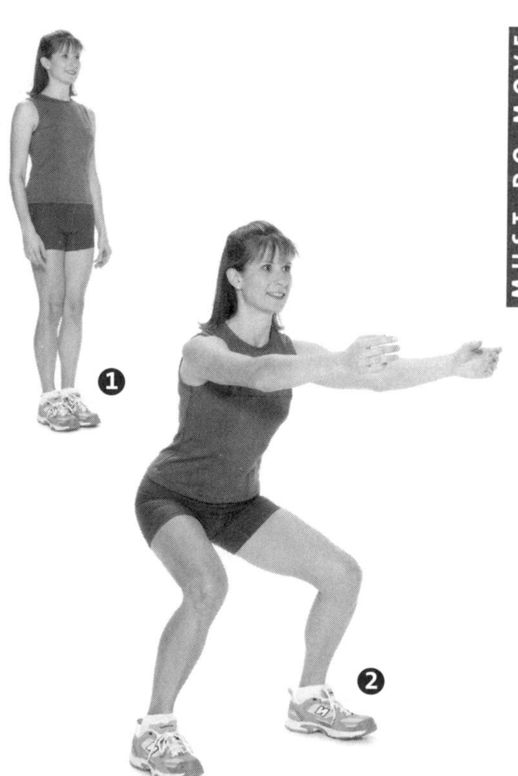

MUST-DO MOVE

Step Squat

Starting position: Stand with your feet together and your hands down at your sides.

Movement: Step your left foot out to the side 2 to 2½ feet. Keeping your back straight, lower yourself, bending from the knees and hips as though you're sitting down, as you inhale. Let your arms come out in front of you to help you balance. Stop just before your thighs are parallel to the floor. Hold for a second and then exhale as you push back up, bringing your left foot back in. Do five or six reps with your left foot and then do five or six reps stepping with your right foot.

Technique: Don't let your knees move forward over your toes. Don't round your back.

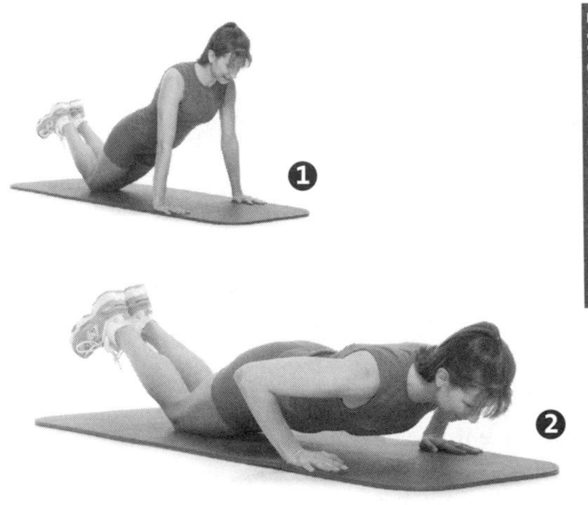

MUST-DO MOVE

Bent-Knee Pushup

Starting position: Lie facedown on the floor. Bend your knees so that your feet are up in the air, and place your palms on the floor near your shoulders so that your elbows are pointing up. Press down with your hands, extend your arms, and lift your body off the floor.

Movement: Keeping your head, back, hips, and knees in a straight line, bend your elbows out to the sides and lower your body as you inhale, until your chest nearly touches the floor. Hold for a second and then exhale as you slowly push back up.

Technique: Don't bend at the hips. Don't arch your back.

MUST-DO MOVE

Back Lunge

Starting position: Stand with your feet together. Hold a dumbbell in each hand, either at shoulder height or at your sides.

Movement: Step your left foot back 2 to 3 feet. Inhale as you bend your right knee and lower your body straight down until your right knee is bent 90 degrees and your left knee nearly touches the floor. Your rear heel will come off the floor. Hold for a second and then exhale as you push yourself back up, bringing your left foot back in. Finish all of your repetitions, then repeat the exercise stepping back with your right foot.

Technique: Don't lean forward. Don't let your front knee move forward over your toes.

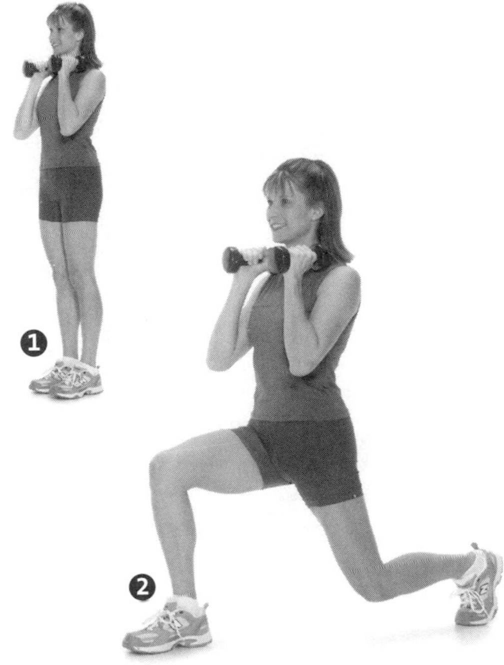

continued

The Workout

Level 1 *continued*

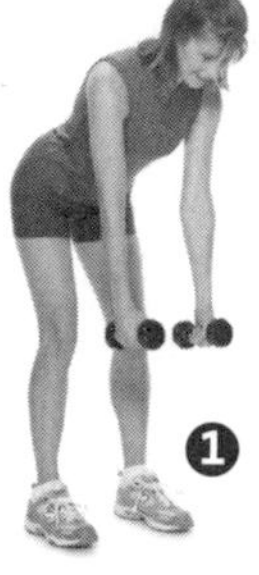

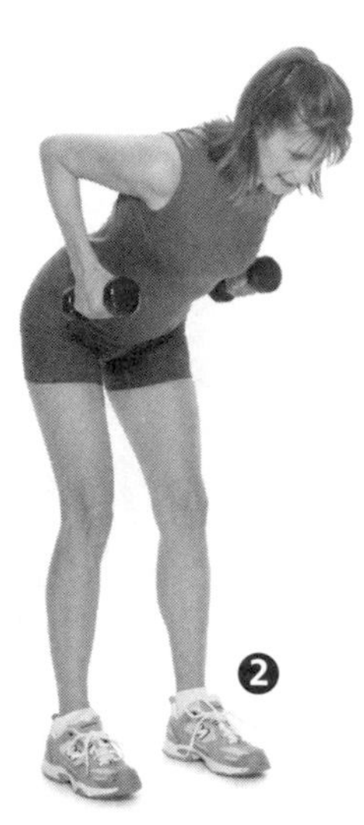

MUST-DO MOVE

Bent-Over Row

Starting position: Stand with your feet shoulder width apart, knees bent slightly. Hold a dumbbell in each hand with your arms at your sides. Keep your back flat, and lean forward, bending at the hips so that the dumbbells are hanging at arm's length in front of you, palms facing each other.

Movement: Bending your elbows back and squeezing your shoulder blades, lift the weights toward your ribs as you exhale, until your elbows are higher than your back. Hold for a second and then inhale as you slowly lower them.

Technique: Don't arch your back. Don't pull your shoulders up toward your ears. Don't raise your torso as you lift the dumbbells.

Alternate move: If you have back problems, support yourself with one hand on a chair and do the rows one arm at a time.

Seated Biceps Curl with a Twist

Starting position: Sit on the edge of a chair with your feet hip width apart. Hold dumbbells at your sides with your palms facing in.

Movement: Bending your elbows and turning your wrists upward, lift the dumbbells toward your shoulders as you exhale. Stop when the dumbbells are at chest height, palms facing your body. Hold for a second and then inhale as you slowly lower them.

Technique: Don't move your upper arms.

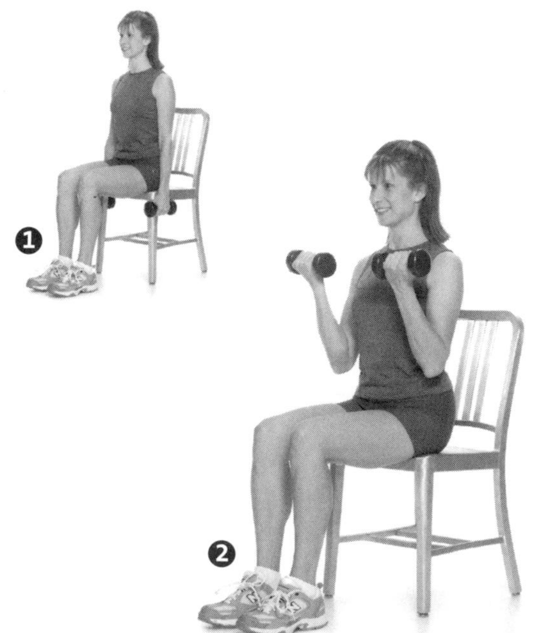

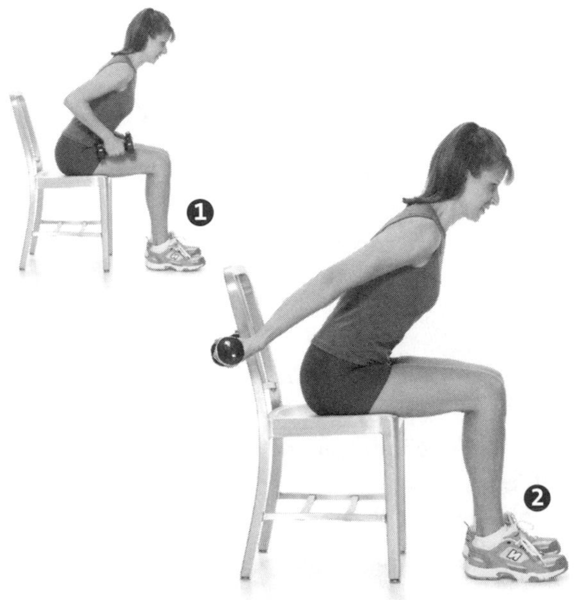

Seated Triceps Kickback with a Twist

Starting position: Sit on the edge of a chair with your feet hip width apart and hold a dumbbell in each hand. Keep your back flat and lean forward, bending at the hips. Bend your arms at about 90-degree angles with your dumbbells at about hip height.

Movement: Without moving your upper arms, press the dumbbells back as you exhale, extending your arms and turning your wrists so that your palms face the ceiling. Hold for a second and then inhale as you slowly lower them.

Technique: Don't move from your shoulders. Don't raise your torso as you lift the dumbbells.

Alternate move: If you have back problems, do the kickbacks one arm at a time and place the forearm of your other arm across your thighs for extra support.

Lateral Raise

Starting position: Stand with your feet shoulder width apart, knees bent slightly. Hold a dumbbell in each hand with your arms at your sides, palms facing in, and elbows bent slightly.

Movement: Exhale as you slowly raise the dumbbells out to the sides until they are at about shoulder height. Hold for a second and then inhale as you slowly lower them.

Technique: Don't lift your shoulders. Don't lift higher than shoulder height.

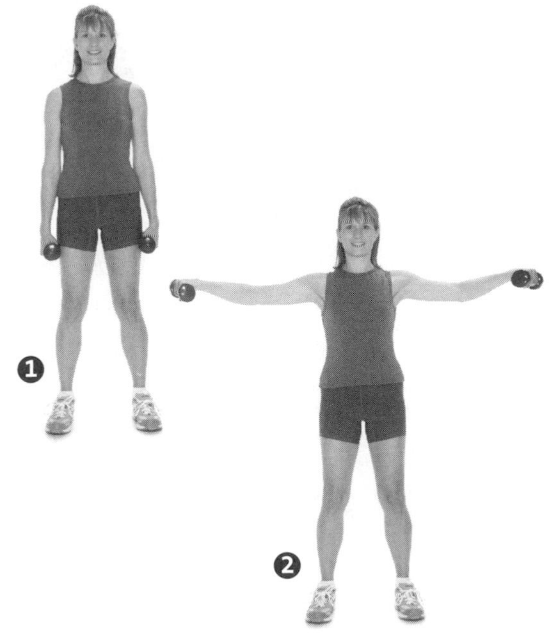

The Workout

Level 2

Easy Walk: 40 Minutes

- 5-minute warmup: Walk 2½ to 3 miles per hour, or 100 to 115 steps per minute.
- 30-minute moderate walk: Increase your speed to 3 to 3½ miles per hour, 115 to 125 steps per minute, or a pace that lets you comfortably carry on a conversation.
- 5-minute cooldown: Slow down to 2½ to 3 miles per hour, or 100 to 115 steps per minute.

High-Rep Strength Training: 30 Minutes

- Do three reps of each exercise. Start to do another rep, but stop at the midpoint of the exercise and pulse, moving in a shorter range of motion, three times. Finish by returning to the starting position. Do this three times for each exercise and repeat the sequence of exercises three times. Use a lighter weight, if needed.
- To warm up, use lighter weights, or none at all, the first time through, and for the squat and lunge exercises, only go partway down.

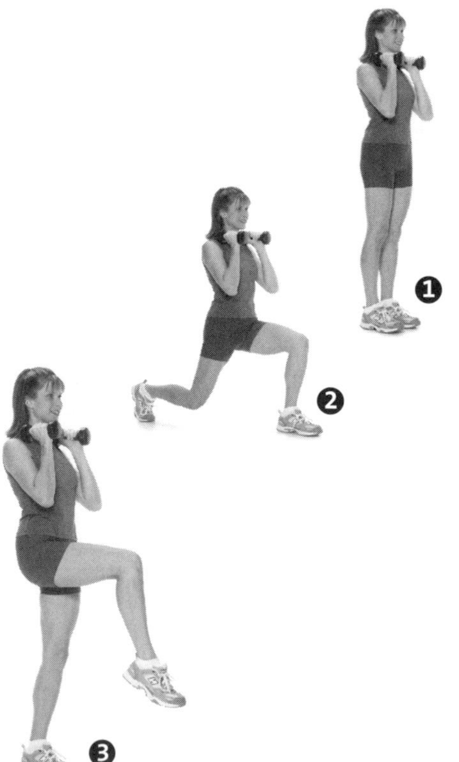

MUST-DO MOVE

Back Lunge with Knee Lift

Starting position: Stand with your feet together. Hold a dumbbell in each hand, either at shoulder height or at your sides.

Movement: Step your right foot back 2 to 3 feet. Inhale as you bend your left knee and lower your body straight down until your left knee is bent 90 degrees and your right knee nearly touches the floor. Your rear heel will come off the floor. Hold for a second and then exhale as you push yourself back up. Lift your right knee up in front of you before bringing it back to the starting position. Finish all of your repetitions, then repeat the exercise stepping back with your left foot.

Technique: Don't lean forward. Don't let your front knee move forward over your toes.

Alternate move: If this move is too challenging, try doing it without dumbbells.

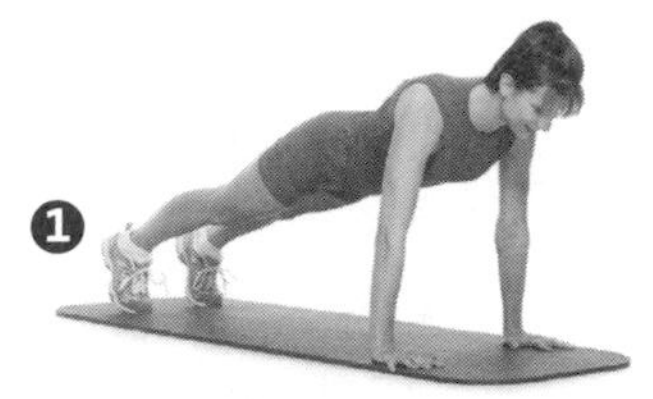

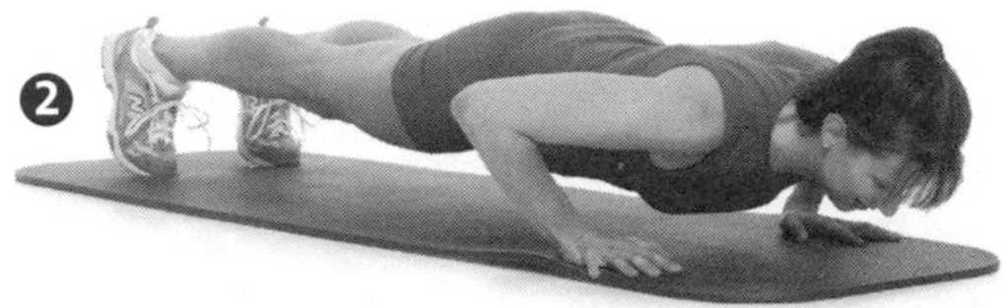

MUST-DO MOVE

Pushup

Starting position: Lie facedown on the floor with your feet flexed and toes tucked. Place your palms on the floor near your shoulders so that your elbows are pointing up. Press down with your hands, extend your arms, and lift your body off the floor so that it forms a straight line from head to toe.

Movement: Keeping your head, back, hips, and legs in a straight line, bend your elbows out to the sides and lower your body as you exhale, until your chest nearly touches the floor. Hold for a second and then exhale as you push back up. If you can't do all the recommended reps in this full pushup position, that's okay. Just drop down onto one or both knees and complete the remaining reps.

Technique: Don't bend at the hips. Don't arch your back.

MUST-DO MOVE

Bent-Over Row

Starting position: Stand with your feet shoulder width apart, knees bent slightly. Hold a dumbbell in each hand with your arms at your sides. Keep your back flat and lean forward, bending at the hips so that the dumbbells are hanging at arm's length in front of you, palms facing each other.

Movement: Bending your elbows back and squeezing your shoulder blades, lift the weights toward your ribs as you exhale, until your elbows are higher than your back. Hold for a second and then inhale as you slowly lower them.

Technique: Don't arch your back. Don't pull your shoulders up toward your ears. Don't raise your torso as you lift the dumbbells.

Alternate move: If you have back problems, support yourself with one hand on a chair and do the rows one arm at a time.

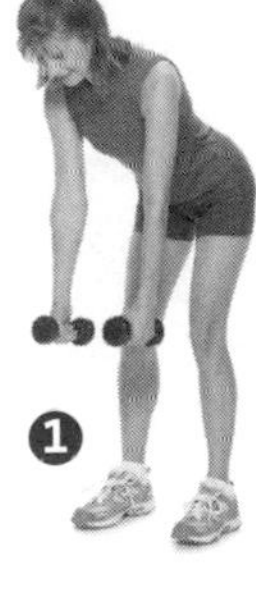

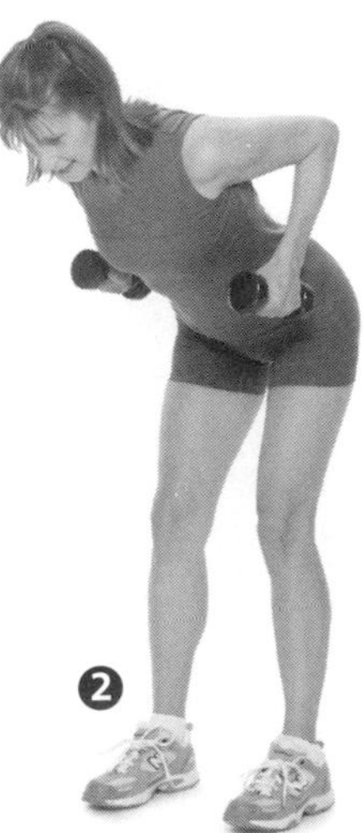

continued

The Workout

Level 2 *continued*

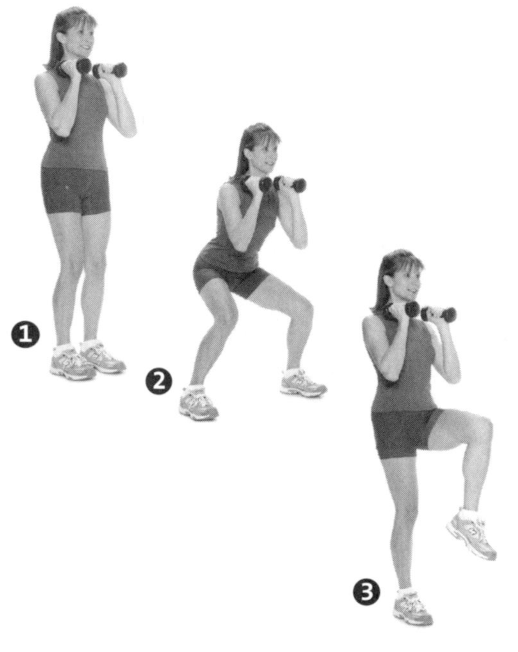

MUST-DO MOVE

Step Squat with Knee Lift

Starting position: Stand with your feet together. Hold a dumbbell in each hand either at shoulder height or at your sides.

Movement: Step your left foot out to the side 2 to 2½ feet. Keeping your back straight, lower yourself, bending from the knees and hips as though you're sitting down, as you inhale. Stop just before your thighs are parallel to the floor. Hold for a second and then exhale as you push back up, lifting your left knee out in front of you before returning to the starting position. Do five or six reps with your left foot and then do five or six reps stepping with your right foot.

Technique: Don't let your knees move forward over your toes. Don't round your back.

Biceps Curl

Starting position: Stand with your feet shoulder width apart, knees bent slightly. Hold a dumbbell in each hand with your palms facing forward.

Movement: Bending your elbows, lift the dumbbells toward your shoulders as you exhale. Stop when the dumbbells are at chest height, palms facing your body. Hold for a second and then inhale as you slowly lower them.

Technique: Don't move your upper arms.

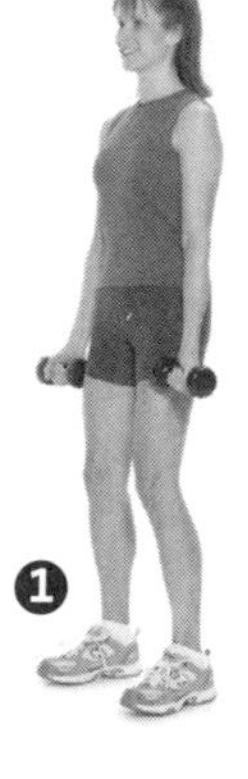

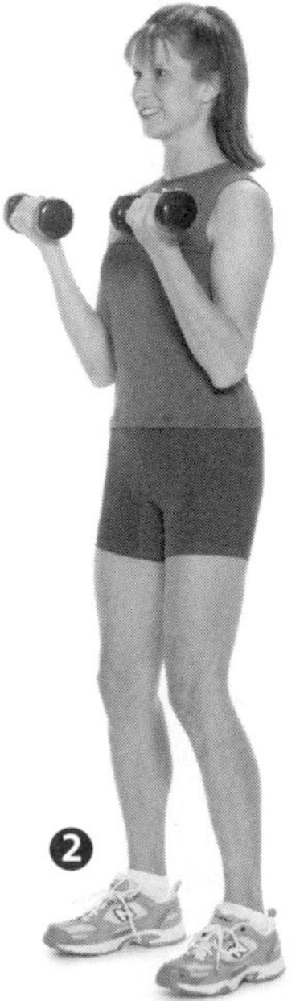

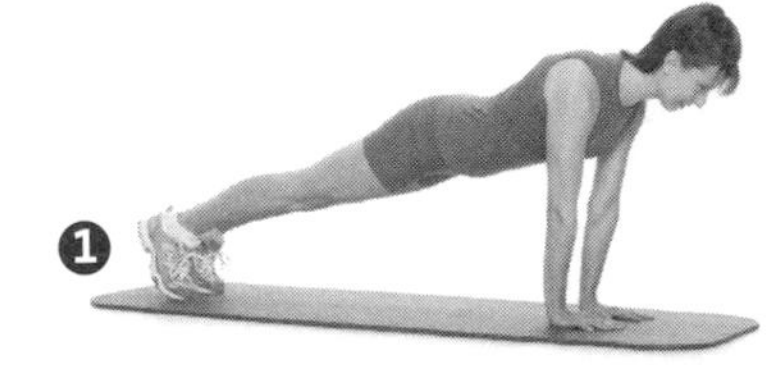

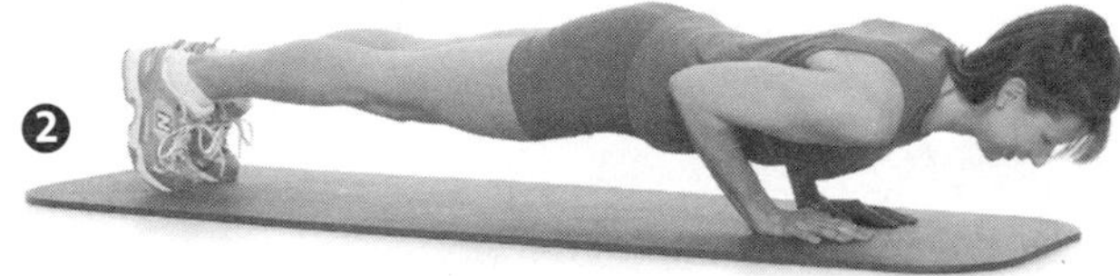

Triceps Pushup

Starting position: Lie facedown on the floor with your feet flexed and toes tucked. Place your palms on the floor close to your ribs so that your elbows are pointing up. Press down with your hands, extend your arms, and lift your body off the floor.

Movement: Keeping your head, back, hips, and legs in a straight line, bend your elbows back, keeping your arms close to your body, as you inhale. Lower your body until your chest nearly touches the floor. Hold for a second and then exhale as you push back up. If you can't do all the recommended reps in this full pushup position, that's okay. Just drop down onto one or both knees and complete the remaining reps.

Technique: Don't let your elbows point out to the sides. Don't bend at the hips. Don't drop your belly toward the floor.

Parallel Overhead Press

Starting position: Stand with your feet shoulder width apart and knees bent slightly. Hold a dumbbell in each hand at shoulder height, palms facing each other and elbows pointing forward.

Movement: Exhale as you slowly press the dumbbells straight overhead without locking your elbows. Hold for a second and then inhale as you slowly lower them.

Technique: Don't arch your back. Don't lift the dumbbells forward or back.

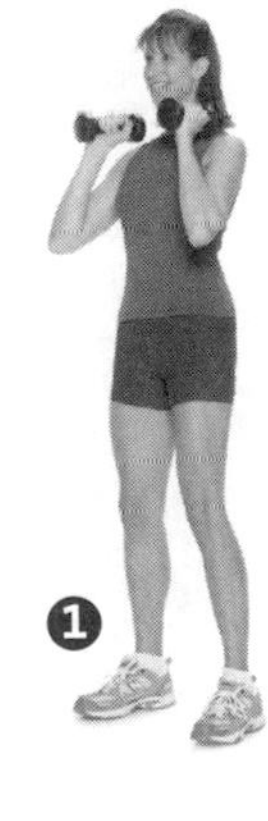

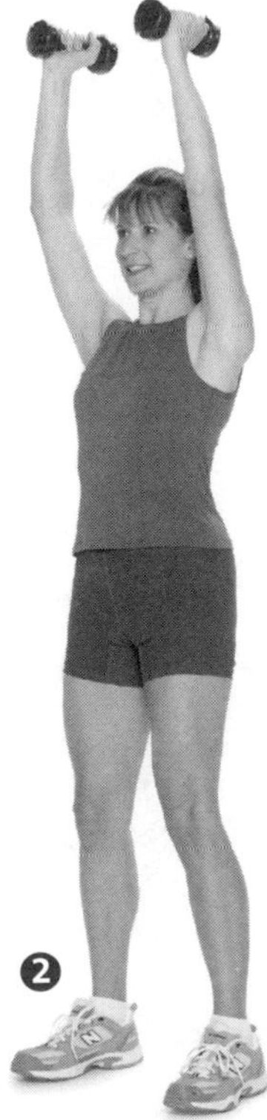

The Workout

Level 3

Easy Walk: 40 Minutes

- 5-minute warmup: Walk 2½ to 3 miles per hour, or 100 to 115 steps per minute.
- 30-minute moderate walk: Increase your speed to 3½ to 4 miles per hour, 125 to 135 steps per minute, or a pace that lets you comfortably carry on a conversation.
- 5-minute cooldown: Slow down to 2½ to 3 miles per hour, or 100 to 115 steps per minute.

High-Rep Strength Training: 30 Minutes

- Do three reps of each exercise. Start to do another rep, but stop at the midpoint of the exercise and pulse, moving in a shorter range of motion, three times. Finish by returning to the starting position. Do this three times for each exercise and repeat the sequence of exercises three times. Use a lighter weight, if needed.
- To warm up, use lighter weights, or none at all, the first time through, and for the squat and lunge exercises, only go partway down.

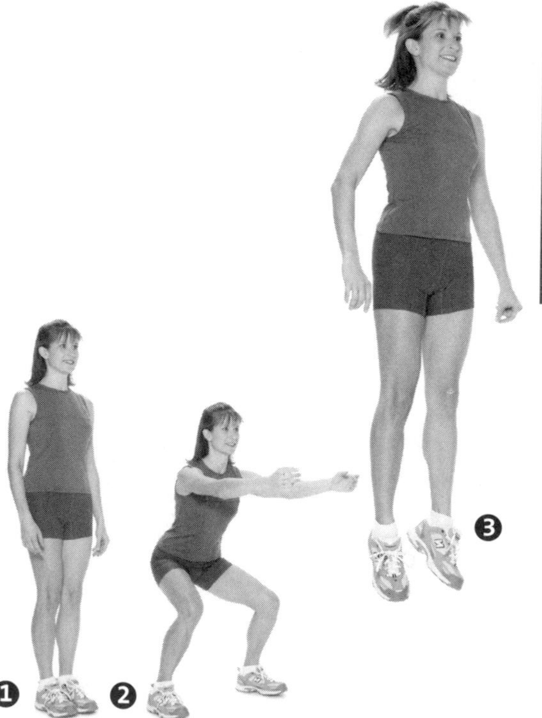

MUST-DO MOVE

Step Squat with Jump

Starting position: Stand with your feet together and your hands down at your sides.

Movement: Step your left foot out to the side 2 to 2½ feet. Keeping your back straight, lower yourself, bending from the knees and hips as though you're sitting down, as you inhale. Let your arms come out in front of you to help you balance. Stop just before your thighs are parallel to the floor. Hold for a second and then exhale as you jump and bring your left foot back to the starting position. Do five or six reps with your left foot and then do five or six reps stepping with your right foot.

Technique: Don't let your knees move forward over your toes. Don't round your back. Don't do this move while holding weights.

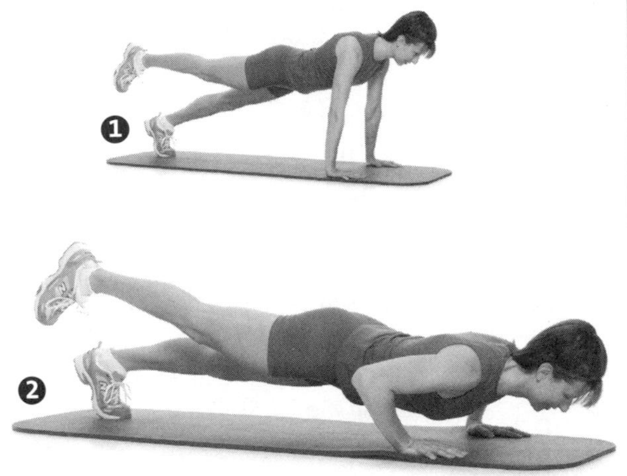

MUST-DO MOVE

One-Leg Pushup

Starting position: Lie facedown on the floor with your feet flexed and toes tucked. Place your palms on the floor near your shoulders so that your elbows are pointing up. Press down with your hands, extend your arms, and lift your body off the floor so that it forms a straight line from head to toe, and lift your right foot off the floor.

Movement: Keeping your head, back, hips, and legs in a straight line, bend your elbows out to the sides and lower your body as you inhale, until your chest nearly touches the floor. Hold for a second and then exhale as you push back up. If you can't do all the recommended reps in this full pushup position, that's okay. Just drop down onto both feet or one or both knees and complete the remaining reps. Do half of the recommended reps with your right leg off the floor and the other half with your left leg off the floor.

Technique: Don't bend at the hips. Don't arch your back.

MUST-DO MOVE

Balancing Bent-Over Row

Starting position: Stand with your right foot in front of your left. Hold a dumbbell in each hand with your arms at your sides. Keep your back flat and lean forward, lifting your back foot off the floor so that your left leg, back, and head are as parallel to the floor as possible. The dumbbells should be hanging at arm's length directly below your shoulders, palms facing each other.

Movement: Bending your elbows back and squeezing your shoulder blades, lift the weights toward your ribs as you exhale, until your elbows are higher than your back. Hold for a second and then inhale as you slowly lower them. Do half of the recommended reps balancing on your right leg and the other half on your left leg.

Technique: Don't arch your back. Don't pull your shoulders up toward your ears. Don't raise your torso as you lift the dumbbells.

Alternate move: If you have back problems, keep both legs down, support yourself with one hand on a chair, and do the rows one arm at a time.

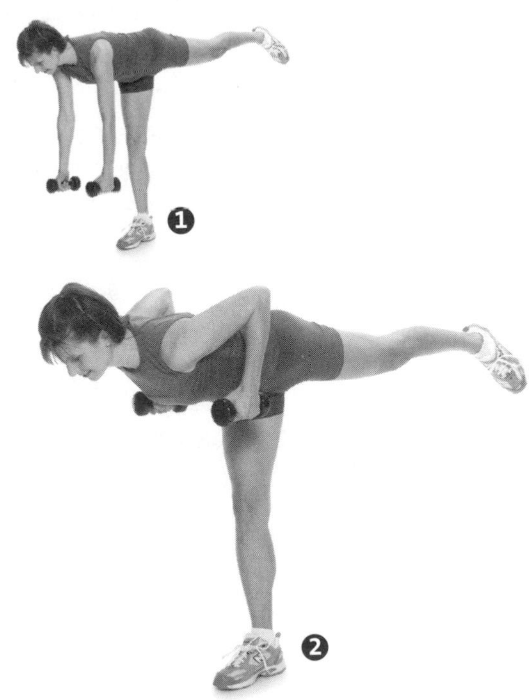

continued

The Workout

Level 3 *continued*

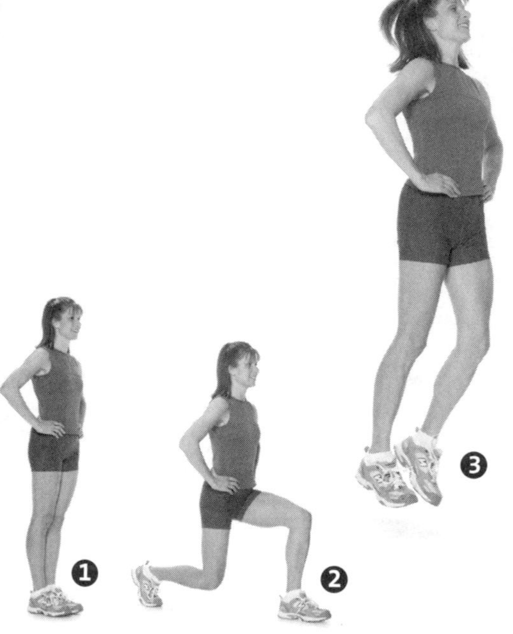

MUST-DO MOVE

Front Lunge with Jump

Starting position: Stand with your feet together and your hands on your hips.

Movement: Step your left foot forward 2 to 3 feet. Inhale as you bend your left knee and lower your body straight down until your left knee is bent 90 degrees and your right knee nearly touches the floor. Your rear heel will come off the floor. Hold for a second and then exhale as you push off with your left foot and jump your feet together. Finish all of your repetitions, then repeat the exercise stepping forward with your right foot.

Technique: Don't lean forward. Don't let your front knee move forward over your toes.

Balancing Biceps Curl

Starting position: Stand with your feet together, knees bent slightly. Hold a dumbbell in each hand with your palms facing forward. Lift your right knee up in front of you so that you're balancing on your left leg.

Movement: Bending your elbows, lift the dumbbells toward your shoulders as you exhale. Stop when the dumbbells are at chest height, palms facing your body. Hold for a second and then inhale as you slowly lower them. Do half of the recommended reps balancing on your left leg and the other half on your right leg.

Technique: Don't move your upper arms.

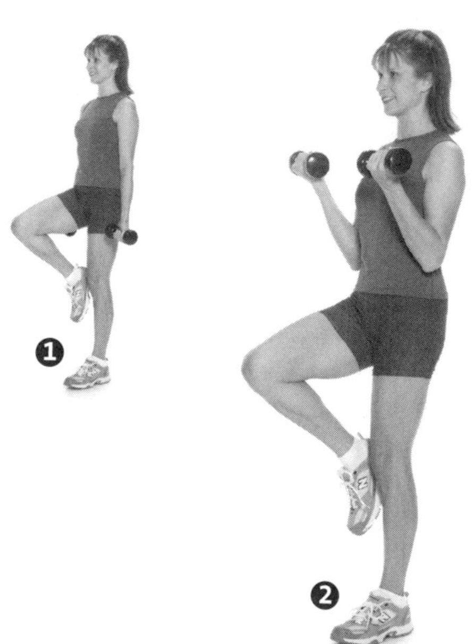

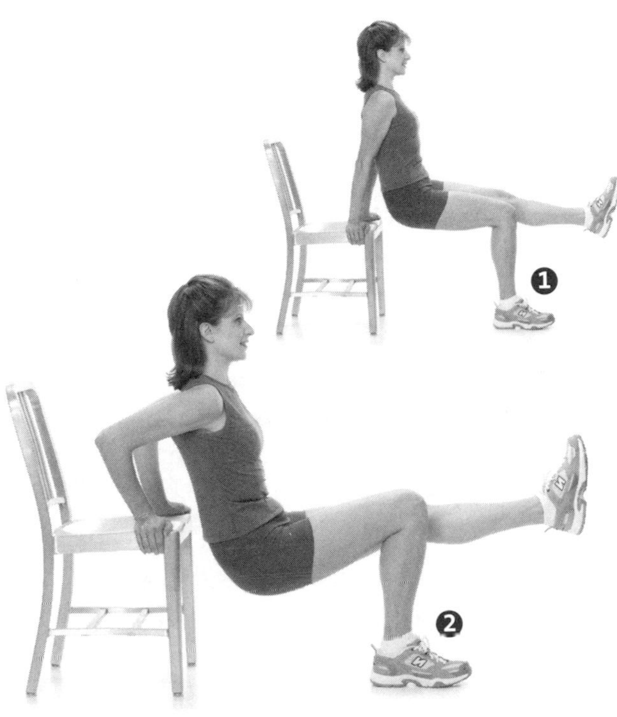

One-Leg Triceps Dip

Starting position: Sit on the edge of a chair, place your hands on either side of you, and grasp the chair seat. Slide your buttocks off the chair, walk your feet out until your legs are bent at about 90 degrees, lift your left foot off the floor, and extend your left leg. You should be balancing on your hands and right foot.

Movement: Bending your arms so that your elbows point behind you, slowly lower your body toward the floor as you inhale. Keep your buttocks as close to the chair as possible. Stop when your elbows are bent about 90 degrees. Hold for a second and then exhale as you press back up. Do half of the recommended reps with your left leg extended and the other half with your right leg extended.

Technique: Don't sink into your arms, allowing your shoulders to come up toward your ears. Don't bend your knees to help lower yourself.

Alternate move: For a more challenging version, extend your legs straight and balance on your heels.

Balancing Overhead Press

Starting position: Stand with your feet together, knees bent slightly. Hold a dumbbell in each hand at shoulder height with your palms facing forward and elbows pointing out to the sides. Lift your right knee up in front of you so that you're balancing on your left leg.

Movement: Exhale as you slowly press the dumbbells straight up overhead. Hold for a second and then inhale as you slowly lower them. Do half of the recommended reps balancing on your left leg and the other half on your right leg.

Technique: Don't arch your back. Don't lift the dumbbells forward or back.

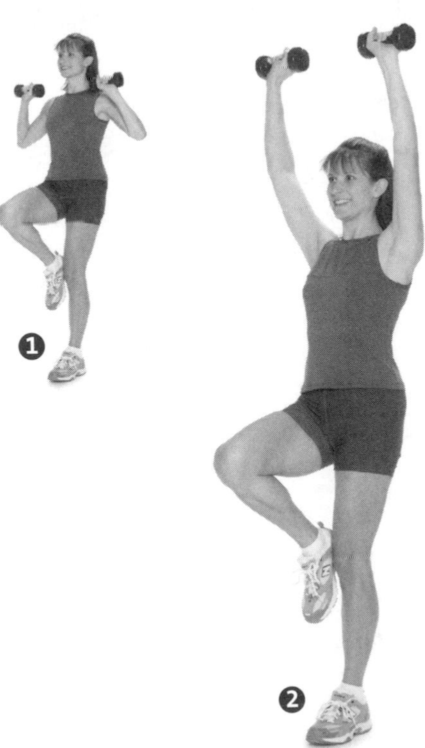

FIRM UP / DAY 18

Avoid Diet Saboteurs

Want to really bring out the worst in people? Lose weight. Ten pounds or a ton, you'll be showered with so much fattening food—by people who claim to love you—that it will send the price of sugarcane and lard futures through the roof.

Diet saboteurs are everywhere. In fact, in one survey, 24,000 overweight women reported that losing weight created problems in their relationships that regaining the weight would have resolved.

The problem usually starts because you're in change mode (and darned happy to be there), but your friends and family aren't. "Rarely would a real friend malevolently undermine your diet," says nutrition professor Audrey Cross, Ph.D., of Rutgers University in New Brunswick, New Jersey. "They just do unconscious things to keep the relationship the way it was."

How do you politely say "back off" to those you love? "It's important to ask for help," says Carlo DiClemente, Ph.D., coauthor of *Changing for Good,* whose strategies for curing drug and alcohol addicts are now being used to help people change the way they eat.

We tend to believe that if people loved us, they'd know what to do. Not true! For some, being constantly asked about how much they've lost may drive them to cheat, while others may find this helpful in keeping them on track. You need to be specific about your needs. Even those closest to you can't read your mind.

And when friends or family are enticing you, offer some compromises.

- Instead of scarfing down wings and blue cheese with friends, try going to a restaurant where they can still get wings and you can get healthier food.
- Instead of taking a 2-hour lunch, try eating a quick lunch, then go shopping or take a walk.
- Instead of doing girls' night out at a restaurant or bar, try getting together at a spa for a manicure and pedicure; you can talk your heads off and have a great time.

FIRM UP TIPS

ON YOUR PLATE	HAVE FUN!
Reflect on your choices. Looking at yourself in a mirror while eating may help you consume 22 to 32 percent fewer calories.	*Grab the kids and play hopscotch on the driveway. A half-hour of jumping from square to square burns 175 calories.*

Meal Plan

Most of these recipes are custom designed to make 1 serving–no fuss, no muss; just fix, eat, and go! If a recipe makes more than 1 serving, it's noted below. Save that extra serving for another meal, or share it with your spouse or your walking buddy.

Breakfast

McDonald's Egg McMuffin: Order it without cheese and get an 8-ounce carton 1% milk to wash it down.

Healthy Snack

Fruit to Go: Have a 4-ounce container (½ cup) fruit (in juice, not syrup). Check labels for about 60 calories per serving, such as single-serve, peel-top cans of Del Monte Fruit Naturals Diced Peaches in Pear and Peach Juice or Dole Pineapple FruitBowls. Serve with 1 slice whole wheat bread topped with 1 slice reduced-fat cheese.

Lunch

Peanut Butter 'n' Banana Sandwich: Spread 2 tablespoons peanut butter on 1 slice toasted whole wheat bread and thinly slice 1 banana to cover the layer of peanut butter.

Indulgent Treat

Dandy Candy: Treat yourself to 1 Milky Way Lite candy bar.

Dinner

Pasta with Chickpeas: Makes 2 servings. Prepare 2 cups cooked pasta (any variety). Toss 2 teaspoons olive oil, 2 tablespoons Parmesan cheese, 1 teaspoon each dried basil and minced garlic with 1 cup canned (rinsed and drained) chickpeas and the cooked pasta. Serve half (save the rest for Friday) with 1 cup cooked spinach with 1 teaspoon trans-fat-free margarine.

Healthy Snack

Pudding and Fruit: Have 1 ready-to-serve fat-free chocolate pudding cup. Serve with ¾ cup blueberries.

Nutrient analysis: 1,667 calories, 65 g protein, 212 g carbohydrates, 57 g total fat, 19 g saturated fat, 258 mg cholesterol, 23 g dietary fiber, 1,920 mg sodium, 1,269 mg calcium

FIRM UP TIP

ENERGY BOOSTER

Laugh it up. "A good laugh has many positive physiological effects," according to Joel Goodman, director of the Humor Project, Inc., in Saratoga Springs, New York, "such as boosting immune function, enhancing respiration, and lowering levels of stress hormones." For a dose of hilarity, check out these Web sites: www.dumb.com and www.brainofbrian.com.

The Workout

Level 1

Interval Walk: About 30 Minutes

- 5-minute warmup: Walk 2 miles per hour, about 95 steps per minute.
- 3-minute moderate pace: Increase your speed to 3 miles per hour, about 115 steps per minute.
- 1-minute speedup: Pick up your pace even more to 3½ miles per hour, about 125 steps per minute.
- Repeat moderate pace/speedup sequence five times.
- 5-minute cooldown: Slow down to 2 miles per hour, about 95 steps per minute.

Core Training: 20 Minutes

- Do the sequence of exercises one time.

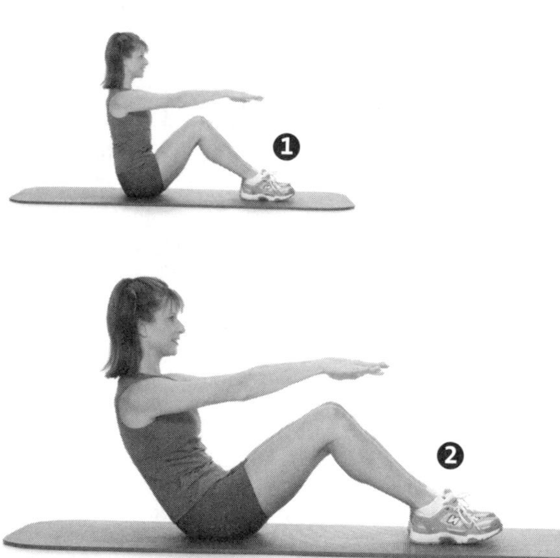

Roll-Down

Starting position: Sit on the floor with your knees bent and your feet flat. Hold your arms out in front of you, parallel to the floor.

Movement: Using your abs, slowly roll down 3 to 4 inches, one vertebra at a time, as you inhale. Hold for a second and then exhale as you slowly roll back up. Do 12 reps.

Technique: Your abs should be powering the move. Don't move quickly.

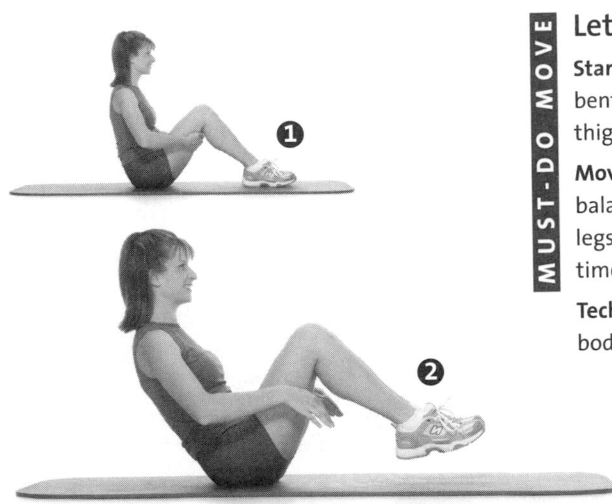

MUST-DO MOVE

Let-Go Balance

Starting position: Sit on the floor with your knees bent and your feet flat. Place your hands behind your thighs.

Movement: Lift your feet off the floor slightly and balance on your sitting bones. Try letting go of your legs. Hold for five breaths and then relax. Do one time only.

Technique: Keep your abs tight and the rest of your body relaxed, especially your shoulders.

Ab Crunch

Starting position: Lie on your back with your knees bent, feet flat on the floor, and hands behind your head.

Movement: Using your abs, slowly raise your head, shoulders, and upper back about 45 degrees off the floor as you exhale. Think of shortening the distance between your ribs and pelvis. Hold for a second and then inhale as you slowly lower yourself. Do 12 reps.

Technique: Don't pull your chin to your chest. Don't arch your back.

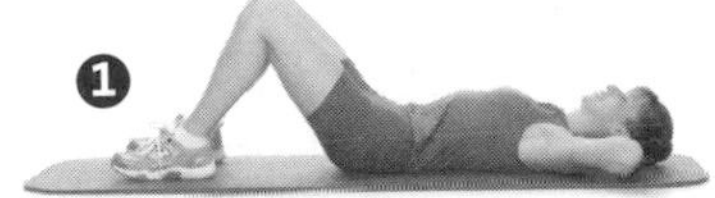

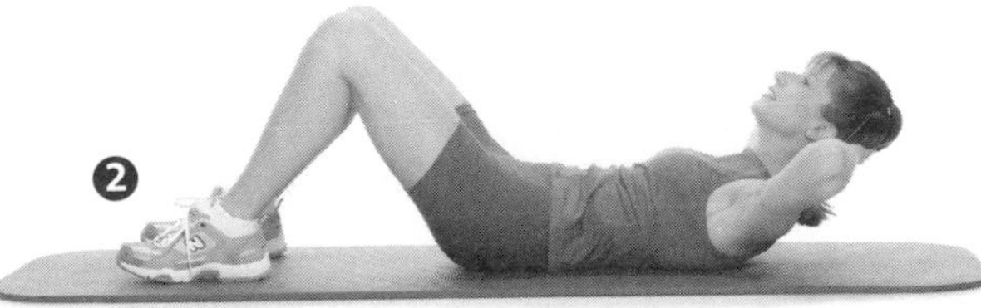

continued

The Workout

Level 1 *continued*

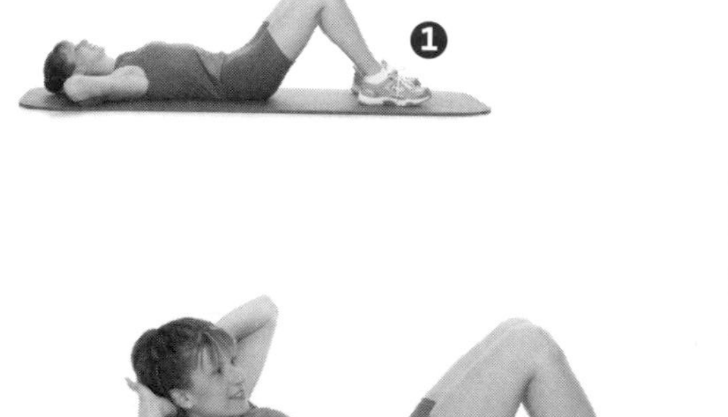

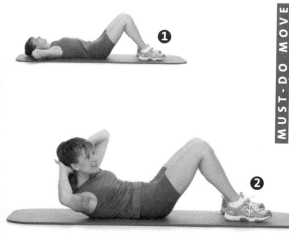

MUST-DO MOVE

Twisting Crunch

Starting position: Lie on your back with your knees bent, feet flat on the floor, and hands behind your head.

Movement: Using your abs, slowly lift your head and left shoulder off the floor, twist to the right, and bring your left shoulder toward your right knee as you exhale. Hold for a second and then inhale as you slowly lower yourself. Repeat, alternating sides. Do a total of 12 reps, 6 reps to each side.

Technique: Don't pull your chin to your chest. Don't arch your back.

MUST-DO MOVE

Bridge with Lift

Starting position: Lie on your back with your knees bent, feet flat on the floor, and arms at your sides, palms facing up.

Movement: Contracting your abs, buttocks, and lower back, press into your feet and lift your butt, hips, and back off the floor as you exhale, to form a straight line from your shoulders to your knees. Lift one foot a few inches off the floor. Hold for three breaths and then lower your foot. Lift the other foot up and hold for three breaths. Lower your foot and then relax. Do one time only.

Technique: Don't lift too high—your upper back and shoulders should remain on the floor. Don't bend at the waist or hips. Don't let your knees fall inward or outward.

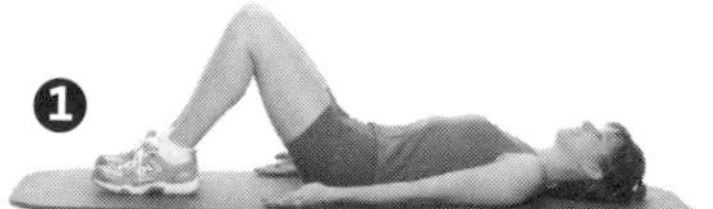

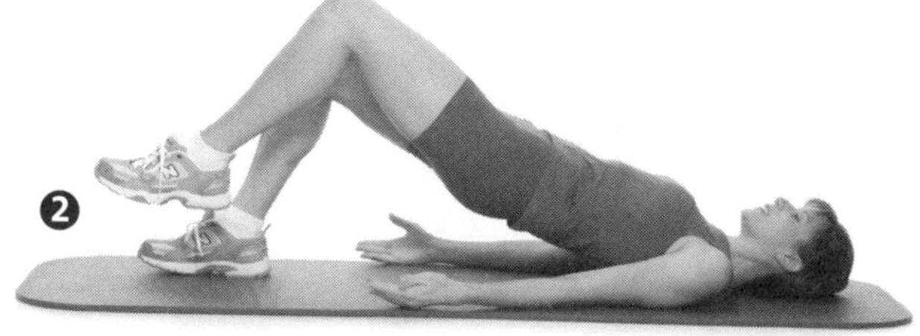

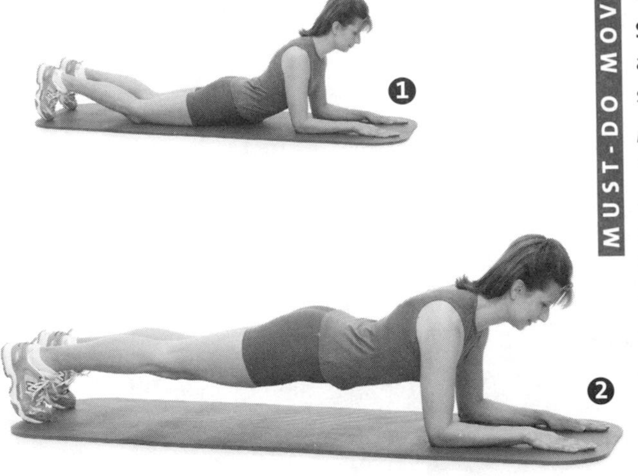

MUST-DO MOVE

Plank

Starting position: Lie facedown with your feet flexed and toes tucked. Your elbows should be under your shoulders and your forearms and palms on the floor.

Movement: Contracting your abs and back, press into your forearms as you exhale and lift your pelvis and legs off the floor so that your back and legs form a straight line. Hold for five breaths and then relax. Do one time only.

Technique: Don't lift your head up or let it drop. Don't bend at the waist or hips. Don't let your belly drop toward the floor.

Kneeling T-Stand with Arm Up

Starting position: Sit on your left hip with your left leg bent, your right leg extended, right arm extended on your leg, and left hand on the floor below your shoulder.

Movement: Using your abs, lift your hips off the floor as you exhale and raise your right arm overhead. Look up toward your right hand. Hold for five breaths, relax, and then repeat on the other side. Do one time only on each side.

Technique: Don't let your body roll forward; think of it as being sandwiched between two walls. Keep everything in line.

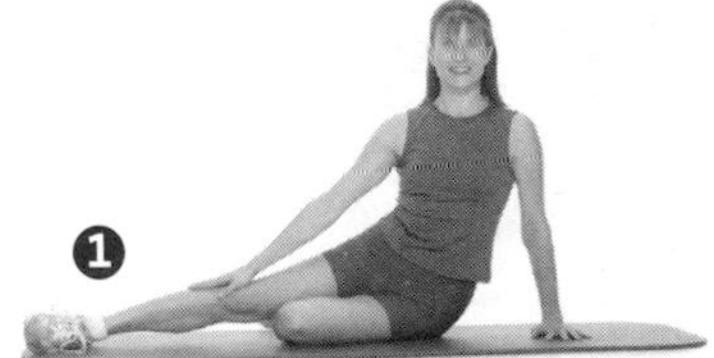

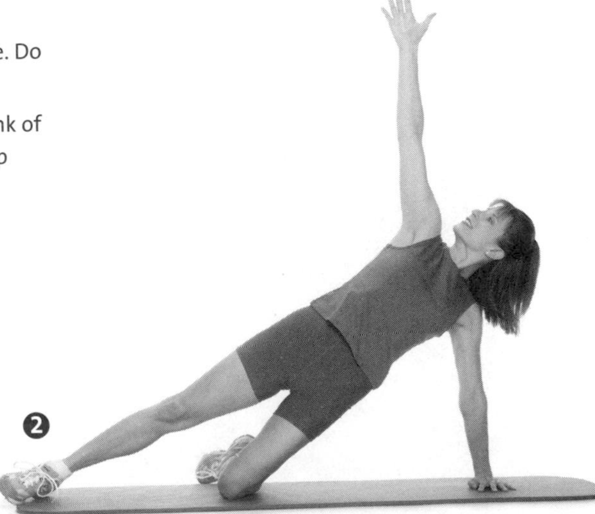

The Workout

Level 2

Interval Walk: About 30 Minutes

- 5-minute warmup: Walk 2½ miles per hour, about 100 steps per minute.
- 4-minute moderate pace: Increase your speed to 3½ miles per hour, about 125 steps per minute.
- 3-minute speedup: Pick up your pace even more to 4 miles per hour, about 135 steps per minute.
- Repeat moderate pace/speedup sequence three times.
- 5-minute cooldown: Slow down to 2½ miles per hour, about 100 steps per minute.

Core Training: 20 Minutes

- Do the sequence of exercises one time.

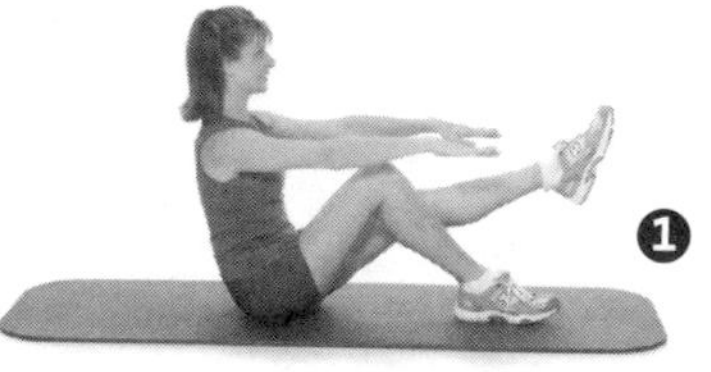

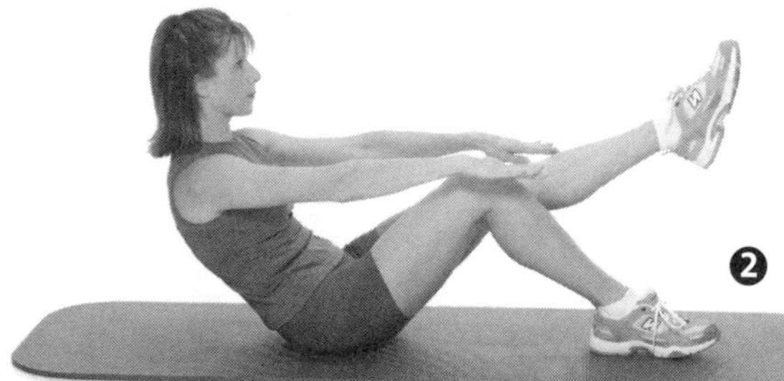

One-Leg Roll-Down

Starting position: Sit on the floor with your knees bent and your feet flat. Lift your left foot off the floor and extend your left leg. Hold your arms out in front of you, parallel to the floor.

Movement: Using your abs, slowly roll down 4 to 5 inches, one vertebra at a time, as you inhale. Hold for a second and then exhale as you slowly roll back up. Do six reps, switch legs, and do six more reps.

Technique: Your abs should be powering the move. Don't move quickly.

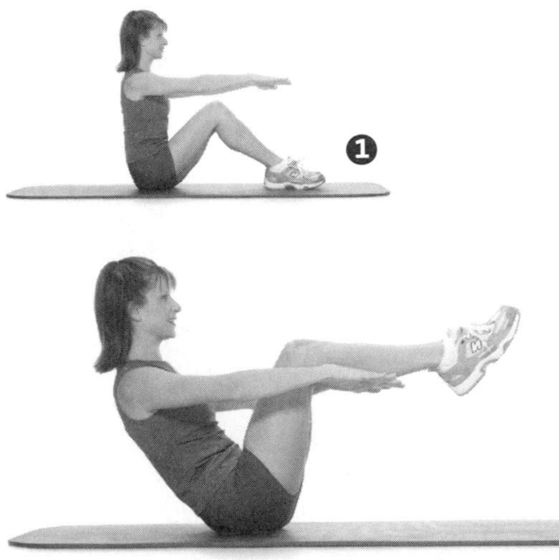

MUST-DO MOVE

Full Balance

Starting position: Sit on the floor with your knees bent and your feet flat. Hold your arms straight out in front of you, parallel to the floor.

Movement: Lift your feet so that your calves are parallel to the floor, and balance on your sitting bones. Hold for five breaths and then relax. Do one time only.

Technique: Keep your abs tight and the rest of your body relaxed, especially your shoulders.

Legs-Up Ab Crunch

Starting position: Lie on your back with your legs in the air and your hands behind your head.

Movement: Using your abs, slowly raise your head, shoulders, and upper back about 45 degrees off the floor as you exhale. Think of shortening the distance between your ribs and pelvis. Hold for a second and then inhale as you slowly lower yourself. Do 12 reps.

Technique: Don't pull your chin to your chest. Don't arch your back.

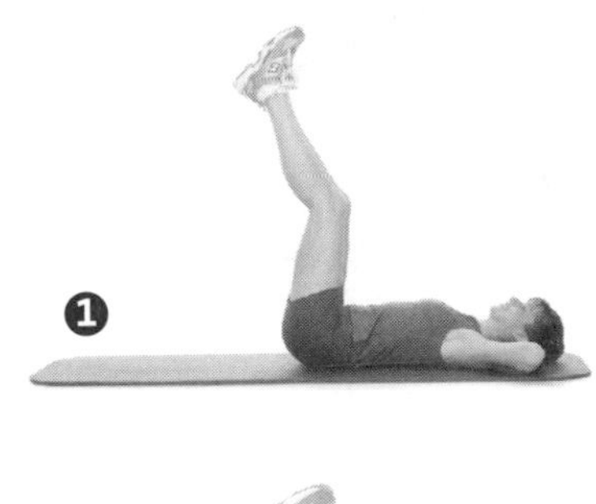

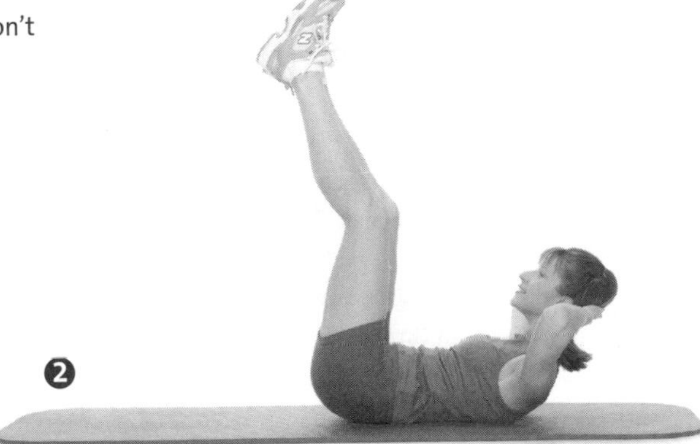

continued

The Workout

Level 2 *continued*

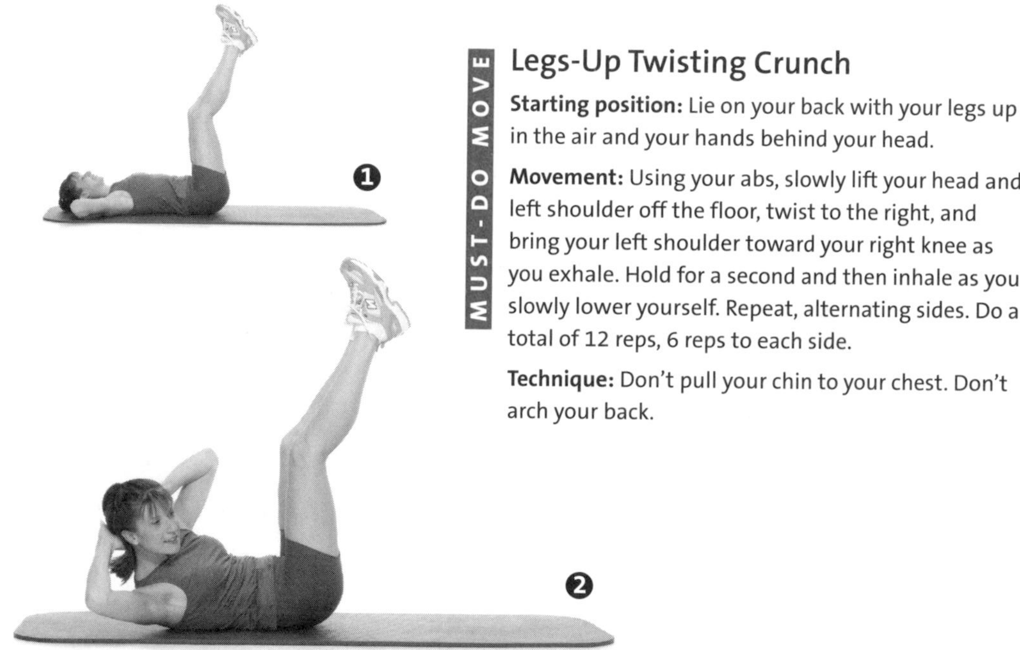

MUST-DO MOVE

Legs-Up Twisting Crunch

Starting position: Lie on your back with your legs up in the air and your hands behind your head.

Movement: Using your abs, slowly lift your head and left shoulder off the floor, twist to the right, and bring your left shoulder toward your right knee as you exhale. Hold for a second and then inhale as you slowly lower yourself. Repeat, alternating sides. Do a total of 12 reps, 6 reps to each side.

Technique: Don't pull your chin to your chest. Don't arch your back.

MUST-DO MOVE

One-Leg Heel Bridge

Starting position: Lie on your back with your knees bent, feet flat on the floor, and arms at your sides, palms facing up. Lift your toes off the floor so that only your heels are touching, and then extend your right leg.

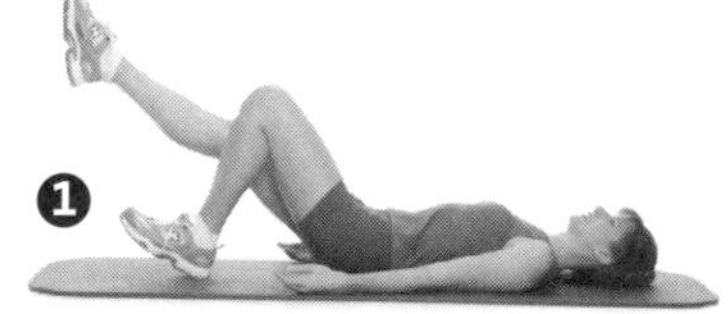

Movement: Contracting your abs, buttocks, and lower back, press into your heel and lift your butt, hips, and back off the floor as you exhale, to form a straight line from your shoulders to your knees. Slowly lower your buttocks toward the floor and then lift back up. Do six lifts, hold for three breaths, and then relax. Repeat with the opposite leg extended. Do one time only.

Technique: Don't lift too high—your upper back and shoulders should remain on the floor. Don't bend at the waist or hips. Don't let your knees fall inward or outward.

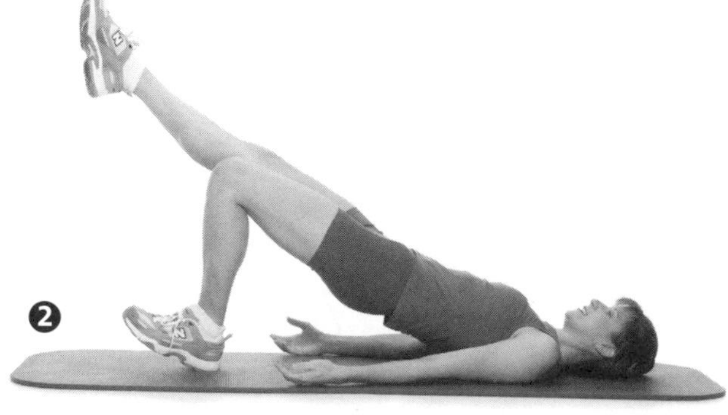

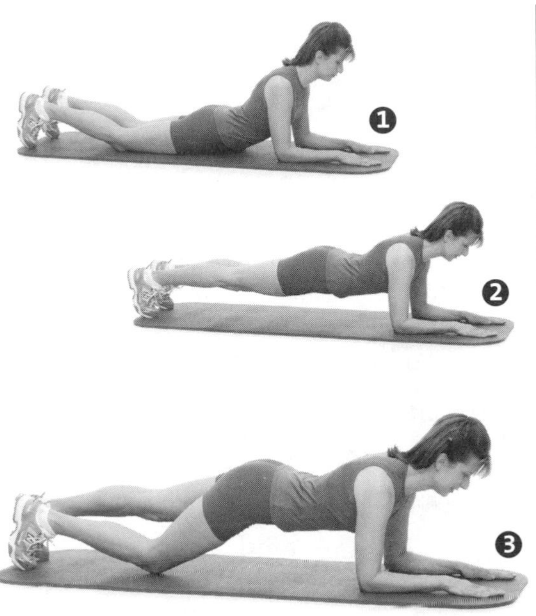

MUST-DO MOVE

Plank with Knee Drop

Starting position: Lie facedown with your feet flexed and toes tucked. Your elbows should be under your shoulders and your forearms and palms on the floor.

Movement: Contracting your abs and back, press into your forearms as you exhale and lift your pelvis and legs off the floor so that your back and legs form a straight line. Slowly drop your right knee toward the floor and then straighten. Do six knee touches with your right leg, hold for three breaths, do six knee touches with your left leg, hold for three breaths, and then relax. Do one time only.

Technique: Don't lift your head up or let it drop. Don't bend at the waist or hips. Don't let your belly drop toward the floor.

T-Stand with Arm Up

Starting position: Sit on your left hip with your legs extended to the side, your right ankle over the left, right arm extended on your leg, and left hand on the floor below your shoulder.

Movement: Using your abs, lift your hips, legs, and ankles off the floor and raise your right arm overhead as you exhale. Look up toward your right hand. Hold for five breaths, relax, and then repeat on the other side. Do one time only on each side.

Technique: Don't let your body roll forward; think of it as being sandwiched between two walls. Keep everything in line. Don't let your ankles touch the floor.

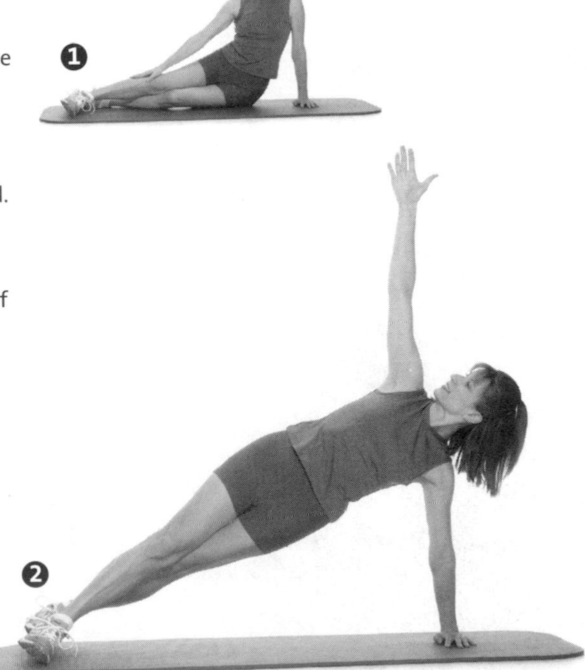

The Workout

Level 3

Interval Walk: About 30 Minutes

- 5-minute warmup: Walk 3 miles per hour, about 115 steps per minute.
- 1-minute moderate pace: Increase your speed to 4 miles per hour, about 135 steps per minute.
- 3-minute speedup: Pick up your pace even more to 4½ miles per hour, about 145 steps per minute.
- Repeat moderate pace/speedup sequence five times.
- 5-minute cooldown: Slow down to 3 miles per hour, about 115 steps per minute.

Core Training: 20 Minutes

- Do the sequence of exercises one time.

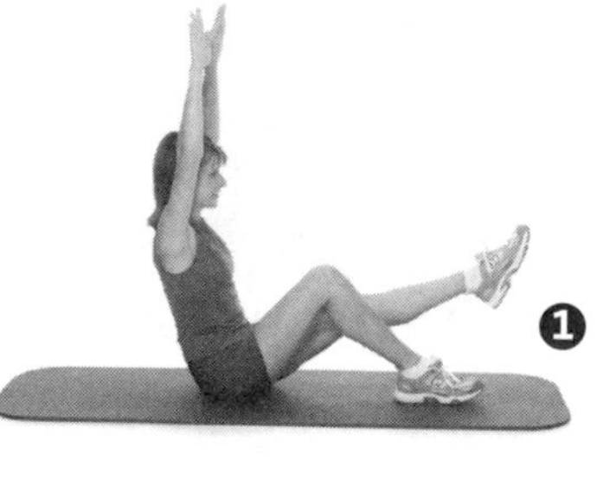

❶

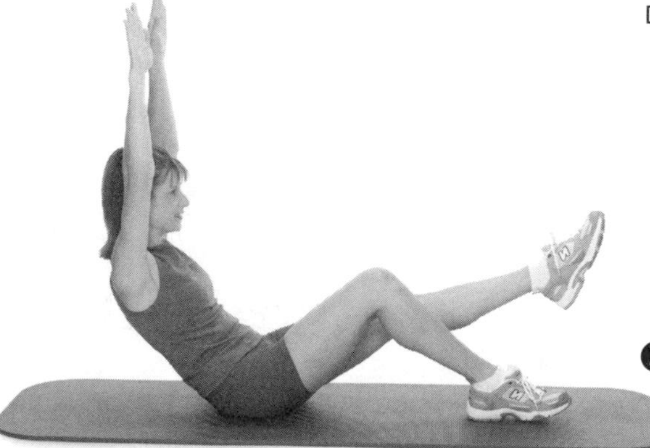

❷

Extended One-Leg Roll-Down

Starting position: Sit on the floor with your knees bent and your feet flat. Lift your left foot off the floor and extend your left leg. Hold your arms up overhead.

Movement: Using your abs, slowly roll down 5 to 6 inches, one vertebra at a time, as you inhale. Hold for a second and then exhale as you slowly roll back up. Do six reps; then switch legs and do six more reps.

Technique: Your abs should be powering the move. Don't move quickly.

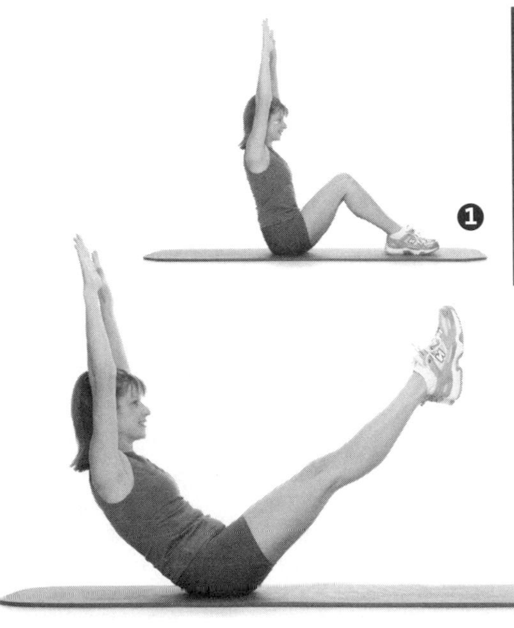

MUST-DO MOVE

Fully Extended Balance

Starting position: Sit on the floor with your knees bent and your feet flat. Hold your arms up overhead.

Movement: Lift your feet off the floor, extending your legs straight, and balance on your sitting bones. Hold for five breaths and then relax. Do one time only.

Technique: Keep your abs tight and the rest of your body relaxed, especially your shoulders.

Reverse Crunch

Starting position: Lie on your back with your legs up in the air and your hands behind your head. Cross your legs at the shins.

Movement: Slowly contract your abs as you exhale, and press your back into the floor, tilting your pelvis and lifting your hips 2 to 4 inches off the floor. Keep your upper body relaxed. Hold for a second and then inhale as you slowly lower. Do 12 reps.

Technique: Don't swing your legs.

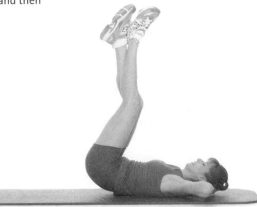

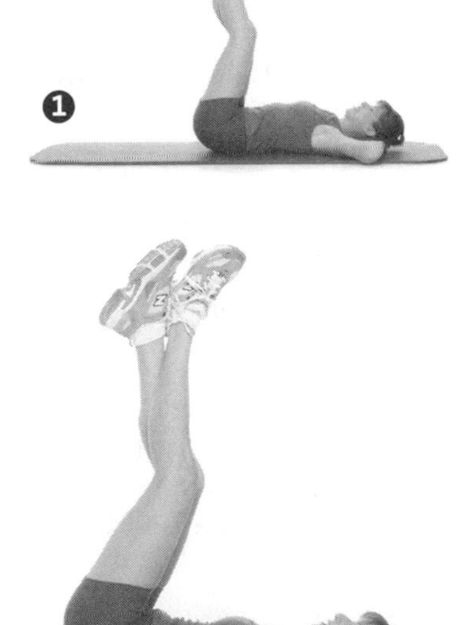

continued

The Workout

Level 3 *continued*

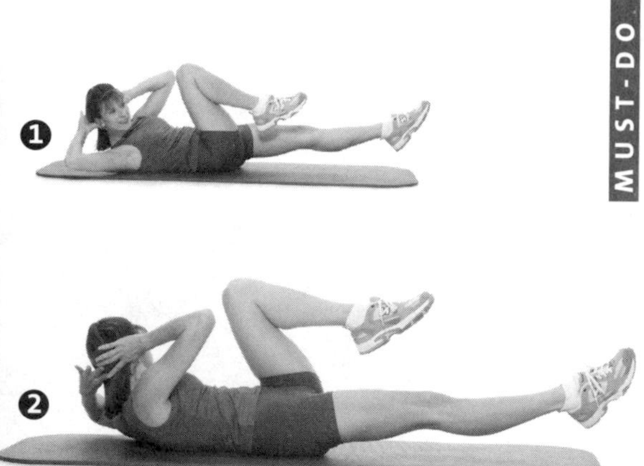

MUST-DO MOVE

Bicycle

Starting position: Lie on your back with your legs bent, feet flat on the floor, and hands behind your head. Lift your head and shoulders off the floor into a crunch position. Lift your feet off the floor, keeping your legs bent about 45 degrees.

Movement: Simultaneously, twist your left shoulder toward your right knee and bend your right knee in toward your chest while straightening your left leg. Then using a bicycle-pedaling motion, straighten your right leg, while bringing the left knee in toward your chest and twisting your right shoulder to the left. That's 1 rep; do 12 reps.

Technique: Don't pull your chin to your chest. Don't arch your back.

MUST-DO MOVE

One-Leg Heel Bridge with Arms Up

Starting position: Lie on your back with your knees bent, feet flat on the floor, and arms extended over your chest. Lift your toes off the floor so that only your heels are touching, and then extend your right leg.

Movement: Contracting your abs, buttocks, and lower back, press into your heel and lift your butt, hips, and back off the floor as you exhale, to form a straight line from your shoulders to your knees. Slowly lower your buttocks toward the floor and then lift back up. Do six lifts, hold for three breaths, and then relax. Repeat with the opposite leg extended. Do one time only with each leg.

Technique: Don't lift too high—your upper back and shoulders should remain on the floor. Don't bend at the waist or hips. Don't let your knees fall inward or outward.

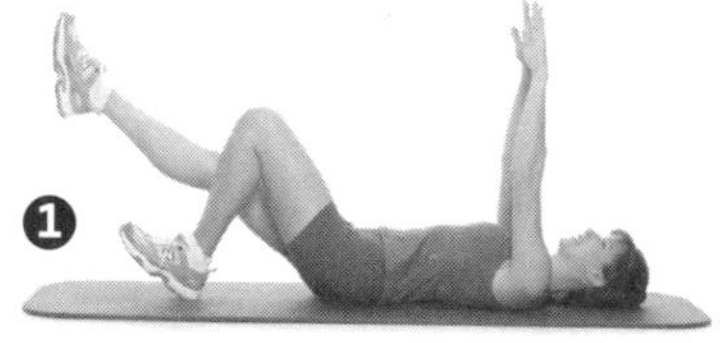

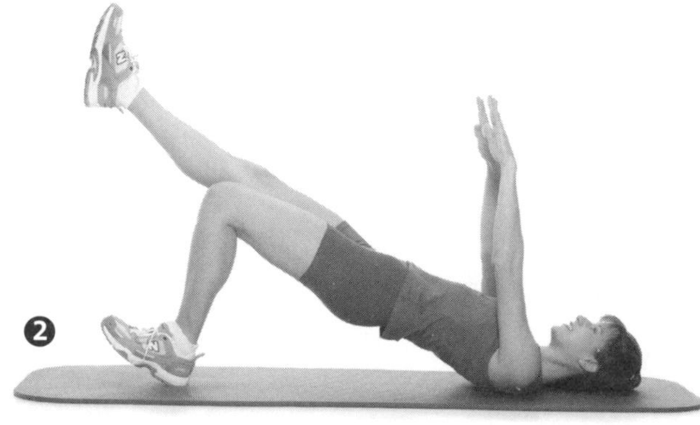

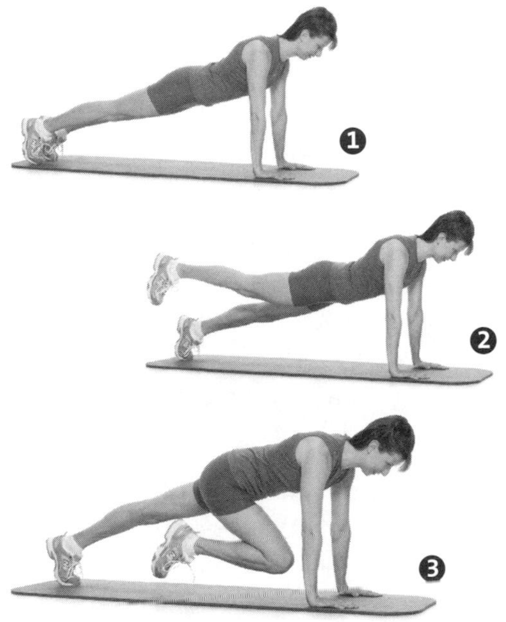

MUST-DO MOVE

Extended Plank with Lift and Bend

Starting position: Lie facedown with your feet flexed and toes tucked. Place your palms on the floor near your shoulders so that your elbows are pointing up. Contracting your abs and back, press into your hands as you exhale, straighten your arms, and lift your torso and legs off the floor so that your head, back, and legs form a straight line.

Movement: Lift your right foot off the floor and hold for three breaths. Next, pull your right knee in toward your chest and press it back out for six reps and then put that foot back on the floor. Lift your left foot off the floor and hold for three breaths. Next, pull your left knee in toward your chest and press it back out for six reps, put that foot back on the floor, and then relax. Do one time only.

Technique: Don't lift your head up or let it drop. Don't bend at the waist or hips. Don't let your belly drop toward the floor.

T-Stand with Arm and Leg Up

Starting position: Sit on your left hip with your legs extended to the side, your right ankle over the left, right arm extended on your leg, and left hand on the floor below your shoulder.

Movement: Using your abs, lift your hips, legs, and ankles off the floor as you exhale; raise your right arm overhead, looking up toward your hand; and lift your right leg up. Hold for five breaths, relax, and then repeat on the other side. Do one time only on each side.

Technique: Don't let your body roll forward; think of it as being sandwiched between two walls. Keep everything in line. Don't let your ankles touch the floor.

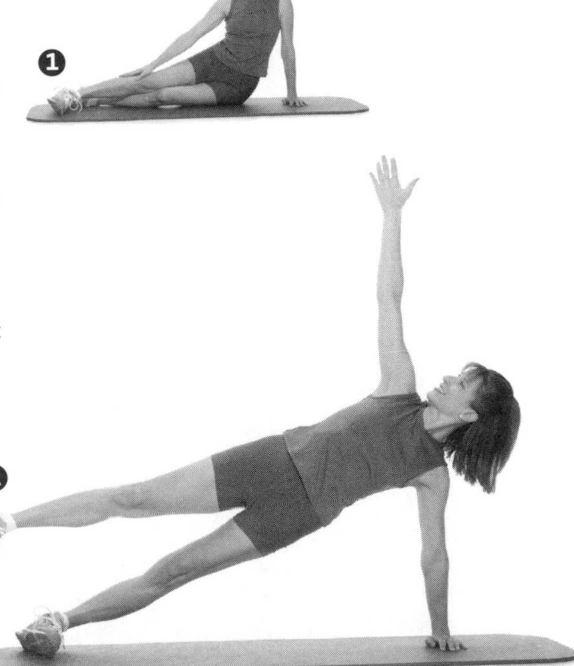

FIRM UP / DAY 19

Sleep It Off

Getting less than 8 hours of shut-eye a night can make controlling your weight more difficult. Sleep deprivation disrupts your body's normal ability to process and control various weight-related hormones (glucose, cortisol, and thyroid hormones). This imbalance encourages cells to store excess fat and lowers your body's fat-burning ability. Lack of sleep may also make it more difficult to control cravings.

But just 9 hours of sleep for three consecutive nights can reverse this, making weight loss easier. Here's how to get enough Zzzs.

Move your body. Regular exercise (30 minutes most days of the week) reduces stress and raises body temperature, which primes you for slumber.

Cut the chemicals. Avoid foods and drinks high in sugar and caffeine. Avoid alcohol as well: It can feel sedating, but it actually disrupts sleep.

Set the stage for sleep. Set standard bedtimes and wake times that allow for 8 to 9 hours of sleep. Each evening, prepare yourself for sleep: Take a bath, read a meditation book, or listen to relaxing music. Also, make sure that your bedroom is dark, cool, and quiet.

Take a siesta. If you don't get a good night's sleep, take a 10-minute nap the next day. It will improve both your mood and your ability to stick to your diet.

Too little sleep can also boost levels of dangerous, inflammation-promoting hormones linked to heart attack, stroke, and high blood pressure.

FIRM UP TIPS

ENERGY BOOSTER	FIT FACT
Dab some peppermint oil on your collar during your workout. In a study at Wheeling Jesuit University in West Virginia, 40 athletes ran faster and did more pushups when exposed to peppermint scent than to other scents or none at all. "Peppermint boosts mood, so you perform better without working harder," says researcher Bryan Raudenbush, Ph.D.	*Even when stressed, physically fit women had a lower rise in blood pressure when stressed than those less fit, according to one small study. One reason for this may be that exercisers have higher levels of a chemical compound called nitric oxide, which helps arteries respond to stress more healthfully.*

Meal Plan

Most of these recipes are custom designed to make 1 serving–no fuss, no muss; just fix, eat, and go! If a recipe makes more than 1 serving, it's noted below. Save that extra serving for another meal, or share it with your spouse or your walking buddy.

Breakfast

Hot Cereal with Apricots: Microwave ½ cup multigrain hot cereal (such as Quaker, Mother's, or any other brand that has about 130 calories per ½ cup uncooked). Follow package directions, but instead of using all water, use half water and half fat-free milk (in most cases, that means ½ cup water and ½ cup fat-free milk to ½ cup dry cereal). Cook with 3 chopped dried apricots (6 halves). It usually takes 1 to 2 minutes to cook. Serve with ½ cup fat free milk and 1 stick reduced-fat string cheese.

Healthy Snack

Vegetables and Dip: Dip 15 baby carrots into 2 tablespoons reduced-fat veggie cream cheese and serve with 1 peach.

Lunch

Taco Bell: Order the Chili Cheese Burrito or the Gordita Supreme Chicken. Bring along a sandwich bag of 1 cup celery and carrot sticks (or other vegetable) and 1 small apple.

Indulgent Treat

Chips with Cheese: Spread 1 small snack-size (¾-ounce) bag tortilla chips on a microwave-safe plate. Top with ¼ cup reduced-fat shredded cheese. Heat 45 seconds to 2 minutes in the microwave until melted.

Dinner

Beef and Vegetables: Microwave according to package directions Uncle Ben's Mexican-Style Rice Bowl Beef Fajita, Lean Cuisine Café Classics Southern Beef Tips, or a similar frozen meal (check the label for 270 to 300 calories and 5 to 9 grams of fat). Add a salad: 1 cup romaine or mixed greens and ½ medium tomato, sliced. Top with 1 tablespoon regular dressing or 2 tablespoons light dressing.

Healthy Snack

Pears Drizzled with Chocolate: Open 1 can pear halves. Drizzle 1½ tablespoons chocolate syrup over 1 canned pear half and top with 1 tablespoon chopped nuts (any type). Serve with ½ cup fat-free milk.

Nutrient analysis: 1,680 calories, 83 g protein, 231 g carbohydrates, 52 g total fat, 16 g saturated fat, 108 mg cholesterol, 25 g dietary fiber, 2,333 mg sodium, 1,284 mg calcium

FIRM UP TIP

ON YOUR PLATE

Expose yourself. Instead of avoiding those doughnuts in the office, look at them and then walk away. Each time you successfully navigate temptations, your self-control gets stronger.

The Workout

Level 1

Easy Walk: 40 Minutes

- 5-minute warmup: Walk 2 to 2½ miles per hour, or 95 to 100 steps per minute.
- 30-minute moderate walk: Increase your speed to 2½ to 3 miles per hour, 100 to 115 steps per minute, or a pace that lets you comfortably carry on a conversation.
- 5-minute cooldown: Slow down to 2 to 2½ miles per hour, or 95 to 100 steps per minute.

Heavy Strength Training: 25 Minutes

- Do four to six reps of each exercise, using a heavier weight. Repeat the sequence of exercises three times.
- To warm up, use lighter weights, or none at all, the first time through, and for the squat and lunge exercises, only go partway down.

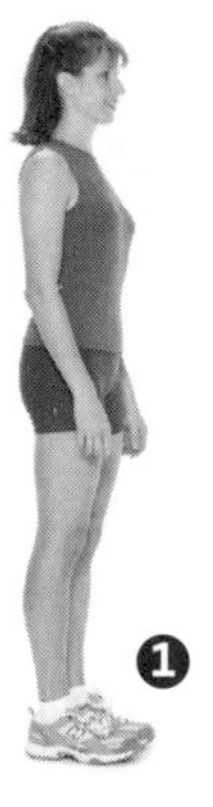

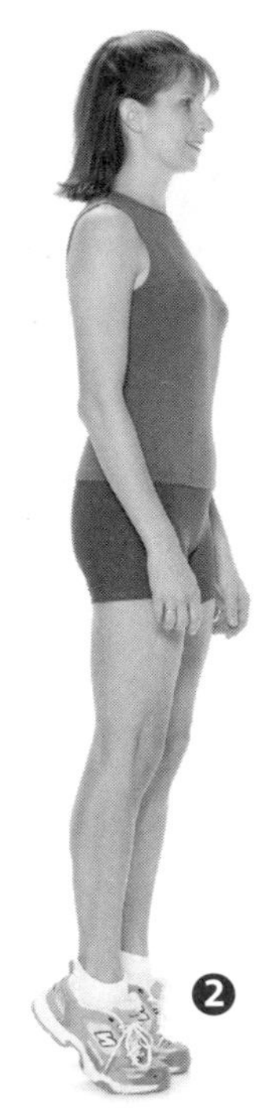

Heel Raise

Starting position: Stand with your feet together. Lightly hold on to a chair or wall with one hand if needed for balance.

Movement: Exhale as you slowly lift your heels off the floor, rolling up onto your toes. Hold for a second and then inhale as you slowly lower them.

Technique: Don't bend at the waist or lean forward, back, or to the side. Don't bend your legs.

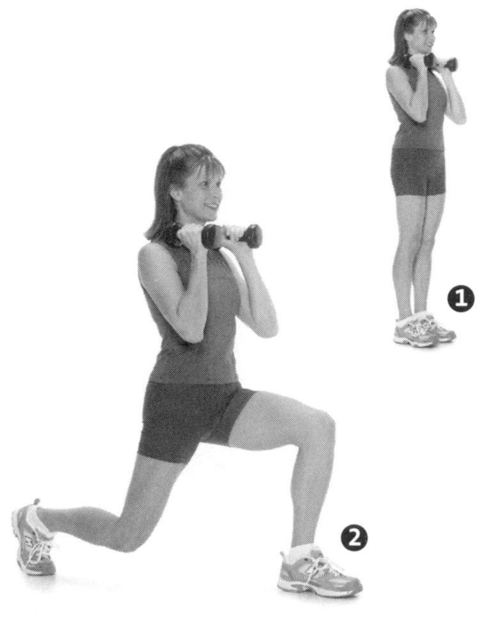

MUST-DO MOVE

Back Lunge

Starting position: Stand with your feet together. Hold a dumbbell in each hand, either at shoulder height or at your sides.

Movement: Step your right foot back 2 to 3 feet. Inhale as you bend your left knee and lower your body straight down until your left knee is bent 90 degrees and your right knee nearly touches the floor. Your rear heel will come off the floor. Hold for a second and then exhale as you push yourself back up, bringing your right foot back in. Finish all of your repetitions, then repeat the exercise stepping back with your left foot.

Technique: Don't lean forward. Don't let your front knee move forward over your toes.

Step Squat

Starting position: Stand with your feet together and your hands down at your sides.

Movement: Step your right foot out to the side 2 to $2\frac{1}{2}$ feet. Keeping your back straight, lower yourself, bending from the knees and hips as though you're sitting down, as you inhale. Let your arms come out in front of you to help you balance. Stop just before your thighs are parallel to the floor. Hold for a second and then exhale as you push back up, bringing your right foot back in. Do five or six reps with your right foot and then do five or six reps stepping with your left foot.

Technique: Don't let your knees move forward over your toes. Don't round your back.

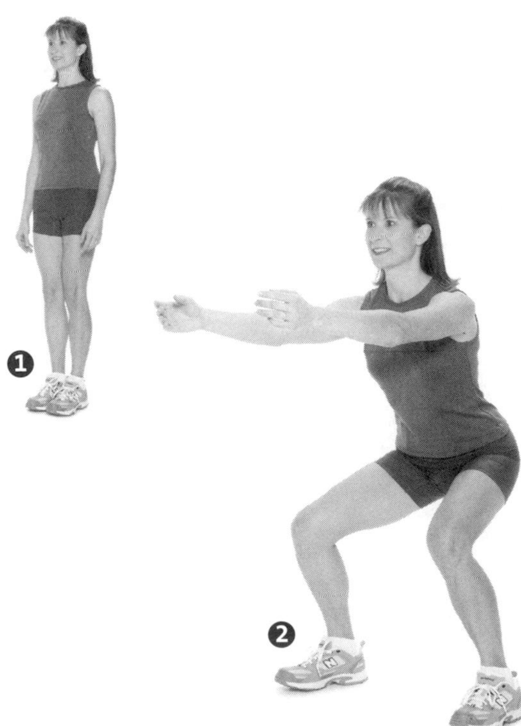

continued

The Workout

Level 1 *continued*

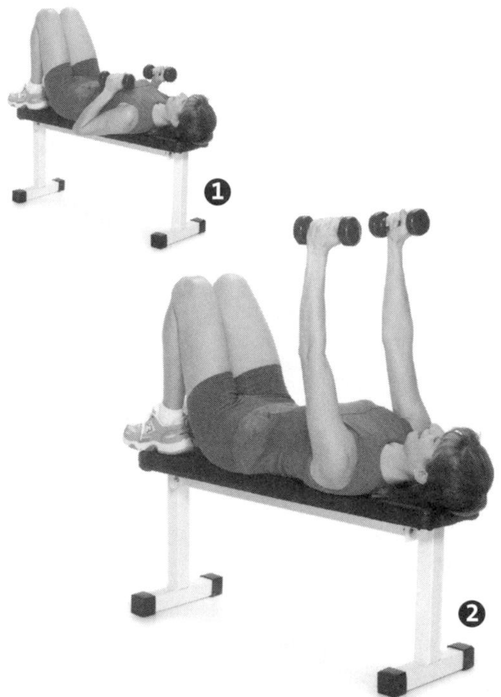

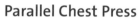

Parallel Chest Press

Starting position: Lying on the floor (or on a bench), hold dumbbells parallel and just above your shoulders; your elbows should be pointing toward your feet.

Movement: Exhale as you press the dumbbells straight up over your chest, extending your arms. Hold for a second and then inhale as you slowly lower them.

Technique: Don't press the dumbbells back toward your head or forward toward your feet: They should go straight up and down. Don't arch your back.

Alternate position: If it's uncomfortable to have your feet on the bench, you can place them on the floor. Make sure your back doesn't arch in that position.

MUST-DO MOVE

Bent-Knee Pushup

Starting position: Lie facedown on the floor. Bend your knees so that your feet are up in the air, and place your palms on the floor near your shoulders so that your elbows are pointing up. Press down with your hands, extend your arms, and lift your body off the floor.

Movement: Keeping your head, back, hips, and knees in a straight line, bend your elbows out to the sides and lower your body as you inhale, until your chest nearly touches the floor. Hold for a second and then exhale as you slowly push back up.

Technique: Don't bend at the hips. Don't arch your back.

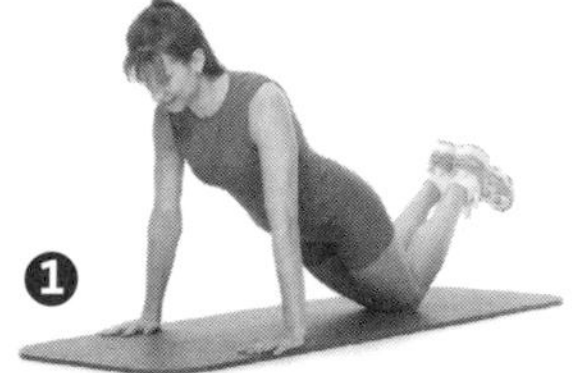

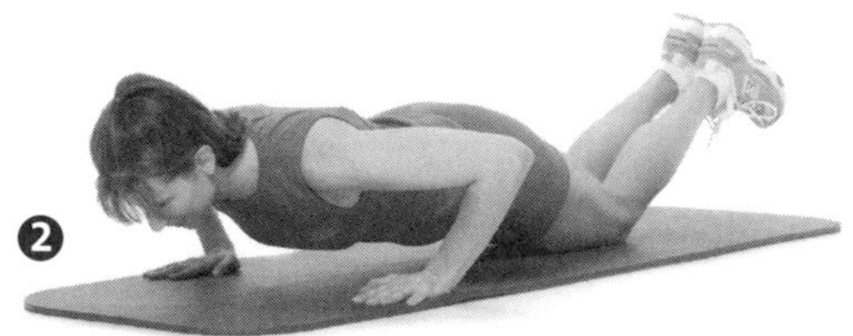

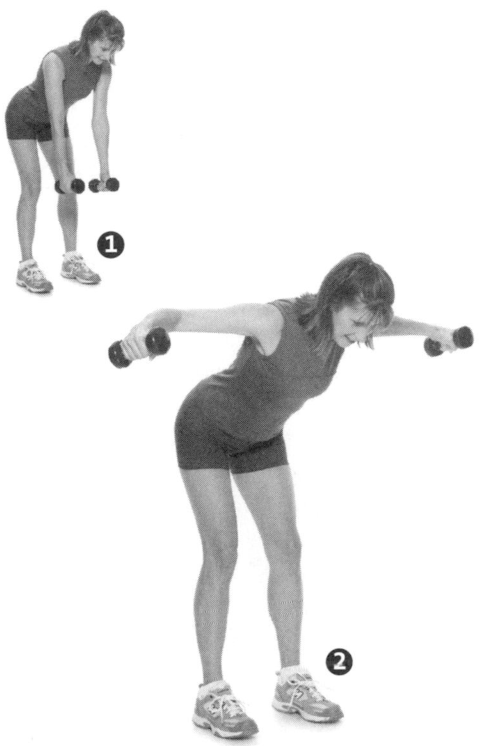

Back Fly

Starting position: Stand with your feet shoulder width apart and knees bent slightly. Hold a dumbbell in each hand with your arms at your sides. Keep your back flat and lean forward, bending at the hips so that the dumbbells are hanging at arm's length in front of you, palms facing each other and elbows bent slightly.

Movement: Keeping your back straight, squeeze your shoulder blades together and lift the dumbbells up and out to the sides as you exhale, pulling your elbows back as far as comfortably possible. Hold for a second and then inhale as you slowly lower them.

Technique: Don't arch your back. Don't raise your torso as you lift the dumbbells.

Alternate move: If you have back problems, support yourself with one hand on a chair and do the flies one arm at a time.

MUST-DO MOVE

Bent-Over Row

Starting position: Stand with your feet shoulder width apart, knees bent slightly. Hold a dumbbell in each hand with your arms at your sides. Keep your back flat and lean forward, bending at the hips so that the dumbbells are hanging at arm's length in front of you, palms facing each other.

Movement: Bending your elbows back and squeezing your shoulder blades, lift the weights toward your ribs as you exhale, until your elbows are higher than your back. Hold for a second and then inhale as you slowly lower them.

Technique: Don't arch your back. Don't pull your shoulders up toward your ears. Don't raise your torso as you lift the dumbbells.

Alternate move: If you have back problems, support yourself with one hand on a chair and do the rows one arm at a time.

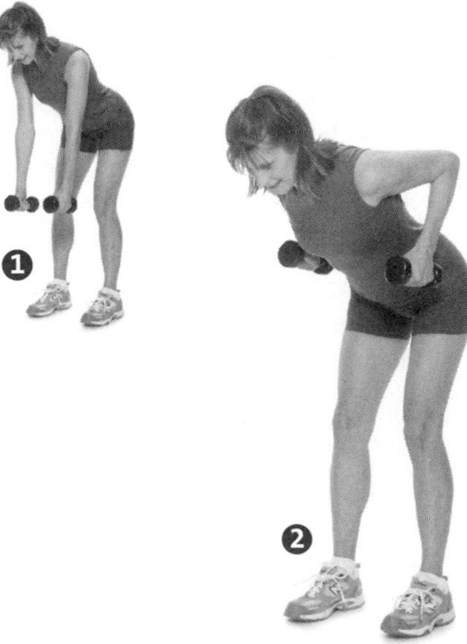

continued

The Workout

Level 1 *continued*

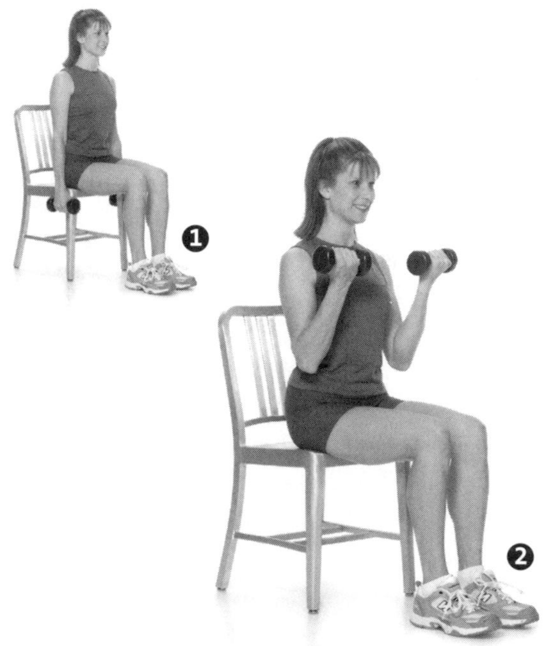

Seated Biceps Curl with a Twist

Starting position: Sit on the edge of a chair with your feet hip width apart. Hold dumbbells at your sides with your palms facing in.

Movement: Bending your elbows and turning your wrists upward, lift the dumbbells toward your shoulders as you exhale. Stop when the dumbbells are at chest height, palms facing your body. Hold for a second and then inhale as you slowly lower them.

Technique: Don't move your upper arms.

Seated Triceps Kickback with a Twist

Starting position: Sit on the edge of a chair with your feet hip width apart and hold a dumbbell in each hand. Keep your back flat and lean forward, bending at the hips. Bend your arms at about 90-degree angles with your dumbbells at about hip height.

Movement: Without moving your upper arms, press the dumbbells back as you exhale, extending your arms and turning your wrists so that your palms face the ceiling. Hold for a second and then inhale as you slowly lower them.

Technique: Don't move from your shoulders. Don't raise your torso as you lift the dumbbells.

Alternate move: If you have back problems, do the kickbacks one arm at a time and place the forearm of your other arm across your thighs for extra support.

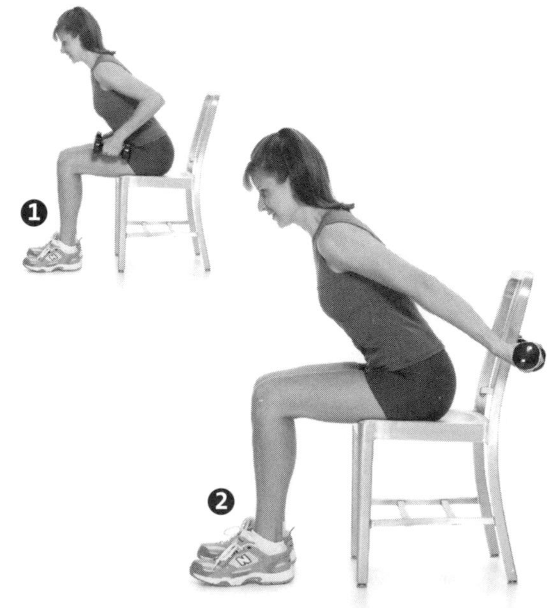

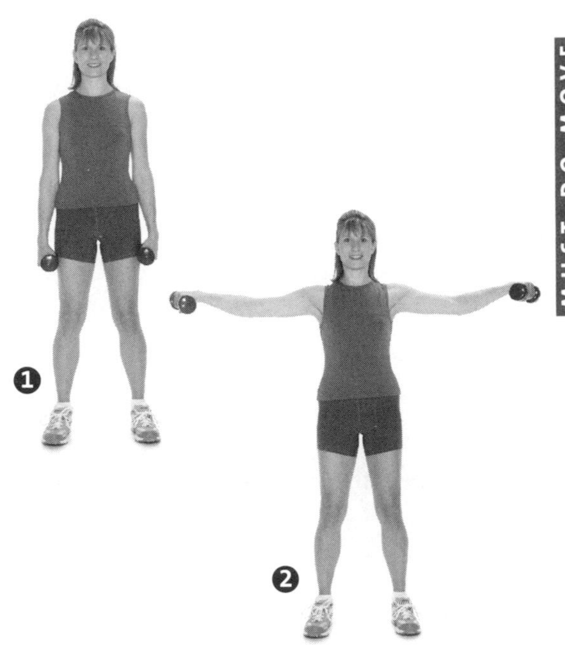

MUST-DO MOVE

Lateral Raise

Starting position: Stand with your feet shoulder width apart, knees bent slightly. Hold a dumbbell in each hand with your arms at your sides, palms facing in, and elbows bent slightly.

Movement: Exhale as you slowly raise the dumbbells out to the sides until they are at about shoulder height. Hold for a second and then inhale as you slowly lower them.

Technique: Don't lift your shoulders. Don't lift higher than shoulder height.

Shoulder Shrug

Starting position: Stand with your feet shoulder width apart, knees bent slightly. Hold a dumbbell in each hand with your arms at your sides, palms facing in.

Movement: Exhale as you slowly lift your shoulders up toward your ears as high as possible. Hold for a second and then inhale as you slowly lower them.

Technique: Don't bend your elbows. Don't use your arms to lift.

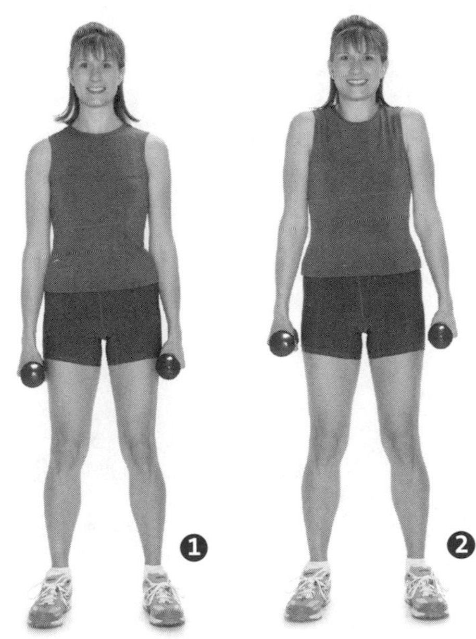

The Workout

Level 2

Easy Walk: 40 Minutes

- 5-minute warmup: Walk 2½ to 3 miles per hour, or 100 to 115 steps per minute.
- 30-minute moderate walk: Increase your speed to 3 to 3½ miles per hour, 115 to 125 steps per minute, or a pace that lets you comfortably carry on a conversation.
- 5-minute cooldown: Slow down to 2½ to 3 miles per hour, or 100 to 115 steps per minute.

Heavy Strength Training: 30 Minutes

- Do four to six reps of each exercise, using a heavier weight. Repeat the sequence of exercises three times.
- To warm up, use lighter weights, or none at all, the first time through, and for the squat and lunge exercises, only go partway down.

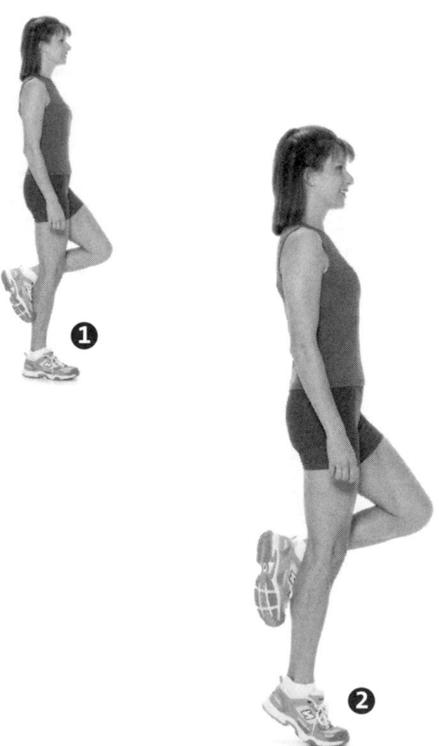

Single-Heel Raise

Starting position: Stand on one foot with the other resting on your calf. Lightly hold on to a chair or wall with one hand if needed for balance.

Movement: Exhale as you slowly lift your heel off the floor, rolling up onto your toes. Hold for a second and then inhale as you slowly lower it. Do the recommended number of reps and then switch feet.

Technique: Don't bend at the waist or lean forward, back, or to the side. Don't bend your supporting leg.

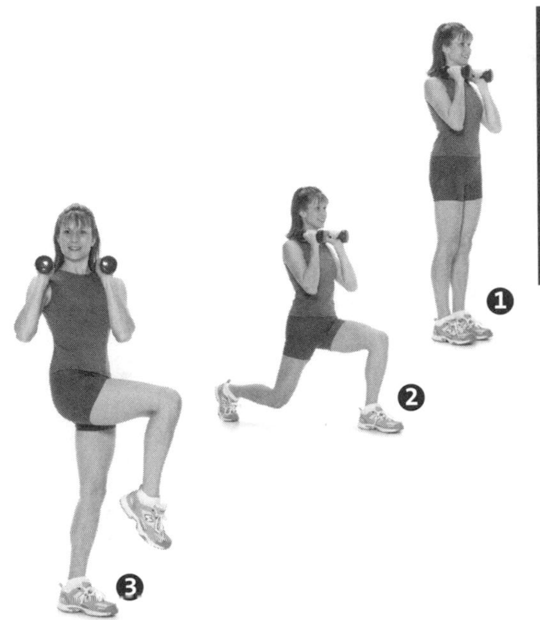

MUST-DO MOVE

Back Lunge with Knee Lift and Twist

Starting position: Stand with your feet together. Hold a dumbbell in each hand, either at shoulder height or at your sides.

Movement: Step your right foot back 2 to 3 feet. Inhale as you bend your left knee and lower your body straight down until your left knee is bent 90 degrees and your right knee nearly touches the floor. Your rear heel will come off the floor. Hold for a second and then exhale as you push yourself back up. Lift your right knee up in front of you as you twist your torso to the right before returning to the starting position. Finish all of your repetitions, then repeat the exercise stepping back with your left foot.

Technique: Don't lean forward. Don't let your front knee move forward over your toes.

Step Squat with Jump

Starting position: Stand with your feet together and your hands down at your sides.

Movement: Step your right foot out to the side 2 to $2\frac{1}{2}$ feet. Keeping your back straight, lower yourself, bending from the knees and hips as though you're sitting down, as you inhale. Let your arms come out in front of you to help you balance. Stop just before your thighs are parallel to the floor. Hold for a second and then exhale as you jump and bring your right foot back to the starting position. Do two or three reps with your right foot and then do two or three reps stepping with your left foot.

Technique: Don't let your knees move forward over your toes. Don't round your back. Don't do this move while holding weights.

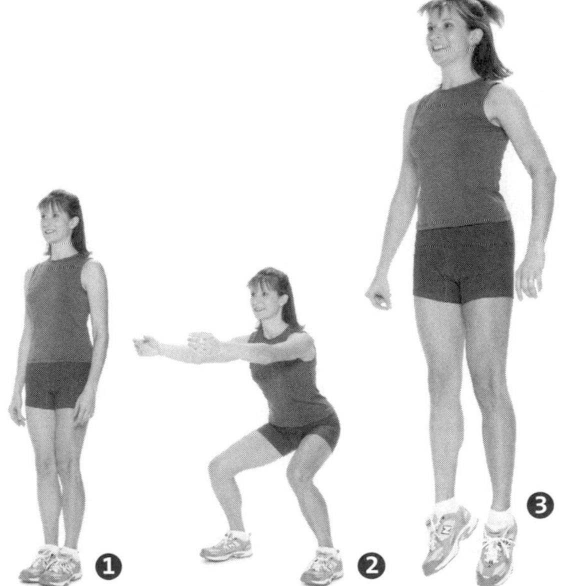

continued

The Workout

Level 2 *continued*

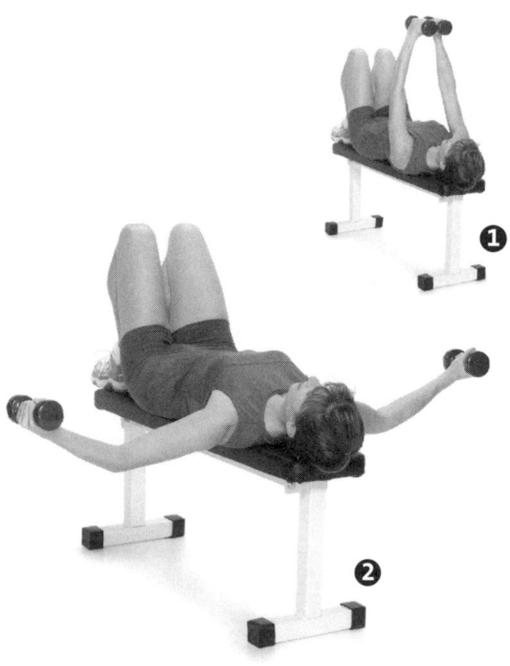

Chest Fly

Starting position: Lie on your back on the floor (or on a bench) with your knees bent and your feet flat on the floor. Hold a dumbbell in each hand above your chest with your palms facing each other and your elbows slightly bent.

Movement: As you inhale, slowly lower your arms out to the sides. Hold for a second and then as you exhale, press the dumbbells back up.

Technique: Don't arch your back. If you're doing this on a bench, don't lower the dumbbells below shoulder height.

Alternate position: If it's uncomfortable to have your feet on the bench, you can place them on the floor. Make sure your back doesn't arch in that position.

MUST-DO MOVE

Pushup

Starting position: Lie facedown on the floor with your feet flexed and toes tucked. Place your palms on the floor near your shoulders so that your elbows are pointing up. Press down with your hands, extend your arms, and lift your body off the floor so that it forms a straight line from head to toe.

Movement: Keeping your head, back, hips, and legs in a straight line, bend your elbows out to the sides and lower your body as you inhale, until your chest nearly touches the floor. Hold for a second and then exhale as you push back up. If you can't do all the recommended reps in this full pushup position, that's okay. Just drop down onto one or both knees and complete the remaining reps.

Technique: Don't bend at the hips. Don't arch your back.

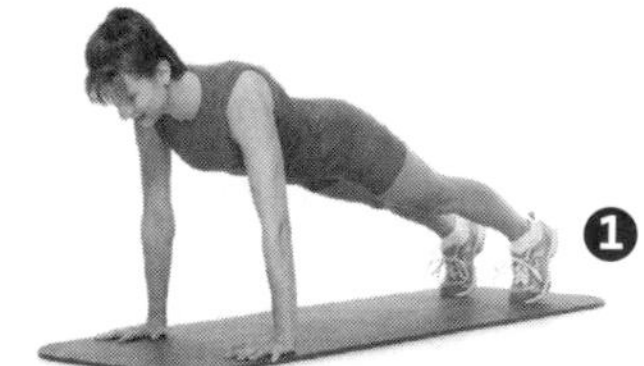

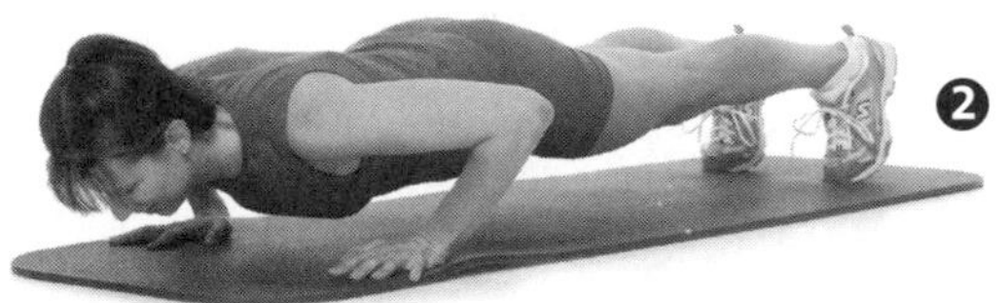

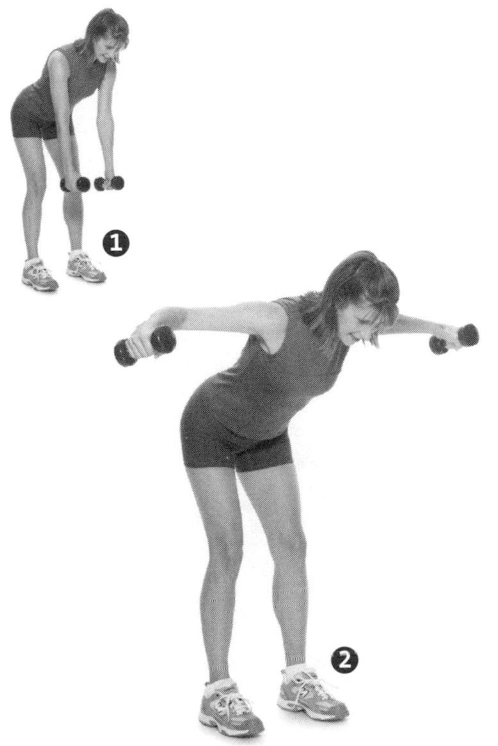

Back Fly

Starting position: Stand with your feet shoulder width apart and knees bent slightly. Hold a dumbbell in each hand with your arms at your sides. Keep your back flat and lean forward, bending at the hips so that the dumbbells are hanging at arm's length in front of you, palms facing each other and elbows bent slightly.

Movement: Keeping your back straight, squeeze your shoulder blades together and lift the dumbbells up and out to the sides as you exhale, pulling your elbows back as far as comfortably possible. Hold for a second and then inhale as you slowly lower them.

Technique: Don't arch your back. Don't raise your torso as you lift the dumbbells.

Alternate move: If you have back problems, support yourself with one hand on a chair and do the flies one arm at a time.

MUST-DO MOVE

Bent-Over Row

Starting position: Stand with your feet shoulder width apart, knees bent slightly. Hold a dumbbell in each hand with your arms at your sides. Keep your back flat and lean forward, bending at the hips so that the dumbbells are hanging at arm's length in front of you, palms facing each other.

Movement: Bending your elbows back and squeezing your shoulder blades, lift the weights toward your ribs as you exhale, until your elbows are higher than your back. Hold for a second and then inhale as you slowly lower them.

Technique: Don't arch your back. Don't pull your shoulders up toward your ears. Don't raise your torso as you lift the dumbbells.

Alternate move: If you have back problems, support yourself with one hand on a chair and do the rows one arm at a time.

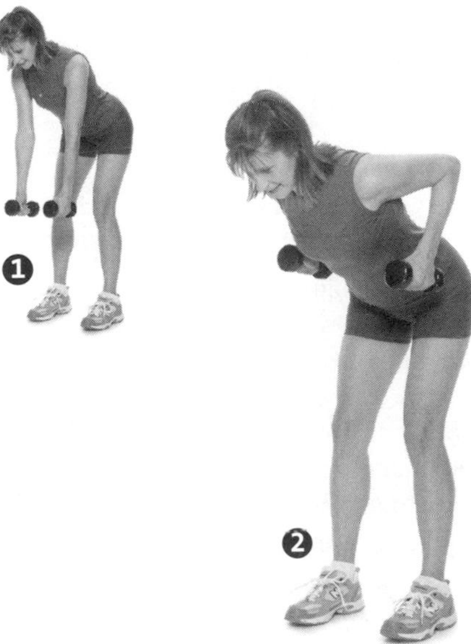

continued

The Workout

Level 2 *continued*

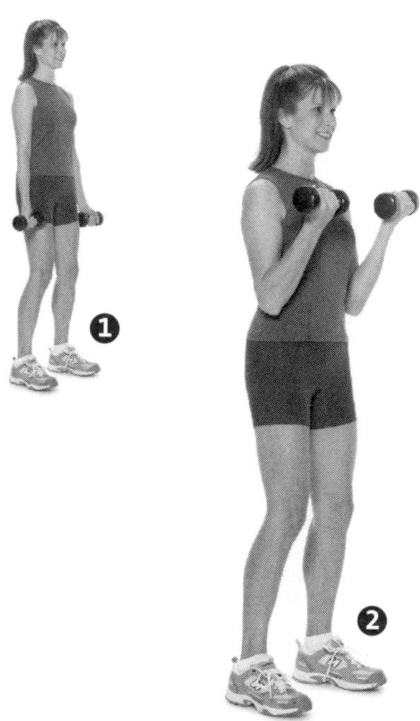

Biceps Curl

Starting position: Stand with your feet shoulder width apart, knees bent slightly. Hold a dumbbell in each hand with your palms facing forward.

Movement: Bending your elbows, lift the dumbbells toward your shoulders as you exhale. Stop when the dumbbells are at chest height, palms facing your body. Hold for a second and then inhale as you slowly lower them.

Technique: Don't move your upper arms.

Triceps Pushup

Starting position: Lie facedown on the floor with your feet flexed and toes tucked. Place your palms on the floor close to your ribs so that your elbows are pointing up. Press down with your hands, extend your arms, and lift your body off the floor.

Movement: Keeping your head, back, hips, and legs in a straight line, bend your elbows back, keeping your arms close to your body, as you inhale. Lower your body until your chest nearly touches the floor. Hold for a second and then exhale as you push back up. If you can't do all the recommended reps in this full pushup position, that's okay. Just drop down onto one or both knees and complete the remaining reps.

Technique: Don't let your elbows point out to the sides. Don't bend at the hips. Don't drop your belly toward the floor.

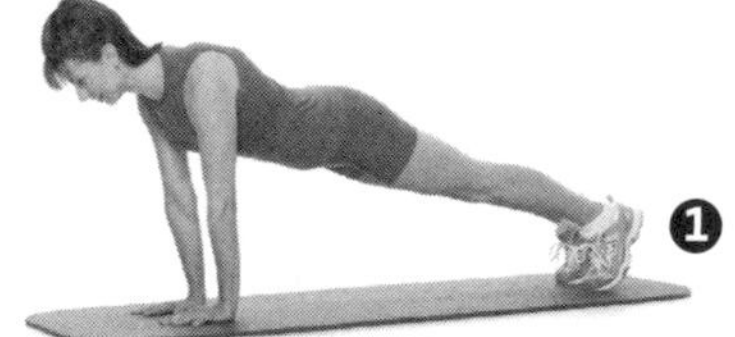

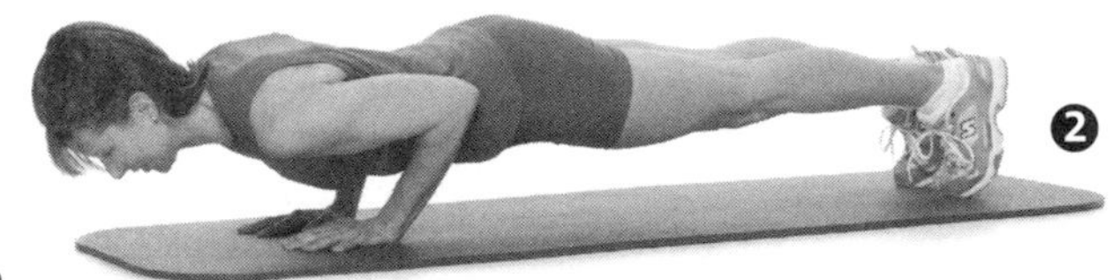

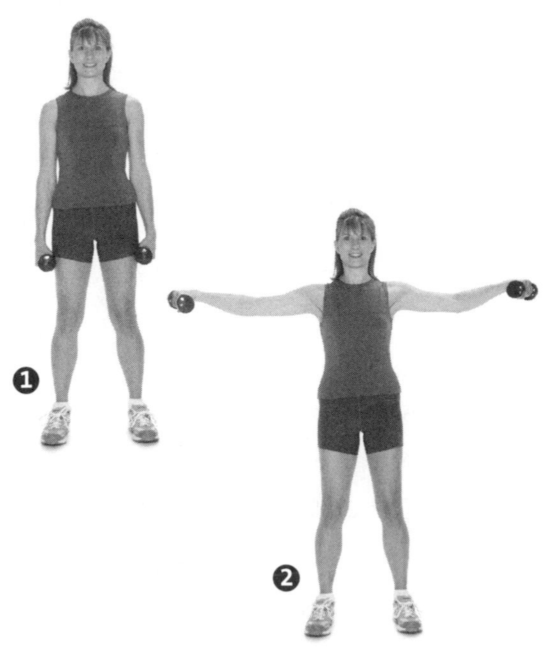

Lateral Raise

Starting position: Stand with your feet shoulder width apart, knees bent slightly. Hold a dumbbell in each hand with your arms at your sides, palms facing in and elbows bent slightly.

Movement: Exhale as you slowly raise the dumbbells out to the sides until they are at about shoulder height. Hold for a second and then inhale as you slowly lower them.

Technique: Don't lift your shoulders. Don't lift higher than shoulder height.

MUST-DO MOVE

Parallel Overhead Press

Starting position: Stand with your feet shoulder width apart and knees bent slightly. Hold a dumbbell in each hand at shoulder height, palms facing each other and elbows pointing forward.

Movement: Exhale as you slowly press the dumbbells straight overhead without locking your elbows. Hold for a second and then inhale as you slowly lower them.

Technique: Don't arch your back. Don't lift the dumbbells forward or back.

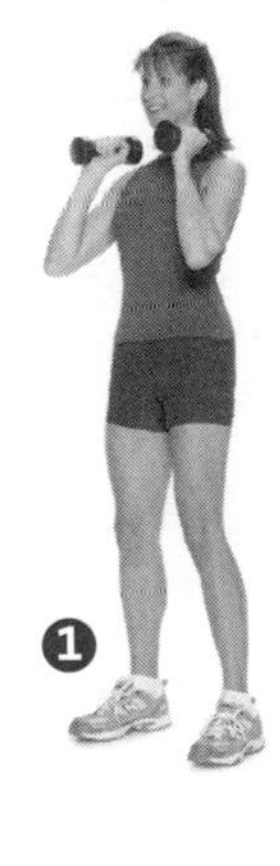

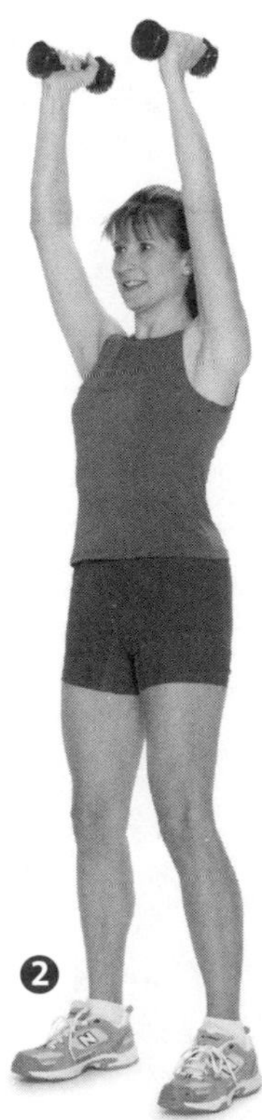

The Workout

Level 3

Easy Walk: 40 Minutes

- 5-minute warmup: Walk 2½ to 3 miles per hour, or 100 to 115 steps per minute.
- 30-minute moderate walk: Increase your speed to 3½ to 4 miles per hour, 125 to 135 steps per minute, or a pace that lets you comfortably carry on a conversation.
- 5-minute cooldown: Slow down to 2½ to 3 miles per hour, or 100 to 115 steps per minute.

Heavy Strength Training: 30 Minutes

- Do four to six reps of each exercise, using a heavier weight. Repeat the sequence of exercises three times.
- To warm up, use lighter weights, or none at all, the first time through, and for the squat and lunge exercises, only go partway down.

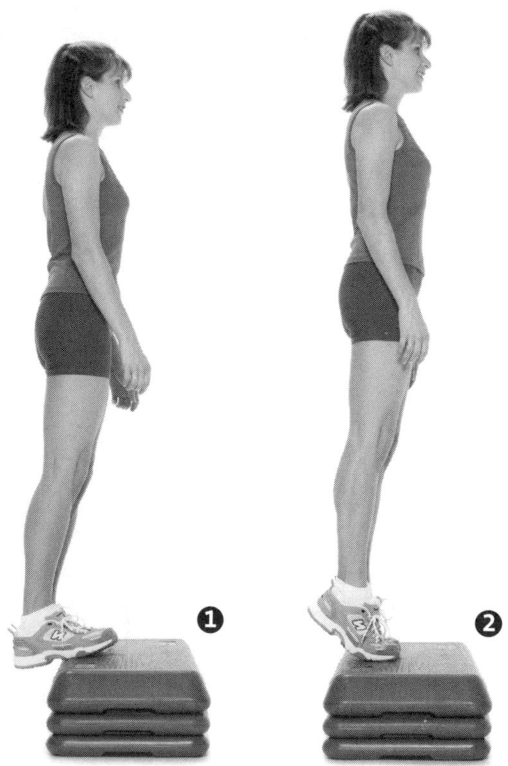

Heel Raise on Step

Starting position: Stand on the edge of a step so that your heels are hanging off. Lightly hold on to the railing, a chair, or a wall with one hand if needed for balance.

Movement: Exhale as you slowly rise up onto your toes. Hold for a second and then inhale as you slowly lower, allowing your heels to drop below the edge of the step.

Technique: Don't bend at the waist or lean forward, back, or to the side.

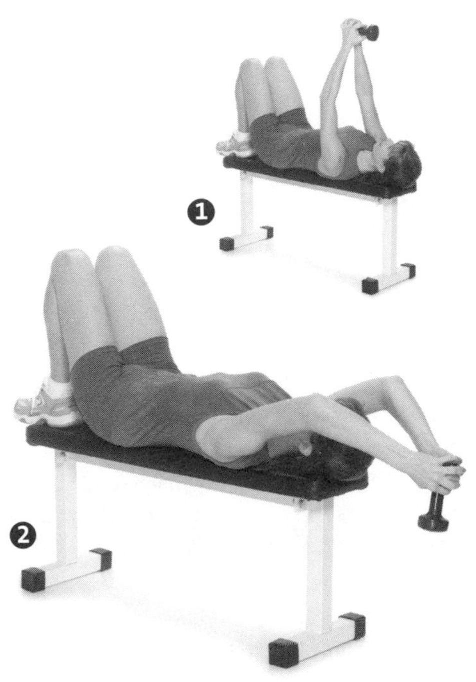

Pullover

Starting position: Lie face up on the floor (or on a bench). Grasp a dumbbell with both hands and hold it above your chest with your elbows bent slightly.

Movement: Inhale as you lower the dumbbell backward over your head as far as comfortably possible without bending your elbows any farther than at the start. Hold for a second and then exhale as you slowly raise it to the starting position.

Technique: Don't arch your back. Don't bend your elbows to lower the weight.

Alternate position: If it's uncomfortable to have your feet on the bench, you can place them on the floor. Make sure your back doesn't arch in that position.

MUST-DO MOVE

One-Leg Pushup

Starting position: Lie facedown on the floor with your feet flexed and toes tucked. Place your palms on the floor near your shoulders so that your elbows are pointing up. Press down with your hands, extend your arms, and lift your body off the floor so that it forms a straight line from head to toe, and lift your left foot off the floor.

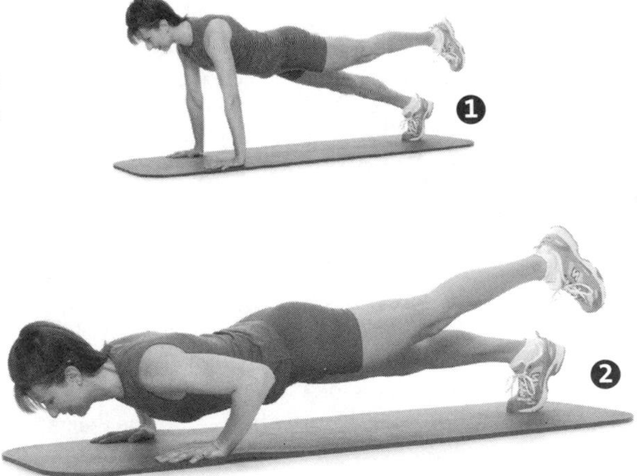

Movement: Keeping your head, back, hips, and legs in a straight line, bend your elbows out to the sides and lower your body as you inhale, until your chest nearly touches the floor. Hold for a second and then exhale as you push back up. If you can't do all the recommended reps in this full pushup position, that's okay. Just drop down onto both feet or one or both knees and complete the remaining reps. Do half of the recommended reps with your left leg off the floor and the other half with your right leg off the floor.

Technique: Don't bend at the hips. Don't arch your back.

continued

The Workout

Level 3 *continued*

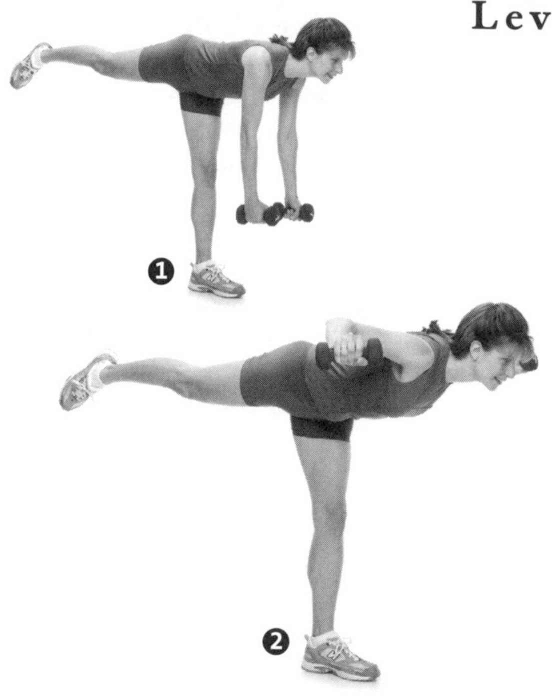

Balancing Back Fly

Starting position: Hold a dumbbell in each hand and lean forward, lifting your right foot so that your left leg, back, and head are parallel to the floor and your arms are below your shoulders, palms facing each other and elbows bent slightly.

Movement: Keeping your back straight, squeeze your shoulder blades together and lift the dumbbells up and out to the sides as you exhale. Hold for a second and then inhale as you slowly lower them. Do half of the recommended reps balancing on your left leg and the other half on your right leg.

Technique: Don't arch your back. Don't raise your torso as you lift the dumbbells.

Alternate move: If you have back problems, keep both legs down and support yourself with one hand on a chair and do the flies one arm at a time.

MUST-DO MOVE

Balancing Bent-Over Row

Starting position: Stand with your right foot in front of your left. Hold a dumbbell in each hand with your arms at your sides. Keep your back flat and lean forward, lifting your back foot off the floor so that your left leg, back, and head are as parallel to the floor as possible. The dumbbells should be hanging at arm's length directly below your shoulders, palms facing each other.

Movement: Bending your elbows back and squeezing your shoulder blades, lift the weights toward your ribs as you exhale, until your elbows are higher than your back. Hold for a second and then inhale as you slowly lower them. Do half of the recommended reps balancing on your right leg and the other half on your left leg.

Technique: Don't arch your back. Don't pull your shoulders up toward your ears. Don't raise your torso as you lift the dumbbells.

Alternate move: If you have back problems, keep both legs down, support yourself with one hand on a chair, and do the rows one arm at a time.

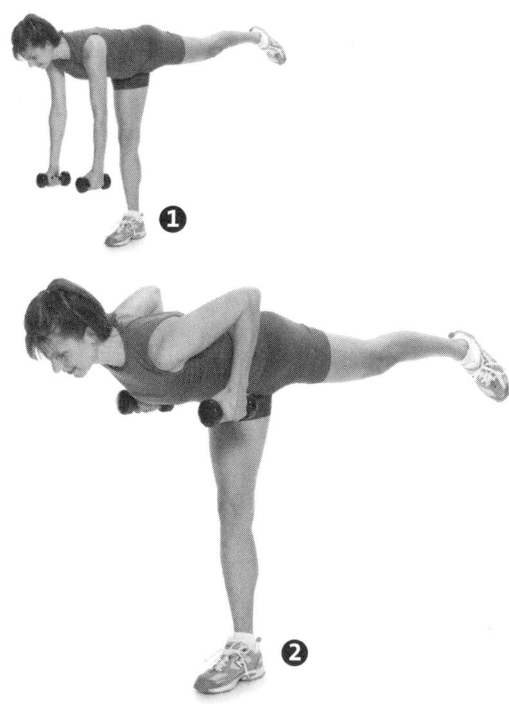

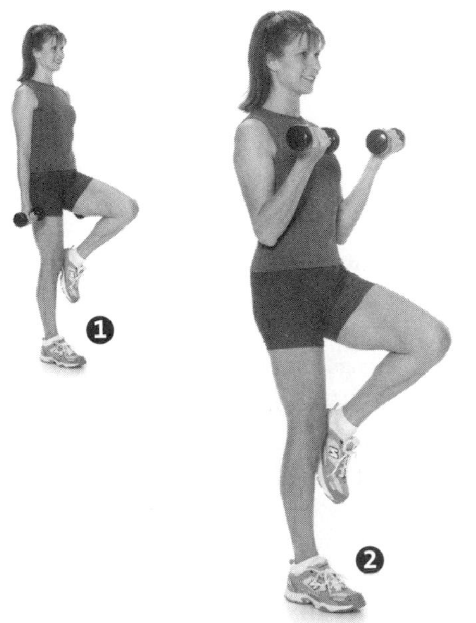

Balancing Biceps Curl

Starting position: Stand with your feet together, knees bent slightly. Hold a dumbbell in each hand with your palms facing forward. Lift your left knee up in front of you so that you're balancing on your right leg.

Movement: Bending your elbows, lift the dumbbells toward your shoulders as you exhale. Stop when the dumbbells are at chest height, palms facing your body. Hold for a second and then inhale as you slowly lower them. Do half of the recommended reps balancing on your right leg and the other half on your left leg.

Technique: Don't move your upper arms.

Lunge Jump

Starting position: Stand with your feet together and your hands on your hips.

Movement: Step your right foot forward 2 to 3 feet. Inhale as you bend your right knee and lower your body straight down until your right knee is bent 90 degrees and your left knee nearly touches the floor. Your rear heel will come off the floor. Hold for a second and then exhale as you push off with your right foot, jump, and switch your legs, landing with your left foot in front. Lunge and then jump again, alternating legs each jump for a total of four to six jumps.

Technique: Don't lean forward. Don't let your front knee move forward over your toes.

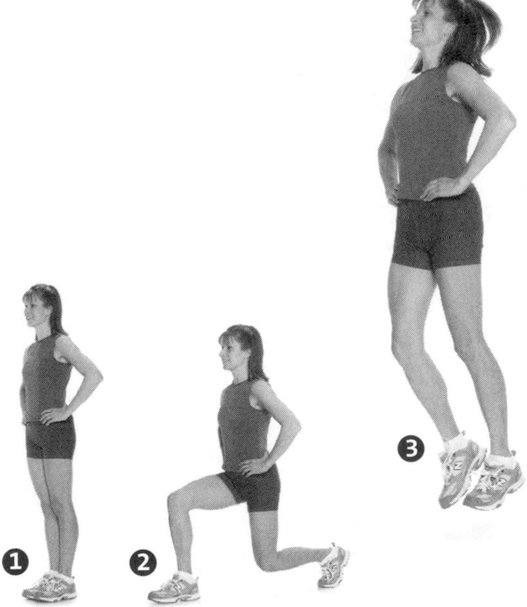

continued

The Workout

Level 3 *continued*

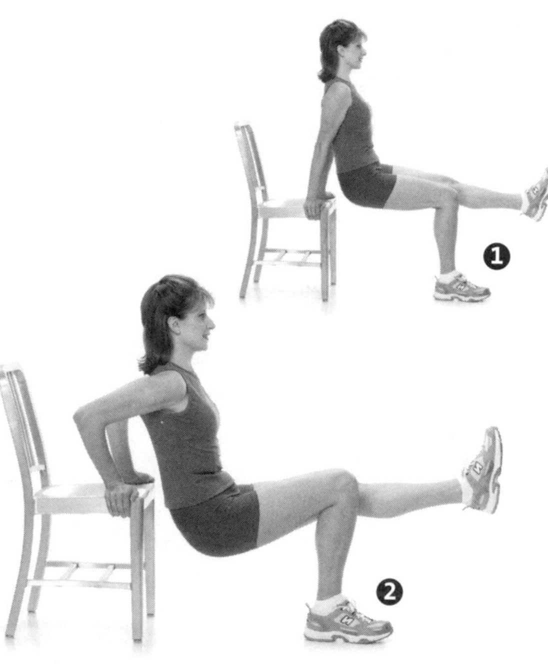

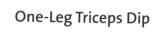

One-Leg Triceps Dip

Starting position: Sit on the edge of a chair, place your hands on either side of you, and grasp the chair seat. Slide your buttocks off the chair, walk your feet out until your legs are bent at about 90 degrees, lift your left foot off the floor, and extend your left leg. You should be balancing on your hands and right foot.

Movement: Bending your arms so that your elbows point behind you, slowly lower your body toward the floor as you inhale. Keep your buttocks as close to the chair as possible. Stop when your elbows are bent about 90 degrees. Hold for a second and then exhale as you press back up. Do half of the recommended reps with your left leg extended and the other half with your right leg extended.

Technique: Don't sink into your arms, allowing your shoulders to come up toward your ears. Don't bend your knees to help lower yourself.

Alternate move: For a more challenging version, extend your legs straight and balance on your heels.

Balancing Lateral Raise

Starting position: Stand with your feet together, knees bent slightly. Hold a dumbbell in each hand with your arms at your sides. Lift your right knee up in front of you so that you're balancing on your left leg.

Movement: Exhale as you slowly lift the dumbbells out to the sides, until they are at about shoulder height. Hold for a second and then inhale as you slowly lower them. Do half of the recommended reps balancing on your left leg and the other half on your right leg.

Technique: Don't lift your shoulders up toward your ears. Don't lift higher than shoulder height.

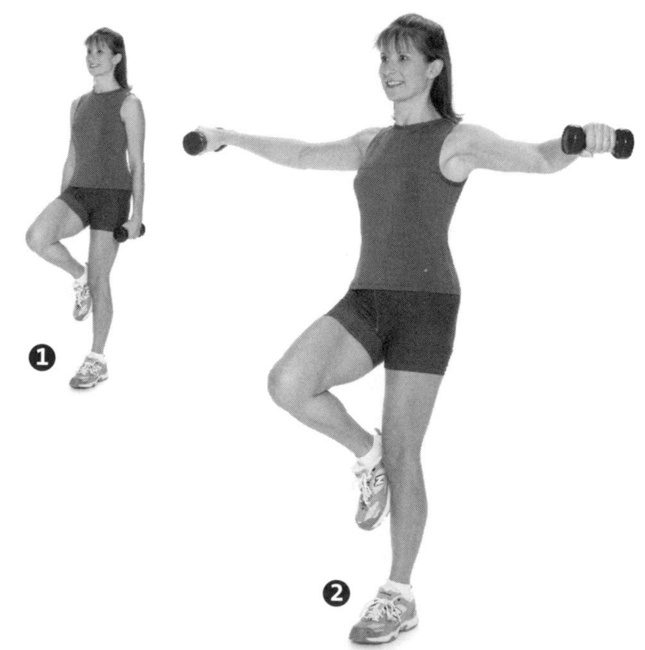

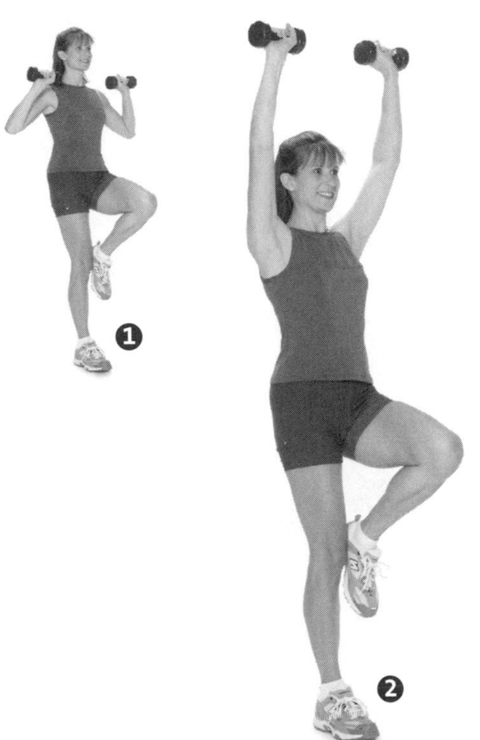

MUST-DO MOVE

Balancing Overhead Press

Starting position: Stand with your feet together, knees bent slightly. Hold a dumbbell in each hand at shoulder height with your palms facing forward and elbows pointing out to the sides. Lift your left knee up in front of you so that you're balancing on your right leg.

Movement: Exhale as you slowly press the dumbbells straight up overhead. Hold for a second and then inhale as you slowly lower them. Do half of the recommended reps balancing on your right leg and the other half on your left leg.

Technique: Don't arch your back. Don't lift the dumbbells forward or back.

MUST-DO MOVE

Squat Jump

Starting position: Stand with your feet together and your hands down at your sides.

Movement: Jump your feet out to the sides 2 to 2½ feet apart. As you land, lower yourself, bending your knees and hips as though you're sitting down. Let your arms come out in front of you to help you balance. Stop just before your thighs are parallel to the floor. Hold for a second and then exhale as you jump and bring both feet back together.

Technique: Don't let your knees move forward over your toes. Don't round your back. Don't do this move while holding weights.

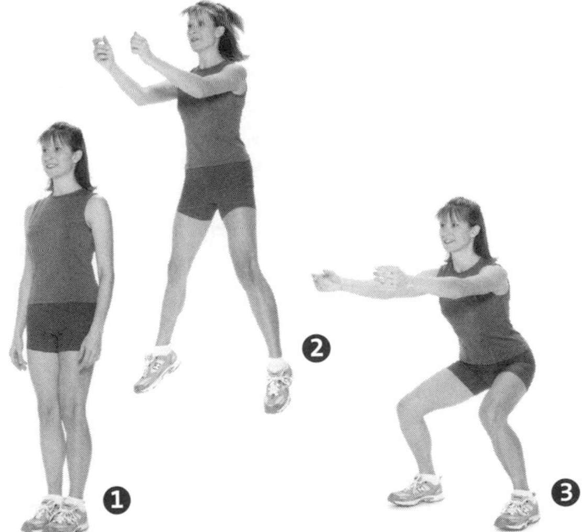

FIRM UP / DAY 20

Real-Life Success Story

When Sue Torpey, 50, of Perkasie, Pennsylvania, joined the *Prevention* program 5 years ago, her travel business specializing in cruises was really starting to grow. And so was her waistline. Hosting one food-filled cruise after another, she was really worried about her weight. "The food is unbelievable on these cruises, and it's available 24 hours a day."

But once Sue started exercising, she lost 14 pounds and discovered that it's possible to keep the weight from coming back. "As long as I stick to lifting weights and eating sensibly at other times, I don't gain weight. Before, I would have put on 10 pounds easily."

To make sure she doesn't miss her morning workouts, Sue prepares ahead of time. "It's hard for me to get going in the morning—even though I enjoy it once I start," she admits. "So I make it as easy as possible. I set out my workout clothes before I go to bed; I put my weights by the treadmill. It's all ready for me come morning.

"Now, I work out 6 days a week," she adds. "I mix it up, doing aerobics and using the elliptical machine, but I always include weights; that's what keeps my fat levels down and my stamina up. Recently, I've been doing hours of manual labor getting ready to open a new business, and I'm outlasting my 20-year-old kids." And when she introduced a friend to the program, her friend lost 42 pounds.

FIRM UP TIPS

ON YOUR PLATE	GET FIRM FASTER
Blot the fat. You can dab off about a teaspoon of oil—or 40 calories and 4.5 grams of fat—from two slices of pizza.	*Pop a piece of gum. Researchers discovered that chewing sugar-free gum all day increases your metabolic rate by about 20 percent. That could burn off more than 10 pounds a year.*

Meal Plan

Most of these recipes are custom designed to make 1 serving–no fuss, no muss; just fix, eat, and go! If a recipe makes more than 1 serving, it's noted below. Save that extra serving for another meal, or share it with your spouse or your walking buddy.

Breakfast

Almond Butter and Apple Sandwich: Open and toast ½ whole wheat pita (6½-inch size). Spread with 1 tablespoon almond butter and stuff with 1 thinly sliced Granny Smith apple. Serve with 1 cup fat-free milk.

Healthy Snack

English Muffin with Peanut Butter: Toast ½ whole grain English muffin and spread with 1 tablespoon peanut butter and 1 tablespoon raisins.

Lunch

Egg Salad with Roasted Red Pepper: Prepare egg salad by combining 2 chopped hard-boiled eggs (discard 1 yolk or cook it and give it to your dog as a healthy treat) with 2 teaspoons horseradish spread, 2 tablespoons light mayonnaise, and ¼ cup chopped roasted red peppers, drained. Add ¼ cup finely chopped celery, if desired. Serve with 1 cup fat-free milk and 17 grapes.

Healthy Snack

Trail Mix: Have 1 serving from the batch you made last week.

Dinner

Tuna and Bean Pasta Salad: Combine tuna from lunch Tuesday with pasta from dinner Wednesday. Serve with 1 cup lettuce with ½ cup sliced cucumber and 1 tablespoon light salad dressing. Serve with 1 apple.

Indulgent Treat

Pepperoni Pizza: Enjoy 1 slice of a medium pie at Little Caesar's. Choose the "Pan! Pan!" variety.

Nutrient analysis: 1,691 calories, 80 g protein, 206 g carbohydrates, 67 g total fat, 15 g saturated fat, 292 mg cholesterol, 24 g dietary fiber, 2,730 mg sodium, 1,038 mg calcium

FIRM UP TIP

MIND OVER MATTER

Think yourself thinner. If you still can't drag yourself out of bed for an early-morning walk, at least imagine yourself hopping out of bed, lacing up your sneaks, and hitting the pavement for an invigorating sunrise jaunt. Mentally rehearsing "thin" habits boosts the belief that you can actually do them. When you're confident that you can do something, you're more likely to succeed.

The Workout

Level 1

Speed Walk: Less Than 20 Minutes

- Follow the same route as the first and second weeks. The goal is to complete the distance in less time.
- 5-minute warmup: Walk 2 miles per hour, about 95 steps per minute.
- Under-10-minute speedup: Starting at the same spot as last week, increase your speed, walking as quickly as you can, until you reach the point where you slowed down last week. You should be able to do the same distance and shave off a few more seconds this week.
- 5-minute cooldown: Slow down to 2 miles per hour, about 95 steps per minute.

Core Training: 20 Minutes

- Do the sequence of exercises one time.

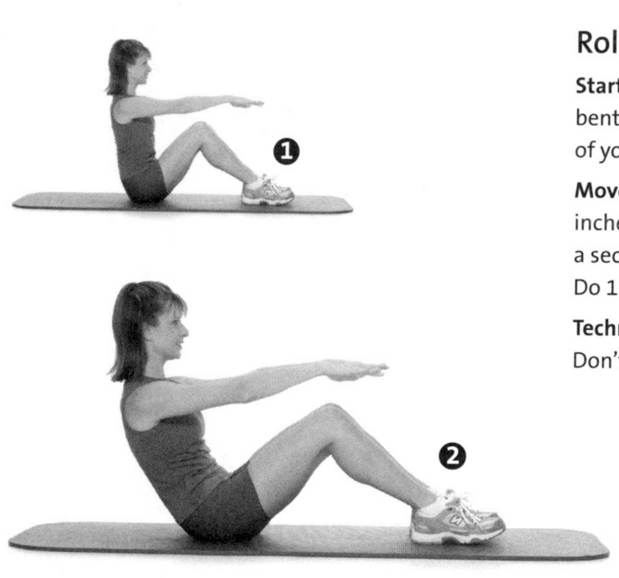

Roll-Down

Starting position: Sit on the floor with your knees bent and your feet flat. Hold your arms out in front of you, parallel to the floor.

Movement: Using your abs, slowly roll down 3 to 4 inches, one vertebra at a time, as you inhale. Hold for a second and then exhale as you slowly roll back up. Do 12 reps.

Technique: Your abs should be powering the move. Don't move quickly.

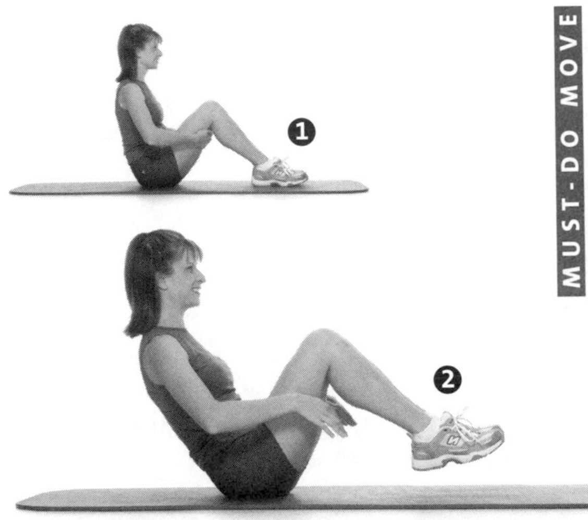

MUST-DO MOVE

Let-Go Balance

Starting position: Sit on the floor with your knees bent and your feet flat. Place your hands behind your thighs.

Movement: Lift your feet off the floor slightly and balance on your sitting bones. Try letting go of your legs. Hold for five breaths and then relax. Do one time only.

Technique: Keep your abs tight and the rest of your body relaxed, especially your shoulders.

Ab Crunch

Starting position: Lie on your back with your knees bent, feet flat on the floor, and hands behind your head.

Movement: Using your abs, slowly raise your head, shoulders, and upper back about 45 degrees off the floor as you exhale. Think of shortening the distance between your ribs and pelvis. Hold for a second and then inhale as you slowly lower yourself. Do 12 reps.

Technique: Don't pull your chin to your chest. Don't arch your back.

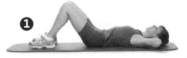

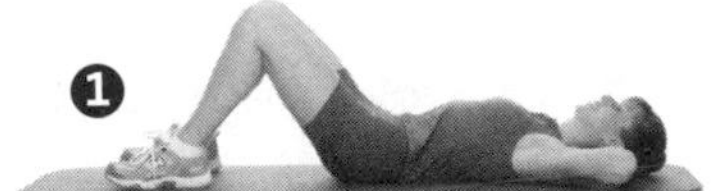

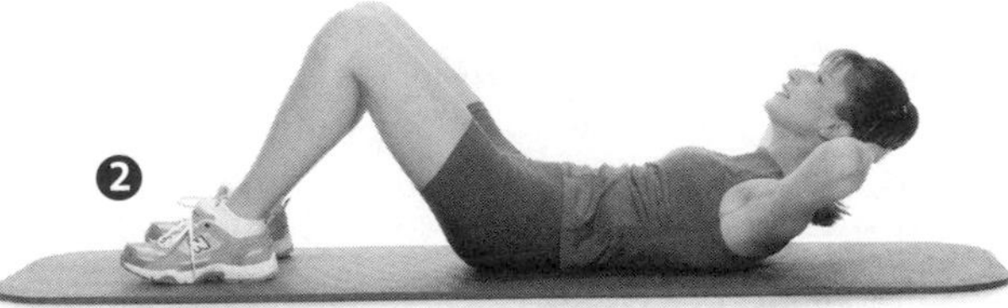

continued

The Workout

Level 1 *continued*

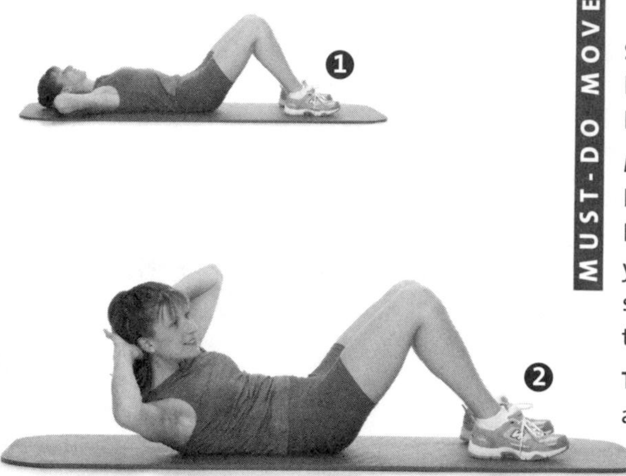

MUST-DO MOVE

Twisting Crunch

Starting position: Lie on your back with your knees bent, feet flat on the floor, and hands behind your head.

Movement: Using your abs, slowly lift your head and left shoulder off the floor, twist to the right, and bring your left shoulder toward your right knee as you exhale. Hold for a second and then inhale as you slowly lower yourself. Repeat, alternating sides. Do a total of 12 reps, 6 reps to each side.

Technique: Don't pull your chin to your chest. Don't arch your back.

MUST-DO MOVE

Bridge with Lift

Starting position: Lie on your back with your knees bent, feet flat on the floor, and arms at your sides, palms facing up.

Movement: Contracting your abs, buttocks, and lower back, press into your feet and lift your butt, hips, and back off the floor as you exhale, to form a straight line from your shoulders to your knees. Lift one foot a few inches off the floor. Hold for three breaths and then lower your foot. Lift the other foot up and hold for three breaths. Lower your foot and then relax. Do one time only.

Technique: Don't lift too high—your upper back and shoulders should remain on the floor. Don't bend at the waist or hips. Don't let your knees fall inward or outward.

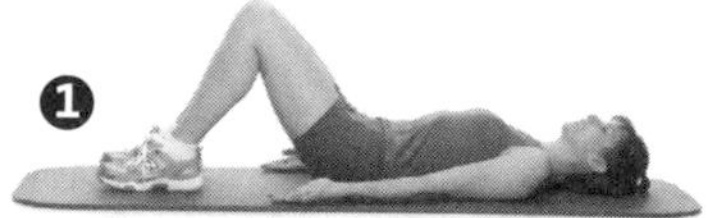

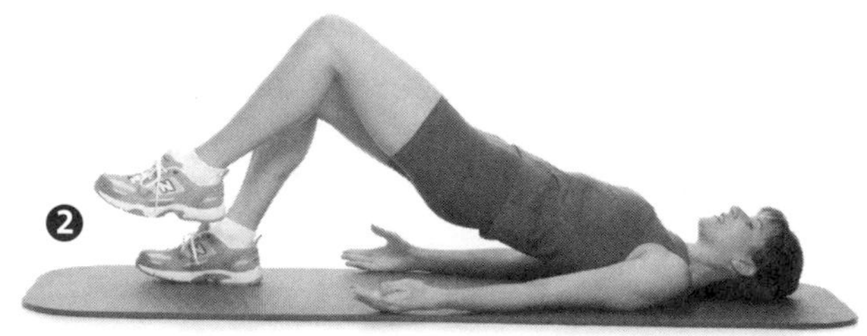

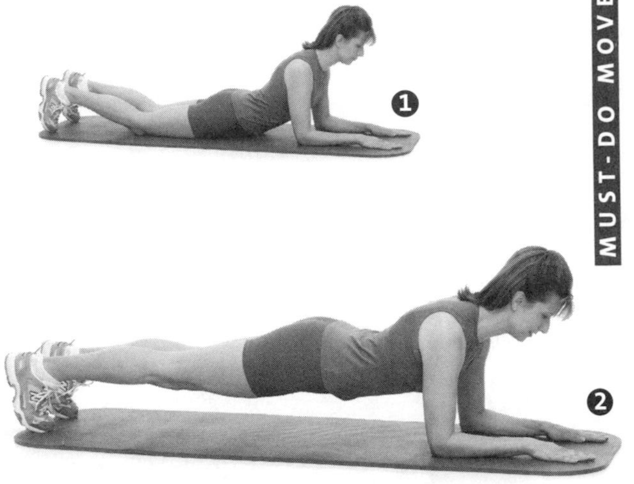

MUST-DO MOVE

Plank

Starting position: Lie facedown with your feet flexed and toes tucked. Your elbows should be under your shoulders and your forearms and palms on the floor.

Movement: Contracting your abs and back, press into your forearms as you exhale and lift your pelvis and legs off the floor so that your back and legs form a straight line. Hold for five breaths and then relax. Do one time only.

Technique: Don't lift your head up or let it drop. Don't bend at the waist or hips. Don't let your belly drop toward the floor.

Chest and Leg Lift

Starting position: Lie facedown on the floor with your arms at your sides.

Movement: Exhale as you lift your head, chest, and legs 5 to 10 inches off the floor. Hold for a second and then inhale as you slowly lower yourself. Do 12 reps.

Technique: Don't lift too high.

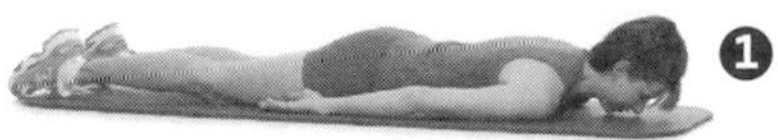

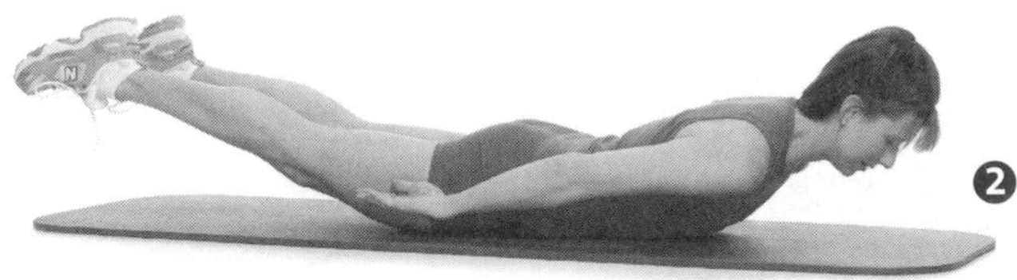

The Workout

Level 2

Speed Walk: Less Than 20 Minutes

- Follow the same route as the first and second weeks. The goal is to complete the distance in less time.
- 5-minute warmup: Walk 2 to 2½ miles per hour, 95 to 100 steps per minute.
- Under-10-minute speedup: Starting at the same spot as last week, increase your speed, walking as quickly as you can, until you reach the point where you slowed down last week. You should be able to do the same distance and shave off a few more seconds this week.
- 5-minute cooldown: Slow down to 2 to 2½ miles per hour, 95 to 100 steps per minute.

Core Training: 20 Minutes

- Do the sequence of exercises one time.

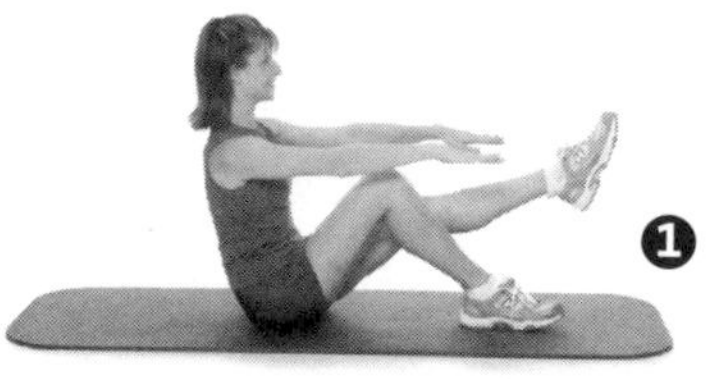

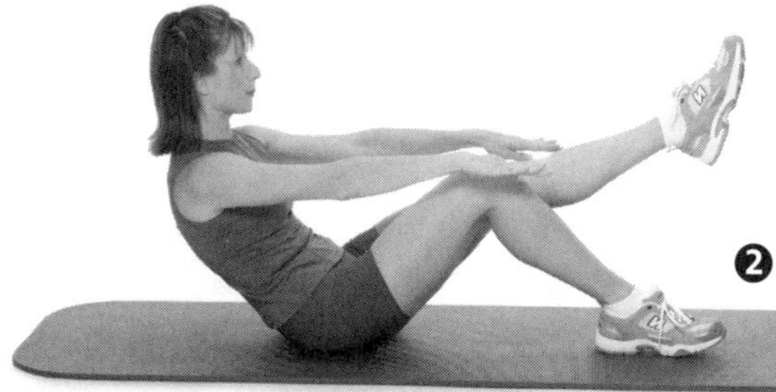

One-Leg Roll-Down

Starting position: Sit on the floor with your knees bent and your feet flat. Lift your left foot off the floor and extend your left leg up. Hold your arms out in front of you, parallel to the floor.

Movement: Using your abs, slowly roll down 4 to 5 inches, one vertebra at a time, as you inhale. Hold for a second and then exhale as you slowly roll back up. Do six reps; then switch legs and do six more reps.

Technique: Your abs should be powering the move. Don't move quickly.

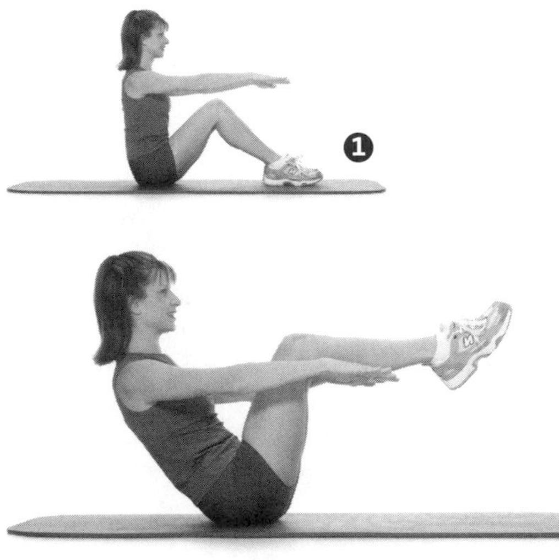

MUST-DO MOVE

Full Balance

Starting position: Sit on the floor with your knees bent and your feet flat. Hold your arms straight out in front of you, parallel to the floor.

Movement: Lift your feet so that your calves are parallel to the floor, and balance on your sitting bones. Hold for five breaths and then relax. Do one time only.

Technique: Keep your abs tight and the rest of your body relaxed, especially your shoulders.

Legs-Up Ab Crunch

Starting position: Lie on your back with your legs in the air and your hands behind your head.

Movement: Using your abs, slowly raise your head, shoulders, and upper back about 45 degrees off the floor as you exhale. Think of shortening the distance between your ribs and pelvis. Hold for a second and then inhale as you slowly lower yourself. Do 12 reps.

Technique: Don't pull your chin to your chest. Don't arch your back.

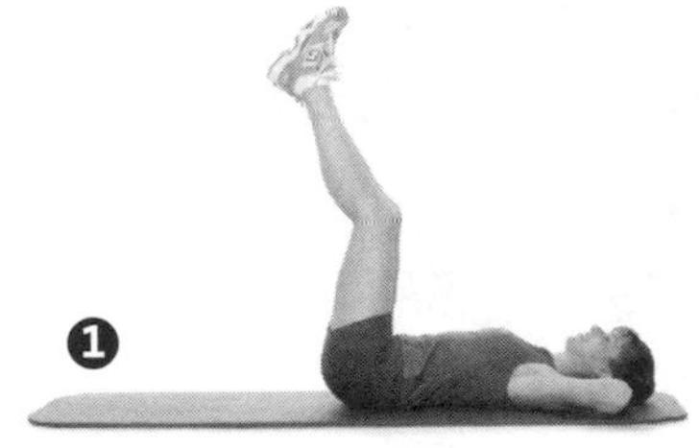

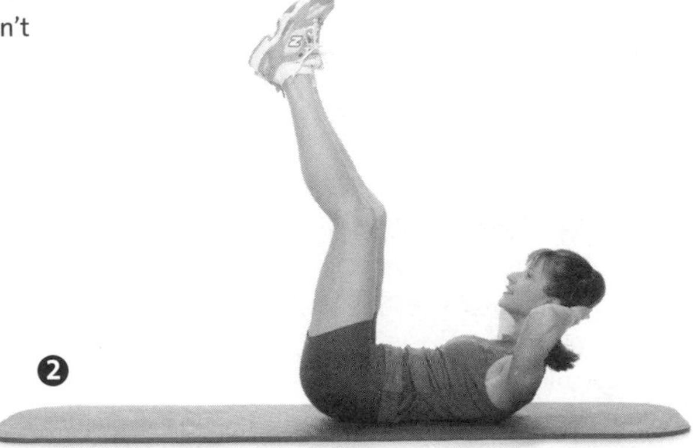

continued

The Workout

Level 2 *continued*

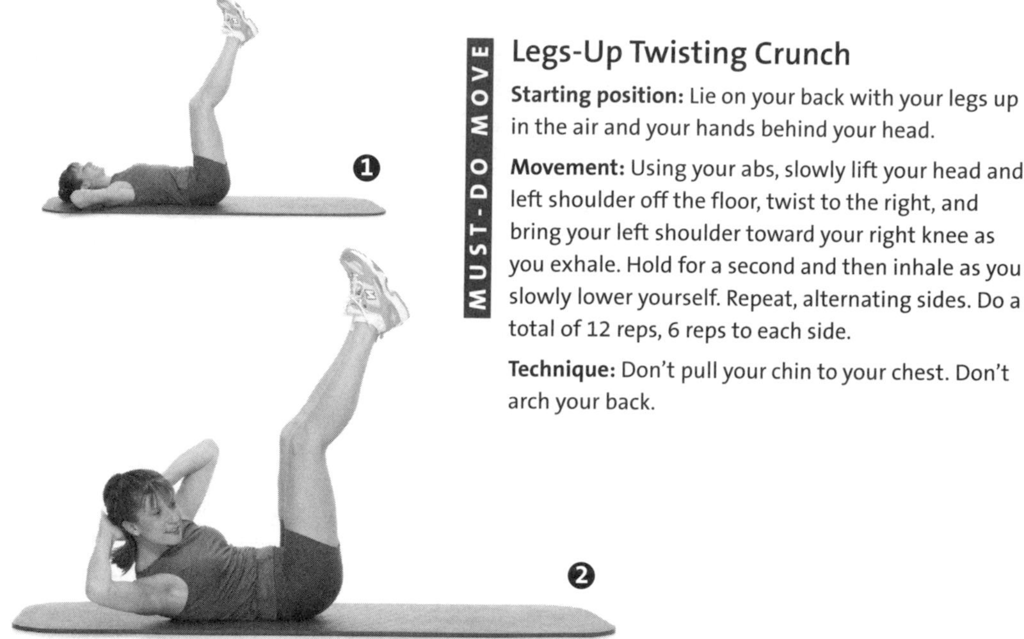

MUST-DO MOVE

Legs-Up Twisting Crunch

Starting position: Lie on your back with your legs up in the air and your hands behind your head.

Movement: Using your abs, slowly lift your head and left shoulder off the floor, twist to the right, and bring your left shoulder toward your right knee as you exhale. Hold for a second and then inhale as you slowly lower yourself. Repeat, alternating sides. Do a total of 12 reps, 6 reps to each side.

Technique: Don't pull your chin to your chest. Don't arch your back.

MUST-DO MOVE

One-Leg Heel Bridge

Starting position: Lie on your back with your knees bent, feet flat on the floor, and arms at your sides, palms facing up. Lift your toes off the floor so that only your heels are touching and then extend your right leg.

Movement: Contracting your abs, buttocks, and lower back, press into your heel and lift your butt, hips, and back off the floor as you exhale, to form a straight line from your shoulders to your knees. Slowly lower your buttocks toward the floor and then lift back up. Do six lifts, hold for three breaths, and then relax. Repeat with the opposite leg extended. Do one time only.

Technique: Don't lift too high—your upper back and shoulders should remain on the floor. Don't bend at the waist or hips. Don't let your knees fall inward or outward.

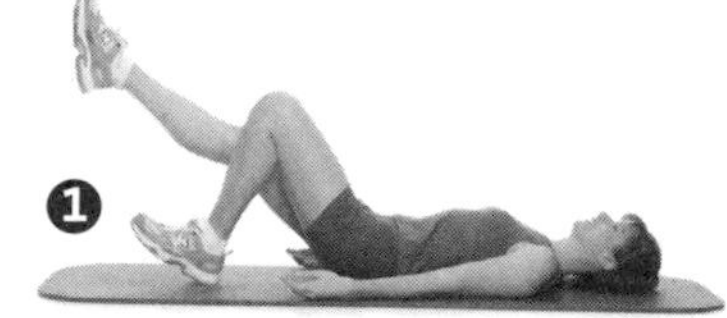

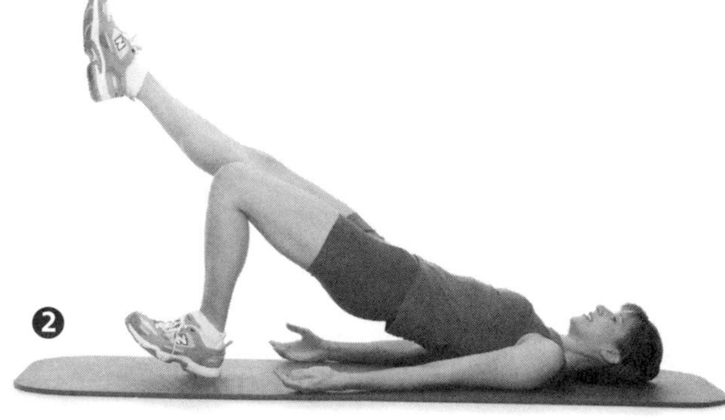

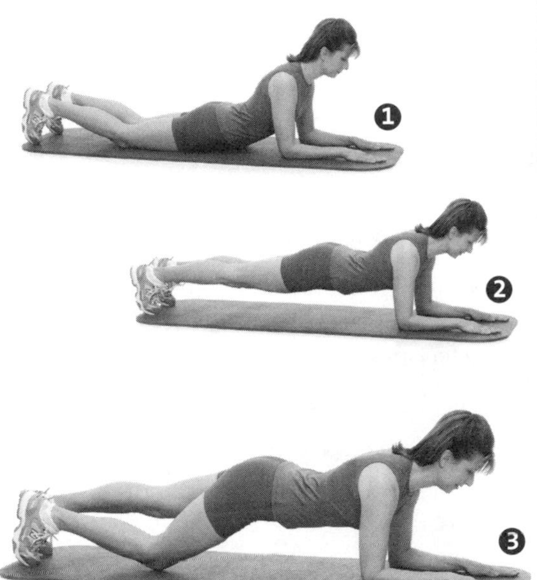

MUST-DO MOVE

Plank with Knee Drop

Starting position: Lie facedown with your feet flexed and toes tucked. Your elbows should be under your shoulders and your forearms and palms on the floor.

Movement: Contracting your abs and back, press into your forearms as you exhale and lift your pelvis and legs off the floor so that your back and legs form a straight line. Slowly drop your right knee toward the floor and then straighten. Do six knee touches with your right leg, hold for three breaths, do six knee touches with your left leg, hold for three breaths, and then relax. Do one time only.

Technique: Don't lift your head up or let it drop. Don't bend at the waist or hips. Don't let your belly drop toward the floor.

Chest Lift with a Twist

Starting position: Lie facedown on the floor with your hands under your chin.

Movement: Exhale as you lift your head and chest 5 to 6 inches off the floor and twist slightly to the right. Hold for a second and then inhale as you slowly lower. Do 12 reps, alternating sides for the twists.

Technique: Don't lift too high.

Alternate move: If this is too challenging, or you have back problems, skip the twist and do only the lift.

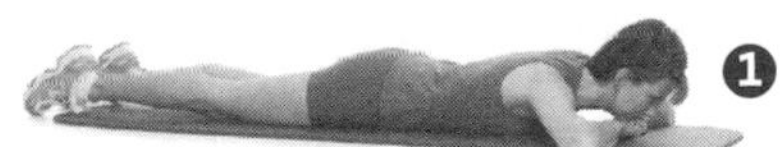

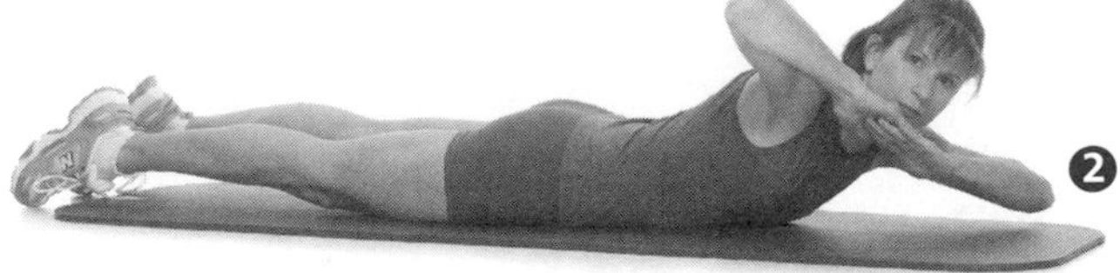

The Workout

Level 3

Speed Walk: Less Than 20 Minutes

- Follow the same route as the first and second weeks. The goal is to complete the distance in less time.
- 5-minute warmup: Walk 2½ to 3 miles per hour, 100 to 115 steps per minute.
- Under-10-minute speedup: Starting at the same spot as last week, increase your speed, walking as quickly as you can, until you reach the point where you slowed down last week. You should be able to do the same distance and shave off a few more seconds this week.
- 5-minute cooldown: Slow down to 2½ to 3 miles per hour, 100 to 115 steps per minute.

Core Training: 20 Minutes

- Do the sequence of exercises one time.

Extended One-Leg Roll-Down

Starting position: Sit on the floor with your knees bent and your feet flat. Lift your left foot off the floor and extend your left leg. Hold your arms up overhead.

Movement: Using your abs, slowly roll down 5 to 6 inches, one vertebra at a time, as you inhale. Hold for a second and then exhale as you slowly roll back up. Do six reps and then switch legs.

Technique: Your abs should be powering the move. Don't move quickly.

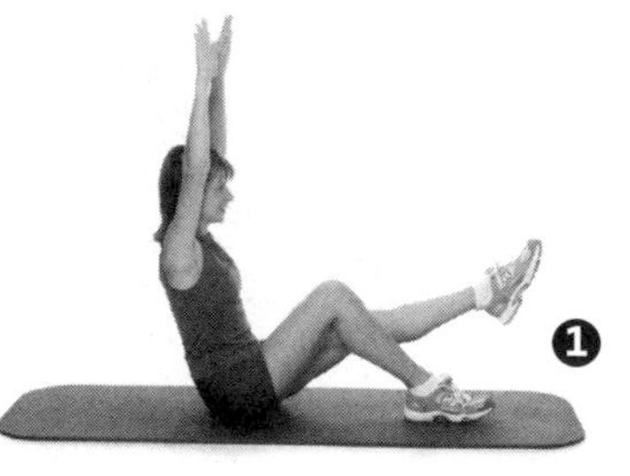

❶

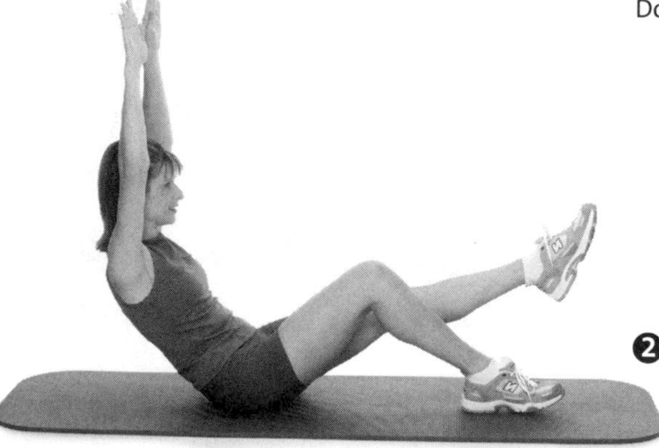

❷

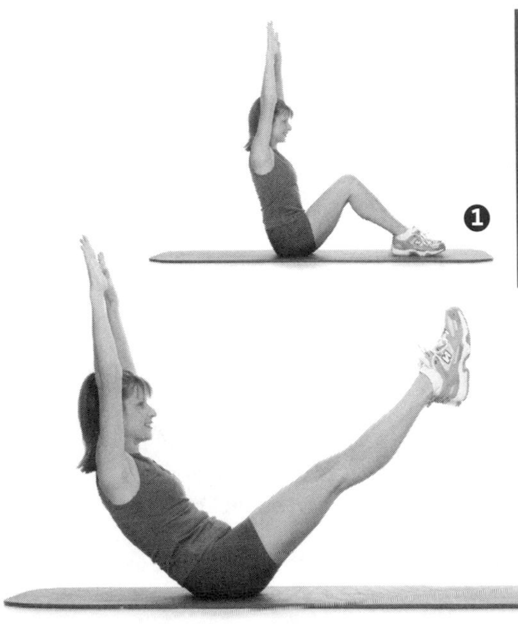

MUST-DO MOVE

Fully Extended Balance

Starting position: Sit on the floor with your knees bent and your feet flat. Hold your arms up overhead.

Movement: Lift your feet off the floor, extending your legs straight, and balance on your sitting bones. Hold for five breaths and then relax. Do one time only.

Technique: Keep your abs tight and the rest of your body relaxed, especially your shoulders.

Reverse Crunch

Starting position: Lie on your back with your legs up in the air and your hands behind your head. Cross your legs at the shins.

Movement: Slowly contract your abs as you exhale, and press your back into the floor, tilting your pelvis and lifting your hips 2 to 4 inches off the floor. Keep your upper body relaxed. Hold for a second and then inhale as you slowly lower. Do 12 reps.

Technique: Don't swing your legs.

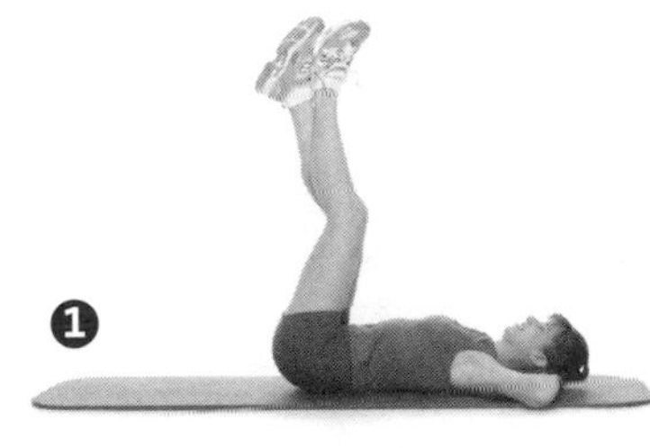

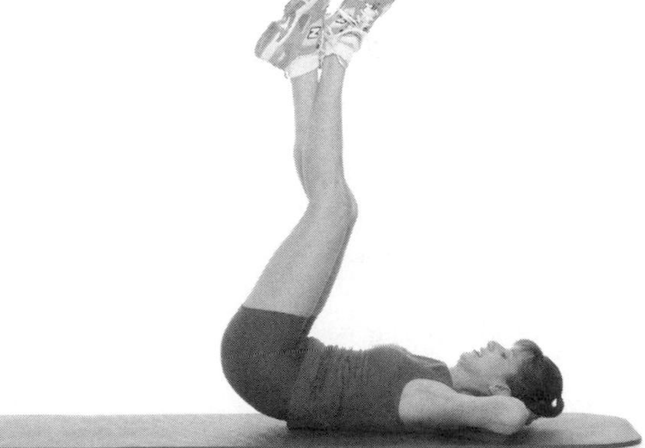

continued

The Workout

Level 3 *continued*

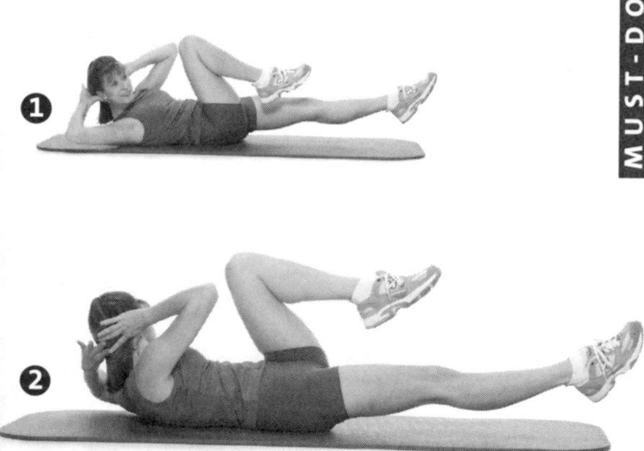

MUST-DO MOVE

Bicycle

Starting position: Lie on your back with your legs bent, feet flat on the floor, and hands behind your head. Lift your head and shoulders off the floor into a crunch position. Lift your feet off the floor, keeping your legs bent about 45 degrees.

Movement: Simultaneously, twist your left shoulder toward your right knee and bend your right knee in toward your chest while straightening your left leg. Then using a bicycle-pedaling motion, straighten your right leg while bringing the left knee in toward your chest and twisting your right shoulder to the left. That's 1 rep; do 12 reps.

Technique: Don't pull your chin to your chest. Don't arch your back.

MUST-DO MOVE

One-Leg Heel Bridge with Arms Up

Starting position: Lie on your back with your knees bent, feet flat on the floor, and arms extended over your chest. Lift your toes off the floor so that only your heels are touching and then extend your right leg.

Movement: Contracting your abs, buttocks, and lower back, press into your heel and lift your butt, hips, and back off the floor as you exhale, to form a straight line from your shoulders to your knees. Slowly lower your buttocks toward the floor and then lift back up. Do six lifts, hold for three breaths, and then relax. Repeat with the opposite leg extended. Do one time only with each leg.

Technique: Don't lift too high—your upper back and shoulders should remain on the floor. Don't bend at the waist or hips. Don't let your knees fall inward or outward.

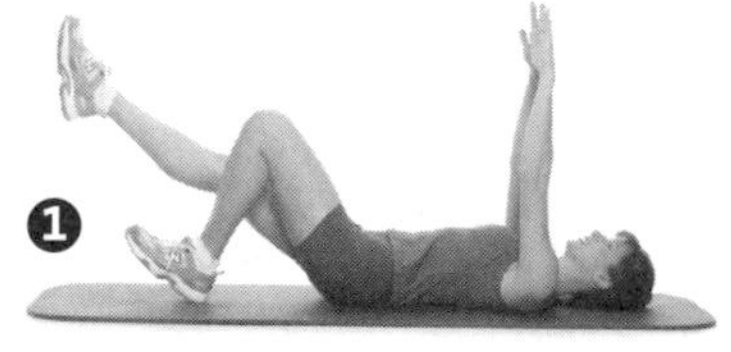

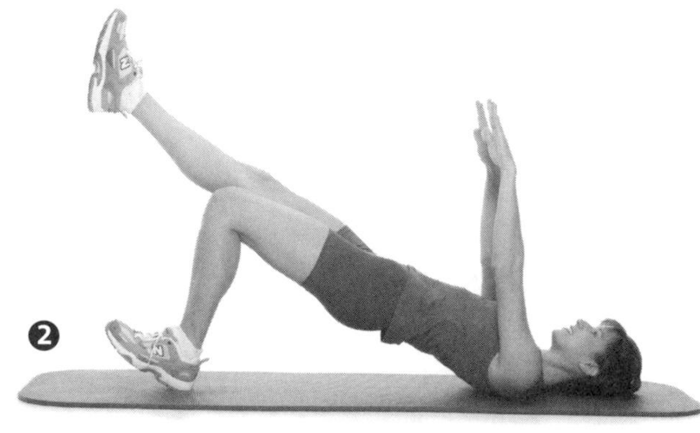

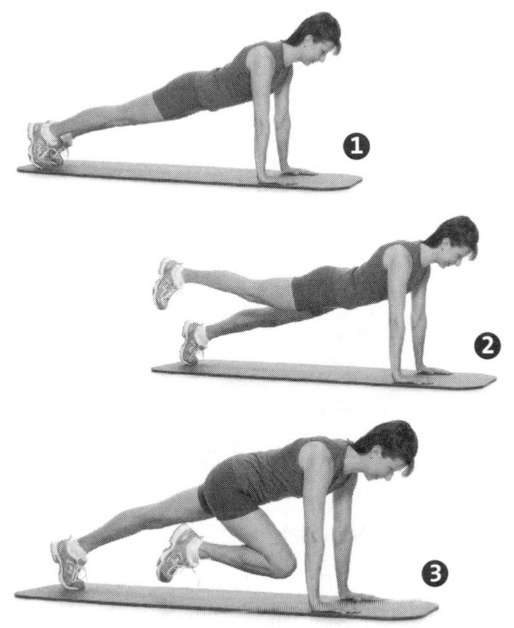

MUST-DO MOVE

Extended Plank with Lift and Bend

Starting position: Lie facedown with your feet flexed and toes tucked. Place your palms on the floor near your shoulders so that your elbows are pointing up. Contracting your abs and back, press into your hands as you exhale, straighten your arms, and lift your torso and legs off the floor so that your head, back, and legs form a straight line.

Movement: Lift your right foot off the floor and hold for three breaths. Next, pull your right knee in toward your chest and press it back out for six reps and then put that foot back on the floor. Lift your left foot off the floor and hold for three breaths. Next, pull your left knee in toward your chest and press it back out for six reps, put that foot back on the floor, and then relax. Do one time only.

Technique: Don't lift your head up or let it drop. Don't bend at the waist or hips. Don't let your belly drop toward the floor.

Swimming Chest and Leg Lift

Starting position: Lie facedown on the floor with your arms extended overhead.

Movement: Lift your arms, head, chest, and legs 5 to 10 inches off the floor. Hold as you swim your arms back to your sides and forward again, as if you were doing the breaststroke, and then slowly lower yourself. Do 12 reps.

Technique: Don't lift too high.

Alternate move: For an easier version, keep your legs down on the floor and lift only your upper body.

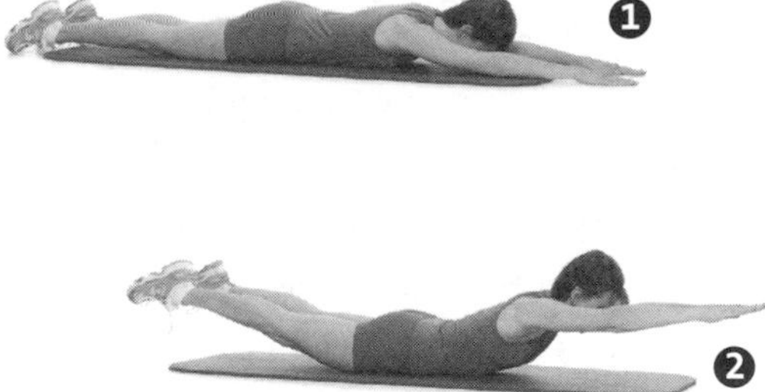

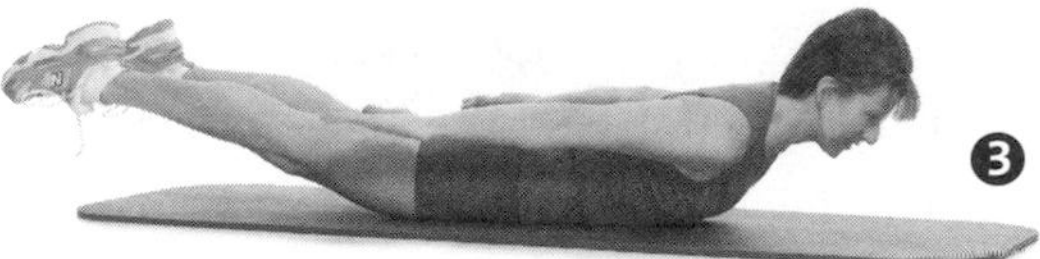

FIRM UP / DAY 21

My Success Story

Congratulations, you've done it! You should be very proud of yourself.

By now, you should definitely be seeing some definition in your arms and legs, be feeling stronger and more energetic, and start noticing that your clothes are a little looser. But this is only the beginning. With a fit mind and body, you can take on anything you put your mind to—losing more weight, starting a new career, or building new relationships.

Whether you plan to continue following *Prevention*'s Firm Up in 3 Weeks Program (see part 5 for guidance) or try something else, challenge yourself to some type of physical goal—a 10-K, half-marathon, or marathon walk or run; a hiking, biking, or walking trip; or even a triathlon. These types of events provide great motivation to continue training and can offer some other wonderful experiences.

About 5 years ago, when my friend Carol, a 3-year breast cancer survivor, learned that her cancer was back, I decided to participate in the Avon Breast Cancer 3-Day—a 60-mile walk to raise money to fight breast cancer. It was also a way for me to take the advice that I often give readers: Challenge yourself by signing up for a charity walk/run/ride that's beyond your current abilities.

The thought of training for several months—during the winter—was daunting. So I recruited my then 60-year-old mom, Rosalie.

We started in the first week of January—just 4 miles at first. During the week, we logged miles separately on our treadmills. On weekends, we'd walk together for up to 6 hours straight, which gave us plenty of time to talk. We reconnected in a way that we hadn't since before I went away to college. I'd tell her all about my life just like I used to do when I came home from school as a child. She would do the same, and then we'd reminisce. We hadn't spent that much time together in about 15 years.

Four months later, we joined 2,800 other walkers for the 3-day event, walking 20 miles each day. Along the way, we met other mothers and daughters walking together—many in honor of loved ones with breast cancer. And we heard inspiring stories of women triumphing over breast cancer and training so that they could join us on this walk.

Walking hand in hand, my mother, the other walkers, and I finished our last mile to the cheers of hundreds of spectators. As I high-fived with each of the 400 breast cancer survivors who walked with us, I cried. I never imagined that meeting such a physical challenge would have such an emotional impact. I was proud of myself—but I was even more proud of my mom and the survivors. I hope if I'm ever faced with the challenge of a life-threatening disease that I have their courage. And I was so happy to have shared this experience with my mom. I hope that when I'm 60, I have her spirit to take on new challenges.

(For information on the Avon Walk for Breast Cancer, call toll-free (877) 925-5286, or go to www.avonwalk.org.)

Meal Plan

Most of these recipes are custom designed to make 1 serving–no fuss, no muss; just fix, eat, and go! If a recipe makes more than 1 serving, it's noted below. Save that extra serving for another meal, or share it with your spouse or your walking buddy.

Breakfast

Bran Muffin and Applesauce: Have 1 small bran muffin (2½-inch diameter, a little smaller than a tennis ball) with 1 cup fat-free milk, 22 peanuts, and ½ cup unsweetened applesauce (such as single-serving, peel-top Mott's Natural Style or any other unsweetened applesauce).

Healthy Snack

Pria Bar and Peanut Butter: Spread 1 tablespoon peanut butter on any variety Pria bar.

Lunch

Spinach Omelet: Heat ½ box (5 ounces) frozen spinach in the microwave. Squeeze out excess water. Mix with ¼ teaspoon salt, ½ teaspoon ground black pepper, and 2 teaspoons minced garlic. Preheat a nonstick skillet over medium heat and coat with olive oil cooking spray. Beat 1 whole egg and 4 egg whites (or ¾ cup Egg Beaters) with 2 tablespoons fat-free milk and ½ teaspoon ground black pepper. Pour into the skillet. Immediately spoon the spinach mixture over the eggs. Serve with 2 Wasa crispbreads and 1 cup fat-free milk.

Healthy Snack

Apricot Indulgence: Have 3 dried apricots (or 6 halves). Serve with 2 graham cracker squares (2½-inch size) spread with 1 tablespoon peanut butter. Serve with 1 cup fat-free milk.

Dinner

Italian Restaurant: Have 1 cup spaghetti with about ½ cup tomato sauce and 2 ounces seafood–about 10 large shrimp, 8 mussels, or 6 clams. Add a side salad (1½ cups mixed greens); use 1 tablespoon reduced-calorie dressing.

Indulgent Treat

Peanut Butter and Chocolate: Scoop 1½ tablespoons peanut butter out of the jar onto a spoon, top the scoop with 1 tablespoon mini chocolate chips, and enjoy right off the spoon!

Nutrient analysis: 1,626 calories, 87 g protein, 185 g carbohydrates, 69 g total fat, 15 g saturated fat, 330 mg cholesterol, 25 g dietary fiber, 2,640 mg sodium, 1,046 mg calcium

FIRM UP TIP

HAVE FUN!

Coach your kid's soccer team. You'll be a good role model, spend more time with your kids, and get a workout. Running around the field and practicing drills with the team zaps 272 calories an hour.

The Workout

Levels 1, 2, and 3

Long Walk: 60 Minutes

- Drive to a different neighborhood or find a trail and walk at a comfortable pace that you can sustain for 60 minutes.

FIRM UP TIPS

ENERGY BOOSTER

Join a group that walks, bikes, runs, pogo-sticks—whatever. You'll get motivation and support to stay active, plus all the health benefits of being connected to other people.

GET FIRM FASTER

Step outside. A stimulating environment distracts you, so you work harder without realizing it. In one study, gardening burned nearly 30 percent more calories than indoor aerobics: 392 calories versus 306. Other research has shown that walkers unconsciously pick up their pace outdoors.

Your Reward Diary

Remember to write down your weekly reward here. What are you doing for yourself this week?

____

____

____

____

____

____

____

____

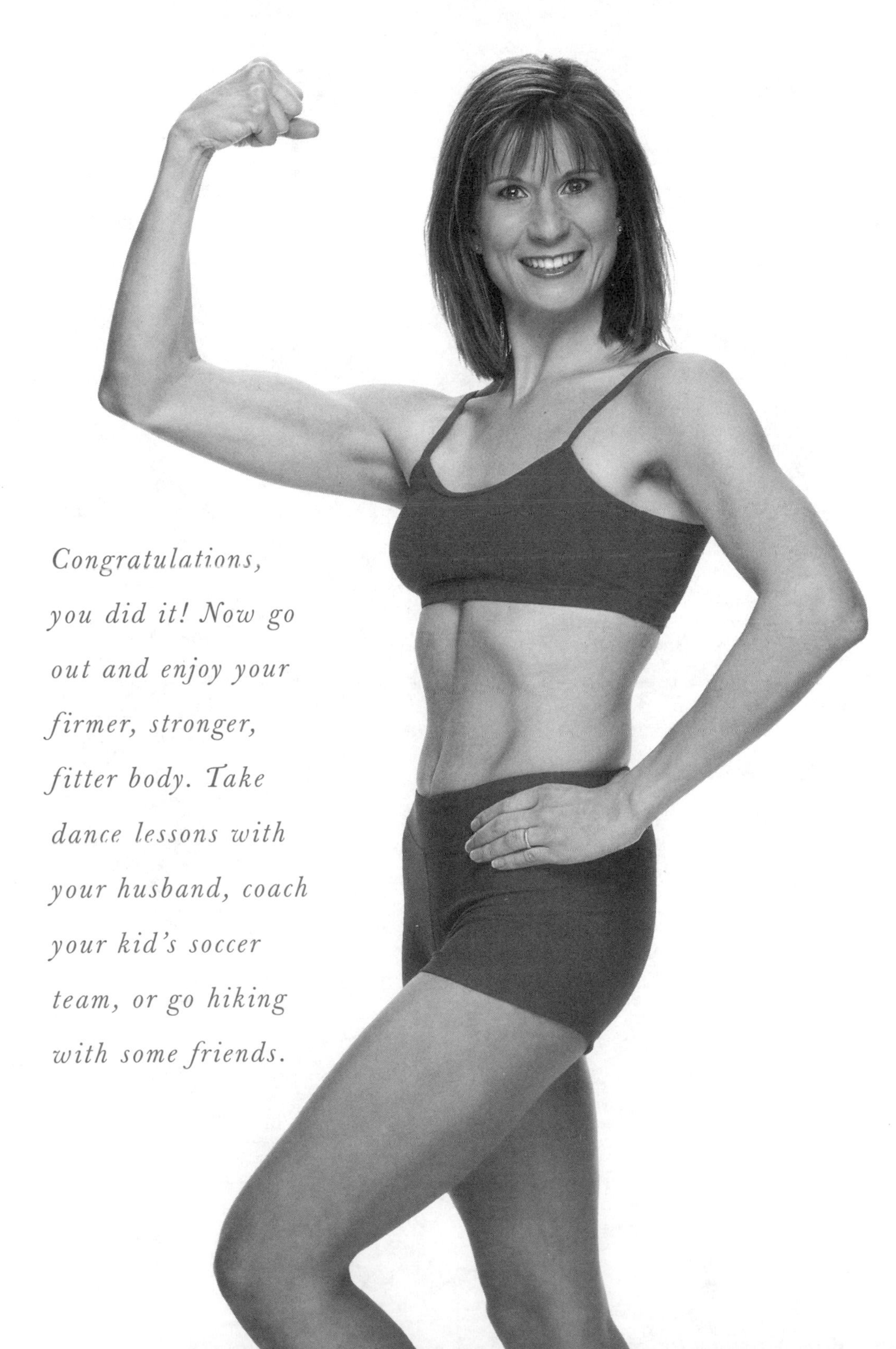

Congratulations, you did it! Now go out and enjoy your firmer, stronger, fitter body. Take dance lessons with your husband, coach your kid's soccer team, or go hiking with some friends.

PART 3

THE FIRM UP DIET

CHAPTER 6

The Science behind the Firm Up Eating Plan

Food and nutrition science is constantly changing. One day high-carb is the diet *du jour,* and the next it's low-carb. To develop the Firm Up Eating Plan, registered dietitians Tracy Gensler and Kristine Napier and I waded through all the research to find the best of the best and put it all together in a diet program that is super-nutritious, easy to follow, enjoyable, and delicious. Not only will it help you drop weight and firm up, but you'll also have more energy and lower your risk of heart disease, diabetes, cancer, and osteoporosis.

The plan is based on 10 simple guidelines:

1. Watch calories.
2. Pump up the volume.
3. Choose fiber-rich foods.
4. Limit refined carbs.
5. Get enough protein.
6. Increase calcium.
7. Beware of beverages.
8. Eat only when hungry.
9. Have smaller meals more often.
10. Don't deprive yourself.

Let's look at each one in more detail.

WATCH CALORIES

If you think you can eat whatever you want and work it off later at the gym, think again. You'd need to walk for about 3½ hours to burn off a small fast-food cheeseburger, fries, and shake. But that's not the only problem. Overeating—even overeating healthy foods—may make it harder for your body to burn fat, suggests preliminary animal research. So your eating habits could negate all those miles and reps you've logged.

QUICK TIP **People who regularly enjoy ready-to-eat breakfast cereal with fruit weigh less than those who either skip breakfast or eat other breakfast foods such as eggs and bacon or bagels, according to one study. Cereal eaters also ate less fat and cholesterol and more fiber during the day.**

That's why keeping an eye on calories—but not obsessing about them—is important. Our 3-week meal plan and mix-and-match meals make it easy. Depending on your calorie goal (we recommend about 1,700 for most women, especially if they're active), you can have one or two healthy snacks a day and still enjoy a daily treat. If you want to cut more calories (we don't recommend going below 1,500), limit the treats to three times a week and have only one healthy snack on those days. The rest of the week, have two healthy snacks and no treats. This will help to ensure that you're getting all the important nutrients you need.

But don't cut your calories below 1,500. Going too low can sabotage your efforts by shifting your body into starvation mode. That means it will start to conserve energy by burning fewer calories—exactly the opposite of what you want to do when you're trying to shed pounds. It can also affect the amount of calories you burn during exercise, according to preliminary research. After 3 days of eating only 1,200 calories a day, you start conserving energy, so the metabolic boost that you would normally get after exercise drops. "This 'withholding' by your body means that you'll miss burning hundreds of calories over time," says study author Nancy Keim, Ph.D., of the Western Human Nutrition Research Center in Davis, California.

A key to keeping calories in check is to keep your portion sizes under control. In our supersized world, however, that's becoming more and more difficult to do. Cookbooks now advise cutting a pan of brownies into 16 pieces instead of the 30 recommended in the 1960s, even though the pan size and ingredients are exactly the same. Car manufacturers are installing larger cup holders in cars to accommodate the increasing size of drive-thru-restaurant beverages. And even diet foods such as frozen meals are getting larger. For guidelines on keeping your portions sensible, see "Avoid Portion Distortion."

Avoid Portion Distortion

HERE'S WHAT SENSIBLE portions should look like.

Food	The Size of . . .
3-oz steak	A deck of cards
1 cup cooked pasta	2 tennis balls
6 oz juice	A small yogurt container
½-oz cookie	Half a yo-yo
2-oz bagel	A credit card's width or smaller
2-oz muffin	A small apple
1 oz cheese	A domino
2 Tbsp peanut butter	A ping-pong ball

PUMP UP THE VOLUME

Calories are only part of the weight-loss story. "It's the volume of food—not the number of calories—that you eat that determines when you're full," says Barbara Rolls, Ph.D., professor of nutrition at Pennsylvania State University in State College and coauthor of *Volumetrics: Feel Full on Fewer Calories*. "You consistently eat about the same volume of food day after day. So you can lose weight by eating more foods that are low on the energy-density scale: those with lots of water, such as fruits, vegetables, and broth-based soups." They help because they're high in volume—meaning that you get lots of mouthfuls—but low in calories. Very energy-dense foods, on the other hand, contain loads of calories crammed into a little package—cheesecake, for example. That's why you can polish off a piece in a snap, but struggle to finish a large salad, says Dr. Rolls. Eating foods that are less energy-dense can naturally reduce the number of calories that you eat by up to 20 percent—without making you feel hungry.

CHOOSE FIBER-RICH FOODS

High-volume foods such as fruits and vegetables are also loaded with fiber. In addition to filling you up for fewer calories, fiber also blocks absorption of some of the calories that you consume by scooting them through your body before they can be absorbed. Experts estimate that each gram of fiber substituted for simple carbohydrates results in a 7-calorie loss. That means upping your daily fiber intake from 14 grams (the average for most women) to 30 grams (the average for our meal plans) would, by itself, result in more than a 100-calorie-a-day drop—or about a 10-pound weight loss in a year.

Fiber may also boost your energy level. In a study of 139 people, those who started eating cereal packed with 6 to 12 grams of fiber daily reported feeling more energetic than those who began eating a look-alike, low-fiber cereal. Asked to rate their energy levels, the high-fiber crowd gave themselves scores 10 percent higher than the low-fiber pack. They also reported feeling better, even thinking more clearly.

The researchers who conducted the study speculate that the extra fiber may help by alleviating that common little problem that no one likes to talk about: constipation. Previous studies have found that people who switch to high-fiber diets and leave constipation in the dust feel more energetic, possibly because they feel lighter and more comfortable. And a high-fiber diet is smart for so many more reasons: It can help lower your risks of diabetes, heart disease, and, possibly, cancer.

To get your daily fiber quota—about 30 grams a day—make sure you're eating plenty of fruits, vegetables, whole grains, and beans.

QUICK TIP **Take a big slice off sandwich calories. Instead of using bread to make a sandwich, cut through a head of iceberg lettuce to make ½-inch-thick slices of 2-calorie "lettuce bread." Fill with reduced-fat cheese, lean deli meat, and your favorite mustard. Saves 120 to 200 calories per sandwich.**

LIMIT REFINED CARBS

Refined carbohydrates such as white bread and white pasta are essentially refined sugars and refined flours. Generally, they are less healthy than unrefined (or complex) carbs such as whole grains, beans, fruits, and vegetables that contain fiber. All carbs are eventually broken down into glucose (blood sugar) in the body, but refined carbs are broken down and absorbed more quickly, so they upset your body's precise blood sugar balance and may cause more glucose to become available to the cells than the body needs. When that happens, you gain weight, because the excess glucose gets turned into fat. To make matters worse, because refined carbs are broken down so quickly and have little fiber, you're soon hungry again.

The best way to avoid refined carbohydrates is to look for whole grain products. But that can be a bit more difficult than it sounds. The "hearty dark rye" or those "seven-grain crackers" that look so convincingly whole grain usually contain mostly refined white flour. To your body, that's the same as sugar.

HOW CAN I TELL IF IT'S WHOLE GRAIN?

The only way to know if something is really a whole grain food is to read the label carefully and apply the rules below. (For brand-specific recommendations, see "A Shopper's Guide to Whole Grains.")

- **Wheat:** If you don't see the word *whole* in the ingredients list, the product is made from refined wheat flour.

- **Oats:** Whether you see the word *whole* or not, the product is made from whole oats. (All oat products are made from whole oats.)
- **Rye:** You must see the word *whole*. Most so-called rye and pumpernickel breads in the United States are made of mainly refined wheat flour.

A Shoppers' Guide to Whole Grains

SO YOU DON'T have to hunt around for the real thing, we've compiled a list of 37 delicious whole grain products. (Bonus: All the products are trans-fat-free. Trans fats have been found to increase bad LDL cholesterol and lower good HDLs, which may increase the risk of heart disease.)

Bread

Alvarado St. Sprouted Sourdough Bread
Goya Corn Tortillas
Matthew's Whole Wheat English Muffins
Mestemacher Three-Grain Bread
Mestemacher Whole Rye Bread with Muesli
Pepperidge Farm 100% Stone-Ground Whole Wheat Bread
Thomas' Sahara 100% Whole Wheat Pita Bread
Wonder Stone Ground 100% Whole Wheat Bread

Cereal

Arrowhead Mills Steel-Cut Oats
General Mills' Cheerios
General Mills' Wheat Chex
Kellogg's Frosted Mini-Wheats
Post Bran Flakes
Post Raisin Bran
Quaker Instant Oatmeal
Quaker Old-Fashioned Oats
Quaker Quick 1-Minute Oats

Crackers

Ak-Mak Stone-Ground Sesame Crackers
Kavli Hearty Thick Crispbread
Ryvita Sesame Rye Crispbread
Wasa Hearty Rye Original Crispbread
Whole Foods Baked Woven Wheats

Pasta

Annie's Whole Wheat Shells and Cheddar
DeCecco Whole Wheat Linguine
Fantastic Whole Wheat Couscous
Hodgson Mill Whole Wheat Bow Tie
Hodgson Mill Whole Wheat Lasagna

Rice

Fantastic Brown Basmati Rice
Kraft Minute Instant Brown Rice
Lundberg Family Farms Wehani Brown Rice
Success 10-Minute Brown Rice
Uncle Ben's Instant Brown Rice
Wegmans Quick-Cook Spanish Brown Rice

Snacks

Bearitos Tortilla Chips
Health Valley Healthy Chips Double Chocolate Cookies
Kashi Seven Whole Grains and Sesame
New Morning Organic Cinnamon Grahams

- **Corn:** Look for the word *whole.* Unfortunately, some whole corn products don't bother to use it.
- **Rice:** You must see the word *brown.* That is, brown basmati rice is whole grain; basmati rice is refined.

GET ENOUGH PROTEIN

Adding some lean protein to your meals can help keep your appetite under control. Researchers from Yale University found that women who had 2 to 3 ounces of protein food (14 to 21 grams) at lunch ate about 20 percent fewer calories at dinner. Protein appears to blunt the appetite by triggering a greater secretion of the hormone cholecystokinin, which, among other jobs, sends a message to your brain that you are satiated. Protein also raises levels of glucagon, another satiety hormone that decreases food intake and, over time, even body weight.

In another study, people who ate high-protein snacks stayed full nearly 40 minutes longer than high-carbohydrate snackers did. But don't go overboard. Too many protein calories can just as easily end up as fat on your thighs. And make sure you're getting your protein from lean sources, such as lean meat, poultry, and fish; low-fat tofu, cheese, and yogurt; and beans. Lean protein sources can help you avoid getting too much artery-clogging saturated fat.

INCREASE CALCIUM

Calcium has long been touted for building strong bones. Now study after study shows it may also play a big role in helping people slim down. In one study, overweight people who took a calcium supplement lost 26 percent more body weight and 38 percent more body fat than others who ate the same reduced-calorie diet minus the supplement. Another group fared even better when they got their calcium from dairy products: They lost a whopping 70 percent more weight and 64 percent more fat on a high-dairy diet (three or four servings of low-fat dairy products totaling 1,200 to 1,300 milligrams of calcium a day). A good proportion of the fat losses were in the belly, too!

Scientists suspect that calcium forces fat out of cells and into the bloodstream, where it's more quickly oxidized, or burned off. If your body doesn't get enough calcium, fat cells retain the fat and can grow steadily. And many women don't get enough: Only 14 percent of women ages 20 to 50 meet the current calcium recommendation of 1,000 milligrams a day, and only 4 percent of women over 50 meet the 1,200-milligram goal. (The average female calcium intake is 652 milligrams.) That's why our diet plan is loaded with calcium—nearly 1,000 milligrams a day on average.

In addition, studies now suggest that calcium helps lower your risk of colon cancer, heart disease, and stroke; lowers blood pressure; and reduces PMS symptoms.

BEWARE OF BEVERAGES

Instead of drinking a can of soda, you might as well just stick it right on your hips, because that's where those 150 calories are likely to end up. "Calories you drink don't help satisfy your appetite," says Richard Mattes, R.D., Ph.D., nutrition researcher at Purdue University in West Lafayette, Indiana. Because you're not satiated, you end up consuming more calories overall. That's why the Firm Up Eating Plan recommends calorie-free beverages such as water, unsweetened tea, diet drinks, and coffee. Why waste calories on something that won't fill you up? Count regular soft drinks, juice, wine, beer, and other sweetened beverages as indulgent snacks, recognizing that enticing high-cal beverages can pile on the same number of calories as you'd get in a fattening dessert.

But don't skimp on fluids, especially water. When researchers followed 20,000 people for 6 years, they found that women who drank at least five glasses of water a day had a 40 percent lower risk of fatal heart attack compared with those who drank two glasses or less or who got most of their daily fluids from soft drinks, juice, coffee, or milk. Water decreases blood's thickness, lowering the risk of developing heart-attack-triggering blood clots. Other beverages seem to increase blood's thickness, because water is drawn out of the bloodstream to help digest them, says researcher Jacqueline Chan, Dr.P.H., of the School of Public Health at Loma Linda University in California.

Staying hydrated can also lower your risk of urinary tract infections, kidney stones, bladder and colon cancer, and constipation.

QUICK TIP A recent study found that compared with juice or water, having one alcoholic drink before a meal led to eating 200 extra calories. (And that's on top of the added calories in the drink itself—up to 500 for a creamy drink like a piña colada.) Subjects ate faster, took longer to feel full, and continued eating even after they were no longer hungry.

EAT ONLY WHEN HUNGRY

Focus on your body's need for food—not just your head's desire to eat what looks good. French researchers recently reported that people who eat snacks when they are already full simply pile on more calories without feeling full for any longer. In other words, the snack did not delay their next meal or reduce the amount they ate.

Most of us are out of touch with our hunger. Instead, we eat because it's time, because everyone else is eating, because we're stressed or depressed, or simply because there is food in front of us. To help you get in touch with true hunger, use a scale from 0 (famished) to 10 (completely stuffed). Stop and evaluate your hunger throughout the day. The goal is to stay between 3 and 7 at all times: 3 is reasonable hunger and a good time to eat; 7 is comfortably full but not stuffed and a good time to stop eating.

HAVE SMALLER MEALS MORE OFTEN

By eating small meals throughout the day, you'll maximize your body's calorie-burning ability. "As you get older, your body's ability to use food decreases," says Melissa Stevens, R.D., of the Cleveland Clinic Foundation. In one study, older women burned about 30 percent fewer calories after eating a 1,000-calorie meal than younger women—187 calories versus 246 calories. Both groups burned similar amounts after 250- and 500-calorie meals—which is why all meals in the Firm Up Eating Plan are under 500 calories. Over time, eating two or three large meals per day (even if you're still eating the same number of calories) could pack on 6 pounds in a year.

DON'T DEPRIVE YOURSELF

Experts call it "forbidden fruit syndrome." "When we tell ourselves we can't have something, we immediately focus our attention on what's forbidden, which increases our desire and chances of losing control," says Marsha Hudnall, R.D., of Green Mountain at Fox Run, a "nondiet" weight-control spa in Ludlow, Vermont.

In one study, researchers assigned 24 obese women to one of two treatment groups: The first group stuck to a traditional diet that restricted calories; the second joined a "behavioral choice"

Foods That Fight Emotional Eating

A STRESSFUL DAY could send anyone on the hunt for chocolate, but if you regularly reach for ice cream, cookies, or cake when you're upset or tense, it may have nothing to do with a lack of willpower. For you, carbohydrates may stimulate an especially powerful release of pleasure-producing hormones in your body. Like a nicotine addiction, such a compulsion is tough to break—but not impossible.

Surprisingly, *food* can help you do it. Sweet-but-nutritious complex carbohydrates such as the foods listed below have the same calming effect. They're less harmful to your waistline, however, because they have fewer calories than the candy bars or other calorie-rich foods you might normally seek, says Leigh Gibson, Ph.D., a senior research fellow at University College in London, who has studied this phenomenon. You'll also be less likely to overeat throughout the rest of the day if you treat your choice like a meal instead of a mindless snack. Find a place away from your office or away from whoever is upsetting you. Then sit down and slowly enjoy your food.

Fresh fruit or canned light fruit
Lightly sweetened whole grain cereals such as Multigrain Cheerios
Multigrain waffle with light syrup
Oatmeal
Sweet potato, or baked potato with light sour cream and chives
Tomato soup
Whole wheat toast with jam

program that taught them how to deal with foods they considered a problem. Although the traditional group lost weight initially, they tended to regain it, while the choice group continued a slow-but-steady weight loss that resulted in twice the lost poundage of the first group a year later.

"Instead of saying to themselves, 'I can't have potato chips,' we asked participants to decide if they really wanted them, to determine a reasonable amount if the answer was yes, and then have them," explains study author Tracy Sbrocco, Ph.D., clinical psychologist at the Uniformed Services University of the Health Sciences in Bethesda, Maryland. "Because nothing is forbidden, the seduction and struggle of resisting certain foods is eliminated. Eventually, you say no–and with less effort." When you eat closer to how you want to and don't feel deprived, you're happier and more motivated. That's why we designed the Firm Up Eating Plan to include a daily 200-calorie treat. Enjoy!

Okay, now you know what our Firm Up Eating Plan contains. And you've mastered the 10 basic principles behind the plan and looked over the study results that prove it works. Here's how to use it: First, turn to the weekly chapters (3, 4, and 5). You'll find a shopping list at the beginning of each chapter that tells you what foods to buy for that week. Next, at the beginning of each day, you'll find a meal plan for that day, with recommendations for breakfast, lunch, dinner, two healthy snacks, and one indulgent treat.

You may use these menus as is–and for the 3 weeks you're on the program, I recommend that you do, to ensure fast results. But if you don't like something on a given day's menu, turn to chapter 7, Mix-and-Match Meals, and substitute any of the 50 breakfasts in that chapter for the breakfast you'd like to replace. The same is true of lunch, dinner, healthy snacks, and indulgent treats (again, there are 50 or so of each to choose from). Not only do these mix-and-match meals give you lots of options while you're on the 3-week program, they're perfect to help you maintain your firmed-up figure once you've finished the program. (You'll find more about that in part 5, Firm Up and Beyond.)

CHAPTER 7

Mix-and-Match Meals

You definitely won't be bored on the Firm Up Eating Plan! Registered dietitians Tracy Gensler and Kristine Napier and I have created at least 50 meal choices each for breakfast, lunch, and dinner. In addition, we've added at least 50 choices each for healthy snacks and indulgent treats, because we don't believe in depriving ourselves–or you. And we've provided options to fit everyone's lifestyle–whether you love to cook or prefer to dine out, whether you dine solo or have lots of mouths to feed, and whether you like to cook from scratch or survive on convenience foods. There's something for everyone, and lots to choose from, so you can stick with the plan well beyond the 3 weeks.

As we've mentioned in chapter 6, depending on your daily calorie goal (we recommend about 1,700 for most women, especially if they're active—which you *will* be if you're following our Firm Up Action Plan), you can have one or two healthy snacks a day and still enjoy a treat every day. If you want to cut calories further (we don't recommend going below 1,500), limit the treats to three times a week and have only one healthy snack on those days. The rest of the week, have two healthy snacks and no treat. This will help to ensure that you're getting all the important nutrients you need.

As added nutritional insurance, we recommend that you take a daily multivitamin/mineral supplement that contains 100 percent of the Daily Value (DV) of most nutrients, plus take 100 to 500 milligrams of vitamin C and 500 milligrams of calcium if you're under 50. Take two 500-milligram doses of calcium (for example, morning and evening) if you're 50 or older.

To make following this plan even easier, here are some of our favorite brands for common items that appear in the meals.

- **Cheese:** Look for Cabot Light Cheddar 50%, Borden's 2% Milk American, Veggie Slices, or a brand with no more than 5 grams of fat per ounce. For shredded cheese, try Kraft 2% Milk Natural Reduced-Fat Shredded Cheese. For cheese sticks, try Healthy Choice or Frigo reduced-fat varieties.
- **Chicken:** Try Perdue Short Cuts or Louis Rich Carving Board Chicken Strips, which are perfect for when you don't have time to cook.
- **Margarine:** Brummel and Brown, SmartBeat Super Light, or I Can't Believe It's Not Butter Light Trans-Fat-Free—all are trans-fat-free.
- **Milk:** Soy milk can be substituted for any milk in the meals. Look for a brand that has about 110 calories per cup and is fortified with 30 to 40 percent of the Daily Value for calcium, such as White Wave Silk or Sun Soy brands.
- **Tofu:** Try Mori-Nu Silken Low-Fat tofu. Be sure to select the firm variety, although the desired firmness generally depends on the recipe.
- **Tortillas:** Choose Goya corn tortillas.
- **Veggie burgers:** Try Boca, the Original Gardenburger, or Amy's California Veggie Burger, or choose patties in the 110- to 130-calorie range.
- **Waffles:** Look for Kellogg's Low-Fat Nutri-Grain or a brand with no more than 170 calories for two waffles.

BREAKFAST CHOICES

Each meal serves one unless otherwise specified. Breakfasts average 330 calories each.

BREADS

1 **Almond Butter and Apple Sandwich:** Open and toast ½ whole wheat pita (6½-inch size). Spread with 1 tablespoon almond butter, and stuff with 1 thinly sliced Granny Smith apple. Serve with 1 cup fat-free milk.

2 **Bagel and Cheese:** Spread ½ bagel (2½- to 3-ounce size, such as Lender's refrigerated honey wheat bagels, 2.85 ounces) with 2 tablespoons farmer's cheese or reduced-fat cream cheese. Serve with ½ cup fat-free milk and ¾ cup honeydew melon pieces.

3 **Bagel, Lox, and Cream Cheese:** Spread ½ bagel (2½- to 3-ounce size, such as Lender's refrigerated honey wheat bagels, 2.85 ounces) with 4 teaspoons reduced-fat cream cheese and 1 ounce (29 grams) smoked salmon (1 to 2 strips of Nova lox–it's lower in sodium). Serve with 1 cup strawberries and 1 cup fat-free milk.

4 **Cinnamon Bread with Raisins and Peanut Butter:** Spread 1 slice Pepperidge Farm Cinnamon Swirl Bread with 1 tablespoon peanut butter, and sprinkle with 2 tablespoons raisins. Serve with 1 cup fat-free milk.

5 **Creamy Ricotta English Muffin:** Combine a 15½-ounce container low-fat ricotta cheese with 2 tablespoons honey and 3 tablespoons smooth or chunky peanut butter. (This recipe makes six ⅓-cup servings. See Breakfast #36 and Healthy Snacks #12, 14, and 32 for more serving ideas. You can keep the filling in the fridge for up to 7 days or freeze single servings for up to 1 month.) Spoon ⅓ cup ricotta mixture onto ½ whole wheat English muffin and serve with 1 cup fat-free milk.

6 **Crumpets and Almond Butter:** Toast 2 whole grain crumpets (Trader Joe's offers many high-fiber varieties), or use a whole wheat English muffin, and spread with 1 tablespoon almond butter. Serve with 10 fresh cherries.

7 **English Muffin and Almond Butter:** Toast ½ whole wheat English muffin, and spread with 1 tablespoon almond butter. Serve with 1 cup fat-free milk and 1 apple spread with 2 tablespoons farmer's cheese or reduced-fat cream cheese.

8 **English Muffin and Fruit:** Toast ½ whole wheat English muffin, spread with 2 tablespoons farmer's cheese or reduced-fat cream cheese, and top with 1 tablespoon chopped walnuts. Serve with 1 cup fat-free milk and 1 cup cantaloupe pieces.

9 **French Toast and Berries:** Dip 1 slice whole wheat bread in ¼ cup Egg Beaters or 1 beaten egg white mixed with 2 tablespoons fat-free milk. Grill in a nonstick skillet coated with cooking spray. Top with 1 teaspoon trans-fat-free margarine and ½ tablespoon maple syrup. Serve with 1 cup blueberries and ½ cup fat-free milk.

10 **Pita with Farmer's Cheese and Fruit Salsa:** Finely chop 1 fresh peach, ¼ avocado, 2 tablespoons red onion, and 1 kiwifruit. Combine with 1 teaspoon olive oil and the juice of 1 lime. (This recipe makes 2 servings. See Breakfast #27 for another serving idea. Store salsa in the refrigerator for up to 3 days.) Toast ½ whole wheat pita (6½-inch size), spread with 2 tablespoons farmer's cheese or reduced-fat cream cheese, and fill with half of the fruit salsa. Serve with 1 cup fat-free milk.

11 **Pita and Hummus to Go:** Split 1 whole wheat pita (6½-inch size) in half along the edge (you'll have two flat ovals). Toast and top each half with 2 tablespoons hummus. Serve with 1 small orange and ½ cup fat-free milk.

12 **Cheese Toast:** In the toaster oven, heat 1 slice whole wheat bread topped with 2 slices reduced-fat cheese until the cheese is slightly melted. Serve with ½ grapefruit and 3 dried apricots (or 6 halves).

13 **Cinnamon Toast:** Toast 1 slice whole wheat bread. Spread with 1 teaspoon trans-fat-free margarine, ½ teaspoon sugar, and a sprinkling of cinnamon. Serve with 1 cup fat-free milk, 1 slice reduced-fat cheese, and 1 medium apple.

14 **Hot Chocolate and Toast:** Have 1 mug hot chocolate (heat 1 cup fat-free milk, then mix in 1 tablespoon chocolate syrup). Serve with 1 slice whole wheat toast spread with 1 tablespoon almond butter. Serve with ½ cup fruit salad, your choice of fruit.

15 **Peanut Butter and Jelly Toast:** Toast 1 slice whole grain bread and spread with 1 tablespoon peanut butter and 2 teaspoons jelly. Serve with 1 cup cut fruit of your choice and 1 cup fat free milk.

16 **Tomato–Feta Cheese Salad on Pumpernickel Toast:** Combine 1 medium tomato, sliced; ½ teaspoon olive oil; ½ teaspoon dried basil; 1 tablespoon sliced black olives; 1 tablespoon finely chopped red onion; and 3 tablespoons reduced-fat feta cheese. Toast 1 slice pumpernickel bread (80 calories per slice) and top with the salad. Serve with 1 cup fat-free milk and 8 medium-size green grapes.

CEREAL, OATMEAL, AND GRITS

17 **Cheese Grits:** Stir 4 tablespoons shredded reduced-fat cheese into ¾ cup hot grits cooked according to package directions. Serve with 1 cup fat-free milk and 1 medium orange.

18 **Cheerios and Blueberries:** Top 1 cup Cheerios (or 100 calories' worth of other whole grain "O"-type cereal) with ½ cup fresh or ¼ cup frozen blueberries, 2 tablespoons chopped almonds, and 1 cup fat-free milk (drink it up if you don't use it all with the cereal).

19 **Bowl of Cherries:** Top ½ cup low-fat granola (such as Healthy Choice) with 2 tablespoons toasted walnuts or almonds, 10 fresh cherries, and ¾ cup fat-free milk (drink it up if you don't use it all with the cereal).

20 **Grape-Nuts:** Have ¼ cup Grape-Nuts cereal with 1 cup fat-free milk (drink all of the milk). Top the cereal with 2 tablespoons chopped almonds. Serve with 1 stick reduced-fat string cheese.

21 **Hot Cereal with Apricots:** Microwave ½ cup multigrain hot cereal (such as Quaker, Mother's, or any other brand that has about 130 calories per ½ cup uncooked). Follow package directions, but instead of using all water, use half water and half fat-free milk (in most cases, that means ½ cup water and ½ cup fat-free milk to ½ cup dry cereal). Cook with 3 chopped dried apricots (6 halves). It usually takes 1 to 2 minutes to cook. Serve with ½ cup fat-free milk and 1 stick reduced-fat string cheese.

22 **Muesli and Apples:** Top ½ cup muesli (such as Kellogg's Mueslix or other muesli with about 150 calories per ½ cup) with 1 small chopped apple and 1 cup fat-free milk. Serve with 1 slice reduced-fat cheese.

23 **Cinnamon Oatmeal:** Cook 1 packet instant plain oatmeal (¾ cup cooked oatmeal) and add water according to package directions. Top with a 0.9-ounce packet of Sunsweet dried plums, 1 tablespoon chopped almonds, a dash of cinnamon, and 1 teaspoon maple syrup or honey. Serve with ½ cup fat-free milk.

24 **Puffed Cereal with Blueberries:** Serve 1 cup puffed, unsweetened whole grain cereal (such as Kashi or one with about 125 calories per cup) with 1 tablespoon chopped walnuts, ½ cup fresh or ¼ cup frozen blueberries, and ½ cup fat-free milk. (Drink any leftover milk or add to coffee or tea.) Serve with 1 stick reduced-fat string cheese.

25 **Raisin Bran and Banana:** Top ½ cup raisin bran (such as Post, Kellogg's, or any other cereal with about 140 calories per ¾ cup) with ½ small chopped banana, 2 tablespoons chopped walnuts, and 1 cup fat-free milk. (Drink any leftover milk or add to coffee or tea.)

26 **Shredded Wheat and Strawberries:** Top 1 cup shredded wheat (such as Post Bite-Size Shredded Wheat 'n Bran or other cereal containing about 160 calories per 1-cup serving) with 1 cup sliced strawberries and 1 cup fat-free milk. (Drink any leftover milk or add to coffee or tea.) Serve with 1 hard-boiled egg.

CRACKERS

27 **Cheese and Crackers with Fruit Salsa:** Finely chop 1 fresh peach, ¼ avocado, 2 tablespoons red onion, and 1 kiwifruit. Combine with 1 teaspoon olive oil and the juice of 1 lime. (This recipe makes 2 servings. See Breakfast #10 for another serving idea. Store salsa in the refrigerator for up to 3 days.) Top 3 Wasa crispbreads with 3 tablespoons crumbled reduced-fat feta cheese and half of the fruit salsa. Serve with 4 large strawberries.

28 **Peanut Butter Crackers and Fruit:** Spread 2 tablespoons peanut butter and 1½ teaspoons jam on 3 Reduced-Fat Triscuit crackers or 2 Wasa crispbreads. Serve with ½ cup honeydew melon pieces.

DRINKS

29 **Soy Surprise Shake:** Combine 4 ounces low-fat firm tofu, ½ teaspoon pure vanilla extract, 1 cup frozen strawberries (thawed), 1 cup fat-free milk, and ½ cup crushed ice. Add 2 tablespoons chocolate syrup. Mix with a hand blender or an electric blender. Top with 2 tablespoons low-fat granola cereal.

30 **Strawberry Slush:** Combine 8 ounces strawberry-flavored fat-free yogurt, ½ cup fresh or ¼ cup frozen strawberries, 1½ teaspoons honey, 4 ounces low-fat firm tofu, and several ice cubes (add cubes one at a time). Mix with a hand blender or electric blender. Serve with 3 Reduced-Fat Triscuit crackers.

EGGS

31 **English Muffin with Scrambled Egg:** Scramble 1 egg (or ¼ cup Egg Beaters) in a nonstick skillet with 1 teaspoon trans-fat-free margarine. Put the scrambled egg on 1 split and toasted whole wheat English muffin. Serve with 1 cup fat-free milk.

32 **Western Omelet:** Coat a nonstick skillet with cooking spray and heat over medium heat. Whisk 1 egg and 2 egg whites (or ½ cup Egg Beaters) with ¼ teaspoon salt, ½ teaspoon ground black pepper, 2 tablespoons fat-free milk, and ½ teaspoon onion powder (if desired). Pour into the skillet and top with ¾ cup chopped vegetables of your choice (tomatoes, peppers, mushrooms, and onions). Serve with 1 cup fat-free milk and 1 slice whole wheat toast spread with 1 teaspoon trans-fat-free margarine.

33 **Healthy Fried Egg:** Heat a nonstick skillet over low to medium heat and add 1 teaspoon trans-fat-free margarine. Carefully crack 1 whole egg into the sizzling margarine. Take 1 teaspoon trans-fat-free margarine and drop it on top of the sizzling egg. Once the egg white is very white and the edges are a little crispy, remove the egg from the skillet with a spatula. Serve with 1 cup fat-free milk and ½ whole wheat English muffin topped with 2 teaspoons jelly.

34 **Sausage and Egg on an English Muffin:** Scramble 1 egg (or ¼ cup Egg Beaters) in a nonstick skillet with 1 teaspoon trans-fat-free margarine. Toast ½ whole wheat English muffin. Heat 1 Morningstar Farm Veggie Breakfast Patty in the microwave oven according to package directions. Top the muffin with the egg and the breakfast patty. Serve with 1 small banana.

35 **Toast and Eggs:** Scramble 1 egg and 1 egg white (or ½ cup Egg Beaters) in a nonstick skillet coated with cooking spray. (Optional: scramble with ¼ cup mushrooms and 1 teaspoon chopped scallions.) Serve with 1 slice whole grain toast spread with 1 teaspoon trans-fat-free margarine, 1 cup fruit salad, and 1 cup fat-free milk.

WAFFLES

36 **Creamy Ricotta on a Toasted Waffle:** Combine a 15½-ounce container low-fat ricotta cheese with 2 tablespoons honey and 3 tablespoons smooth or chunky peanut butter. (This recipe makes six ⅓-cup servings. See Breakfast #5 and Healthy Snacks #8, 12, 14, and 32 for more serving ideas. You can keep the mixture in the fridge for up to 7 days or freeze single servings for up to 1 month.) Top a toasted whole grain waffle with ⅓ cup ricotta mixture and serve with 1 cup fat-free milk.

37 **Waffle with Peanut Butter:** Toast 1 frozen whole grain waffle. Spread with 1½ tablespoons peanut butter. Serve with 1 cup fruit of your choice and ½ cup fat-free milk.

38 **Waffle and Strawberries:** Toast 1 frozen whole grain waffle. Top with 2 tablespoons peanut butter and ¾ cup fresh or ⅓ cup frozen unsweetened strawberries, smashed. Serve with ½ cup fat-free milk.

YOGURT

39 **Apple Yogurt:** Top 8 ounces (1 cup) fruit-flavored fat-free yogurt with 1 medium chopped apple. Serve with 1 stick reduced-fat mozzarella cheese and ½ cup fat-free milk.

40 **Fruit 'n' Yogurt Spread on a Toasted Crumpet:** Toast 1 whole grain crumpet. (Trader Joe's offers many high-fiber varieties, or use a whole wheat English muffin.) Mix 1 cup

low-fat yogurt (any flavor) with 1 cup chopped firm fruit (such as an apple) and spread on your crumpet. Serve with 1 cup fat-free milk.

41 **Graham Crackers and Yogurt:** Spoon 4 ounces (½ cup) fat-free yogurt (any flavor) into a cereal bowl. Crumble 2 graham cracker squares (2½-inch size) over the yogurt, and add 1 tablespoon chopped almonds or walnuts. Serve with ¾ cup blueberries.

42 **Yogurt with Granola and Bananas:** Top 8 ounces (1 cup) fat-free fruit-flavored yogurt with ½ cup low-fat granola (without raisins, such as Healthy Choice), 2 tablespoons chopped walnuts, and ½ small banana, sliced.

ON-THE-GO

43 **Bran Muffin and Applesauce:** Have 1 small bran muffin (2½-inch diameter, a little smaller than a tennis ball) with 1 cup fat-free milk, 22 peanuts, and ½ cup unsweetened applesauce (such as single-serving, peel-top Mott's Natural Style or any other unsweetened applesauce).

44 **Cheese and Crackers:** Take along 3 Wasa crispbreads, 1 stick reduced-fat string cheese, and 1 small peach. Serve with 1 cup fat-free milk.

45 **Diner Breakfast:** Order 1 toasted English muffin with 2 servings Egg Beaters prepared in very little margarine (it doesn't hurt to ask). Also, order 1 cup fruit salad and 1 glass fat-free milk.

46 **Energy Bar:** Have 1 Luna bar, ½ cup fat-free milk, ⅛ cup pistachios, and a 0.9-ounce package Sunsweet dried plums.

47 **McDonald's Egg McMuffin:** Order it without cheese and get an 8-ounce carton 1% milk to wash it down.

48 **McDonald's Fruit 'n' Yogurt Parfait:** Choose the standard size and ask for it without the granola topping (save a whopping 100 calories). Instead, bring along 1 tablespoon chopped almonds to sprinkle on.

49 **Oatmeal:** Prepare an instant packet of regular oatmeal. Top with 1 tablespoon chopped nuts. Serve with 1 cup fat-free milk and 1 individual container unsweetened applesauce (or ½ cup any unsweetened applesauce).

50 **Smoothie to Go:** Have 1 Yoplait Nouriche smoothie, any flavor. Serve with 8 peanuts. (This is a healthy smoothie, but it is packed with a hefty dose of refined sugar, so limit to one or two a week.)

LUNCH CHOICES

Each meal serves one unless otherwise specified. Lunches average 370 calories each.

BURGERS, HOT DOGS, AND SUBS

1 **Veggie Burger with Baked Fries and Steamed Fresh Baby Spinach:** Bake ½ cup Ore-Ida shoestring-style fries in the toaster oven according to package directions—no oil or spray necessary. While they are baking, heat a nonstick skillet coated with cooking spray over low to medium heat. When the skillet is hot, toss in 2 cups loose baby spinach leaves and 1 teaspoon minced garlic; gently toss for 2 minutes. The leaves should be a little wilted but not mushy.

Top the leaves with 1 to 2 tablespoons balsamic vinegar. Heat a veggie burger in the microwave according to package directions and serve with 2 to 3 tablespoons ketchup, if desired. Skip the bun.

2 **Hot Dog and Baked Beans:** Microwave a 1-ounce 97%-reduced-fat beef hot dog and serve sliced with yellow or Dijon mustard. Rinse a 16-ounce can vegetarian baked beans. Mix half of the can with 2 teaspoons barbecue sauce and 1 teaspoon Dijon mustard. Serve with 10 medium-size red grapes.

3 **Meatball and Cheese Sub:** Heat 3 (1-ounce) turkey meatballs (see Dinner #10 for the recipe) with ¼ cup spaghetti sauce topped with ⅛ cup reduced-fat shredded cheese. Serve on 1 toasted whole grain hamburger roll with 1½ cups romaine lettuce and ½ chopped paste (Roma-style) tomato, topped with 2 tablespoons light salad dressing.

CHICKEN

4 **Mexican Chicken Wrap:** Preheat a toaster oven to 300°F. Combine 3 ounces canned chicken breast (drained) with 1 tablespoon light mayonnaise, 2 teaspoons Dijon mustard, and ½ teaspoon ground black pepper. Put the mixture onto a 6½-inch whole wheat tortilla, top with ¼ cup reduced-fat shredded cheese and 3 to 5 strips roasted red peppers from a jar (drained), and roll. Heat for 5 minutes and top with ⅓ cup salsa. Serve with 1 cup cantaloupe cubes.

5 **Sizzling Stir-Fry:** Heat a nonstick skillet over medium heat and add 2 teaspoons olive oil. Add ⅓ cup raw or frozen sliced peppers; ⅓ cup raw or frozen broccoli, cauliflower, and carrots; and ¼ cup raw or frozen edamame (sweet green soybeans). Add 3 ounces (½ cup) cooked, sliced chicken strips. Top with 2 teaspoons light soy sauce and continue heating until thoroughly warmed.

6 **Angel Hair Pasta and Chicken:** Heat a nonstick skillet coated with cooking spray over medium heat. Slice 3 ounces chicken breast (about the size of your palm) and combine with ¼ cup Campbell's Healthy Request Cream of Mushroom soup and 2 tablespoons white cooking wine in the skillet. Sauté the chicken until nearly done. Meanwhile, cook ¾ cup frozen vegetables, such as sliced mushrooms or cut leaf spinach. Top 1 cup cooked angel-hair pasta with the chicken mixture and the vegetables.

FROZEN FOODS

7 **Bean Burrito:** Microwave according to package directions Amy's Bean and Rice Burrito, Amy's Bean and Cheese Burrito, or Don Miguel's Lean Olé! Bean and Rice Burrito, or Don Miguel's Chicken and Black Bean Burrito (check the label for 260 to 280 calories and 6 to 9 grams of fat). Serve with 1 cup celery sticks stuffed with 2 tablespoons reduced-fat cream cheese.

8 **Beef Entrée:** Microwave according to package directions Lean Cuisine Café Classics Southern Beef Tips or a similar frozen meal (check the label for 260 to 280 calories and 6 to 9 grams of fat). Add 1 cup raw vegetables of your choice dipped in 1 tablespoon light dressing, and serve with 1 cup fat-free milk.

9 **Chicken Entrée:** Microwave according to package directions a chicken-based frozen entrée such as Smart Ones Fire-Grilled Chicken

and Vegetables or a similar frozen meal (check the label for 260 to 280 calories and 5 to 9 grams of fat). Add 1 cup cooked sugar snap peas topped with 1 tablespoon chopped walnuts. Serve with 1 cup fat-free milk.

10 **Italian for Lunch:** Microwave according to package directions Lean Cuisine Everyday Favorites Cheese Ravioli or a similar frozen meal (check the label for 260 to 280 calories and 6 to 9 grams of fat). Have 1 cup raw vegetables of your choice (baby carrots work well) dipped in 2 tablespoons reduced-fat veggie cream cheese. Serve with 1 cup fat-free milk.

11 **South of the Border:** Microwave according to package directions Lean Cuisine Chicken Enchilada Suiza with Mexican-Style Rice, Smart Ones Chicken Enchilada Suiza, Smart Ones Fajita Chicken Supreme, Amy's Black Bean Enchilada Whole Meal, or a similar frozen meal (check the label for 270 to 280 calories and 6 to 9 grams of fat). Serve with 1 cup sliced cucumber dipped in 1 tablespoon light salad dressing, and $\frac{1}{2}$ cup mandarin oranges topped with 1 tablespoon chopped walnuts.

12 **Stuffed Pockets and Soup:** Microwave according to package directions Lean Pockets (Turkey, Broccoli, and Cheese; or Chicken Broccoli Supreme) or Amy's Vegetarian Pizza in a Pocket, Amy's Broccoli and Cheese in a Pocket, or Amy's Soy Cheeze Veggie Pizza in a Pocket (check the label for 250 to 280 calories and 7 to 10 grams of fat). Serve with $\frac{2}{3}$ cup lentil soup (canned is fine), heated, and 1 cup fresh spinach (get prewashed, bagged spinach for convenience) with 1 tablespoon light dressing.

13 **Veggie Cheeseburger:** Microwave a veggie burger according to package directions. When nearly cooked, top the burger with 1 slice reduced-fat cheese and melt. Place on a whole grain bun spread with mustard and ketchup to taste. Add 3 slices tomato and some romaine lettuce. Serve with $\frac{1}{2}$ cup red pepper strips or other vegetable of your choice.

MEATLESS MEALS

14 **Baked Potato, Broccoli, and Cheese:** Top 1 baked potato (roughly $2\frac{1}{3}$-inch diameter × $4\frac{3}{4}$-inch length) with 4 tablespoons shredded reduced-fat Cheddar cheese and 1 cup cooked broccoli florets (microwaved frozen broccoli is fine). If you're eating out, ask for less cheese, no margarine or butter, and double the broccoli. Serve with $\frac{1}{2}$ cup canned pineapple chunks.

15 **Bean Burrito:** Top 1 warmed whole wheat tortilla with $\frac{1}{3}$ cup canned (rinsed and drained) pinto or black beans, partly mashed; 4 tablespoons shredded reduced-fat Cheddar cheese; and 3 tablespoons salsa. Roll and serve. Add 1 cup baby carrots and 2 tablespoons light dressing for dipping.

16 **Chili Tortilla:** Warm 1 whole wheat tortilla. Top with $\frac{3}{4}$ cup vegetarian chili (such as Natural Touch Low-Fat Vegetarian Chili), 1 tablespoon light sour cream, and $\frac{1}{8}$ cup shredded reduced-fat cheese. Serve with $\frac{3}{4}$ cup fat-free milk.

17 **Loaded Yogurt:** Have an 8-ounce fat-free vanilla yogurt topped with 1 tablespoon chopped almonds, walnuts, or pecans; 3 tablespoons low-fat granola; and 1 tablespoon

unsweetened dried fruit. Serve with 1 medium cucumber, sliced.

18 **Ravioli and Fresh Fruit:** Serve 1 cup cooked low-fat ravioli (such as Contadina Light Cheese Ravioli) topped with ⅓ cup spaghetti sauce. Serve with ½ cup fat-free milk and 1 cup raw broccoli with 2 tablespoons balsamic vinegar for dipping.

19 **Spinach Omelet:** Heat ½ box (5 ounces) frozen spinach in the microwave. Squeeze out excess water. Mix with ¼ teaspoon salt, ½ teaspoon ground black pepper, and 2 teaspoons minced garlic. Heat a nonstick skillet over medium heat and coat with cooking spray. Beat 1 whole egg and 4 egg whites (or ¾ cup Egg Beaters) with 2 tablespoons fat-free milk and ½ teaspoon ground black pepper. Pour into the skillet. Immediately spoon the spinach mixture over the eggs. Serve with 2 Wasa crispbreads and 1 cup fat-free milk.

20 **Vegetarian Chili:** Open 1 can vegetarian chili (such as Natural Touch Low-Fat Vegetarian Chili). Warm 1 cup chili topped with ⅓ cup shredded reduced-fat cheese. Serve with 1 cup strawberries and ½ cup fat-free milk.

PIZZA

21 **Pita Vegetable Pizza:** Slice a 6½-inch whole wheat pita lengthwise to produce 2 rounds. Spread each round with 1½ tablespoons pizza sauce or thick spaghetti sauce; ¼ cup chopped mushrooms, zucchini, peppers, or other vegetables; and 4 tablespoons reduced-fat shredded mozzarella cheese. Heat in an oven or toaster oven at 350°F for 8 minutes, or until the cheese just melts. Serve with 1 cup cooked broccoli.

22 **Pizza and Broccoli:** Heat 1 slice pizza from Dinner #31 or 32. Serve with 1 cup cooked broccoli florets topped with 1 tablespoon chopped walnuts.

SALADS

23 **Chicken Salad:** Makes 2 servings. Mix a 6-ounce can chicken breast meat with 2 teaspoons horseradish spread, 2 tablespoons light mayonnaise, ½ cup finely chopped celery, 10 sliced baby carrots, and 7 halved grapes. Spread half of the mixture on 1 toasted whole grain hamburger roll. Serve with 1 cup fat-free milk.

24 **Egg Salad with Roasted Red Pepper:** Prepare egg salad by combining 2 chopped hard-boiled eggs (discard 1 yolk or cook it and give it to your dog as a special treat) with 2 teaspoons horseradish spread, 2 tablespoons light mayonnaise, and ¼ cup chopped roasted red peppers from a jar (drained). Add ¼ cup finely chopped celery, if desired. Serve with 1 cup fat-free milk and 17 grapes.

25 **Fruit Salad:** Combine 2 cups of your favorite chopped fruit (suggest 1 banana and 1 kiwifruit) with 1 tablespoon chopped nuts (walnuts, pecans, or almonds work well) and 1 teaspoon shredded coconut. Serve with ½ cup 1% cottage cheese (sprinkled with cinnamon if you like) and 20 baby carrots.

26 **No-Mayo Tuna Pasta Salad:** Makes 2 servings. Combine 6 ounces water-packed tuna with 4 tablespoons white wine vinegar, 2 teaspoons olive oil, 4 tablespoons each finely chopped celery and sweet red pepper, and 1 teaspoon ground black pepper. Mix half of the

tuna mixture (check out Dinner #40 to use up the rest) with 1 cup cooked spiral pasta. Serve with 1 medium tomato, sliced and sprinkled with ground black pepper (if desired), and 1 fresh peach.

27 **Spinach–Blue Cheese Salad:** Toss together 2 cups spinach and 1 small tomato cut into wedges or 6 cherry tomatoes. Top with 2 tablespoons crumbled blue cheese, 1 sliced hard-boiled egg, and 1½ tablespoons light salad dressing. Serve with 2 Wasa crispbreads topped with 1 tablespoon hummus and 1 slice (1 ounce) turkey breast.

28 **Taco Salad:** Begin with 2 cups romaine lettuce. Top with ½ cup canned (rinsed and drained) black beans, ¼ cup reduced-fat shredded cheese, 2 tablespoons sliced black olives, ⅓ cup salsa, and 2 tablespoons light sour cream. Crumble 9 baked tortilla chips over all. Top with 2 tablespoons light dressing.

29 **Tuna, Bean, and Corn Tossed Salad:** In a plastic container with a lid, combine half of a 6-ounce can drained water-packed tuna with ⅓ cup canned (rinsed and drained) beans (chickpeas and cannellini beans are good choices) and ⅓ cup canned or frozen corn. Add ½ cup sliced tomatoes, ½ cup chopped green or red pepper, and 1 stick string cheese, chopped. Toss with 1 tablespoon light dressing. (Optional: Add 1 to 2 tablespoons fresh parsley, basil, or dill.)

SANDWICHES AND WRAPS

30 **Grilled Cheese and Tomato Sandwich:** Between 2 slices whole wheat bread, place 2 slices reduced-fat cheese and 3 slices tomato. Grill in a nonstick skillet coated with cooking spray or in the toaster oven until melted. Serve with 1 cup raw vegetables of your choice (such as cherry tomatoes, sliced green or red peppers, or baby carrots).

31 **Ham and Cheese on Rye:** Spread 2 slices rye bread with mustard to taste. Fill your sandwich with 3 ounces lean ham sliced for lunchmeat (about 3 slices) and 1 slice reduced-fat cheese, 3 slices tomato, and romaine lettuce. Serve with ½ cup baby carrots dipped in 1 tablespoon light salad dressing.

32 **Peanut Butter 'n' Banana Sandwich:** Spread 2 tablespoons peanut butter on 1 slice toasted whole wheat bread and thinly slice 1 banana to cover the layer of peanut butter.

33 **Peanut Butter and Jelly:** Spread 1 slice whole wheat bread with 1½ tablespoons peanut butter and 1 tablespoon jelly or jam. Serve with 1 tangerine, and 1 cup celery sticks and baby carrots dipped in 2 tablespoons reduced-fat veggie cream cheese.

34 **Roast Beef Sandwich:** Spread 2 slices whole wheat bread with 1 tablespoon reduced-fat mayo each, plus mustard to taste (horseradish mustard tastes even better with this sandwich). Fill with 3 ounces lean roast beef sliced for sandwiches (usually 3 slices), 4 slices tomato, and romaine lettuce. Serve with an 8-ounce can V8 vegetable juice.

35 **Sandwich and Fruit Pudding:** Spread 2 teaspoons Dijon or yellow mustard, if desired, on 1 slice whole wheat bread. Top with 3 ounces sliced lean lunchmeat (usually 3 slices) and 1 slice reduced-fat cheese. Prepare instant pudding (any flavor) with fat-free milk. (Make

half of the box at one time and store the remaining half in a tightly sealed plastic bag on your pantry shelf.) Serve ½ cup pudding topped with ¾ cup fresh berries (any variety). Also serve 1 cup sliced cucumber.

36 **Smoked Turkey and Cranberry Sandwich:** Spread 1 slice whole wheat bread with 1 tablespoon reduced-fat mayo. Fill with 3 ounces smoked turkey (usually 3 slices), 2 tablespoons cranberry sauce, and romaine lettuce. Serve with 1 cup sliced cucumber and 1 apple spread with 1 tablespoon peanut butter for dessert.

37 **Soup and a Half-Sandwich:** Heat ½ cup chicken noodle, chicken rice, beef noodle, chicken gumbo, or 100 calories' worth of any similar soup (such as Campbell's Healthy Request Chicken Noodle soup) with ½ cup water. Spread 1 slice whole wheat bread, cut in half, with mustard to taste. Pile on 2 slices turkey breast (2 ounces) and 1 slice reduced-fat cheese. Serve with 1 cup fresh broccoli florets dipped in 2 tablespoons light ranch dressing.

38 **Tuna Salad Sandwich on English Muffin:** Combine 1 tablespoon reduced-fat mayo and 1 teaspoon spicy mustard with half of a 6-ounce can drained water-packed tuna. Make a sandwich with 1 toasted whole wheat English muffin, 2 slices tomato, ¼ cup roasted red peppers from a jar (drained), and romaine lettuce. Serve with an 8-ounce can V8 vegetable juice and 1 kiwifruit.

39 **Turkey, Avocado, and Bacon Wrap:** On a 6½-inch whole wheat tortilla, place 3 ounces turkey breast sliced for sandwiches (usually 3 slices); 1 strip bacon, crumbled (save time by microwaving precooked bacon, such as Oscar Mayer Ready-to-Serve Bacon); 2 tablespoons diced avocado; and 2 slices tomato (optional: 1 tablespoon salsa). Roll and serve with ½ cup baby carrots and ½ cup mandarin oranges.

SOUP

40 **Black Bean Soup with Sour Cream:** Heat 1½ cups canned black bean soup. Top with 2 tablespoons reduced-fat sour cream. Serve with 1 cup baby carrots, 4 Reduced-Fat Triscuit crackers (or 65 calories' worth of another whole wheat cracker), and 1 slice reduced-fat Cheddar cheese.

41 **Creamy Tomato Soup:** Mix ½ cup Campbell's Reduced-Sodium Tomato soup with ¾ cup fat-free milk. Heat in a microwave oven to the desired temperature, and stir thoroughly. Top with 1 tablespoon (½ ounce) soy nuts. Serve with ½ small banana and 1 slice whole wheat French bread (about the size of your palm).

EATING OUT

42 **Arby's:** Order the Junior Roast Beef Sandwich and a side salad. Use 2 tablespoons reduced-calorie dressing.

43 **Fast-Food Hamburger (Burger King, Wendy's, Hardee's, or McDonald's):** Order the smallest hamburger on the menu, which usually means the "regular" size, with mustard and ketchup, but no mayo. And order a small orange juice. Bring along a sandwich bag

of 1 cup raw vegetables for munching, or order the side salad with 1 packet fat-free vinaigrette.

44 **Grilled Chicken Caesar Salad:** Many restaurants use about 6 ounces chicken; you want to eat 3 ounces, about the size of a deck of cards. (In most cases, that means you'll have chicken to take home. Those chicken slices will come in handy for some of the other lunches and dinners in this plan.) Eat 2 or more cups of salad greens. Ask for dressing on the side and use 2 tablespoons. Top with 3 tablespoons croutons (2 tablespoons if they're the really greasy type). Have ½ cup fruit for dessert.

45 **Grilled Chicken Sandwich:** Have Wendy's Grilled Chicken Sandwich or McDonald's Chicken McGrill without the mayo spread. If you must have mayo, ask for just a dab or use ½ tablespoon, max. Bring along a sandwich bag of 1 cup sliced red pepper (or other vegetable) and ¾ cup fresh blueberries.

46 **Pizza and Crunchy Vegetables:** Have 1 slice of a large (14-inch) pizza or 1½ slices of a medium (12-inch) pizza. Choose plain cheese or, better yet, top with 2 vegetables, such as mushrooms and green pepper. (Choose only medium- or thin-crust pizza, such as Domino's Hand-Tossed Pizza). Serve with 1 cup sliced red, yellow, or orange pepper and 1 small red apple.

47 **Salad Bar:** Take 1 cup mixed greens or romaine lettuce and 1½ cups chopped raw (plain, not marinated) vegetables of your choice (such as tomatoes, shredded carrots, or sliced cucumber); toss with 1½ tablespoons regular dressing or 3 tablespoons reduced-calorie dressing. Choose either ½ cup cottage cheese or a heaping ½ cup tuna (plain, no mayo). Top with 2 tablespoons chopped egg or 2 tablespoons shredded cheese. Serve with 1 small slice whole grain bread or French bread (about the size of your palm). Eat with 2 tablespoons raisins.

48 **Subway Sandwiches:** Order a 6-inch Subway Veggie Delite on wheat bread with 2 servings (4 triangles) cheese of any type and 1 tablespoon light mayo, honey mustard, or Southwest dressing. Ask them to stuff your sandwich with veggies, such as tomatoes and peppers. Or have the Subway Turkey Breast and Bacon Wrap with a Veggie Delite salad and use 1 tablespoon fat-free Italian dressing. Or have the Subway Deli Tuna Sandwich (deli sandwiches are on smaller rolls than subs) with a Veggie Delite salad and use 1 tablespoon fat-free Italian dressing.

49 **Taco Bell:** Order the Chili Cheese Burrito or the Gordita Supreme Chicken. Bring along a sandwich bag of 1 cup celery and carrot sticks (or other vegetable) and 1 small apple.

50 **Vegetarian Salad Bar:** Take 1 cup mixed greens or romaine lettuce and ½ cup beans (such as chickpeas or pinto beans); ¼ cup plain or marinated tofu (not deep-fried); 1½ cups chopped raw (plain, not marinated) vegetables of your choice (such as tomatoes, shredded carrots, or sliced cucumber); and 1½ tablespoons regular dressing or 3 tablespoons reduced-calorie dressing. Serve with 1 small slice whole wheat bread or French bread (about the size of your palm).

DINNER CHOICES

Each meal serves one unless otherwise specified. Dinners average 400 calories per serving.

BEEF

1 **Beef and Rice:** Prepare ⅓ cup cooked brown rice. In a nonstick skillet over medium heat, cook nearly halfway through 3 ounces crumbled raw 93% lean ground beef. In a bowl, combine ½ cup canned sliced mushrooms (rinse thoroughly and drain), ½ cup raw or frozen chopped onions, ½ cup low-fat/low-sodium cream of mushroom soup, and 1 teaspoon minced garlic. Pour over the ground beef and cook, covered, until the beef is cooked thoroughly. Serve over the brown rice. Have 1½ cups raspberries for dessert.

2 **Hamburger with Vegetables:** Serve a 3-ounce cooked hamburger on a wheat roll loaded with spinach leaves, sliced tomato, and sliced onion. Top with 2 to 3 tablespoons ketchup, if desired. Serve with 1 cup cooked green beans topped with 1 teaspoon chopped almonds.

3 **Barbecue Beef and Pasta:** In a nonstick skillet over medium-high heat, cook 2 tablespoons chopped white onion in 1 teaspoon olive oil. Cook for 1 minute, then reduce heat to medium. Add 2 teaspoons Worcestershire sauce, cover, and cook for 5 minutes. Add 4 ounces 92% lean ground beef and cook for 1 minute. Add 1 tablespoon barbecue sauce and ½ can (15-ounce size) crushed tomatoes, and continue to simmer until the beef is thoroughly cooked. Serve over 1 cup cooked pasta, any variety.

4 **Beef and Barley in the Slow Cooker:** Makes 3 servings. Combine in a slow cooker 12 ounces round, sirloin, or flank steak cut into 1-inch pieces with ½ cup quick barley, 1 can Campbell's Healthy Request Cream of Mushroom soup, 1 cup water, 1½ cups sliced mushrooms (fresh, frozen, or canned), 1½ cups frozen carrots, ½ teaspoon salt, ¼ teaspoon black pepper, and ½ teaspoon dried thyme. Mix well, cover, and cook on low for 7 to 8 hours.

CHICKEN AND TURKEY

5 **Apricot Chicken in the Slow Cooker:** Makes 4 servings. Pour ½ cup apple juice and ½ cup water into a slow cooker. Place 4 frozen 4-ounce boneless chicken breasts (one 4-ounce frozen breast is slightly larger than the size of a deck of cards) into the slow cooker. In a small bowl, mix together ¼ cup all-fruit style apricot jelly with ¼ cup Russian dressing and 1 teaspoon onion powder. Top the chicken breasts with the mixture. Cook on low for 5 to 6 hours. Serve each piece of chicken over ⅔ cup cooked rice or 1 cup cooked pasta.

6 **Chicken and Baked Beans:** Dark-meat lovers: Have a thigh, no skin. White-meat lovers: Have 1 whole 3-ounce skinless breast (about the size of a deck of cards). To save time, go with rotisserie chicken from the supermarket. Add ¾ cup canned baked beans, heated, and 1 heaping cup steamed matchstick-cut or baby carrots.

7 **Chicken Quesadilla:** Preheat oven to 400°F. Place ½ whole wheat tortilla on a cookie sheet. Spray the tortilla for 2 to 3 seconds with cooking spray. Top with 1 chopped paste (Roma-

style) tomato, 1/4 cup raw or frozen chopped onion, 3 ounces (about 1/2 cup or the size of a deck of cards) chicken breast strips, 1/4 cup shredded reduced-fat cheese, 1 tablespoon sliced black olives, and 1 teaspoon minced garlic from a jar. Cover with the other half of the tortilla. Spray for 2 to 3 seconds with cooking spray. Bake for 10 to 12 minutes. Top with 2 to 3 tablespoons salsa.

8 **Faux Fried Chicken:** Marinate a 3-ounce (about the size of a deck of cards) skinless chicken breast in 1/2 cup buttermilk for 1 hour in the refrigerator. (To make buttermilk, add 1 tablespoon lemon juice to 1/2 cup fat-free milk.) Mix 1/8 cup dried potato flakes with 2 tablespoons all-purpose flour, add 1/4 teaspoon each ground black pepper and salt, and dredge the chicken in the mixture to coat (discard any remaining buttermilk marinade). Spray a nonstick skillet with cooking spray and heat over medium heat with 2 teaspoons canola oil. Pan-fry the chicken until golden brown and cooked through. Serve with 1/2 cup mashed potatoes (made from potato flake mix) and 1 cup salad topped with 2 teaspoons lemon juice, 1 tablespoon balsamic vinegar, and 1/4 teaspoon black pepper.

9 **Grilled Chicken Caesar Salad:** Begin with 2 cups romaine lettuce. Warm 3 ounces (about 1/2 cup) chicken strips. Top the salad with 2 tablespoons light Caesar dressing and 15 seasoned croutons (skip the cheese-flavored ones; they're higher in calories). Serve with 1 apple. (To make homemade croutons: Spread 1 slice pumpernickel bread with 1 teaspoon trans-fat-free margarine and sprinkle on 1 teaspoon Italian-style bread crumbs. Spray with cooking spray for 1 to 2 seconds. Toast in a toaster oven. Slice into chunks.)

10 **Pasta and Turkey Meatballs:** Prepare 1 cup cooked pasta, any type. Simmer 3 (1-ounce) turkey meatballs in a nonstick skillet containing 1/2 inch water (replenish water if needed during cooking). To make turkey meatballs, combine 1 pound turkey breast meat with 1/3 cup Italian-style bread crumbs and 1 egg; mix thoroughly. (Freeze extras in a tightly sealed plastic bag for future meals.) Top with 1/4 cup spaghetti sauce and serve with 2/3 cup cooked green beans.

11 **Roasted Chicken with Brown Rice:** Prepare 2/3 cup cooked brown rice. Serve with a 3-ounce (about the size of a deck of cards) roasted chicken breast, 1 ear fresh corn (or 1/2 cup cooked frozen corn), and 1 cup cooked broccoli florets topped with 1 teaspoon trans-fat-free margarine.

12 **Tossed Salad with Roasted Chicken and Feta:** Toss 2 cups lettuce (suggest romaine) with 5 chopped baby carrots; 1 tablespoon sliced black olives; 1 medium tomato, sliced; 1/4 avocado; 1/4 cup chopped red onion; and 2 tablespoons crumbled feta cheese. Toss with 2 teaspoons olive oil and a generous amount of balsamic vinegar. Top with 3 ounces (about 1/2 cup) cold chopped roasted chicken and serve with 7 strawberries.

13 **Zucchini and Chicken Pasta:** Serve 1/2 cup cooked pasta (any variety) with 1/4 cup spaghetti sauce and 2 ounces (about 1/4 cup) cooked chicken strips. Chop 3/4 cup zucchini and place in a colander. Cook the zucchini by pouring the hot pasta water over it when you drain the cooked pasta into the colander. Mix all the ingredients together and serve.

FROZEN FOODS

14 **Beef and Vegetables:** Microwave according to package directions Uncle Ben's Mexican-Style Rice Bowl Beef Fajita, Lean Cuisine Café Classics Southern Beef Tips, or a similar frozen meal (check the label for 270 to 300 calories and 5 to 9 grams of fat). Add a salad: 1 cup romaine lettuce or mixed greens and ½ medium tomato, sliced. Top with 1 tablespoon regular dressing or 2 tablespoons light dressing.

15 **Fettuccini Alfredo:** Microwave according to package directions Lean Cuisine Everyday Favorites Chicken Fettuccini or a similar frozen meal (check the label for 270 to 280 calories and 6 to 10 grams of fat). Steam or microwave ¾ cup fresh or frozen broccoli. Pour chicken the fettuccini over the broccoli. Serve with 7 frozen red grapes.

16 **Macaroni and Cheese:** Heat Amy's Macaroni and Soy Cheeze according to package directions and serve with 2 cups romaine lettuce topped with 1 teaspoon olive oil and 2 tablespoons balsamic vinegar.

17 **Seafood Dinner:** Microwave according to package directions Lean Cuisine Café Classics Baked Fish, Healthy Choice Lemon Pepper Fish, or a similar frozen meal (check the label for 290 to 320 calories and 6 to 8 grams of fat). Add 1 cup steamed or microwaved vegetables (fresh or frozen) tossed with a spritz of lemon and 1 teaspoon olive oil.

18 **Spinach Lasagna:** Microwave 1 single-serving Cascadian Farm Spinach Lasagna according to package directions. Set aside, covered. Serve with 1 cup steamed sugar snap peas topped with 2 teaspoons trans-free margarine, and ½ cup cantaloupe cubes.

19 **Tortellini, Manicotti, or Lasagna:** Microwave according to package directions Healthy Choice Manicotti with Three Cheeses or Cheese Ravioli, Amy's Tofu Vegetable Lasagna, or a similar frozen meal (check the label for 300 to 330 calories and 9 to 12 grams of fat). Toss 1 cup romaine lettuce or mixed greens and ½ cup chopped vegetables of your choice (such as tomato or cucumber) with 1½ tablespoons light salad dressing and 1 tablespoon chopped almonds.

20 **Veggie Burger on the Ranch:** Grill or microwave a veggie burger according to package directions. Serve on a whole grain bun spread with 1 tablespoon reduced-calorie ranch (or Caesar) dressing. (Optional: Instead of dressing, use mustard and ketchup to taste). Add 2 thick slices tomato and romaine lettuce. Serve with ½ cup raw veggies (such as carrot and celery sticks) and ½ cup vegetarian baked beans. (Rinse a 16-ounce can vegetarian baked beans. Mix half of the can with 2 teaspoons barbecue sauce and 1 teaspoon Dijon mustard.)

MEATLESS

21 **Breakfast for Dinner:** Make 2 eggs (or ½ cup Egg Beaters) your way: poached, soft-boiled, or scrambled in a nonstick skillet with 1 tablespoon trans-fat-free margarine and coated with butter-flavored cooking spray (if desired). Serve with 1 slice whole wheat toast with 2 tea-

spoons jam or jelly. Add a 6-ounce glass of tomato juice.

22 **Cereal for Dinner:** In a big bowl, put 200 calories' worth of your favorite cereal (that's a scant cup raisin bran, 1¾ cups Cheerios, 1¾ cups Wheat or Corn Chex, or 1¼ cups Shredded Wheat 'n Bran; for other cereals, check labels to figure out what 200 calories translates to in cups). Add 1 tablespoon roasted sunflower seeds and 1 cup fresh or ½ cup frozen blueberries, and top with 1 cup fat-free milk. Drink all of the milk.

23 **Cheese Omelet with Tomatoes:** Coat a nonstick skillet with cooking spray and heat over medium heat. Beat 1 whole egg and 2 egg whites (or ½ cup Egg Beaters) with 2 tablespoons fat-free milk and ½ teaspoon ground black pepper. Mix thoroughly and pour into the skillet. Top with ¼ cup reduced-fat shredded cheese, 1 chopped paste (Roma-style) tomato, and ⅛ cup chopped sweet onion (if desired). Serve with 1 cup fat-free milk and 1 slice whole wheat toast topped with 1 teaspoon trans-fat-free margarine.

24 **Ravioli and Garlic Spinach:** Heat an entire box (10 ounces) spinach in the microwave oven. Squeeze out excess water. Mix with ¼ teaspoon salt, ½ teaspoon ground black pepper, and 2 teaspoons minced garlic. Prepare refrigerated low-fat ravioli such as Contadina Light Cheese Ravioli according to the package directions. Serve ¾ cup ravioli topped with ⅓ cup spaghetti sauce. Serve with half of the garlic spinach and 1 small orange, sliced.

25 **Vegetarian Chili with Cornbread:** Heat 1 cup canned vegetarian chili. Serve with a 2 × 3-inch piece of cornbread (about 1½ ounces or 42 grams; check your supermarket bakery department) or 1 serving Pillsbury Cornbread Twists (in refrigerated cans).

26 **Veggie Stir-Fry:** Heat a nonstick skillet coated with cooking spray and 2 teaspoons olive oil. Pan-fry 6 ounces low-fat firm tofu in block form for 2 minutes on each side. Break up the tofu into smaller pieces in the skillet and add 2 ounces low-sodium tomato soup and 2 ounces water. Continue cooking for 6 to 8 minutes. Scoop out the tofu and set aside. Using the remaining liquid in the skillet, stir-fry 1 cup fresh or frozen broccoli florets and ½ cup fresh or frozen snow peas with ½ teaspoon each cumin and coriander. Add 2 tablespoons water at a time if needed during cooking. Mix with the tofu and serve in 1 whole wheat tortilla. Have 1 cup chopped fresh fruit (such as 1 peach and 5 strawberries) for dessert.

27 **Waffles Florentine:** Makes 2 servings. Toast 4 whole grain frozen waffles and microwave a 9-ounce microwave-ready bag fresh baby spinach (or 2 cups frozen chopped spinach). Fry 4 eggs in a nonstick skillet coated with cooking spray. Top each waffle with 1 egg, one-quarter of the spinach (about ½ cup), and 1 tablespoon grated Parmesan cheese.

PASTA

28 **Asparagus Pasta:** Prepare 1 cup cooked penne pasta. Whisk together 1 teaspoon olive oil, 1 teaspoon minced garlic, 2 tablespoons white cooking wine, and ¼ teaspoon each ground

black pepper and salt. Pour over the pasta. Cook 8 large frozen or fresh asparagus spears and slice into the pasta mixture. Top with 2 ounces (about ⅓ cup) leftover cooked chicken breast strips.

29 **Italian Pasta Salad:** Cook 1 cup spiral pasta. Add ¼ teaspoon ground black pepper to 2 tablespoons Italian dressing. Toss the pasta with the dressing. Slice 1 medium tomato. Cut 2 ounces (about 2 slices) lean ham deli meat and 1 slice reduced-fat cheese into strips. Top the pasta with the tomato, ham, cheese, and 1 tablespoon sliced black olives.

30 **Pasta with Chickpeas:** Makes 2 servings. Prepare 2 cups cooked pasta, any variety. Toss 2 teaspoons olive oil, 2 tablespoons Parmesan cheese, and 1 teaspoon each dried basil and minced garlic with 1 cup canned (rinsed and drained) chickpeas and the cooked pasta. Serve half (check out Dinner #40 to use up the rest) with 1 cup cooked snow peas with 1 teaspoon trans-fat-free margarine.

PIZZA

31 **Homemade Pizza:** Top 1 large Neopolitan-style pizza crust with 1¼ cups spaghetti sauce and 1¾ cups (7 ounces) reduced-fat shredded cheese. Top with any vegetables you choose, such as thinly sliced fresh red pepper, thawed frozen (or raw) chopped onion, chopped fresh tomato or a small can stewed tomatoes, and a small can mushrooms (all drained). Remember that the vegetables add only 25 calories per ½ to 1 cup, so be generous. Bake the pizza at 400°F for 12 to 15 minutes. Cut the pizza into 8 equal slices. Serve 1 slice with 2 cups bagged baby spinach leaves tossed with 2 tablespoons light salad dressing and 2 tablespoons chopped walnuts. Store the remaining 7 slices in the refrigerator for up to 3 days or freeze to eat later.

32 **Take-Out Pizza:** Have 1 slice of a large (14-inch) pizza or 1½ slices of a medium (12-inch) pizza topped with 2 vegetables, such as mushrooms and green pepper. (Use only medium- or thin-crust pizza, such as Domino's Hand-Tossed Pizza.) For frozen pizza, check labels and have 265 to 280 calories' worth. Serve with a salad: 1 cup mixed greens and ½ cup chopped vegetables of your choice (such as tomatoes, peppers, and carrots) with 2 tablespoons reduced-calorie dressing.

PORK

33 **Chinese Pork in the Slow Cooker:** Makes 4 servings. Start by putting 1 cup uncooked rice into a slow cooker and cover with 3 cups water. Combine ½ teaspoon salt, 1 teaspoon curry powder, and 3 tablespoons olive oil, and brush the oil mixture on both sides of a 16-ounce (1-pound) pork tenderloin. Place the pork into the slow cooker and pour in 1 can Campbell's Healthy Request Cream of Mushroom soup and 4 cups frozen Chinese vegetables. If desired, top with 4 tablespoons light soy sauce. Cook on low heat for 8 hours. Before serving, turn the cooker to the high-heat setting and boil for 10 minutes.

34 **Pork Tenderloin with Apple Butter:** Preheat oven to 350°F. Mix together ⅛ teaspoon ground cinnamon, 1 tablespoon brown sugar, 2 tablespoons apple butter, 3 tablespoons

apple juice, and if desired, ⅛ teaspoon ground cloves. Place a 4-ounce (slightly larger than the size of a deck of cards) pork tenderloin in a covered baking dish and bake for 25 minutes. Remove from oven, uncover, top with the apple butter mixture, and continue baking, uncovered, for 10 minutes. Serve with ½ cup brown rice and 1 cup cooked snow peas topped with 1 teaspoon trans-fat-free margarine.

SEAFOOD

35 **Broccoli Rice with Shrimp:** Makes 3 servings. In a medium pot, cook according to package directions 1 box (6.2-ounce size) Uncle Ben's Long Grain and Wild Rice Fast-Cook Recipe, using 1 tablespoon trans-fat-free margarine. As soon as it starts to simmer, add 1½ cups fresh broccoli, chopped in small pieces, but do not stir it into the rice until the rice is cooked. While the rice is cooking, add 1 tablespoon olive or canola oil and 1 clove minced garlic (or 1 teaspoon garlic powder) to a large nonstick skillet over medium heat. Sauté the garlic for 30 seconds, then add about 30 large or 36 medium peeled shrimp (7 ounces), either fresh or frozen and thawed. Cook until the shrimp turn pink, about 4 to 5 minutes, stirring constantly. Serve one-third of the broccoli-rice mixture with one-third of the shrimp.

36 **Grilled Lobster:** Makes 2 servings. Begin with a 10-ounce rock lobster tail. Prepare your indoor or outdoor grill for high heat. Whisk together 1 tablespoon olive oil, 1 tablespoon lemon juice, ¼ teaspoon salt, and ½ teaspoon each paprika and ground black pepper to make a marinade. Split the lobster tail and brush the meat side of the tail with marinade. Place meat side down on the grill for 5 to 6 minutes. Turn and cook another 5 minutes. Serve with 1 cup sliced green squash, grilled, and 1 small (1-ounce) French roll.

37 **Salmon with Parmesan Spinach:** Makes 2 servings. Microwave a 9-ounce microwave-ready bag (2 cups cooked) fresh baby spinach (such as Ready Pac brand) according to package directions (about 3 minutes). Carefully remove the hot spinach from the bag, dividing into 2 microwave-safe bowls. In each bowl, add ½ cup (3 ounces) cooked salmon (or ½ cup cooked chicken strips) and sprinkle on 3 tablespoons Parmesan cheese. Microwave each bowl for 30 to 45 seconds, until the cheese begins to melt. Accompany each serving with 2 slices French bread (each about the size of your palm).

38 **Salmon, Rice, and Asparagus:** Makes 2 servings. Preheat oven to 350°F. In a 1½-quart baking dish, pour 1 cup white wine and 1 cup water. Add 5 peppercorns, 2 bay leaves, and 1 peeled clove garlic. Place in the oven. When it comes to a simmer, add 2 pieces (3 ounces each) of boneless salmon fillet. Cook skin side down for 8 minutes, or until cooked all the way through. With a slotted spoon, remove the salmon from the liquid. Serve each piece of salmon with 1 cup cooked flavored rice (such as Uncle Ben's Chef Recipe Chicken and Harvest Vegetable Pilaf) and 1 cup steamed or microwaved asparagus with a spritz of lemon.

39 **Shrimp and Vegetable Stir-Fry:** Prepare ⅔ cup cooked brown rice. Set

aside. Heat a nonstick skillet on the stove over medium heat with 1 teaspoon olive oil. Add 2 cups frozen mixed vegetables and sprinkle with 1 teaspoon Cajun spice seasoning, if desired. In a bowl, coat 16 large or 20 medium peeled shrimp (4 ounces) with ½ teaspoon ground black pepper and 1 teaspoon Cajun spice seasoning. Pour 3 ounces low-sodium, fat-free chicken or vegetable broth into the skillet. Add the shrimp to the skillet once the vegetables are nearly cooked. Cook the shrimp until no longer translucent. Serve the shrimp over rice.

40 **Tuna and Bean Pasta Salad:** Combine tuna from Lunch #26 with pasta from Dinner #30. Serve with 1 cup lettuce with ½ cup sliced cucumber and 1 tablespoon light salad dressing. Serve with 1 apple.

41 **Crab Cakes:** Makes 2 servings. Combine ½ pound fresh lump crabmeat with ⅔ cup soft bread crumbs, ½ cup raw or frozen chopped onion, 1 tablespoon lemon juice, 1 tablespoon fat-free milk, ¼ teaspoon each salt and pepper, and 2 slightly beaten egg whites. Heat 1 tablespoon canola oil in a nonstick skillet over medium-high heat. Form the crab mixture into patties and cook on both sides until golden. Serve with ⅔ cup cooked orzo seasoned with 2 teaspoons lemon juice and ½ teaspoon parsley flakes.

42 **Broiled Scallops:** Makes 2 servings. Preheat oven to 350°F. Rinse 1 pound fresh scallops and place in a shallow baking pan. Sprinkle with 2 teaspoons garlic salt, 2 tablespoons melted trans-fat-free margarine, and 2 tablespoons lemon juice. Broil for 8 minutes, or until the scallops turn golden brown. Serve with 1 slice French bread (about the size of your palm) and 1 cup cooked spinach seasoned with ½ teaspoon ground black pepper and 2 teaspoons lemon juice.

43 **Salmon and Cucumber Pasta Salad:** Toss 1 cup cooked pasta with 2 tablespoons reduced-fat sour cream, 1 tablespoon light mayonnaise, and the juice of 1 lime (about 1½ tablespoons). Add ½ cup chopped cucumber and 3 ounces flaked cooked salmon.

44 **Grilled Maple-Marinated Tuna:** Marinate 4 ounces (uncooked) tuna steak in 1 tablespoon maple syrup, 2 tablespoons orange juice, and freshly ground black pepper (to taste) for 20 minutes. Remove from the marinade and grill or broil approximately 3 minutes on each side. Serve with ½ large baked potato topped with 2 tablespoons reduced-fat sour cream and 8 large asparagus spears topped with 1 teaspoon trans-fat-free margarine.

SOUP

45 **Lentil Soup and French Bread:** Heat 1 cup lentil soup (canned is fine). Serve with 1 large slice (about 6 inches long) warm French bread (such as one-sixth of Pillsbury's Refrigerated Crusty French Loaf) spread with ½ cup roasted red peppers from a jar (drained) and 1 ounce reduced-fat cheese.

46 **Tomato Soup and Grilled Cheese:** Heat 1 cup tomato soup (such as Campbell's Reduced-Sodium Tomato soup). Grilled cheese sandwich: Spread 2 slices whole wheat bread with 1 teaspoon trans-fat-free mar-

garine each. With buttered sides out, place 2 slices reduced-fat cheese between the bread slices. Grill in a nonstick skillet coated with cooking spray or in toaster oven until cheese melts. Serve with 8 baby carrots.

EATING OUT

47 **Au Bon Pain:** Have half the huge Fields and Feta Wrap (share with a friend), plus a medium serving of Tomato Florentine Soup.

48 **Chicken Restaurant (such as Boston Market or Chicken Out):** Order a Quarter Dark-Meat Chicken (leave off the skin) or a Quarter White-Meat Chicken (leave off the skin). Have a side of the red-skin mashed potatoes or mashed sweet potatoes (6 ounces). Add a side of steamed vegetables or coleslaw. Skip the bread that comes with the meal.

49 **Chinese Restaurant:** Order beef, chicken, or shrimp with broccoli. Or order one of these same dishes with mixed vegetables instead of broccoli. Ask for more vegetables than beef, chicken, or shrimp, and ask to have it stir-fried in very little oil. Have 1¼ cups entrée with ¾ cup steamed rice. If the restaurant won't accommodate your requests for less oil and more veggies, then order them steamed with the sauce on the side and use only 4 tablespoons sauce.

50 **Greek or Middle Eastern Restaurant:** Order a chicken and vegetable kebab. Have all the skewered vegetables and about 2½ ounces chicken (usually about ⅓ of the serving). Take the leftover chicken home (it will work perfectly in other dinners). Have a side of Greek salad (with 1½ cups greens and no feta cheese; order dressing on the side and use 1 tablespoon) and 1 cup rice.

51 **Italian Restaurant:** Have 1 cup spaghetti with about ½ cup tomato sauce and 2 ounces seafood–about 10 large shrimp, 8 mussels, or 6 clams. (Take the leftovers home.) Add a side salad (1½ cups mixed greens) and use 1 tablespoon reduced-calorie dressing.

52 **Olive Garden:** Order the Chicken Giardino (vegetables and chicken tossed with pasta in a lemon-herb sauce); leave about a fifth of it on your plate. Or order Shrimp Primavera, eat half, and take the rest home. The entrée comes with a side salad; use 1 tablespoon reduced-calorie dressing.

53 **Schlotzsky's Deli:** Have the small-size Chicken Dijon sandwich from the Light and Flavorful menu and a side garden salad with 1 tablespoon light Italian dressing (no more than ⅓ packet).

54 **T.G.I. Friday's:** Order the Jack Daniel's Salmon (tell your waiter not to bring extra sauce). Have a piece of salmon no bigger than a deck of cards (take the rest home–use it to make Dinner #43). This comes with chef's vegetables; request that they be cooked in minimal oil. Also, ask for your baked potato plain, and eat only half. Use the same strategy when ordering salmon in other restaurants.

55 **Wendy's:** Have the large-size chili and the side salad. Use ⅓ packet of fat-free French dressing.

HEALTHY SNACK CHOICES

Each snack serves one. Snacks average 200 calories each.

BARS

1 **Luna Bar and Fruit:** Serve 1 Luna bar (any flavor) with ½ orange.

2 **Kellogg's Nutri-Grain Cereal Bar and Nuts:** Have your choice of Kellogg's Nutri-Grain Cereal Bar or Twists Cereal Bar with 10 peanuts.

3 **Slim-Fast Bar and Nuts:** Have your choice of any variety Slim-Fast bar with ⅛ cup pistachios.

4 **Pria Bar and Peanut Butter:** Spread 1 tablespoon peanut butter on any variety Pria bar.

BREAD

5 **Cinnamon Bread with Peanut Butter:** Toast 1 slice Pepperidge Farm Cinnamon Swirl Bread and top with 2 teaspoons peanut butter. Serve with ½ cup fat-free milk.

6 **English Muffin with Peanut Butter:** Toast ½ whole wheat English muffin and spread with 1 tablespoon peanut butter and 1 tablespoon raisins.

7 **Pumpernickel Bread with Fruit and Cheese:** Spread 1 tablespoon reduced-fat cream cheese or farmer's cheese on 1 slice pumpernickel bread (toast the bread if you'd like). Serve with 1 small apple.

8 **Ricotta Spread with English Muffin:** Combine a 15½-ounce container low-fat ricotta cheese with 2 tablespoons honey and 3 tablespoons smooth or chunky peanut butter. (This recipe makes six ⅓-cup servings. See Breakfast #36 and Healthy Snacks #12, 14, and 32 for more serving ideas. You can keep this mix in the fridge for up to 7 days or freeze single servings for up to 1 month.) Top ½ whole wheat English muffin with ⅓ cup ricotta cheese spread.

9 **Waffle with Peanut Butter Sprinkled with Peanuts:** Toast 1 whole grain waffle. Top with 1 tablespoon peanut butter and 4 peanuts.

CHEESE

10 **Cottage Cheese and Almond Milk:** Add a few drops almond extract to 1 cup fat-free milk, cold or heated. Serve with ½ cup fat-free or 1% cottage cheese topped with a sprinkle of cinnamon.

CRACKERS

11 **Crackers and Almond Butter:** Top 1 Wasa crispbread with 2 teaspoons almond butter. Serve with 1 cup fat-free milk.

12 **Crackers and Dip:** Dip 2 Wasa crispbreads into ⅓ cup ricotta cheese spread. To make the spread: Combine a 15½-ounce container low-fat ricotta cheese with 2 tablespoons honey and 3 tablespoons smooth or chunky peanut butter. (The recipe makes six ⅓-cup servings. See Breakfasts #5 and 36 and Healthy Snacks #8, 14, and 32 for more serving ideas. You can keep this mix in the fridge for up to 7 days or freeze single servings for up to 1 month.)

13 **Oh, Baby!:** Open 1 jar baby-food peaches or other baby-food fruit (check the label for no more than 70 calories per serving). Serve with 1 Wasa crispbread topped with 1 slice reduced-fat cheese.

14 **Ricotta Spread Surprise and Chocolate Milk:** Mix 1 cup cold fat-free milk with ½ tablespoon chocolate syrup. Serve with a 2½-inch graham cracker square crumbled into ⅓ cup ricotta cheese spread. To make the spread, combine a 15½-ounce container low-fat ricotta cheese with 2 tablespoons honey and 3 tablespoons smooth or chunky peanut butter. (The recipe makes six ⅓-cup servings. See Breakfasts #5 and 36 and Healthy Snacks #8, 12, and 32 for more serving ideas. You can keep this mix in the fridge for up to 7 days or freeze single servings for up to 1 month.)

DRINKS

15 **Banana Soy Smoothie:** In an electric blender (or with a hand blender), combine until smooth: 4 ounces low-fat firm silken tofu with ½ ripe banana, ½ teaspoon pure vanilla extract, and 8 ounces fat-free milk. Blend in 1 or 2 ice cubes.

16 **Berry Smoothie:** In an electric blender (or with a hand blender), combine 1 cup thawed frozen berries, 1 teaspoon vanilla extract, and 1 cup fat-free milk. Slowly add 1 cup crushed ice after the other ingredients.

17 **Café au Lait and Muffin:** Mix together 1 cup hot brewed or instant coffee (regular or decaf), 1 cup hot fat-free milk, and 1 teaspoon sugar (if desired). Serve with a mini blueberry muffin (such as a Hostess Blueberry Mini Muffin).

18 **Hot Chocolate:** Heat 1 cup fat-free milk. Add ½ tablespoon chocolate syrup. (Optional: Add a few drops vanilla extract and top with 2 tablespoons light whipped cream.) Serve with a 2½-inch graham cracker square topped with 1 tablespoon almond butter.

19 **Iced Coffee:** Mix together 1 cup cold fat-free milk with 1 cup room-temperature brewed coffee. Add ice and 1 teaspoon sugar, if desired. Serve with 1 fig cookie.

20 **Maple Milk and Crackers with Almond Butter:** Heat 1 cup fat-free milk. Stir in 1 teaspoon maple syrup. Serve with 4 Reduced-Fat Triscuit crackers topped with 2 teaspoons almond butter.

21 **Peach Slush:** In an electric blender (or with a hand blender), combine 8 ounces peach-flavored fat-free yogurt (check labels for about 120 calories per cup) with 1 peeled and sliced ripe peach or ½ cup canned peaches (in juice, not syrup). Add ½ cup seltzer or club soda. Add 1 or 2 ice cubes and blend until smooth. (For variety, make a slush with berry-flavored yogurt and fresh or frozen berries.) Enjoy with ⅓ cup fat-free or 1% cottage cheese.

22 **Strawberry Milk and Crackers:** Mix 1 cup cold fat-free milk with 2 teaspoons strawberry powder (such as Nesquik). Serve with 4 Reduced-Fat Triscuit crackers topped with 2 tablespoons farmer's cheese or reduced-fat cream cheese.

23 **Strawberry Smoothie:** In an electric blender (or with a hand blender), combine until smooth 1 cup fat-free milk, ½ ripe banana, and ¼ cup fresh or frozen strawberries. Top with 2 tablespoons low-fat granola and eat with a spoon.

24 **Tangy Thirst Quencher:** Drink a 6-ounce can grapefruit juice. Serve with 1

Wasa crispbread topped with 2 tablespoons farmer's cheese or reduced-fat veggie cream cheese.

FRUIT

25 **Apples with Peanut Butter:** Have 1 apple topped with 2 teaspoons peanut butter. Serve with 1 cup fat-free milk.

26 **Applesauce:** Try convenient single-serving peel-top containers with ½ cup applesauce (such as Mott's Natural Style or Mott's Healthy Harvest–any flavor). Serve with 20 peanuts.

27 **Apricot Indulgence:** Have 3 dried apricots (or 6 halves). Serve with 2 graham cracker squares (2½-inch size) spread with 1 tablespoon peanut butter. Serve with 1 cup fat-free milk.

28 **Banana and Chocolate Dip:** Prepare a dip using 2 tablespoons reduced-fat sour cream, ¼ teaspoon vanilla extract, and 1 tablespoon chocolate syrup. Serve with 1 sliced banana. Spear each banana slice with a toothpick for dipping.

29 **Frozen Grapes:** Put 1 cup grapes in the freezer for several hours. Eat right out of the freezer; they're like candy. Serve with 1 stick reduced-fat string cheese or 1 Wasa crispbread topped with 1 tablespoon feta cheese.

30 **Fruit and Almond Butter:** Slice a ripe pear or apple and spread with 2 tablespoons almond butter.

31 **Fruit and Cheese:** Slice a ripe pear or apple and eat it with 1 slice (1 ounce) reduced-fat cheese.

32 **Fruit Cocktail Surprise:** Have ¾ cup (6 ounces) fruit cocktail, drained (canned in juice, not syrup). Mix into ⅓ cup ricotta cheese spread and enjoy. To make the spread, combine a 15½-ounce container low-fat ricotta cheese with 2 tablespoons honey and 3 tablespoons smooth or chunky peanut butter. (This recipe makes six ⅓-cup servings. See Breakfasts #5 and 36 and Healthy Snacks #8, 12, and 14 for more serving ideas. You can keep it in the fridge for up to 7 days or freeze single servings for up to 1 month.)

33 **Fruit to Go:** Have a 4-ounce container (½ cup) fruit (in juice). Check labels for about 60 calories per serving, such as single-serve, peel-top cans of Del Monte Fruit Naturals Diced Peaches in Pear and Peach Juice or Dole Pineapple FruitBowls. Serve with 1 slice whole wheat bread topped with 1 slice reduced-fat cheese.

34 **Fruit with Toasted Nuts:** Serve 2 cups cut fruit (suggest honeydew) with 1½ tablespoons toasted chopped nuts (any variety).

35 **Make It Melon:** Serve 1 cup watermelon with 1 slice (1 ounce) reduced-fat Cheddar cheese on 3 Reduced-Fat Triscuit crackers.

36 **Peanut Butter and Banana Slices with Chocolate Milk:** Slice ½ small banana, top with 2 teaspoons peanut butter and serve with a toothpick for sticky-free eating. Drink ½ cup fat-free milk mixed with 2 teaspoons chocolate syrup.

37 **Pears Drizzled with Chocolate:** Open 1 can pear halves. Drizzle 1½ tablespoons chocolate syrup over 1 canned pear half

and top with 1 tablespoon chopped nuts (any type). Serve with ½ cup fat-free milk.

MEAL-TYPE SNACKS

38 **Cobb Salad:** Combine 2 cups romaine lettuce leaves and ½ chopped paste (Roma-style) tomato, and toss with 1 tablespoon light salad dressing. Top the salad with ⅛ cup reduced-fat shredded cheese, 1 chopped hard-boiled egg, and 1 ounce (usually 1 slice) turkey breast cut into strips.

39 **Leftover Pasta Snack:** Serve ⅓ cup cooked pasta with ¼ cup spaghetti sauce. Top with 1 tablespoon Parmesan cheese and 3 sliced medium olives.

40 **Pizza Muffin:** Toast 1 whole wheat English muffin topped with ¼ cup spaghetti sauce and 1 stick reduced-fat string cheese chopped into ½-inch slices.

NUTS

41 **Raisin-Nut Cluster:** Mix 2 tablespoons raisins with ⅛ cup chopped walnuts, 2 teaspoons honey, and 1 teaspoon maple extract. Place in a small paper cup and top with ½ teaspoon granulated sugar. Freeze and serve slightly thawed.

42 **Trail Mix:** Enjoy 2 tablespoons dried sweetened cranberries, 2 tablespoons raisins, and 2 tablespoons peanuts.

PUDDING

43 **Pudding and Fruit:** Have 1 ready-to-serve fat-free pudding cup (any flavor). Serve with ¾ cup blueberries.

44 **Chocolate Pudding with Peanut Butter:** Melt 1 tablespoon peanut butter in the microwave (heat for 30 to 35 seconds on 50 percent power) and immediately mix into 1 Jell-O brand fat-free chocolate pudding cup.

VEGETABLES

45 **Cheese and Crunch:** Have 1½ slices reduced-fat cheese wrapped around a stick of celery. (Optional: Dip in hot and spicy mustard.) Serve with ½ cup fresh strawberries.

46 **Cheese and a Pickle:** Have 3 tablespoons farmer's cheese or reduced-fat veggie cream cheese on 2 Reduced-Fat Triscuit crackers (or 33 calories' worth of another whole grain cracker) with a pickle of your choice. Serve with 7 grapes.

47 **Vegetables and Dip:** Dip 15 baby carrots into 2 tablespoons reduced-fat veggie cream cheese and serve with 1¼ cups fresh strawberries.

48 **Vegetables and Hummus:** Enjoy 8 baby carrots and ½ cup sliced cucumber with 3 tablespoons hummus. Serve with 1 slice (1 ounce) reduced-fat cheese.

YOGURT

49 **Nutty Yogurt:** Top 8 ounces (1 cup) fat-free yogurt (any flavor–check labels for no more than 120 calories per cup or less) with 2 tablespoons chopped walnuts.

50 **Real Raspberry Yogurt:** Mix ½ cup fresh or ¼ cup thawed frozen raspberries with 8 ounces (1 cup) fat-free berry-flavored yogurt (check labels for no more than 120 calories per cup). Serve with 1 slice reduced-fat cheese.

51 **Tropical Yogurt:** Stir 2 tablespoons tropical dried-fruit mix into an 8-ounce (1 cup) fat-free pineapple- or apricot-flavored yogurt (check labels for no more than 120 calories per cup). Mix in a few drops coconut extract. Top with 1 tablespoon chopped walnuts.

INDULGENT TREATS

Each indulgent treat serves one. Treats average 200 calories each.

APPETIZERS

1 **Fried Shrimp:** Indulge in 10 small fried shrimp.

2 **Buffalo Wings:** Treat yourself to 6 small Buffalo-style chicken wings.

3 **Potato Skins:** Enjoy 2 potato skins topped with cheese, sour cream, chives, and bacon.

4 **Double Dip:** Have 1 cup fresh vegetables with ½ cup creamy spinach artichoke dip.

CAKES, COOKIES, BREADS, NUTS, AND CEREAL

5 **Candied Pecans:** Enjoy 1 ounce praline pecans.

6 **Cheese Crackers with Peanut Butter:** Stop by the convenience store for a 6-piece pack of cheese crackers sandwiched with peanut butter.

7 **Cinnamon Bread with Chocolate Filling:** Preheat the toaster oven to 250°F. Spread 2 teaspoons peanut butter on 1 slice Pepperidge Farm Cinnamon Swirl Bread, then top with 1 tablespoon mini chocolate chips. Bake for 4 to 6 minutes and enjoy!

8 **Cookies:** Have 4 Oreo Chocolate Sandwich Cookies or 4 Chips Ahoy! Real Chocolate Chip Cookies.

9 **Cookies at the Mall:** At Mrs. Fields, have 4 Bite-Size Nibbler Chewy Chocolate Fudge Cookies.

10 **Doughnut and Cider:** Have 8 ounces hot or cold apple cider with 1 Hostess Powdered Sugar Donette.

11 **Kid's Cereal:** Have 1¼ cups Lucky Charms or Froot Loops cereal with ½ cup fat-free milk. Drink all the milk.

12 **Little Debbie Snack:** Treat yourself to 1 Little Debbie Brownie Lights brownie.

13 **S'mores:** Preheat the toaster oven to 250°F. Set out 4 graham cracker squares (2½-inch size). Put 1 tablespoon mini chocolate chips on 2 squares, top with 1 large marshmallow each, then top with another graham cracker square. Bake for 4 to 6 minutes. Let cool for 1 to 2 minutes and enjoy. The snack includes 3 additional 2½-inch graham cracker squares.

14 **Toaster Treat:** Enjoy 1 Brown Sugar Cinnamon Pop Tart.

15 **Twinkie:** Enjoy 1 regular Twinkie (43-gram size).

CANDY

16 **Bit-O-Honey:** Have a 1.7–ounce Bit-O-Honey bar.

17 **Candy Corn Frenzy:** Have 36 pieces (40 grams) candy corn.

18 **Chewy Candy:** Enjoy a 2.25-ounce box Dots candy, any flavor.

19 **Jelly Bean Bonanza:** Have ⅓ cup Starburst jelly beans.

20 **Licorice Break:** Have 1 vending-machine-size package (50 grams) red or black Twizzler licorice.

21 **Milk Maids:** Chew on 4 pieces (40 grams) caramel candy.

22 **Old-Fashioned Treat:** Enjoy a 6-piece Chuckles candy or 6 Circus Peanuts.

CANDY—CHOCOLATE

23 **Dandy Candy:** Indulge in 1 Milky Way Lite candy bar.

24 **Halloween Fun-Size Candy:** Have 200 calories' worth of fun-size candy bars (such as 2 Butterfinger, 2 Three Musketeers, 2 Baby Ruth, or 4 Nestlé Crunch).

25 **M&Ms:** Have a 1½-ounce bag M&Ms Crispy Chocolate Candy.

26 **Dove Chocolate Bar (Dark or Regular Chocolate):** Enjoy a full-size (36.9-gram) Dove chocolate bar for a luscious treat.

27 **Chocolate-Covered Peanuts or Raisins:** Have 16 pieces chocolate-covered peanuts or 40 pieces chocolate-covered raisins.

28 **Malted Milk Balls:** Have 17 malted milk balls.

29 **Raspberries with Melted Chocolate:** Melt 2 tablespoons mini chocolate chips in the microwave (heat in a glass container on 50 percent power for about 50 seconds). Drizzle over 1½ cups fresh raspberries.

CHIPS, POPCORN, AND FRIES

30 **Chips with Cheese:** Spread 1 small snack-size (¾-ounce) bag tortilla chips on a microwave-safe plate. Top with ¼ cup reduced-fat shredded cheese. Heat 45 seconds to 2 minutes in the microwave until melted.

31 **French Fry Fix:** Order a small-size McDonald's french fries and a diet soda.

32 **Frito Fun:** Have 1 snack-size bag (1.25-ounce) corn chips, any variety.

33 **Potato Chips:** Enjoy 1 snack-size bag (1.25-ounce) potato chips, any variety.

34 **Popcorn:** Have 1 mini bag (about 5 cups popped) Orville Redenbacher Movie Theater Butter Popcorn.

35 **Purple Passion:** Serve 8 ounces Minute Maid Grape Soda with ½ ounce purple Terra chips "Terra Blues" (8 or 9 chips).

DRINKS

36 **Cream Soda:** Have 12 ounces of your favorite full-calorie cream soda.

37 **Ice Cream Shake:** Scoop ½ cup Healthy Choice ice cream, any flavor. Mix in a blender with ½ cup fat-free milk and 1 cup crushed ice, if desired. Top with 1 tablespoon chopped nuts.

38 **Wine and Cheese:** Enjoy 4 ounces wine with 1 Wasa crispbread spread with 1 tablespoon farmer's cheese or reduced-fat cream cheese.

39 **Wine and Chocolate:** Indulge in 4 ounces wine with 1 Dove miniature dark chocolate bar.

ICE CREAM

40 **Banana Split:** Slice 1 banana in half lengthwise. Top with ⅓ cup Healthy Choice ice cream, any flavor, and 2 tablespoons Cool Whip Lite.

41 **Ice Cream Cone:** Serve ¾ cup Edy's Blackberry Swirl or French Vanilla ice cream or a kiddie-size (½ cup) Soft-Serve (any flavor) on a wafer cone.

42 **Ice Cream with Chocolate and Nuts:** Serve ½ cup Edy's Neopolitan ice cream with 1 tablespoon chopped almonds and 1 tablespoon mini chocolate chips.

43 **Ice Cream Sundae:** Serve ½ cup Healthy Choice ice cream (any variety), Edy's regular chocolate or coffee ice cream, or Baskin-Robbins Cherries Jubilee ice cream with 1½ tablespoons chopped walnuts and 2 tablespoons light whipped topping.

44 **McDonald's Ice Cream Cone:** Order 1 vanilla reduced-fat ice cream cone.

45 **Silhouette Ice Cream Sandwich:** Serve 1 Silhouette ice cream sandwich with a 2½-inch graham cracker square topped with 2 teaspoons peanut butter.

MEAL-TYPE INDULGENCES

46 **Chicken McNuggets:** Order a 4-piece Chicken McNuggets at McDonald's with your choice of sauce. Have with 1 cup raspberries.

47 **Fried Rice:** Have the smallest portion (about ¾ cup) of fried rice at your favorite Chinese restaurant.

48 **Pepperoni Pizza:** Enjoy 1 slice of a medium pie at Little Caesar's. Choose the "Pan! Pan!" variety.

PEANUT BUTTER AND CHOCOLATE

49 **Graham Crackers with Chocolate and Peanut Butter:** Preheat the toaster oven to 250°F. Set out 4 graham cracker squares (2½-inch size). Spread 1 tablespoon mini chocolate chips on 2 squares. Bake for 4 to 6 minutes. Let cool for 1 to 2 minutes. Spread the remaining 2 squares with 1 tablespoon peanut butter. Press one of each together and enjoy.

50 **Peanut Butter and Chocolate:** Scoop 1½ tablespoons peanut butter out of the jar onto a spoon, top the scoop with 1 tablespoon mini chocolate chips, and enjoy right off the spoon!

PART 4

THE FIRM UP COMPONENTS

CHAPTER 8

Get a Winning Attitude

The difference between success and failure at this or *any* program can be summed up in one word: attitude. That's why I've made it the first of the Firm Up components. This chapter presents my favorite ways to firm up your attitude as you firm up your body.

A few years back, several *Prevention* magazine editors were waiting in a conference room to meet with the magazine's editor in chief at that time. We sat around for about 10 minutes, and when he still hadn't arrived, I offered to check with his assistant. As I headed for the door, another editor called out to me, "There's a phone!" Without even thinking I replied,

"That's okay; I'll walk over to his office." While striding down the hall, it dawned on me that we had a major difference in our attitudes toward movement.

- My impulse was to move–getting up to see what was going on.

  This is an energy-burning attitude.

- Her reaction was to stay seated–using a device to get the job done.

  This is an energy-saving attitude.

Frankly, for most of humanity's existence, the other editor's energy-saving attitude was probably healthiest. When our lives were filled with hard work in the fields, on the hunt, and in factories, we needed to conserve our energy. Throughout civilization, finding ways to free ourselves from physical labor has been a major quest and has led us to important advances–from the wheel to the computer.

But today, this energy-saving attitude is just plain out-of-date. In the 21st century, we live in a push-button, drive-thru, remote-control world that is so filled with laborsaving devices that we've almost totally engineered physical activity out of our days. It's a sad fact of modern life that the vast majority of us spend the vast majority of our days on our increasingly vast behinds. Many times we can't even use our muscles if we want to! Doors fly open automatically; escalators are prominent, while stairs are hidden; people movers whisk us through airports.

QUICK TIP **The less you sit and the more you move, the more fit—and healthy—you'll be.**

Adding Some Action

HERE ARE SOME easy ways to get more activity into your days.

- Use the bathroom that's farthest away from you.
- Take a hike around the block or the field while you wait for your kids to finish piano lessons or soccer practice.
- Instead of e-mailing a coworker, get up and go to her office to talk.
- Skip drive-thrus at banks and restaurants. Instead, park your car and go inside.
- Walk a lap in the grocery store or the mall before you begin to shop.
- If you have a desk job, set a timer to alert you hourly. When it goes off, get up and take a walk, or simply stretch for a minute or two.
- Walk inside to pay for gas.

That's why, if we really want to get fit, we need a major attitude adjustment–one that embraces every possible opportunity to be active, even if it's just walking down the hall. The human body is made to move, and a growing body of research shows that the unnatural state of sitting all day leads to disease. Your risk of developing virtually every chronic ailment–from heart disease and diabetes to depression, osteoporosis, and certain cancers–is increased by being sedentary and reduced by being physically active.

ACTIVATE YOUR LIFE

Adopting an energy-burning attitude goes beyond making a commitment to working out. Yes, formal exercise is important–and by "formal" exercise, I mean the change-your-clothes-and-do-a-workout kind of scheduled, planned physical activity. These workouts are essential and make up the majority of the Firm Up Action Plan (see chapters 3, 4, and 5 for each week's workouts).

Most people understand the importance of formal exercise–even though the majority of Americans don't do it. What most people *don't* understand is the importance of *informal* exercise: moving in your daily life–walking to the mailbox, taking the stairs, carrying your groceries, throwing a ball with the kids. Solid research shows that these types of lifestyle activity can provide health benefits similar to a traditional gym workout. In other words, every step you take counts toward good health and fitness.

Unfortunately, this message still hasn't reached most people–and not just the couch potatoes either. Surprisingly, even committed exercisers who have an energy-burning attitude during their workouts often revert to an energy-saving attitude outside the gym. If you want hard evidence, watch the parking lot at a health club. You'll see people fight for the closest parking space, then go inside and walk on the treadmill. It's not uncommon to see someone drive around for 5 minutes to get a "good" parking spot–then rush in so they won't be late for aerobics class. I've even seen people take the elevator a few floors to work out on the stairclimber!

These contradictory behaviors make it alarmingly clear that our ancient energy-saving attitude is still hot-wired into many people's brains. But if you want to firm up and be fit, you must flip your mental switch over to the energy-burning mode. Thirty minutes–or even an hour every day–of exercise isn't enough to combat 23 hours on your rear end.

ATTITUDE ADJUSTMENT #1:

Adopt an **energy-burning attitude** and get going!

BOTTOMS UP

Another way of thinking about this energy-burning mentality is to adopt a "bottoms up" approach to life. With this outlook, you're always eager to get up and go, whether it's to walk down the hall to see a colleague or to stand up and stretch while you're on the telephone.

Finding ways to move in our energy-saving culture can be challenging–but it's possible.

Fit Fact

IN ONE STUDY of 40 women, those who lost weight by increasing everyday activities such as gardening, walking the dog, and taking the stairs actually maintained their weight loss better than those who lost weight by only participating in structured aerobics classes.

(You'll find daily suggestions on how to incorporate movement into your daily activities throughout the Firm Up Action Plan.) Fortunately, attitudes toward activity are changing as our culture recognizes the health hazard of sedentary habits and tries to make our environment more movement-friendly. Forward-thinking corporations are locating parking lots far from their buildings and installing slow elevators to encourage employees to take the stairs.

Some experts liken our society's attitude toward movement to the way we thought about smoking a generation ago. In the 1970s, we were just beginning to wake up to the dangers of cigarettes and starting to design spaces and create laws to protect people from smoke. Back in our parents' day, who would have thought we would have banned smoking in workplaces, in restaurants, and on public transportation? Yet look how far we've come in making our environment smoke-free! Maybe a generation from now, our children will have accessible stairs and walking paths everywhere—as well as daily, active recess for everyone of all ages.

RESTORE THAT RECESS FEELING

Remember that feeling as a child when the school bell rang and freed you to rush out onto the playground, where you could jump and run and swing to your heart's content? Somewhere on the journey toward adulthood, many of us lost this joy of movement. In fact, a main reason some people don't exercise is that they consider it hard, painful "work"—an unpleasant chore that's "good for them." Say the word *exercise,* and you'll often see people cringe guiltily, shrugging that they just don't have time. Yet Americans watch an average of 4 hours of TV a day. So you know that lack of time is an excuse—because people make time to do things they enjoy.

A central, and often unrecognized, problem here is attitude: If you consider exercise something distasteful but healthy that you should force yourself to endure (like tasteless tofu or nasty medicine), you probably won't stick with an exercise routine.

So the second major attitude adjustment is to think of exercise as fun. That's easier to do if you find an activity you enjoy. Think back to some activities you loved as a child—dancing, swimming, riding your bike—and try them again. Stop worrying if you're "good enough" at the activity and give yourself permission to simply move your body in the spirit of play. In fact, stop viewing your exercise as a workout and start thinking of it as playtime—a welcome recess that frees your body from the confines of its chair. Now, *there's* a word filled with positive associations and joy! Just remember that your daily "recess" isn't simply one more chore to get crossed off your list, but an exhilarating opportunity to move purposefully, breathe deeply, and relieve stress.

ATTITUDE ADJUSTMENT #2:

Put yourself in recess mode and think of exercise as fun.

REPLACE NEGATIVITY WITH THANKS

One reason many of us have lost the joy of motion relates to negative associations linked to exercise. People who lack athletic prowess may still feel the sting of being picked last for a team or being ridiculed by the Gym Teacher from Hell. And even those who are athletically gifted may mistakenly feel that they're not good enough. For some driven athletes, exercise may be a reminder of stressful competitions where they "only" came in second or third. In our "winning is everything" culture, some people have evolved the sad attitude that if they can't come in first, they shouldn't play at all.

Negative attitudes also may be linked to a dissatisfaction with our bodies and a tendency to be self-critical. Even healthy, fit women tend to find fault with certain body parts—frequently the thighs, belly, butt, and breasts. Since being self-critical can dampen the joy of motion, the third major attitude adjustment is to replace negativity with gratitude. Any time you hear yourself mentally "trash-talking" yourself, *stop* and take a deep breath. Then find something to be grateful for concerning that same body part or attribute.

For example, instead of always thinking, "My thighs are too fat," be thankful that you have two strong legs you can walk on. Your perception defines your reality. If you have a critical attitude that always finds flaws, you'll never be satisfied. So instead of constantly looking for what's wrong in every situation, adjust your attitude and start looking for what's right. Hold your head up, smile, and project a healthy, confident attitude. That's what other people will see—and that's how you'll feel.

An added bonus is that liking your body can more than double your chances of getting slimmer. Researchers at Stanford University School of Medicine found that people who started a weight-loss program feeling happiest with their bodies were more than twice as likely to lose weight as their counterparts who were least satisfied with their bodies.

ATTITUDE ADJUSTMENT #3:

Replace negativity with gratitude.

"CAN'T" IS A FOUR-LETTER WORD

In the martial arts studio—or *dojo*—where my colleague Carol Krucoff earned her black belt, the word *can't* was prohibited. New students who used the word—for example, to say, "I can't move that fast" or "I can't do that movement"—were politely told this attitude was unacceptable. Instead, they were instructed to rephrase their comment by eliminating the word *can't*: "I'm having a problem moving that fast" or "I'm finding it difficult to do that movement."

While the difference may seem subtle, in reality it's quite profound. Everyone wants to be right—so when you say, "I can't," you're sending yourself a powerful message that whatever you're attempting is impossible. Simply put, if you say, "I can't," you won't.

In contrast, if you're having a problem doing something or finding it difficult to do something, that's fixable. With time, practice, and patience, you can solve your problem, overcome that difficulty, and succeed. Eliminating the word *can't* is a powerful attitude adjustment that is essential for success.

Carol learned the importance of eliminating doubts when she had to break concrete blocks for her black-belt test back in 1997. At 5 feet 4 inches and 115 pounds—and raised in a generation when ladies didn't sweat, let alone make fists—Carol was 43 years old and terrified that she'd break her ankle rather than the concrete block. So despite years of training and the confidence of her instructor, those doubts and fears caused her to slam her heel painfully into the block rather than break it on her first few attempts.

It was only after serious soul-searching—where she faced her fears and made the commitment to success—that she was able to kick *through* the concrete. Carol broke five 1½-inch-thick concrete blocks with five different kinds of kicks to earn her black belt. And she discovered that the only difference between smashing her heel against the block and sailing her heel right through it was attitude: the elimination of doubts and fears and the total mental commitment to success.

ATTITUDE ADJUSTMENT #4:

Eliminate *can't* from your vocabulary, and you'll find that you can!

Like Carol, you can succeed when you adjust your attitude to focus on success. And soon you'll be looking better and enjoying the benefits of feeling firmer, fitter, and healthier. So up your attitude for even greater benefits that can last a lifetime.

CHAPTER 9

Strength Training: The Firm Up Secret Weapon

Strength training may be the single most important kind of exercise you can do for the way your body looks, feels, and performs right now *and* as you get older. As I mentioned in chapter 1, women in midlife trade up to 1 pound of neglected muscle for up to 2 pounds of fat every year. That loss lowers your metabolic rate—your body's ability to burn calories—which explains why losing weight gets tougher as you get older.

Strength training, more than other types of exercise, helps preserve your precious muscles. Here's how it works: With every squat, curl, and press, you challenge your muscles and create microscopic tears in the tissue. Your body comes to the rescue, filling the gaps with protein and creating new, stronger muscle tissue.

BIG BENEFITS

By replacing lost muscle tissue, not only do you burn more calories–even when you're just sitting around reading or watching TV–you also help prevent a host of diseases that are associated with low muscle mass. Here are just a few of strength training's benefits to your health, appearance, fitness, energy level, and attitude.

- **A flat belly.** Lean muscle helps burn heart disease–triggering abdominal fat. When researchers at the University of Alabama put 26 men and women on a total-body strength-training program for 25 weeks, they found that the women lost a significant amount of dangerous belly fat.
- **Strong bones.** You can start losing bone by your midthirties–a loss that accelerates as you get older, with bone mass plummeting as much as 20 percent in the 5 to 7 years following menopause. Strength training builds bone. In one study, postmenopausal women increased bone density by lifting weights just twice a week for a year.
- **Reduced diabetes risk.** Lean muscle tissue helps your body metabolize blood sugar, or glucose, lessening your risk for diabetes.
- **A healthy heart.** Harvard researchers found that men who strength-trained for 30 minutes or more per week reduced their risk of heart disease by 23 percent. Experts believe women can get significant heart protection, too.
- **Less cellulite.** Reducing lower-body dimples is a matter of replacing lumpy fat with smooth muscle. When renowned researcher and *Prevention* advisor Wayne Westcott, Ph.D., put 16 women, ages 26 to 66, on a strength-training program for 8 weeks, all of them reported having less cellulite at the end of the program. And 70 percent of them reported a *lot* less.
- **Increased energy.** More muscle means everyday tasks are easier, leaving you with more energy at the end of the day to spend on having fun.
- **Protection from free radicals.** Naturally produced unstable oxygen molecules, called free radicals, contribute to everything from wrinkles to heart disease as we age. Strength training may offer protection. When researchers tested 62 people, those who lifted weights three times a week for 6 months showed less evidence of free-radical damage. The group that did no exercise had a 13 percent increase in damage, but the exercising group had increases of only 2 percent.
- **Super confidence.** "Women who lift weights build self-esteem," says exercise physiologist Katherine Coltrin, co-owner of Back Bay Fitness, a health club in Costa Mesa, California. "They stand taller, feel more independent, and exude confidence."

If you like the benefits but are afraid that strength training will make you big and bulky, stop worrying. Women don't have the right hormones to get huge, she says. "The only women I've seen get big, bulging muscles take steroids and lift 4 hours a day." Strength training just puts back the tight, compact muscle you had when you were younger. "Immediately after you lift, you may notice your muscles are bigger, because they're flushed with blood," she notes. "But that effect is temporary."

Q&A STRENGTH TRAINING

If you're new to weight training, you may have a question or two in mind. Here are the answers to a couple of common concerns.

Q. Won't lifting weights make me heavier?

A. If you're already at your ideal weight, you may see the scale's needle inch up slightly when you start strength training. You won't need a bigger pair of jeans, however, because though muscle weighs more than fat, it takes up less space and looks better, too. If you have a few pounds to lose when you start lifting, the first changes you'll be likely to notice will be a smaller waistline and looser clothing. Then, as your new muscle starts burning more calories, those excess fat pounds will come off, and your weight will drop.

Q. Will my muscles be sore every time I lift weights?

A. Forget all that "no pain, no gain" nonsense. Though you will be a little sore when you first start lifting—and anytime you make your workout harder by upping your weights or adding sets—you should never be so sore that it's debilitating, cautions Vincent Perez, P.T., director of sports therapy at the Sports Medicine Center at Columbia-Presbyterian Eastside Hospital in New York City. "Pushing too hard too soon is a common mistake," he says. "Then women get hurt or are sore for days and never lift again. The first couple of times you do a workout, use weights that don't feel too taxing, so your body has a chance to acclimate."

GEAR UP TO GET STRONG

Just as there are a variety of terms for this type of exercise–weight training, resistance training, weight lifting, bodybuilding, pumping iron–there are a variety of ways that you can strength-train. Here are the pros and cons of the most common methods.

DUMBBELLS

These handheld weights range from 2 to 90 pounds. Dumbbells are the focus of the Firm Up Action Plan, but many of the exercises in the program can also be performed using other strength-training equipment.

Pros: Dumbbells are probably the most versatile strength-training equipment. You can use them to strengthen every muscle. They also help train muscles in a full range of motion.

Cons: Women's smaller, sometimes weaker hands can limit the dumbbell weight they can lift. And dumbbells require good coordination to use safely and correctly.

BARBELLS

These are weighted bars to which you can add weight plates for increased resistance.

Pros: Weight is evenly distributed, making it easier to do squats and other lower-body exercises. Since you use both hands, barbells are easier to use than dumbbells for heavy-weight moves.

Cons: Barbells take up more room and are less convenient to store than dumbbells. They also put more stress on wrists and elbows than dumbbells because those joints are locked into one position. Plus, they can be awkward for beginning exercisers to use.

ANKLE WEIGHTS

Ankle weights are weighted bands that strap around your ankles. Many are adjustable to make them lighter or heavier, from 1 to 10 pounds.

Pros: Ankle weights are easy to use. They're good for toning lower-body muscles.

Cons: There are limited uses for ankle weights. They can strain knee and hip joints if used improperly.

BANDS AND TUBING

Elastic rubber bands and tubes (some even with handles) provide resistance as you stretch them.

Pros: They're extremely portable. Bands and tubes are great for toning exercises like leg lifts. And they're good for beginners.

Cons: Bands and tubing don't challenge muscles as well as free weights (barbells and dumbbells). Because they don't provide constant tension, they can make it difficult to maintain proper form throughout exercises.

MACHINES

Exercise machines are made of a stacked-weight-and-cable apparatus, like the Nautilus. They're often found in gyms. Some machines, such as Universal Systems, can be used for a variety of exercises, from biceps curls to leg lifts, while others are used for specific exercises: one machine for chest flies and another for chest presses, for example.

Pros: These machines build good muscle development, especially for beginners. They support your body while isolating the specific muscle being worked.

Cons: Machines are cumbersome and expensive. They limit your range of motion during exercise, which can be uncomfortable or painful. And they're not ideal for balanced, full-body development.

MEDICINE BALLS

These weighted balls range from 1 to 30 pounds.

Pros: Medicine balls make workouts fun. You can use them to train for everyday activities like picking up kids or lifting luggage. They're great for core (ab, back, hip) muscle development.

Cons: They require proper instruction to use safely. You'll need a set of balls for a full-body workout.

STABILITY BALLS

These large, inflated rubber balls are typically used to strengthen stabilizing muscles, especially those of the abs and back. For advanced Firm Up moves using a stability ball, see page 410.

Pros: Stability balls are excellent for developing core muscles and improving balance and coordination.

Cons: The balls can be tricky to get used to. They're not easy to store. And you still need weights for muscle development.

NO EQUIPMENT

You can do strength-training exercises without equipment by using your own body weight for resistance, as in pushups. This is the basis of the core-training component of the Firm Up Action Plan.

Pros: This approach is cheap and always available. These techniques are great for upper-body toning.

Cons: These techniques can be very difficult for beginners. It's hard to fully challenge lower-body muscles.

When setting up your own home gym, you can invest in all or almost none of the above, barring the bare minimum. With three sets of dumbbells, you can do all the exercises you'd ever need. For recommended weights, see page 18.

STRENGTH TRAINING 101

Lift the weight. Lower the weight. Repeat. That's the essence of strength training. But, of course, it's not quite that simple. How much weight you lift, how quickly or slowly you lift, how many sets and repetitions you perform, and even what exercise order you use all affect the outcome of your efforts. Here's a primer for getting started.

LEARN THE LINGO AND LIFT

If you've ever been to a gym class, you've probably heard at least some of these phrases, but you might not be clear on their meanings. Let's begin with a quick refresher. Next time you work out, you'll feel like a pro!

Reps and sets. *Reps* is short for repetitions. Each time you lift and lower, it's considered one repetition. Generally, you perform high reps (12 to 14) for lighter-weight workouts and lower reps (4 to 6) for heavier-weight workouts. A full number of repetitions is called a set. Generally, you do one to three sets of an exercise.

Circuit or linear workout. You can perform a strength-training routine a few ways. The most common way is in a linear fashion, that is, completing all your sets and reps of one exercise before moving on to the next. Or you can perform them in a circuit, completing one set of one exercise, then immediately moving on to the next, repeating the circuit until you have done the desired number of sets for each move. This is the format for the Firm Up Action Plan, because it offers the benefits of performing multiple sets in a minimum amount of time.

Light, medium, or heavy lifting. How much weight you lift depends on the strength of the muscle you're working as well as the desired result. As a rule of thumb, the weight you lift should be heavy enough so that the last repetition in a set is difficult. Using weight that is heavy enough is essential for developing lean muscle tissue. In general, you'll be using heavier weights for large muscle groups, such as your chest, upper back, and legs; lighter weights for small muscles, such as those in your shoulders; and medium weights for midsize muscles, such as those in your arms.

Speed. It's important to lift weights in a controlled manner so that you use your muscles, and not momentum, to do the work. Most experts recommend lifting to a count of 2 or 3, pausing, and then lowering to a count of 3 or 4 for optimum results. You can make any move more challenging, so that you build more muscle and get stronger, by performing the reps more slowly. One advantage: You don't have to lift heavier weights. The disadvantage: It takes longer to do.

Rest and recovery. Rest is the amount of time you take between sets. Recovery is how much time you allow between strength-training bouts. Generally, you should take 30 seconds to a minute of rest before starting the second set of an exercise (you need no rest between exercises in a circuit). Allow 1 day of recovery between strength-training sessions to give your muscles time to repair and rebuild.

Breathing. Though it's tempting to hold your breath while you lift, you'll lift better if you breathe through it. For the best results, exhale during the working phase of an exercise and inhale as you return to the starting position.

Warmup and cooldown. Avoid injury by always warming up your muscles before lifting weights. Do 10 minutes of stationary cycling, light calisthenics, or any activity that will elevate your body temperature. Always stretch your muscles after you've finished working out to cool down.

FIRM TO THE CORE

The hottest trend in strength training today is "core training," performing extensive exercises that strengthen and firm the center-body muscles, especially the abs, obliques (the muscles that run down the sides of your torso), back, and hips.

"Your core is where all your strength comes from," says Troy Weaver, executive director of the YMCA of Central Maryland in Baltimore. Core training is important for stabilizing your back during exercise as well as for performing day-to-day activities like lifting groceries and shoveling snow, he says. "It's crucial for avoiding lower-back problems."

Pilates is one of the most popular forms of core training today. The core training in the Firm Up Action Plan incorporates elements of Pilates, yoga, and traditional calisthenics. But this type of routine doesn't replace traditional weight training for building muscle and bone overall. So for maximum results, the Firm Up Action Plan integrates core training into your strength-training routine by performing the core exercises and weight-lifting moves on alternate days. You'll find the specific 3-week program beginning in chapter 3 on page 23. For sources of equipment, see "Products" in Firm Up Resources on page 418.

I'll bet you're starting to feel stronger just reading about lifting weights. Excellent! Now it's time to get moving–walking, that is. If you're serious about firming up, there *is* a right way to walk. In the next chapter, read about how to do it correctly, choose the gear you need, and get the most from each walk you take.

CHAPTER 10

Walk Off Pounds and Inches

Strolling is better than sitting in front of the TV. But to really slim down, get toned, and boost energy, fitness walking is the answer. By adding a little technique, speed, and distance, you'll see results faster. In this chapter, you'll learn about the walking basics you need to get up to speed.

It all starts with the right equipment–in this case, shoes and socks. Then you need to learn the right way to walk. (And it's probably *not* the way you're walking now.) Once you've corrected your walking form, you'll find out the best ways to walk for maximum calorie burn and muscle toning. And again, you're going to be in for a few surprises. When you have the burn going, I'll show you how to avoid the five biggest problems walkers encounter, how to stay cool in the heat and warm in cold weather, and how to stay safe after dark. Finally, I'll introduce you to the walker's best friend—the treadmill—and tell you how to make sure the treadmill you use is going to be good for your body.

STEPPIN' OUT

One of the great things about walking is that you don't need to invest in a lot of gear—but there is one very important piece of equipment you'll need (well, actually, two): a pair of good walking shoes. They will be your best walking buddies—for 6 months to a year, anyway. So choose them with care.

GET THE RIGHT FIT

There is a shoe out there for everybody—or, more precisely, for every foot. You just need to know a few facts to make sure you get the right fit. Shoes that best support your particular foot type will feel better and last longer, because you'll put less stress on both feet and shoes. You can determine your foot type using the wet test. Here's how to do it.

Dip your bare feet in a pan of water. Then, applying your full weight, step onto concrete, wood, or a piece of brown paper—anywhere you'll leave footprints. Repeat until you get a nice, crisp pattern of your foot. Match your prints to those pictured below. (If yours is somewhere between neutral and flexible, use neutral as your guide. If yours falls between neutral and rigid, choose rigid. If your footprints are different patterns, aim to fit the more flexible one.)

Neutral Print

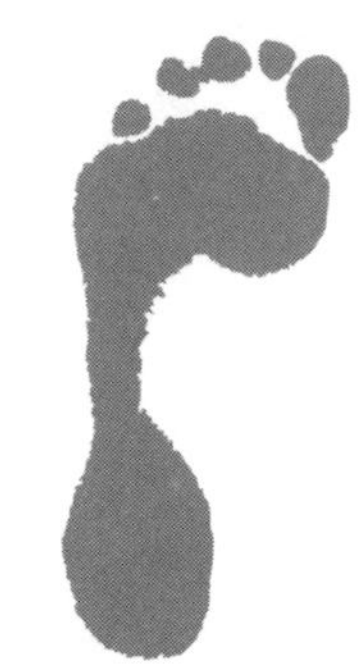

If your footprint is neutral, you'll see about a 1-inch strip of wetness in the midfoot (arch) area.

How you tread: Your foot is well-balanced with normal mobility. (It rolls on the ground, or pronates, almost perfectly.) The foot lengthens and spreads out about half a shoe size when you stand. Your foot absorbs shock well and has good stability.

How to fit: Yours is the easiest foot to fit. You'll do well in soft as well as supportive shoes.

Rigid Print

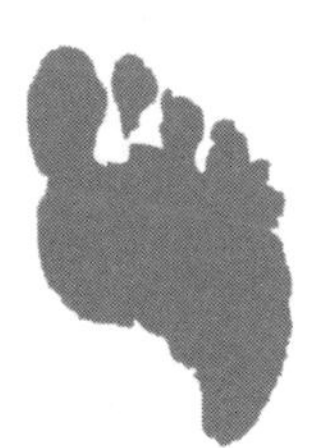

If your footprint is rigid, your arch is so high that you may not see any imprint in the midfoot area.

How you tread: Your foot rolls inward very little during walking (it underpronates) and tends to be stiff, so it doesn't absorb shock very well. (Flexibility allows your foot to become loose to absorb the impact with the ground.)

How to fit: You need soft shoes that are well-cushioned. Go for a roomy upper to accommodate your high arch and instep. A higher heel is good if you have a tight Achilles tendon. Your foot will tend to curve, so look for a shoe that does likewise.

Flexible Print

If your footprint is flexible, your foot will leave the fullest imprint, with the arch area showing the most contact with the paper.

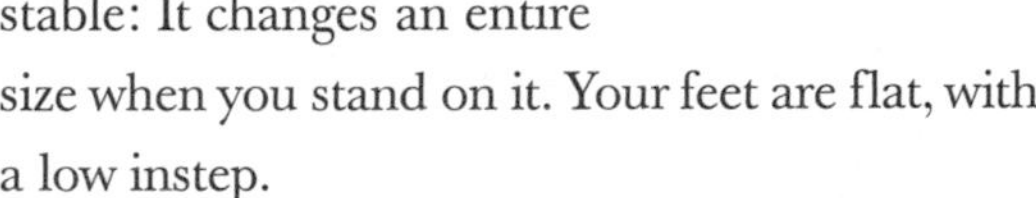

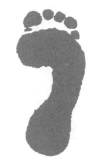

How you tread: Your foot rolls in too much (overpronates) when you walk. Because your foot is very mobile, it absorbs shock well, but it's also unstable: It changes an entire size when you stand on it. Your feet are flat, with a low instep.

How to fit: You need a shoe with "low volume," shorter inside from the laces to the sole. You don't need a ton of cushioning, but you do need good arch support. Also, a lower-heeled shoe will help keep your foot more stable when you walk.

SHOE-SHOPPING CHECKLIST

Now that you know your foot type, it's time to go shopping. Follow these guidelines to help you find the perfect match for your feet.

- Shop at the end of the day, when your feet are largest.
- Go to a store that carries a wide variety of brands and styles so that you have the best chance of finding the right shoes for your feet.
- Tell the salesperson your foot type and how often and how far you'll be walking (or running).
- Wear your walking socks. Some styles are really thick, so you may need to choose a shoe that's a half-size larger than you normally wear, to accommodate them.

Selecting Foot-Friendly Socks

SOCKS ARE THE next most important piece of walking gear. A lousy pair of socks can make a great pair of shoes feel awful. Many stores carry dizzying displays of socks in all brands, colors, sizes, and styles. Some are thick; some are thin. Some support your arch; others pad your bunion. Many footwear manufacturers offer socks bearing the same brand names as their shoes.

As a rule, socks made from synthetic fabrics are best. A little cotton is okay, but all-cotton socks get soggy, lose their shape and softness, and wear through faster. Try a variety of brands and styles until you find one that you really like. Then buy a whole bunch, so you always have a clean pair waiting for you.

- Get your feet measured if possible. As you get older, your feet tend to flatten out, which may affect your shoe size.
- When you try on shoes, make sure there's plenty of room—at least one finger's width—beyond the end of your longest toe (usually the big toe). Measure this space when you're standing up rather than sitting down. Ideally, you should have someone else measure for you. Footwear that's too small can cause all kinds of problems.
- Spend some time in the shoes you are trying on. Walk around the store. If you're in a mall, ask if you can take a few laps around the inside corridors. The shoes should feel great; never buy a pair that you have to break in. In addition, a skilled shoe salesperson should be able to watch you walk and assess whether or not the shoes are giving you enough support.

Q&A WALKING VERSUS RUNNING SHOES

Q. Can I wear running shoes for walking?

A. If you plan to do any running or jogging during your walk, definitely wear running shoes. Running requires far more cushioning and stability for your feet than walking, and running shoes are specifically designed for this.

That doesn't mean you can't wear running shoes if you're just walking. The fit is what counts. Running shoes are usually more readily available than walking shoes, so you have more brands and styles to choose from. On the downside, running shoes tend to have thicker soles than walking shoes. They'll make you taller, but they may also make you more prone to tripping. So be careful!

Walking shoes are specifically designed to help propel you through the heel-to-toe motion of the proper walking technique. While runners land flat-footed, walkers land on their heels. So the heels of walking shoes are often beveled to increase stability. And that stability is equally important when you roll your foot forward and push off with your toe. But if you can't find a walking shoe that fits, by all means, try a running shoe.

WALK THIS WAY

To change your everyday stroll into a pound-shedding stride, you need proper walking form.

"When people start fitness walking for weight loss, they often overstride, taking exaggeratedly large steps to pick up the pace," says former *Prevention* walking editor Maggie Spilner. "That's a mistake. They bounce too much and stress their joints, and it actually slows them down. The farther out your leg is, the more it acts as a break. Short, quick steps, rolling from heel to toe, are safer and allow you to move faster."

You can find your proper stride length with this exercise: Stand with your feet parallel and walking distance (about hip width) apart. Balance on one foot as you raise the opposite knee straight up to waist level. Then, plant the heel of your raised leg straight down. That's your stride length.

Perfect Your Walking Posture

TO CHECK YOUR form, have a friend watch you walk, or walk on a treadmill in front of a mirror. Here are the key points for good walking posture.

- **Stand tall:** Imagine a wire attached to the top of your head, pulling it upward.
- **Head:** Keep your chin up and your ears in line with your shoulders.
- **Eyes:** Look 6 feet in front.
- **Shoulders:** Keep them relaxed and down.
- **Chest:** Imagine that there's a headlight in your breastbone—shine it forward, not down on the ground.
- **Arms:** Relax and swing from the shoulders. Pump your arms forward and back; don't "chicken-wing" them across your body.
- **Elbows:** Bend at 85- to 90-degree angles.
- **Hands:** Cup them loosely. Pump forward, not across your body.
- **Abdominals:** Keep them firm.
- **Back:** Stand straight; don't arch.
- **Pelvis:** Tuck slightly by pulling your belly button back toward your spine.
- **Hips:** Swivel them.
- **Knees:** Keep them soft and pointing forward.
- **Feet:** Point your toes forward, keeping your feet parallel to each other.
- **Front foot:** Plant your heel first; don't let your foot fall inward or outward.
- **Back foot:** Roll forward, pressing into the centerline of your foot; push off with your toes.

QUICK TIP **Wearing a hat, visor, or pair of sunglasses can improve your posture. When the sun is shining brightly, many people tilt their heads forward to avoid the glare, putting extra strain on the neck and upper back. When you wear a hat, visor, or sunglasses, however, you keep your chin up.**

As you walk, roll from heel to toe, pressing into the centerline of your foot, and push off with your toes. This technique automatically incorporates your hips and buttocks, creating a powerful stride that shapes your entire leg, tightens your butt, and trims your waistline.

To make good technique second nature, try these warmup exercises from Suki Munsell, Ph.D., a movement therapist and developer of Dynamic Walking. The Dynamic Walking program is designed to maximize the benefits of walking while minimizing pain and injury. It achieves this through restoring your body's natural, balanced posture. (For more information on the Dynamic Walking system, go to www.dynamicwalking.com.)

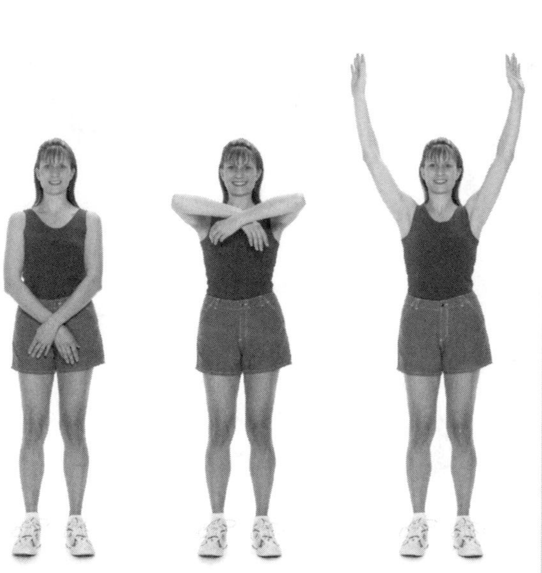

Shirt pull (lengthens your spine to prevent slumping): Cross your arms at the wrists in front of your waist. Now raise your arms as if you're pulling a shirt up and over your head. Grow taller as you reach up. Then lower your arms, letting your shoulders drop into place. Repeat frequently during a walk to help you maintain good posture.

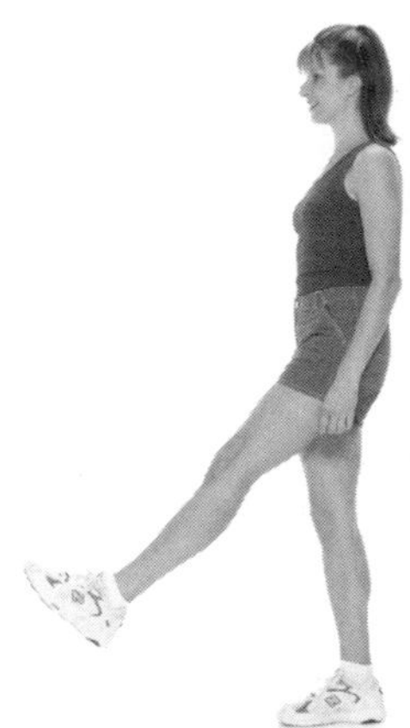

Pendulum swing (keeps your hips lifted so your stride is smooth): While holding on to something for support, balance on your right leg and swing your left leg forward and backward 8 to 10 times without scuffing the ground. Repeat on the other side.

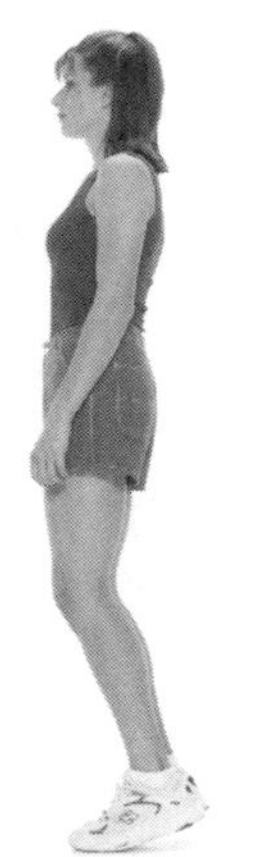

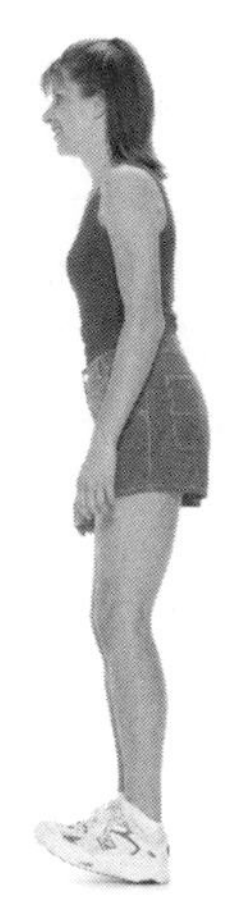

Heel-toe roll (realigns your feet and knees): Stand with your feet parallel, one shoe width apart. With your knees slightly bent, roll from heel to toe 8 to 10 times, rocking back and forth down the center of your feet.

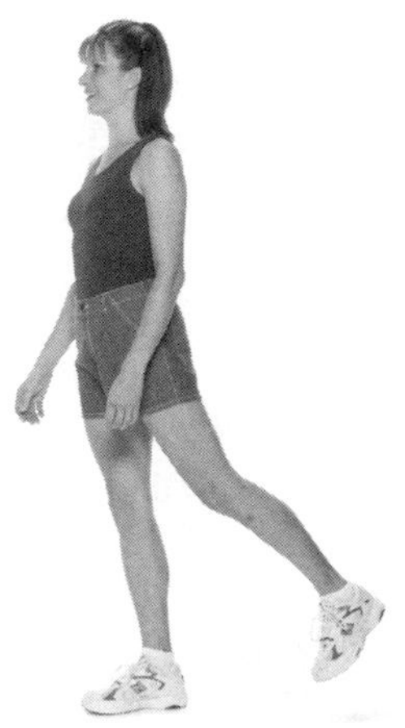

Kick sand (increases push-off power): Standing tall, scrape the ground with one foot as you kick behind you, like a dog digging a hole. Use your whole leg, from the hip to the toes. Don't lean forward too much. Repeat six times on each side.

BURN MORE CALORIES

You'll reap terrific benefits with any walking program. But for faster results, better stamina, firmer muscles, and a greater calorie burn–pick up the pace. Really push it, and you can actually burn more calories walking than jogging–but only if you want to.

Walking at speeds of 5 miles per hour (a 12-minute mile) or faster burns more calories and boosts fitness faster than jogging at the same speed. In fact, every minute you shave off your pace helps. Increasing from a moderate 3½ miles per hour (17-minute mile) to a brisk 4½ miles per hour (13½-minute mile) can shed an extra 10 pounds in a year. Going from 20-minute miles (3 miles per hour) to 15-minute miles (4 miles per hour) could help you lose an extra 7 pounds. (Calculations are based on a 150-pound person walking 1 hour, four times a week.)

The easiest way to gauge your speed without wearing a pedometer–or getting in your car and measuring mileage–is to count the number of steps you walk per minute.

- About 95 steps per minute equals 30 minutes per mile, or 2 miles per hour. This is a leisurely stroll. You'll burn about 3.2 calories a minute.
- About 115 steps per minute equals 20 minutes per mile, or 3 miles per hour. This is a comfortable speed for most people. You'll burn about 4.1 calories a minute.

- About 135 steps per minute equals 15 minutes per mile, or 4 miles per hour. This is considered brisk. It feels challenging. You'll be breathing noticeably faster, but you'll still be able to carry on a simple conversation. You'll burn about 6.4 calories a minute.
- About 155 steps per minute equals 12 minutes per mile, or 5 miles per hour. This is fast. Your breathing will be heavier, and about the only talking you'll feel like doing are one- or two-word responses. At this speed, walking starts to become inefficient from a biomechanical standpoint–it would be easier for your body to break into a jog than to continue walking–which is why you get a greater calorie burn. You'll burn about 8.2 calories a minute.

If you pay attention to your steps, after a while you'll be able to estimate your pace fairly accurately without bothering to count.

BOOSTING THE BURN

One of the best ways to increase your speed is to do it in spurts. Walk at your usual pace and then pick it up for 15, 30, or 60 seconds at a time. Or go faster for the distance from one telephone pole to the next, then ease up and repeat when ready. Take shorter–not longer–steps. Bend your arms at 90-degree angles and swing them forward and back. Focus on pushing off more strongly with your back toes. And go!

You can also up your intensity by adding some elevation to your walk with stairs or hills. From a calorie-burning perspective, 15 minutes of stair- or hill-climbing can burn as many calories as a 30-minute moderately brisk walk. It's also a great way to tone your legs and butt, and a perfect alternative when you're short on time.

Both hill-climbing and stair-climbing burn about 6.8 calories per minute (based on a 150-pound person) if you're going up and down. Stick to going up only–for stair-climbing, take the stairs in a tall building, then go back down on the elevator, or for hill-walking, use a treadmill–and you'll increase to 10.2 calories per minute. One caution: Take it easy on the descents. Going down stairs or down hills can be tough on your knees, so go slow, or better yet skip the down part. Because these are high-intensity activities, start slowly by adding just short bouts.

GREAT GADGETS

You can get more out of your walks by getting your upper body in on the act. Here are two gadgets that can help you burn more calories without having to walk faster.

Q&A HAND WEIGHTS

Q. Will carrying hand weights while I walk increase my calorie burn?

A. It will, but the risk of injury is greater than the few extra calories you'll burn. Swinging extra weight from your arms can cause wrist, elbow, or shoulder injuries such as bursitis. Part of the problem is that when you get tired, you can't put the weights down. So save the hand weights for strength training at home or in the gym.

PowerBelt. This portable device wraps around your waist like a belt. It has two handles that you hold while you walk, swinging your arms back and forth. The handles are attached to cords, which are wound around disks that provide resistance when you pull on the handles. This not only increases your heart rate but also tones the muscles in your shoulders, arms, and back.

Unlike hand weights, the PowerBelt doesn't strain your joints. If your arms get tired, just let go of the handles–they pop right back into place on the belt. Once your arms have rested a bit, just grab the handles and start swinging again.

PowerBelts are available at the Walker's Warehouse. (To order, see the Walker's Warehouse on page 418 of Firm Up Resources.)

Walking poles. These look similar to ski poles, but they have large rubber tips on the bottom. As you plant and press down with the poles, you work your chest, back, abdominal, and arm muscles hundreds of times per mile.

If you have painful knees or achy hips, walking poles can make exercise less painful by transferring force from your legs to the poles and easing the impact on your joints. For example, the average woman walking at 3 miles per hour may experience 190 pounds of force (or 1 to 1½ times her body weight) each time her foot strikes the ground. That could add up to 425,856 pounds every mile! Walking poles could reduce that impact by up to 5 percent, a savings of 6 tons per mile.

Poles are available at sporting goods stores or the Walker's Warehouse, whose contact information is located on page 418 of Firm Up Resources.

AVOID FIVE COMMON PROBLEMS

Although walking is a low-impact sport, injuries and annoying conditions can still arise. Here are five common ones and what you can do to avoid them.

SWOLLEN HANDS

Swelling in your hands is normal. When you swing your arms, blood rushes down into your fingers. It isn't harmful, but it can be uncomfortable, especially if you wear rings. It's a good idea to take off your rings before you go walking.

If the swelling bothers you, try squeezing your hands into fists from time to time while you walk. This helps push blood back from the fingers. Keeping your elbows bent as you swing your arms can also minimize swelling. If that's not enough, try this move: As you walk, reach your left arm to the sky for a few seconds while you tuck your right elbow to your side, bending it to touch your fingers to your right shoulder. Switch sides and repeat, raising your right arm and bending your left. Repeat 5 to 10 times with each arm when needed.

SIDE STITCH

This sudden, stabbing pain in your side results from a spasm of the diaphragm, the muscle that separates your chest and abdomen. It's crying out for oxygen because your expanded lungs and contracted abdomen are blocking normal blood flow. This sounds serious, but it's not.

At the first sign of a side stitch, stop walking. Using three fingers, massage the area where the pain is most severe until you feel relief. Do not hold your breath. As your breathing slows to its normal rate, the pain should subside. Then you can resume your walk. Like any muscle, your diaphragm cramps when it isn't warmed up properly. So remember to start out easily. (For more advice, see page 208.)

SHINSPLINTS

This burning pain in your shins is often the result of doing too much too soon and is especially common among beginners. To avoid shinsplints, increase your distance and pace gradually, and always take time to warm up before doing any speedwork. When you walk, remember to land on the center of your heel (not the outer edges). Replace worn shoes with a new pair that has good arch support and even heels. To strengthen your shins and prevent pain, walk on your heels a few minutes a day.

If you're already in pain, try slowing your pace and stretching your calf muscles. Stand facing a wall with one foot in front of the other. Then with your palms against the wall, lean forward, bending your front knee and keeping your heels flat on the ground. Still in pain? Apply ice for 15 minutes. Be sure to wrap the ice in a towel to protect your skin.

HEEL PAIN

Often, heel pain results from a condition called plantar fasciitis—that's inflammation of the plantar fascia, a sheath of connective tissue that runs along the bottom of the foot. As this tissue becomes overstretched and inflamed, it produces sharp pain, especially first thing in the morning when you get out of bed. (I know, because I've had it.) The pain eases as you walk around, but it can come back, especially if you sit for a long time.

Stretching may help (see plantar fasciitis stretch on page 401). If it doesn't, you may need better walking shoes or special shoe inserts (called orthotics) to keep your ankles from rolling inward (overpronating), which may overstretch and inflame the plantar fascia. If you don't get relief within a week or two, schedule an appointment with a podiatrist.

BLISTERS

A bad case can knock a beginning walker right off her feet. More experienced walkers who step up their workouts or switch to hiking can encounter problems, too. Here's how to keep your feet blister-free.

- When you feel a "hot spot" on your foot, act right away. Take off your shoe and apply moleskin or an adhesive bandage over the affected area.
- Make sure that your shoes fit both feet. Often one foot is larger than the other. The friction created by wearing the wrong-size shoe—whether it's too small or too large—can lead to blisters.
- Wear high-tech socks made from fibers that wick away moisture. Skip the cotton and look for synthetic blends such as CoolMax or Wonderspun.

KEEP YOUR COOL IN THE HEAT

Heat can be dangerous, and some days it may be hotter outside than you think. The combination of humidity and air temperature is known as apparent temperature. And as it rises, so does your risk of heat exhaustion or heatstroke, which can be life-threatening.

Heat-related health problems most often affect people who are older and/or have chronic medical conditions. (If you have any kind of medical condition, you need to ask your doctor whether you should exercise indoors or forgo your workout altogether when the temperature and humidity start soaring.) But even the fittest among us can fall victim to the heat if we overexert ourselves or become dehydrated.

So when the mercury is rising, use "Your Hot-Weather Workout Guide" on page 374 to determine whether to do your walking outside or inside (preferably in air-conditioning).

If you decide that the conditions outside are suitable for walking, you still want to make sure that you're prepared. Here are some of the best ways to keep your cool.

Go early or late. Plan to walk in the early morning or in the evening to avoid the steamiest temperatures. Direct sun can make the temperature feel up to 15°F higher than it really is. For safety tips, see "Be Safe after Dark," on page 376.

Switch shoes. Choose lightweight, light-colored, ventilated walking shoes and socks that wick away sweat. If you have two pairs of shoes, alternate between them every day so that each pair has a chance to dry out completely between uses. This helps you avoid blisters and stinky feet.

Dress lightly. The more skin is exposed, the better sweat can evaporate, and that helps keep you cool.

Lotion up. Remember to wear sunscreen and, strange as it may sound, apply it underneath your shirt, as the garment may not block the sun's harmful ultraviolet rays. For the most protection, put your sunscreen on 15 to 30 minutes before heading out, and reapply every 2 hours if you're out for a very long walk.

Get wet. If it's really hot, or if you don't like wearing tank tops, mist your shirt with a spray bottle of cool water. The dampness acts like air-conditioning when you're out walking.

Wear a hat. A visor protects your face, but your head can still get hot. Instead, choose a hat that's made from a breathable fabric, such as cotton or a cotton-synthetic blend. If you can, soak it in cool water before putting it on.

Drink, drink, drink. Keep a half-full water bottle in the freezer and top it off just before you head out. Take sips regularly while you're walking. Six to 8 ounces of water for every 15 minutes of walking should be enough.

Listen to your body. It will tell you when you can push yourself and when you need to coast. If you develop a headache or become dizzy or weak, stop exercising and head for a cool place. Drink plenty of cool fluids while you're resting.

Your Hot-Weather Workout Guide

TO DETERMINE THE apparent temperature on any given day, find the environmental temperature (that is, the temperature of the outside air) at the top of the chart and the relative humidity on the left-hand side. Then locate the number where the respective column and row meet. That's the apparent temperature.

Relative Humidity	Environmental Temperature (in Fahrenheit)							
	75°	80°	85°	90°	95°	100°	105°	110°
	Apparent Temperature (in Fahrenheit)							
0%	69	73	78	83	87	91	95	99
10%	70	75	80	85	90	95	100	105
20%	72	77	82	87	93	99	105	112
30%	73	78	84	90	96	104	113	123
40%	74	79	86	93	101	110	123	137
50%	75	81	88	96	107	120	135	150
60%	76	82	90	100	114	132	149	
70%	77	85	93	106	124	144		
80%	78	86	97	113	136			
90%	79	88	102	122				
100%	80	91	108					

Once you find the day's apparent temperature, check it against the recommendations below.

- 90°F and below: Head for the great outdoors.
- 91° to 104°F: Proceed with caution.
- 105° to 129°F: Consider indoor options unless you're acclimated to these conditions.
- 130°F and above: Stay indoors.

STAY WARM IN WINTER

For most people, exercising outdoors may be safer in cooler weather than on hot, humid days, because it's easier to regulate your internal temperature. If you get too hot, slow your pace, open your jacket, or take off your hat or gloves. You'll solve the problem instantly.

However, take your workout indoors if there's a risk of frostbite (temperatures around −20°F, including any windchill) or if it's icy. If you have any chronic health problems, such as heart disease, diabetes, or asthma, you need to check with your doctor before you exercise in the cold. She can tell you what precautions to take, if any. Or she may advise you to do your walking indoors.

Go high-tech. Leave that old college sweatshirt in the closet. Instead, treat yourself to some new high-tech synthetic fabrics; they're worth the investment. You'll be warm and dry instead of sweaty and chilled. And you won't be so bundled up that you look like the Abominable Snowman.

Dress in layers. That way, you can adjust your attire as you go, according to the weather and your level of activity. For the innermost layer (the one closest to your skin), choose light garments made from a synthetic fabric such as polypropylene, which wicks away perspiration from your body. That should be topped off with an insulating layer (or two, if it's really cold) for warmth. Look for fleece fabrics such as Polartec. For the outermost layer, or shell, you want a garment that protects you from wind and rain. The fabric should be waterproof, as opposed to water-resistant (which is designed to keep you dry in a light mist). It should also be breathable—meaning that it allows water vapor to escape without actually letting water in—like Gore-Tex. And don't forget a hat and gloves.

Prepare your feet. Often, all you need is a pair of walking shoes and a thick pair of socks. Then as you warm up, your feet warm up, too. Just make sure that your shoes can accommodate your socks, or your feet will get cold from lack of circulation. To keep your feet toasty on bitterly cold days—or for navigating sidewalks that are wet, icy, or slushy—you may want more rugged footwear such as hiking shoes. They have heavy-duty soles that grip better on sloppy or uneven terrain, and they're often waterproof, or at least water-resistant. (To get a pair that fits well, follow the shoe-buying guidelines on page 364.)

Shield your face. First, apply sunscreen and allow it to dry, then add a thick layer of a protective moisturizer, petroleum jelly, or hand cream. Wear a scarf or mask loosely over your nose and mouth to prevent the sting of icy cold air when

QUICK TIP **Most places now have leash laws, so free-roaming dogs are less of a threat to walkers than they once were. But it's smart to be prepared. Protect yourself from loose dogs by tying a sweatshirt around your waist, wearing a fanny pack, carrying an umbrella or walking stick—anything that you can put between you and a dog if one tries to bite you.**

you inhale. This is especially important if you have asthma or heart problems.

Get warm first. Allow at least 10 minutes to warm up. When it's cold outside, your heart and muscles need more time to get ready.

BE SAFE AFTER DARK

Walking alone at night or early in the morning can be risky. It's more difficult for cars to see you, and fewer people are around to deter criminals. But if that's the best time for you to work out, here are some safety tips that will keep you striding confidently.

Don't go alone. I put fliers in 35 mailboxes in my neighborhood to recruit some walking partners for nighttime strolls.

Be visible. Reflective clothing and accessories make it easier for motorists to see you–and being reflective all over is better than having just a few glowing stripes. Reflective clothing is available at sporting goods stores.

Let there be light. Walk in well-lit areas that are free of a lot of bushes and shrubs or other concealing cover.

Play defense. Always watch out for traffic, use sidewalks, pay attention to headlights, and be extra careful around alleys, where vehicles can appear quite unexpectedly.

Walk briskly and with confidence. A confident posture and athletic stride may deter a would-be assailant. Carrying a walking stick may also be a deterrent.

Keep 'em guessing. Don't walk at the same time or along the exact same route every day. Ask your local recreation department for recommendations on safe parks and paths. Or drive to a well-lit, safe-looking neighborhood that you're familiar with.

Walk indoors. Walking at the mall not only is a good way to keep safe–it also keeps you out of weather extremes and storms.

Introduce yourself. Say hello to neighbors and store owners that you see along your route. Chances are they'll watch out for you if you're in the vicinity regularly.

Carry a flashlight. You'll see better, and others will see *you* better.

Arm yourself. Carry some type of safety device, such as an alarm, pepper spray, or both, in case you're attacked. A cell phone is a good idea, too, in case you're injured (which can happen even if you're not attacked) and need to call for help.

TREADMILLS: THE ULTIMATE WALKING GEAR

Your best walking partner may be a treadmill. In one study, women who had a treadmill at home lost twice as much weight as those without one. Rather than skipping your walk if the weather's bad or when it's dark outside, you can hop on a treadmill anytime, even if you have only a few minutes.

A treadmill also takes the guesswork out of working out. You can be accurate on how fast and far you're walking, which allows you to better gauge your calorie burn and track your progress.

Treadmills range in price from $500 to $5,000. Before you buy, put on your sneakers and try out several brands. But skip the nonmotorized ones. Though these machines tend to be cheaper and quieter than motorized models, they are more difficult to use.

To help you start out smoothly and safely, use this step-by-step approach suggested by Mark Bricklin, former editor in chief of *Prevention* magazine and an avid 'miller.

1. Plant your feet on the side rails and grip the handrails. To avoid motor strain, don't step on the belt until the speed reaches about 1 mile per hour (unless your directions tell you otherwise).

2. Keep a light grip on the handrails for a while. Many beginners feel unsteady or disoriented with the belt moving beneath their feet. Once you're comfortable, let your arms swing naturally at your sides.

3. Slowly increase the speed until you're walking at a comfortable, no-hurry pace—as you would at the mall.

4. After a few minutes, with the incline set flat, increase the speed a tad. Keep swinging those arms. You've left the mall, and now you're walking in the park.

5. Position yourself so that the control panel is within easy reach. *Never* let yourself drift backward—some people have been flipped off the back of these machines.

6. Listen to your feet: Are they going *poom, poom, poom*? If so, you're landing flat-footed. That's a no-no. Try landing on your heel and rolling your foot forward.

7. Check where your feet are pointing. If they're aiming outward, try to position them so that they're straight ahead.

8. If you're in front of a mirror, watch your head. If not, have someone else watch and give you feedback. Are you bobbing up and down, like a bicycle with square wheels? If so, your stride is probably too long. Shorten it and aim for a smooth, gliding walk.

9. Make sure that you're not leaning forward from your waist. It only strains your back.

10. Maintain a pace that leaves you feeling invigorated—not panting, aching, or sweating a lot.

11. If your treadmill has an incline function, use it to add oomph to your workout in short bursts—anywhere from 30 seconds to 3 minutes. When walking becomes laborious or you start losing good form, return to a flat position. Or you can slow your pace to adjust to the incline, just as you do when you're walking outdoors.

12. When you're ready to stop, ease up your pace and walk slowly for a few minutes. Then continue to slowly reduce your speed until the belt stops. When you get off, you may feel a little unstable. That's natural. Grab a drink of water and allow yourself a few minutes to regain your "shore legs."

Ready to head for the treadmill right now? (Or the track or the nearest sporting goods store to buy shoes?) Great! But before you go, read the next chapter. It's on stretching. Believe it or not, stretching is one of the most important, but one of the most overlooked, parts of any exercise program. A few good stretches can keep you injury-free and feeling great as you go through the Firm Up Program.

CHAPTER 11

Stretching: The Gentle Way to Feel Good and Look Great

Imagine not being able to bend down to pick up your dropped car keys—or worse, not even being able to turn your head to back out of the garage. It sounds impossible when you're young, but that's the kind of functional loss you could be facing by the time you're a grandmother—*if* you're not careful.

"The average sedentary person will lose 20 to 30 percent of his or her range of motion between ages 30 and 70," says exercise physiologist Katherine Coltrin, co-owner of Back Bay Fitness, a health club in Costa Mesa, California. That's the difference between being able to bend down to tie your shoes and being relegated to a lifetime of slip-ons.

"I've seen people who have worked desk jobs all their lives lose as much as 75 percent of their normal motion by age 60," adds Vincent Perez, P.T., director of sports therapy at the Sports Medicine Center at Columbia-Presbyterian Eastside Hospital in New York City.

WHAT HAPPENS—AND WHY WE NEED TO FIGHT IT

Why the dramatic loss? Like your skin and hair, your body's muscles and connective tissues change over time, explains Marilyn Moffat, P.T., Ph.D., past president of the American Physical Therapy Association. For one thing, your muscles hold less fluid, causing them to become more tough and fibrous. They also have a tendency to shorten and tighten as they lose elasticity. As these tissues grow tighter, it's harder for blood to flow in and deliver nutrients and carry out waste, so calcifications (those hard knots in your back and shoulders) form, further restricting your movement. Making matters worse, your muscle spindles–little sensors that protect your muscles from overstretching–become desensitized, says Katherine Coltrin. "They aren't detecting length and tension the way they once did, which allows your muscles to shorten even further."

The worst part is that loss of mobility may become a self-fulfilling cycle: The more restricted your motion becomes, the more sedentary you're likely to become. "Activity is harder when your muscles are tight, so people will try a new aerobics class or go out dancing, then find that it's difficult and it hurts and never do it again," says Vincent Perez.

On top of how bad poor flexibility makes you feel, it can make you look even worse. The droopy shoulders and hunched back we blame on aging can actually be attributed to short, tight muscles. "Poor flexibility has a tremendous effect on your posture, which in turn leads to back pain, headaches, breathing difficulties, and a host of aches and pains," he adds.

The big lie is that all this is inevitable, says Kevin Steele, Ph.D., vice president of health services at 24 Hour Fitness, a health club in San Ramon, California. "Contrary to what most people believe, our range of motion doesn't have to suffer major deterioration as we age," he says.

Inactivity, more than age, is to blame for the lion's share of our stiffness. "People who exercise regularly take their muscles through their full range of motion almost every day, which helps maintain flexibility," adds Vincent Perez.

Those who don't move much tend to have much greater losses in mobility. No matter what your exercise habits are, if you specifically allocate time to stretch, range of motion can be maintained or in some cases actually improved over time, regardless of your age, says Dr. Steele.

STRETCH ESSENTIALS

There are nearly as many techniques for improving flexibility as there are muscles that need stretching. Though there's more than one "right" way to stretch, experts agree that a consistent routine and proper form are essential to increase your range of motion without risking injury.

Whichever type of stretching you do, you'll notice the benefits right away. Not only will your muscles feel better immediately afterward, you'll also make noticeable improvements in your range of motion in a matter of weeks. In one small study, 10 men and women who performed yoga stretches just twice a week for 8 weeks improved their ability to bend forward by almost 15 percent and their ability to bend backward by a whopping 188 percent. Even stretching just 5 to 10 minutes a day can increase the average person's general range of motion by about 10 percent in 8 to 12 weeks, experts say.

Let's talk about the six most common stretching techniques, from static and ballistic stretching to yoga and tai chi. There is no one best technique for every person, so you should choose the method or methods that work well for you based on your lifestyle and activity level, and that you enjoy most. Read on for the pros and cons of these stretching techniques.

STATIC STRETCHING

This is the flexibility technique most of us know best: slow, controlled stretching, where you reach the end of your range of motion and hold it for a certain amount of time. An example is propping your heel on a step and bending slowly from the hips to stretch the back of your leg.

Pros: Static stretching is superior for improving flexibility and enhancing range of motion. It suppresses the protective "stretch reflex," which causes muscles to tighten if they sense they're being stretched too far. So the muscles gradually adapt to this newly stretched position. Done after exercise, it speeds the delivery of important nutrients into the muscles to promote recovery. It's easy to do; requires minimal, if any, equipment; and can literally be done almost anywhere, anytime. Static stretching is widely recommended by experts and is unlikely to cause injury.

Cons: It takes patience to hold each stretch for the appropriate amount of time–a full 30 seconds–and some people find it boring. Because you're isolating one muscle group at a time, some experts believe it is less effective than techniques more geared to stretching the total body.

BALLISTIC STRETCHING

Once the fitness standard, ballistic stretching is now considered a no-no except among athletes in explosive sports like basketball and tennis. Ballistic stretching involves rapid, uncontrolled bouncing for a short-duration, high-force stretch, such as sitting with your legs straight out in front of you and bobbing your torso up and down toward your knees.

Pros: It may help prevent injury among athletes in high-intensity sports, such as football, by conditioning their muscles to respond to high-speed, ballistic movements.

Cons: Ballistic stretching can actually leave you feeling tighter by overstimulating the muscles' protective stretch reflex and by not allowing

Q&A STRETCHING

Conflicting information has left many people confused about stretching. Here are answers to the most commonly asked questions.

Q. What is the best time of day to stretch?

A. You can stretch practically anytime, anywhere. There are certain times of the day when your body is more receptive to a concentrated stretching routine, however. Stretching after exercise is ideal for increasing flexibility, because your muscles are already warm and supple from your activity. Stretching then also promotes recovery and prevents muscle soreness. Likewise, people tend to be more limber in the afternoon than in the morning, since their muscles are warmed up from the day's activity, so they are more supple and easier to stretch to their fullest extent. If stretching in the morning is your preference, that's okay. Just start slowly with gentle moves to get your circulation flowing.

Q. How often should I stretch?

A. At least 3 to 5 days a week if you want to see results. The more often you can fit it in, the better your benefits. If you have lost significant amounts of flexibility, aim for 10 to 15 minutes every day. Or take a yoga or tai chi class 3 days a week for longer, more structured sessions.

Q. How long do I hold a stretch?

A. Thirty seconds is the optimum length to hold a static stretch for maximum benefits. Experts find that few people actually hold a stretch that long, however. If you don't have the patience for a half-minute hold, try holding it for 10 seconds, releasing for 5 seconds, and repeating the sequence a total of six times. Researchers at the Medical College of Ohio in Toledo found that men and women who held a hamstring stretch six times for 10 seconds had equal improvements in range of motion as those who held the stretch twice for 30 seconds.

Q. How many times should I do each stretch?

A. For the best results, treat stretching as you would strength training, and perform at least two reps of each stretch if you're holding each one for 30 seconds. You'll need to do more reps if you hold your stretches for less time.

Q. Should stretching hurt?

A. Hurt, no. Be slightly uncomfortable, yes. You should stretch until you feel tension in the muscle and hold it at that point. Ideally, as you progress in your stretching regimen, you'll be able to pull the stretch a little farther before feeling tension. If you feel shooting pain or tenderness in a specific spot, that's a sign of injury. You should see a doctor.

Q. Does stretching protect me from injury?

A. Not as much as once thought. Studies show that stretching before exercise provides no injury protection and, in some cases, even seems to contribute to injury. The best way to prevent strains and sprains while you play is by warming up properly. Perform the activity you're preparing for at a low intensity, such as easy volleying to get ready for a tennis match.

the muscles time to adapt to the stretched position. And there's a high potential for injury if the stretches are done improperly.

DYNAMIC STRETCHING

Not to be confused with ballistic stretching, dynamic stretching involves active flexibility exercises that are performed in a controlled manner. The goal is to move multiple muscle groups through an extended range of natural motion. Doing slow windmills with your arms would be one example.

Pros: Provides "functional" flexibility, because the movements mimic everyday motions. Moving multiple muscle groups in unison improves balance and stability.

Cons: Dynamic stretching is slightly more risky than static stretching if not done carefully. And it may not be as effective at increasing overall range of motion as static stretching.

PNF STRETCHING

Proprioceptive neuromuscular facilitation (PNF) stretching is as complex as it sounds. Developed by doctors and physical therapists for use in rehab, PNF stretching is designed to stimulate special nerve endings in the muscles, tendons, and joints known as proprioceptors. These sensors detect changes in muscle tension during activity. Through a series of muscle contractions and stretches (usually with the assistance of an expert), PNF stretching is designed to provide a deep, effective stretch.

Pros: PNF appears to provide greater gains in mobility than any other stretching technique.

Cons: PNF is too difficult to do without a trained professional's assistance. (To find one, call a physical therapy office in your area.) Some people find it more uncomfortable than static stretching.

YOGA

Yoga is thousands of years old but is only recently being appreciated in the Western world as a way to improve flexibility and enhance mobility. The most widely practiced forms of yoga consist of moving through and holding a series of postures that strengthen and stretch muscles and connective tissues. The poses include a wide range of motions such as rotation, forward, backward, and diagonal movements.

Pros: This discipline provides a complete, full-body stretching routine and helps strengthen muscles and relieve stress. It's more interesting than static stretching, and you can choose from many different varieties.

QUICK TIP **The Firm Up Program incorporates both static and dynamic stretching. But no matter which technique you use, don't make this common mistake: I often see people holding their breath when they're stretching. This can make stretching uncomfortable and keep you from enjoying the relaxation it can offer. If you find yourself doing this, try counting aloud as you hold a stretch. You can't talk and hold your breath at the same time!**

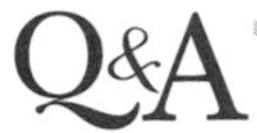

FLEXIBILITY

One glance at the yoga gurus twisted like braided pretzels will tell you that flexibility is not the same for everyone. Here's the lowdown on being limber.

Q. What determines how flexible I am?

A. Lots of factors affect your general flexibility. Women tend to be much more flexible than men (perhaps to make childbirth easier). Children have more elastic connective tissue, so they are more flexible than adults. If you've had an injury to a joint, that can decrease your range of motion or flexibility. There's also genetics. Some people are simply born with greater flexibility than others. But everyone can improve.

Q. How much can I improve my flexibility?

A. A minimum amount of stretching, such as 10 minutes a day, can increase flexibility about 10 percent in 8 to 12 weeks. More concerted efforts, such as regular participation in yoga or structured stretching routines, can produce more dramatic results.

Q. Do strong muscles make you less flexible?

A. Well-toned muscles actually enhance flexibility, since strong muscles mean you're actively using your body in ways that promote circulation and maintain your range of motion. Many people think that overdeveloping muscles through extreme bodybuilding can hinder flexibility, but studies show that U.S. Olympic weight lifters rank a close second to gymnasts in joint range-of-motion tests.

Q. What does being double-jointed mean?

A. *Double-jointed* is a colloquial term for having unusually flexible joints that can bend abnormally far. Unusual flexibility in a finger or a certain joint is common. Some people have extreme flexibility throughout their bodies, which allows them to contort into strange positions, such as bending over backward and touching head to butt. That's obviously not something everyone can achieve!

Cons: Yoga is more time-consuming than static stretching. It can be challenging to practice on your own without learning proper technique in a class or with professional guidance.

TAI CHI

This ancient martial-arts-based discipline uses slow, gentle, deliberate movements to improve balance, flexibility, stamina, and coordination. The fluid movements take the body through a full range of motion.

Pros: Tai chi increases circulation, which may stimulate the repair of damaged joints. Studies show that it helps reduce the pain of arthritis and improves balance. It also relieves tension.

Cons: It's difficult to practice tai chi without professional instruction. It's also more time-consuming than static stretching.

CHAPTER 12

Keep Your Motivation Strong

Just as having the right attitude is essential to success, it's important to keep yourself motivated. Knowing how to stick with the program when times get tough can help you avoid being one of the 50 percent of people who begin an exercise program and drop out within the first 6 months.

"Motivation ebbs and flows like the tides," explains Howard Rankin, Ph.D., clinical psychologist for the weight-loss program Take Off Pounds Sensibly (TOPS). "You go into your closet and find that you can't fit into your favorite pants. At that moment, you're highly motivated. But then you pull on another pair and go about your day, and motivation fades. That cycle is very common."

But it doesn't have to be that way. By employing some strategies to keep exercise meaningful—and most of all, enjoyable—you can stay motivated to stick with your healthy lifestyle changes not only to meet your short-term goals but also to stay fit and healthy for a lifetime.

THE BIG WHY

Experts agree that the most important aspect of staying motivated is understanding *why* you're working out in the first place. "It is critical to understand the why of what you're doing. If you're not really, truly clear on why being more physically active is important to you, then your chair—or your pillow—will win the battle," says personal trainer Charles Stuart Platkin, author of *Breaking the Pattern* and founder of the Nutricise Weight Loss Program. "Just telling yourself, 'I have to go work out,' is not a compelling reason to leave a warm bed. Why is it important to you? What is your reward?"

Too often people answer, "I want to lose weight" or "I want to look better." "But those are superficial things, not the deep motivation," says Dr. Rankin. "*Why* do you want to lose weight? To have more energy, so you can be a better mom? To lower your blood pressure, so you can live to see your grandkids grow up? There's always something more important lurking below the surface. That's the true motivation."

THREE KEYS TO BOOSTING YOUR MOTIVATION

Once you've determined your big why, the key is to always be aware of it, says Dr. Rankin. "Otherwise, motivation will fade." Here are some strategies to help you stay motivated.

Create a "life preserver." "I tell clients to create a detailed visual image of their future selves, after they've reached their goal. It's what I call a 'life preserver,'" says Charles Platkin. "Create a whole screenplay. What are you wearing? How do you feel? Imagine yourself bumping into an old flame. Replaying this scene in your head will help you through the rough times when you'd rather reach for a Hershey bar than a barbell."

Put a positive spin on it. Many big whys are rooted in fear, says Dr. Rankin. "People are often motivated to exercise and eat right because they want to avoid bad things like heart attacks." That's a perfectly good reason. But since it's human nature to avoid thinking of scary things, it may not be the best motivation. "Try to put a positive spin on it, like 'I want to have a strong, healthy heart.'"

Carry a concrete reminder. With the hectic pace and full schedules of daily life, it's easy for your motivation—no matter how compelling—to slip from your consciousness, says Dr. Rankin. To keep it in focus on a daily basis, write a slogan that captures your motivation, like "I want to be a healthy role model for my daughter." Then post it somewhere prominent, like on your bathroom mirror or on the refrigerator. Or find a symbolic image that prompts your memory.

Real-Life Success Story

My biggest inspiration for exercising is seeing the look on people's faces when I tell them I have six children, ages 6 to 16," says Lynn Schultz, of Catonsville, Maryland, who at 5 feet 1 and a fit 102 pounds, typically gets stares of disbelief.

An exerciser in college, Lynn stopped working out when she became pregnant with her first child. "I gained 50 pounds and hated how I felt," she recalls. "So I started exercising again, lost the weight, and decided to make daily workouts a priority in my life."

Every morning, Lynn heads down to her basement playroom and does about 30 minutes of aerobics, either with a workout video or on her elliptical trainer. Every other day, she adds about 20 minutes of strength training, using dumbbells. "When the kids were younger, I'd set them up with markers and crayons to keep them busy," she notes.

In addition to liking how exercise makes her look and feel, Lynn works out to set a good example for her kids. "I want them to understand how important exercise is to good health."

You might wear a heart-shaped pendant if your goal is a strong, healthy heart. When your motivation is right in front of your face, it's harder to forget.

WHO CARES?

Sure, your own health (or fitting into those size 8 jeans) is reason enough to hit the dumbbells, but no woman is an island, and your enthusiasm can fade quickly when you're going it alone. To keep your motivation high, you need the support of those around you—and to be accountable to someone, says certified trainer and sports medicine expert Gillian Hood-Gabrielson, who applies her motivational strategies as a master Fitness by Phone coach.

"When you know someone's checking in on you or depending on you, that alone is enough to boost your motivation when you feel like throwing in the towel," she says.

We also care what others think of us, which can be a powerful motivator, adds Dr. Rankin. "Even the most independent people care how others perceive them." Here's how to use that social dependence to your advantage.

Rally the troops. It's no surprise that support from others can help you stick with an exercise program. But now scientists say *where* that support comes from may be equally important. In a study of more than 900 men and women, researchers at Ohio State University in Columbus found that men were more likely to stay active if they had support from friends, and women exercised more when their families encouraged them. "Having your husband and kids helping you out, asking how your routine is going, and especially exercising with you can be a big help," says lead researcher Lorraine Silver Wallace, Ph.D., now assistant professor at the University of Texas at Tyler.

Partner up. The benefits of enlisting a buddy to work out with you are well-documented. Exercise is more fun—and it's almost impossible to just hit snooze and roll over if you know someone is waiting for you. But pick your buddy wisely, advises Gillian Hood-Gabrielson. "It can be counterproductive to pair up with a good friend, especially if you're both just starting out, because it can be too easy to talk each other out of exercising," she says. "Be sure it's someone you will feel accountable to."

Go pro. Even if you already have a program, hiring a personal trainer can boost your confidence and provide a sense of accountability whether you're just starting out or have been exercising for years. A fitness professional can ensure that you're doing the moves correctly and may push you a little harder than you might otherwise work. Even a few sessions can make a difference.

To find certified trainers in your area, contact any of these organizations: American College of Sports Medicine, (317) 637-9200, www.acsm.org; American Council on Exercise, (800) 825-3636, www.acefitness.org; IDEA Health and Fitness Association, (800) 999-4332, www.ideafit.com; and the National Strength and Conditioning Association, (800) 815-6826, www.nsca-lift.org.

Get Firm Faster

DON'T FEEL LIKE exercising today? Practice the rule of 10. Set your watch alarm or minute timer for 10 minutes at the start of your walk or aerobics video. If you want to quit after 10 minutes, go ahead. Chances are, you'll feel so good that you'll keep going.

ENJOY YOURSELF

Men and women with an alphabet soup of degrees behind their names are forever researching what keeps human beings motivated. The one point on which they all agree is that if you enjoy what you're doing and find it rewarding, you'll ultimately stay motivated to do it for the sake of doing it, without a whole lot of prodding.

"It's critical to enjoy exercise if you're going to stick with it," says Charles Platkin. That may sound like bad news if you're not much of an exercise lover. But the good news is that there are plenty of ways, from the type of music you play to the people you work out with, to make exercise a pleasant experience you look forward to, he says. Here are six great tricks to add enjoyment to *your* exercise routine.

Get organized. Charities and clubs host thousands of organized walking, running, and bicycling events each year. Sign up for a 5-K to benefit your favorite charity. It'll give you something to train for. And the festive, social atmosphere surrounding these events makes them

Get In the Mood to Move

NO MATTER HOW much you love your exercise routine, it can be hard to get yourself out the door when there's been another round of layoffs at work or your mother's ill. "Lots of people skip working out when their mood isn't ideal, because they don't have the mental energy to switch gears," says mental health and exercise expert Jack Raglin, Ph.D., of Indiana University in Bloomington. "But the trick lies in finding the right workout to match the mood you're in." For example, some workouts have a calming effect, while others are stimulating. Here's what Dr. Raglin recommends.

Got the blues? "Studies have shown that even mild exercise—at about 40 percent of your max heart rate—can lift your mood," says Dr. Raglin. "So if you're not up for the usual high-energy stuff, do some leisure activity you enjoy, such as digging in your garden or walking in a park. View it as mental recreation, not exercise."

Is your temper flaring? "As tempting as it may be, skip the kickboxing," he advises. "You can't punch away anger. Instead, do something that involves your mind and keeps you from ruminating on what has you angry. Play racquetball or take an aerobics class you've never tried. Learning new moves will free your mind from what's been upsetting you."

Feeling bored? "Being around people is a quick and easy way to beat boredom. Playing a sport with them is even better," says Dr. Raglin. "Try some tennis or golf. Get together with a group that walks or goes for bike rides on a regular basis. Being outside with other people is invigorating and engages your mind."

Are you stressed-out? "When your brain is overwhelmed and anxious, you need to turn to a mindless activity to settle it down. Something repetitive, such as swimming or walking on a treadmill, requires little mental input and is most effective at reducing feelings of stress and anxiety and increasing calmness," he says.

Walking on sunshine? A happy mood can sideline a workout as easily as a sad one, especially if you feel too "up" to do your same old routine. "Take advantage of good moods to go out and challenge yourself. See if you can run 1 more mile than usual or add another set to your weight routine. Use that energy to feel even better," advises Dr. Raglin.

If you don't have the time or opportunity to do something new, alter your usual workout, such as walking in a different neighborhood or trying some new strength-training moves.

Let your mood be your guide.

positively addictive. To find an event in your area, check out the Web site www.active.com.

Make it a game. Pedometers, which track the steps you take each day, make getting more exercise easy and fun and act as a motivational tool by providing immediate feedback. "Most people are shocked to realize that they're sitting 12 to 14 hours a day and taking an average of only 2,000 to 3,000 steps (about 1 to 1½ miles)," says Andrea Dunn, Ph.D., of the Cooper Institute for Aerobics Research in Dallas. "The pedometer makes it a game to get you moving." Your goal should be 10,000 or more steps a day, which has been shown to boost your health and promote weight loss. And it really isn't difficult to get there. Try walking a few steps more each day. It also provides instant gratification by showing you that taking the stairs or parking in the farthest space really does add up. Pedometers are available at most sporting goods stores, or go online to www.walkerswarehouse.com.

Play outside. Doing your cardio in the beautiful outdoors may inspire you to work harder without even realizing it. A recent study of 15 runners found that they ran faster for a 3-mile-plus run outside than when they ran the same mileage indoors on a treadmill, even though their average heart rate was unchanged. That means they were running faster without working harder, which makes increasing the mileage easier.

Jazz it up. "Music distracts you from thinking about how hard you're working. It also boosts your mood, making you more likely to keep going," according to Robert T. Herdegen, Ph.D., Elliott professor of psychology at Hampden-Sydney College in Virginia. In his study, 12 college students "traveled" 11 percent farther on exercise bikes while listening to music than when they did their pedaling in silence. But just remember to keep the headphones off when you need to hear what's going on in your surroundings to stay safe.

Find active friends. When you're making healthful changes in your life, it's important to be selective about your social circles. "If you hang out with people who are averse to exercise and critical of eating healthfully, they will squelch your motivation," says Dr. Rankin. "You don't have to swear off your old friends, but you'd be wise to find some enthusiastic exercisers to socialize with as well."

Think, "Yes, I can." Insulting yourself (saying, for example, "I'm clumsy" or "I'm terrible at . . . "), as many new exercisers do, won't get you motivated to keep exercising, says exercise psychologist Judy Van Raalte, Ph.D., of the Center for Performance Enhancement and Applied Research at Springfield College in Massachusetts. "The more negative talk people use, the worse they perform." Instead, think, "I'm strong. I'm able. I can do this." It really helps.

PART 5

FIRM UP AND BEYOND

CHAPTER 13

The Stay Firm Plan

You did it! You've completed *Prevention*'s Firm Up in 3 Weeks Program. So now what do you do? That depends on your goals.

If you want to lose more inches, get firmer, or drop more pounds, then repeat the 3-week program. You can either repeat the same level workout you just did or move up to the next level if you're ready for a new challenge. As long as your body continues to respond to a particular level, you can keep doing that one. At the first signs of a plateau–for example, being unable to increase the amount of weight you're lifting, seeing no new definition or firming, or not losing any more pounds or inches–move to the next level. Your body needs a new challenge. If you start with Level 1 and progress through all the levels, you could theoretically have a 9-week program (or continue even longer).

If you're happy with your body and just want to maintain your new figure, you can move on to our Stay Firm Plan. Pick a walking workout level and a strength-training level that you're comfortable with and follow this routine.

- Easy walk–2 days a week
- Interval walk–2 days a week
- Basic weight workout–2 days a week
- Core training–1 day a week

WORKING IT OUT

At the right are some sample workout schedules. There's one if you prefer exercising a little bit every day, and another if you prefer fewer but longer workouts.

HELP WHEN IT HURTS

When life gets really crazy–a huge project at work, a spouse away on business, or a sick relative who needs help–it's all too easy to let exercise and eating right get squeezed out. But even if you can't keep up your full exercise routine during a "crazy time," squeeze in a little time to lift weights, at the very least. When 30 women were put on a 12-month strength-training program with no aerobic requirement and no diet, twice-weekly weight workouts alone were enough to prevent fat gain. And not seeing the needle on the scale go up will make

DAILY WORKOUT SCHEDULE

	Aerobic	Strength
Sunday	Easy walk	–
Monday	–	Basic weights
Tuesday	Interval walk	–
Wednesday	–	Core training
Thursday	Easy walk	–
Friday	–	Basic weights
Saturday	Interval walk	–

4-DAY WORKOUT SCHEDULE

	Aerobic	Strength
Sunday	Easy walk	Basic weights
Monday	–	–
Tuesday	Interval walk	Core training
Wednesday	–	–
Thursday	Easy walk	Basic weights
Friday	–	–
Saturday	Interval walk	–

it easier for you to get back on track when life settles down.

If you *do* notice your clothes getting tighter, add in a few more workouts or go back to the 3-week Firm Up Action Plan. And don't forget to check your eating habits. Many times, you unconsciously start eating more when you've reached your goal. You've worked really hard to get to where you are. Don't throw in the towel now! According to one study, successful dieters say that it gets easier to maintain their new figures over time.

In the next chapter, I'll share some secrets to help you maintain your success so that you can stay firm forever. And then I'll give you some surefire exercises to take your firmness to the next level. Let's go!

FIRM UP TIPS

MYTH BUSTER	ENERGY BOOSTER
Before-bed workouts won't disrupt your sleep if you don't have sleep problems. In fact, they may help you fall asleep faster. When 10 nonexercisers worked out at different times of the day (7:40 to 8:40 A.M., 4:30 to 5:30 P.M., and 8:30 to 9:30 P.M.), they fell asleep two to three times faster when they exercised later in the evening than when they worked out at the other times, according to a Japanese study. Participants also reported that they slept better after their evening workout.	*Stop doing and just be. "Too often when we're tired, we reach for something, such as food or coffee, to cover it up," says Judith Hanson Lasater, Ph.D., a San Francisco physical therapist and yoga instructor who holds a doctorate in East-West psychology. "But what we really need at times like that is to give in to the fatigue so that we can release it." Lie on your back—with your legs resting up on a wall if you'd like—and relax all of your muscles, letting the weight of your body melt into the floor. Take deep abdominal breaths and totally give yourself over to the experience of letting go for 5 to 10 minutes.*

CHAPTER 14

Stay Firm Forever

Want to stay firm? You've worked so hard to achieve a great-looking, healthy body–don't let all your efforts go down the drain now. While you don't have to be as vigilant to stay in shape as you were to get in shape, you can't just slack off and sit around, watch TV, and overeat either. Your biggest challenge will be steering clear of common obstacles that can sabotage all your hard work. The sad fact is that half the people who start a new exercise program drop out in 6 months. To make sure *you* don't become one of those unfortunate statistics, here's a guide to common pitfalls–such as slipups, plateaus, injuries, and boredom–and how to avoid them.

SLIP BUT DON'T FALL

In a moment of weakness, you gorge on nachos or devour a huge slice of cheesecake. Or your child comes down with the flu, and you can't get out to walk all week. If you're like many people, these types of setbacks can prompt you to throw in the towel.

But the reality is that temptations and responsibilities inevitably will lead to some lapses—that's a normal part of shaping up. Fortunately, diet and exercise slipups don't have to become weight-loss disasters. It's what you do *afterward* that determines how quickly you'll recover and get back on track.

> ***QUICK TIP*** **The next time you slip, skip the guilt, enjoy your time off, and then get back on your program.**

"It's not the breaks that hurt weight-loss efforts," explains Rena Wing, Ph.D., of Brown University School of Medicine in Providence, Rhode Island, who has studied diet and exercise lapses. "It's the negative reactions to the breaks—and the subsequent downward spiraling."

SMART STRATEGIES TO GET BACK ON TRACK

Here are five strategies to help you rebound from an exercise or diet disaster.

1. Find the reason behind your slipup. Ask yourself what that pepperoni pizza or hot fudge sundae represented. If it was comfort food because you were feeling overwhelmed at work, talk out your frustration with someone instead. And if you back up a step before the episode occurred, and then keep going back step by step, the situation that caused you to feel overwhelmed may emerge. For example:

- You ate the pizza because you were frustrated and angry.
- You were frustrated and angry because you had to stay late at work and miss your exercise class.
- You had to stay late because your boss overwhelmed you with requests.
- You let yourself get overwhelmed because you didn't want to say no—even though you were doing as much as possible.

Once you've thought it through, you can discuss your responsibilities and career goals with your boss—not with the pizza.

2. Become a matter-of-degree thinker. Unlike a rigid all-or-nothing thinker, who considers any slipup a failure that makes it pointless to continue eating right and exercising, a matter-of-degree thinker assesses the damage and compensates. Here's how it works: If a this type of thinker eats a small plate of nachos at a party, she'll quantify it by attaching a number, such as 200 calories. She then accommodates it by cutting back on her drinks for the evening or walking an extra 20 minutes over the next 2 days. Or, if the slip is skipping her regular evening walk for a week, she'll fit in a few extra morning or lunchtime strolls the following week.

3. Nip a small weight gain in the bud. To help you stay on track, watch your weight. By weighing yourself regularly (once or twice a week at the same time of day is generally enough), you can correct any slacking off. Research from the National Weight Control Registry shows that 75 percent of successful weight-loss maintainers weigh themselves at least once a week. Don't get upset by natural fluctuations of a pound or so. But if you see the numbers steadily going up, it's time to get serious. Other ways to monitor yourself: Record your eating and exercise habits in a food diary or exercise log, try on your jeans (you know when they're getting tight), or check your mirror to see if anything jiggles that nature didn't intend.

4. Plan for future slips. In a world filled with Krispy Kreme doughnuts and all-you-can-eat buffets, it's essential to have a plan for dealing with situations that have been a problem in the past. "It's not about staying on a diet or constant denial," says Howard J. Rankin, Ph.D., author of *Inspired to Lose*. "It's about developing reasonable alternatives that you can live with." For example, if you know your favorite éclairs are served at Monday-morning staff meetings, plan to cut one in half, enjoy it, and let that be your treat for the day—or several days, depending on your progress and goals.

QUICK TIP Give it a rest. Allow yourself permission to skip a day now and then. "It's okay to think 6 instead of 7 days a week," says Franca Alphin, R.D., of the Duke Diet and Fitness Center in Durham, North Carolina. "Just knowing you can take a break is motivating."

5. Cut yourself some slack. Rather than beating yourself up and giving up after a lapse, relax. Recognize that it's only one day, and it won't really matter in the long run as long as you get back to your healthy eating and exercise program—quickly.

PUSH PAST A PLATEAU

One of the most dangerous exercise drop-out zones is the dreaded "plateau"—where you feel like you're on a hamster wheel, thinking you're doing everything right but getting nowhere.

Plateaus can be particularly frustrating for novice exercisers, who become hooked on the dramatic changes generally experienced during the first 6 weeks to 3 months of a new exercise program. But the truth is, once your body gets accustomed to your routine, you'll see diminishing returns for the time and muscle spent.

That's because humans improve physically by the overload principle, which means your body adapts to a new stimulus by getting stronger. Over time, however, your body becomes efficient at doing that activity. So when the stimulus is no longer new, improvements level off.

REENERGIZE YOUR PROGRAM

Since most people adapt to an exercise routine in about 6 weeks, that's a good time to change your workout. But you don't have to make drastic alterations to push past a plateau. Something as simple as walking a different route or changing the order of your strength-training circuit can help throw your body a curve that will reignite your progress.

Here are three basic ways to reenergize your program.

1. Try a new activity. Walking is the primary aerobic activity for the Firm Up Action Plan, but that doesn't mean you can't try something new. And when you hit a plateau, it is often a signal that you *need* to mix things up. Alternate walking with something new, such as inline skating, cycling, or salsa dancing. This technique of alternating activities is known as cross-training. Working different muscle groups in different ways can help you achieve better results and more well-rounded fitness while reducing your risk of injury and boredom.

2. Stick with the basics, but do them in different ways. Find a hilly route to walk or add some speed walks or long walks from the Firm Up Action Plan back into your routine. For strength training, put some high-rep or heavy-weight workouts back into your schedule.

3. Add an inspiring new element. Listening to motivational music, getting advice from a coach or trainer, or exercising with a fitness buddy can all provide the spark to push past a plateau.

The point is to get out of the rut of always doing the "same old same-old."

PLATEAU-BUSTING QUESTIONS

If you're still stuck, ask yourself the following questions to make sure you aren't slacking off. That often happens when you've reached your goal: You think you can loosen up a bit (and you can, to a point), but over time, you get a little too loose.

- **Are you using a heavy enough weight?** Pick one that works your muscle to fatigue—which typically means that you can do from 8 to 15 reps with good technique. Once you're able to do 15 repetitions with a weight for three sets in a row, move up to a weight that's heavier.

- **Are you working out enough?** Exercise is always one of the first things to go when life gets hectic. Walks get shorter, slower, or even skipped more often than they should. Start tracking your workouts to see how much you're *really* doing—you may be surprised.

- **Are you eating too much?** Mindless munching and forgotten nibbling can undermine diet success. Even "tastes"—like having a handful of a friend's popcorn at the movies or licking the bowl while cooking—can rack up a few hundred uncounted calories, which can pile on pounds quickly. Write down what you eat for a few days to make sure you're not consuming more than you think you are. And to avoid unaware eating, chew gum while cooking or cleaning up from meals, keep your hands busy with needlework while watching TV, and eliminate unnecessary distractions—such as the TV or a book—while you're eating.

It's important to recognize, too, that your fitness gains will be affected by your genetic potential. Once you've been exercising consistently for a year or more, you may reach a "happy plateau," where you've come close to your genetic potential for fitness and can move your training into maintenance mode.

OUCH! THAT HURTS

The "no pain, no gain" exercise theory is out. But occasional aches and pains are part of an active lifestyle. To reduce your chances of an injury–which can be a surefire way to sidetrack your efforts–follow these tips.

- Start warm and limber. Like taffy, muscles are brittle when cold and pliable when warm. Exercise lightly at first and stretch a little.
- Ease into higher intensities. There are many ways you can make your workout more challenging–go faster, walk farther, lift more weight, work out more often. But only increase one component of your workout at a time to avoid overdoing it and risking an injury.
- Add variety. Alternate activities to avoid overusing certain body parts.
- Alternate intensity. If you worked out hard yesterday, go easier today.

TAKE THIS TEST

If something starts to hurt, you need to listen to your body. Here's how to tell if your ache needs expert attention.*

1. How does it feel?
   a. Like a dull ache
   b. Like a sharp or shooting pain
2. Where is it?
   a. In a muscle
   b. Near or in a joint
3. How does it feel when you exercise?
   a. It becomes less painful
   b. There's no improvement or it gets worse
4. When did you notice the pain?
   a. The next day
   b. During a workout or immediately following one

If you answered all A's: It's probably okay to work through this type of pain. If it doesn't clear up in a day or two, however, you may need to cut back your workout.

If you answered any Bs: Take a few days off and ice the pain. If it doesn't go away, see a doctor.

*These are general guidelines for healthy individuals. If you have any type of chronic joint or muscular condition, consult your doctor.

GETTING HELP

Sometimes you need a little help from the experts to get over a hump. Here's a rundown of professionals who can help with a variety of obstacles.

Podiatrists. Trained to handle any foot-related condition–from simple corns to serious infections–podiatrists are not M.D.'s, but they must complete a 4-year course of study to earn a doctor of podiatric medicine (D.P.M.) degree. They must also be licensed by the state in which they practice. The American Podiatric Medical Association (APMA) offers information about

> ***QUICK TIP*** **In a society where most people gain at least a pound a year, recognize that keeping yourself at a healthy weight and fitness level is a major accomplishment.**

Exercises for Strong, Supple Feet

A LOT OF foot pain can be avoided (and alleviated) by strengthening and stretching the muscles in your feet and legs. Here are four exercises to the rescue! Do these exercises in bare feet.

HEEL RAISE/TOE POINT

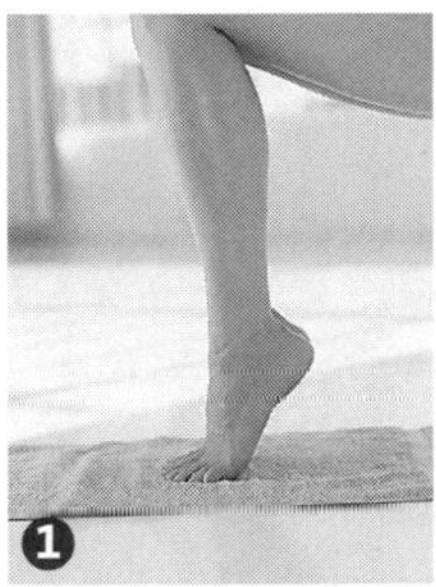

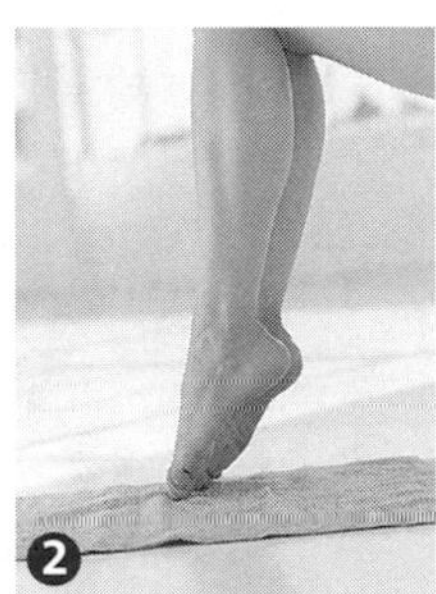

While seated, (1) rise onto the balls of your feet, (2) go up onto your tiptoes, and curl your toes under (not shown). Hold each position for 5 seconds. Repeat 10 times every day. It's good for people with hammertoes, toe cramps, and arch pain.

TOWEL SCRUNCHES

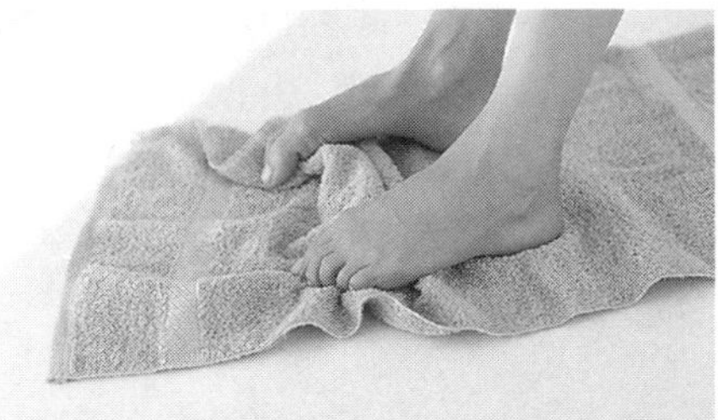

Sit and place a medium-size towel on the floor in front of your feet. By scrunching your toes, pull the towel inch by inch into the arch of your feet. Do this exercise one to three times daily. It strengthens the whole foot.

PLANTAR FASCIITIS STRETCH

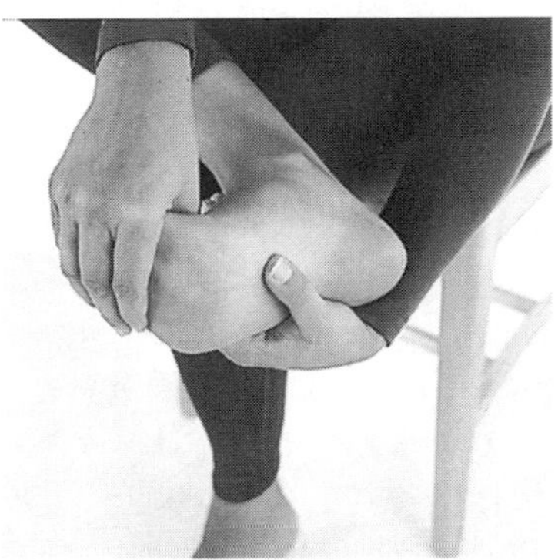

Sit in a chair and place the ankle of your injured foot across the opposite thigh. With the same-side hand, pull your toes toward your shin until you feel a stretch in your arch. Run your opposite hand along the sole of your foot; you should feel a taut band of tissue down the center. Do 10 stretches, holding each for 10 seconds. Repeat the stretches at least three times a day, especially before getting out of bed in the morning and before standing up after any prolonged sitting, such as riding in a car or sitting at a desk. (In a study of 101 adults who had plantar fasciitis, 83 percent who performed this stretch had no heel pain or less pain after 8 weeks.)

Avoid This Common Problem

WAKING UP WITH achy, stiff muscles is usually a signal that you overdid it. But instead of hitting the couch, get off it. Moving appears to be one of the best ways to relieve soreness. It works by pumping the excess fluid that's contributing to the pain out of the muscles. Take care to avoid more damage by choosing a low-intensity activity such as easy walking or gentle stretching. To avoid further soreness, ease up a bit.

foot health and referrals to podiatrists in your area on its Web site, www.apma.org, and by phone at (800) 366-8227. In addition, the American Academy of Podiatric Sports Medicine is a nationwide organization of podiatrists with a special interest in sports injuries. For information and referral, visit its Web site, www.aapsm.org, or call (888) 854-3338.

Dietitians. Registered dietitians (R.D.'s) are food and nutrition professionals who have–at minimum–a bachelor's degree in the field and who have completed an accredited preprofessional experience program and passed a national examination. Some R.D.'s also hold certifications in specialized areas of practice, such as pediatric nutrition or diabetes education. R.D.'s can help you meet a specific objective–like losing weight or reducing high blood pressure–by designing a personalized nutrition program. For referral, visit the American Dietetic Association's Web site at www.eatright.org or call (800) 877-1600.

Orthopedists. Medical doctors specializing in the diagnosis, care, and treatment of musculoskeletal disorders, orthopedists focus on conditions affecting the bones, joints, ligaments, muscles, and tendons. Look for orthopedists who are fellows of the American Academy of Orthopaedic Surgeons (AAOS), which means that–in addition to 4 years of medical school–the doctor has completed at least 5 years of an approved residency in orthopedics. For information and referral, contact the AAOS at its Web site, www.aaos.org, or by phone at (800) 346-2267.

Physical therapists. Trained to examine, evaluate, and treat people with health conditions resulting from injury or disease, physical therapists have extensive education in anatomy and body mechanics. They administer a variety of techniques to enhance recovery, such as therapeutic exercise, massage, ultrasound, and heat and cold applications. In most states, you need a doctor's referral to see a physical therapist, who typically has a degree in the field (often a master's degree) and is licensed by the state. Many also specialize in areas, such as geriatrics, orthopedics, pediatrics, and sports medicine. For information and referral, visit the American Physical Therapy Association's Web site, www.apta.org, or call them at (800) 999-2782.

Personal trainers. In the unregulated field of personal training, consumers need to be cautious, since certifications are available from more than 250 organizations of varying quality.

Credentials range from little more than having big biceps to holding advanced degrees in exercise science. To distinguish the emerging breed of well-educated exercise specialists from unqualified "gym rats," top professional organizations have begun offering new certification programs designed to teach trainers how to work with clients who have chronic health conditions such as diabetes, arthritis, asthma, high blood pressure, pregnancy, osteoporosis, and lower-

Ice or Heat?

ONE OF THE most common sports-medicine questions is whether to chill out or warm up an injury. Both heat and ice can boost healing by manipulating blood flow. Ice restricts blood flow, which reduces inflammation and pain. Heat increases circulation, which boosts the supply of oxygen to the site, accelerating the removal of waste products. The trick is knowing when to use each.

This "cheat sheet" was created by our sister publication, *Runner's World,* with expert input from Carl Nissen, M.D., of the University of Connecticut Health Center in Farmington, and Christine Worsley, assistant athletic trainer at the Rochester Institute of Technology in New York.

CHOOSE ICE

After an injury: Within the first 24 to 48 hours, apply for 20 minutes, then remove for 20 minutes. Repeat often. Try to apply within 20 minutes of sustaining an injury.

How to apply: Place a thin towel over your skin for protection, then wrap the ice pack tightly around the area. Or try an ice massage: Freeze a paper cup full of water, tear off the top rim to expose the ice, and move the ice continuously over the injury.

Precautions: Those with Raynaud's disease or former frostbite sufferers should not use ice on affected body parts.

CHOOSE HEAT

After an injury: Apply for 20 minutes at a time 24 hours after a minor injury (or 48 hours after an acute injury).

How to apply: Place the heat pack on top of the injured area. Do not apply body weight. (Don't sit the injured area on top of the heat pack.)

Precautions: Do not apply heat to injured areas with broken skin.

COMBINE ICE AND HEAT

Use a combination of ice and heat about 48 hours after an injury. Either alternate cold and hot packs for 10 minutes, or try a contrast bath. Fill two buckets, one with cold water and some ice, and the other with tolerably hot water. Soak the area in the cold bucket for 2 minutes, then switch to the hot bucket for 2 minutes. By alternating, you keep the swelling down with the cold, while you keep the blood and its nutrients circulating through the injured area with the heat.

back pain. For example, the American Council on Exercise now certifies qualified personal trainers as "clinical exercise specialists." And IDEA Health and Fitness Association, the world's leading membership organization for health and fitness professionals, has a new personal-fitness-trainer recognition system that identifies trainers as professional, advanced, elite, or master trainers. They offer referrals on their Web site, www.ideafit.com.

The following are among the most respected organizations offering certifications for personal trainers and other exercise specialists.

- The American College of Sports Medicine, PO Box 1440, Indianapolis, IN 46206-1440; Web site, www.acsm.org.
- The American Council on Exercise, 4851 Paramount Drive, San Diego, CA 92123; Web site, www.acefitness.org; phone number, (800) 825-3636.
- The Cooper Institute for Aerobics Research, 12330 Preston Road, Dallas, TX 75230; Web site, www.cooperinst.org.
- The National Strength and Conditioning Association, 1885 Bob Johnson Drive, Colorado

Got Pain? Try This Doctor

WHEN I WAS sidelined with a foot injury a few years ago, I went to a podiatrist, who wanted to operate, and an orthopedist, who told me to stop running and doing aerobics. I finally got the help I needed from a physiatrist (pronounced *fizz-EE-at-trist*), a medical doctor who specializes in physical medicine and rehabilitation.

Instead of just looking at my feet, he checked my leg strength, flexibility, and the way I walked and ran. In addition to a chronic foot problem, he discovered that my hip muscles were tight and weak. This was aggravating my foot problem every time I tried to resume exercising. Now I do stretches and strengthening exercises for these areas, and I've been able to prevent or manage any pain.

Physiatrists focus on getting you back to previous activity levels without surgery. They use therapies such as exercise, biofeedback, massage, heat and cold, electrotherapy, hydrotherapy—and prescription medication when needed. In addition to treating acute conditions, a physiatrist aims to prevent future problems.

Besides exercise-related problems or injuries, physiatrists also treat other medical problems that can impair function, such as back pain, arthritis, carpal tunnel syndrome, multiple sclerosis, osteoporosis, and stroke.

To find a physical medicine and rehabilitation doctor in your area, contact the American Academy of Physical Medicine and Rehabilitation at (312) 464-9700 or www.aapmr.org.

Springs, CO 80906; Web site, www.nsca-lift.org; phone number, (800) 815-6826.

- The Aerobics and Fitness Association of America, 15250 Ventura Boulevard, Suite 200, Sherman Oaks, CA 91403; Web site, www.afaa.com; phone number, (877) 968-7263.

TOO MUCH OF A GOOD THING

Although it's rarely a problem for the average exerciser, if you're taking your workout to a higher level–such as training for a race or competition–you could fall prey to overtraining problems.

After a tough workout, your body needs time to rebuild. In fact, it's this very process of stressing a muscle, then letting it rest and repair, that helps you get stronger. This is why experts recommend waiting 48 hours between weight-training workouts. Yet overenthusiastic exercisers may mistakenly believe that "more is better," and engage in intense training that undermines their ability to repair and strengthen.

Overtraining leads to fatigue, reduced performance, and often, difficult-to-treat injuries, such as stress fractures. Generally, warning signs precede overtraining problems. Common symptoms are excessive fatigue, difficulty sleeping, unusual irritation, loss of appetite, or lack of motivation. If you think overtraining is the problem, take these pulse tests.

Morning pulse. Check your resting pulse rate as soon as you wake up in the morning–before you get out of bed–and learn what is normal for you. An increase of more than five beats per minute that doesn't return to normal in a few days could signal a problem.

Training pulse. If you feel unusually tired during a workout, take your pulse. If it's higher than usual and doesn't return to normal during your next workout, your body is telling you something.

If you experience any of the symptoms mentioned above, try these four strategies.

1. Cross-training. Alternate between two or more activities that use different muscle groups, for example, an impact activity like walking and a nonimpact activity like cycling or swimming.

2. Hard/easy workouts. If you want to do the same activity every day, alternate high-intensity, shorter workouts with easier, longer ones.

3. Upper/lower body training. If you want to strength-train every day, focus on your upper body one day and lower body the next.

4. Rest. Take a day off each week to rest. You don't have to flop on the couch–just avoid stressful physical activity. Depending on your fitness level, it may be restful to do light gardening, stroll with your spouse, or play ping-pong with your kids.

If you cut back on your exercise and your symptoms persist, see your doctor. There may be an underlying medical problem that's making you feel bad.

COMBATING BOREDOM

"If I have to get on that treadmill one more time, I'm going to scream!" Sound familiar? Since nobody's holding a gun to your head and making you exercise or eat a healthy diet, it's easy–all too easy–to decide that you're bored to tears with your routine. But before you give up on it, ask yourself: Are you really bored? Boredom is actually easy to fix. Maybe you just need to vary your walking route, walk with a friend, or take up a new form of exercise. It may be as simple as changing the CD you listen to while you work out. If you're bored with your diet, maybe you've been eating the same breakfast every day for a month and need a little variety.

First, make sure that boredom really is the issue. When you start to think about it, you may discover that you're upset about something, or you just don't feel motivated the way you did when you were doing the Firm Up Program. If boredom isn't the core problem, try one (or all) of these tips to rekindle your drive.

- Reread chapter 8, Get a Winning Attitude, and/or chapter 12, Keep Your Motivation Strong.
- If you think the problem is that you need a strong structure to stay with the plan, go back to week 1 and do the program again.
- If it's frustration rather than boredom that's tripping you up–walking and exercising seem to be taking up so much of your precious "free" time–consider investigating time management. Take a class, read a book, hire a pro for a consultation. See where you can save time and apply those newfound hours, quarter-hours, and so on to the other things you feel that you're missing.
- Turn back to "Find the reason behind your slipup," on page 397, and reread the section on how to get back to the heart of the issue. The technique will work just as well now. Keep digging deeper until you get to the real reason you want to give up.

> ***QUICK TIP*** **Boredom is really easy to fix! Try something new, or do something old in a new way. You're only limited by your imagination.**

BEATING BOREDOM

Okay, you've checked it out, and you know that the problem really *is* boredom. What to do? Try our "Boredom Busters" below for a start. Make it a game, and soon you'll be coming up with all sorts of boredom busters of your own. Don't forget to ask your friends, family, and coworkers what they do when their exercise routines start to bore them. You may be surprised at how creative they are!

Boredom Busters: Walking

Here are seven ways to put some fun back into your walks.

1. Make walking a family affair. Ask your parents or grandparents to walk with you, and record them as they talk about their life. Walk with your kids and listen to what's on their minds. Walk hand in hand with your spouse.

2. Turn your walk into a game. Walk as long as it takes to spot, say, three red cars. Then set a new game objective and keep on walking.

3. Dust 'em. Pick a walker on your path who seems a bit fitter and faster than you. Then try to pass her.

4. Enjoy a mini-getaway. Plan an itinerary that takes you and a friend on a brisk, hour-long walk ending at a coffee shop or flea market.

5. Create a walking book club. Instead of discussing a book over dessert, meet your group on a weekend morning to walk and talk.

6. Explore new places. Get a map of area trails from your local department of parks and recreation. Walk a different path each week.

7. Expand your circle of walking buddies. It'll offer you more lively conversations and a backup partner if one can't make it.

Boredom Busters: Strength Training

Use these eight techniques to add some spark to your strength-training routine.

1. Create a competition. Even if you and your buddy can't work out at the same time, you can have a little fun with this idea. Get together for a workout and record how much each of you can lift for various exercises. Then do it again in a month or two to find out who improved the most. Wager $20, a video, or anything else that will motivate you.

2. Try a circuit. Break up your weight-lifting routine with bouts of aerobic activity. Do a set of bench presses. Next, hop on the stationary bike for a brisk 2½-minute spin; then it's back to the weights. Keep repeating this cycle until you've finished your weight workout.

3. Get with a group. Most gyms offer group strength-training classes. The upbeat music and group energy make the time fly. If your gym doesn't offer this type of class or you prefer to work out at home, join us with *Prevention*'s strength-training video. (To order, see the Walker's Warehouse on page 418.)

4. Stay focused. Pay attention to your body. When possible, put your hand on the muscle that you're targeting and feel it contract and relax. Focus on your breathing. Before you know it, you'll be finished.

5. Play some ball. Use a stability ball—a large, inflatable exercise ball—in place of a bench to sit or recline on for exercises such as biceps curls, bench presses, and chest flies. (For descriptions of some of these exercises, see page 409.) It takes more concentration to keep your balance. (Tip: Start with a lighter weight than you're used to lifting.) Exercise balls are available at many major sporting goods stores, or see "Products" in the Firm Up Resources on page 418.

6. Join a gym. You may develop some new friendships, which will also make you want to go to the gym. One caution: You may spend more time chatting than lifting. Don't forget the workout!

7. Hire a personal trainer. They're not as expensive as you think, especially if you persuade a friend to join you. Many trainers will offer group sessions at reduced rates, and you don't have to use a trainer constantly. Go regularly for a few sessions, and then when you're on track, go back once a month or so for some fine-tuning and reinforcement.

8. Lift by the tube. If all else fails, do your workout while you watch TV.

Boredom Busters: Eating

Try these four tactics to help liven up your meals.

1. Get out of that rut. If you're eating the same breakfasts and lunches, or are cooking the same dinners week after week, you need a change. Check out the mix-and-match meals in chapter 7, buy a new cookbook, or ask a friend to share some of her favorite recipes with you to give you new meal ideas.

2. Explore exotic tastes. Wander around a gourmet or ethnic store and try something new, such as baba ghannouj or sag paneer. Many Indian and Middle Eastern dishes feature delicious spices and wholesome ingredients, so you can enjoy them without guilt. Just use good portion control!

3. Take a detour at the grocery store. Most shopping trips are very automatic: You grab the same items off the same shelves every week without giving the other shelves or aisles a glance. Slow down, check out what you've been missing, and vow to pick up something new—a fruit or veggie you've never tried or some of the new ethnic frozen meals—during every visit. In no time, you'll find some new favorites to add to your regular meals.

4. Sign up for a cooking class. Explore new flavors with Thai or Indian cooking. It may be just what you need to spice up your tastebuds.

Now that you've beaten your Firm Up saboteurs and are motivated to keep going, I'd like to introduce you to the next level of exercises. They keep me fit and firm, and I know they'll work for you. Turn to chapter 15 and check them out!

FIRM UP TIP

MIND OVER MATTER

Look for the good things in life. Keep a "gratitude diary." At the end of every day, list the things for which you're grateful: the butterfly that paused by your window, the puppy who licked your hand, the friend who brought you daffodils, the tick of a grandfather clock that kept time for your mother and grandmother before you, the baby who opened his eyes and looked at the world for the very first time. Remembering all these blessings is the best anti-anxiety agent of all.

CHAPTER 15

Stay Firm Moves

When you're ready for a new challenge, I've created modifications of 11 exercises from the Firm Up Action Plan. Simply swap them into that particular week's routine. All of these moves are done on a stability ball—a large, inflatable exercise ball that adds an element of instability to your workout. Doing exercises on a stability ball forces many of the core muscles in your torso to work overtime to stabilize you atop the ball.

Stability balls cost about $30 and can be found at many major sporting goods stores, or see "Products" in Firm Up Resources on page 418. Here are general guidelines for getting the right size ball.

When you're sitting on the ball, your knees and hips should be in line so that your thighs are parallel to the floor. That's why getting a ball that's the right size (see "Get on the Ball") is so important. One size does *not* fit all!

The more inflated the ball is, the more difficult it will be to balance. So if you're new to stability-ball exercises, don't inflate the ball all the way.

QUICK TIP **Replace your desk chair or recliner with a stability ball. You have to engage your core muscles to maintain your balance, so you get a workout while you're sitting.**

GET ON THE BALL

If You're . . .	Buy This Ball . . .
Under 5'1"	45 cm
5'1"–5'7"	55 cm
5'7"–6'2"	65 cm
Over 6'2"	75 cm

THE NEXT LEVEL

Exercises using the stability ball are challenging and fun. (You may be tempted to bounce around on the ball a little bit just for the heck of it, too. Go for it!) These 11 exercises will take your firmness to the next level and increase your agility while building your balance. And they're a great way to get some variety in your strength-training program.

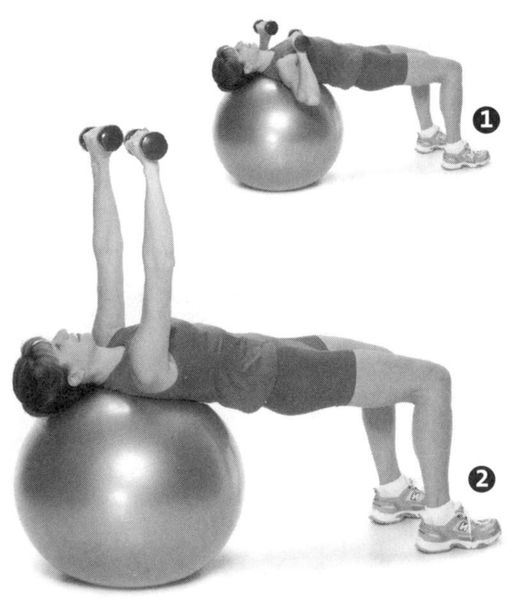

Chest Press

Starting position: Lie on a stability ball so that it's supporting your head and upper back. Your feet should be flat on the floor and your hips and thighs parallel to the floor. Hold dumbbells end to end and just above your shoulders. Your elbows should be pointing out to the sides.

Movement: Exhale as you press the dumbbells straight up over your chest, extending your arms. Hold for a second and then inhale as you slowly lower.

Technique: Don't let your buttocks drop toward the floor.

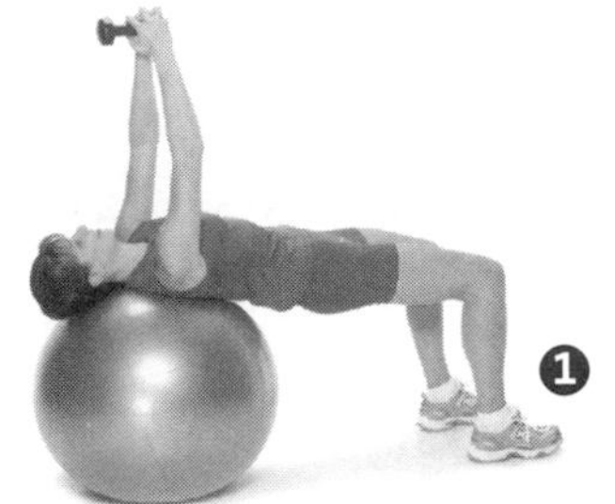

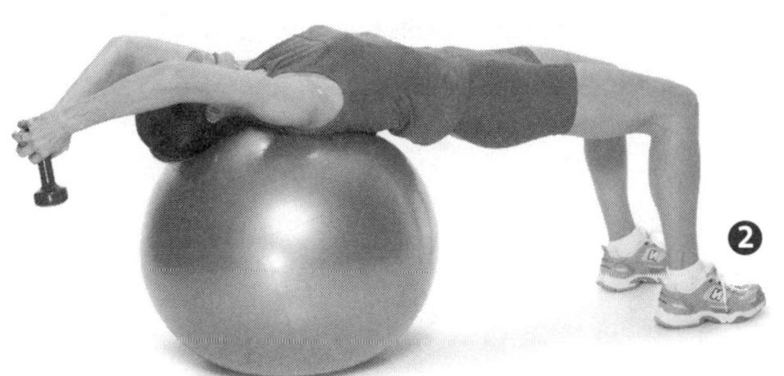

Pullover

Starting position: Lie on a stability ball so that it's supporting your head and upper back. Your feet should be flat on the floor and your hips and thighs parallel to the floor. Grasp a dumbbell with both hands and hold it above your chest. Keep a slight bend in your elbows.

Movement: Inhale as you lower the dumbbell backward over your head as far as is comfortably possible without bending your elbows any farther than at the start. Hold for a second and then exhale as you slowly raise it to the starting position.

Technique: Don't let your buttocks drop toward the floor.

FIRM UP TIP

GET FIRM FASTER

Hit the stairs for a quick calorie blaster. Five 2-minute bouts of stairclimbing is equivalent to about 36 minutes of walking. When researchers tested 15 healthy but inactive young women (average age 18) for 8 weeks, those who worked up to climbing 199 steps in about 2 minutes, five times a day, posted a 17 percent increase in cardio fitness levels compared with women who did nothing. This is a big change for a modest effort.

continued

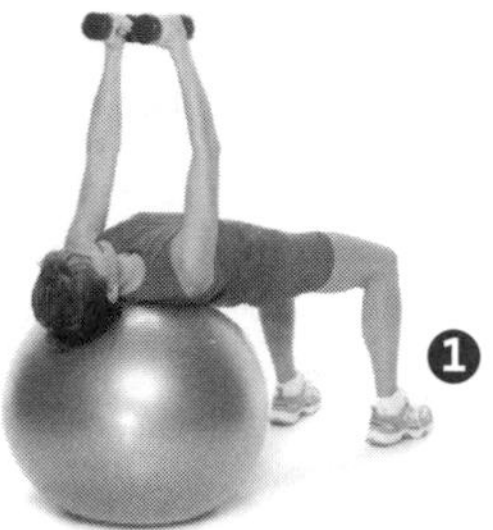

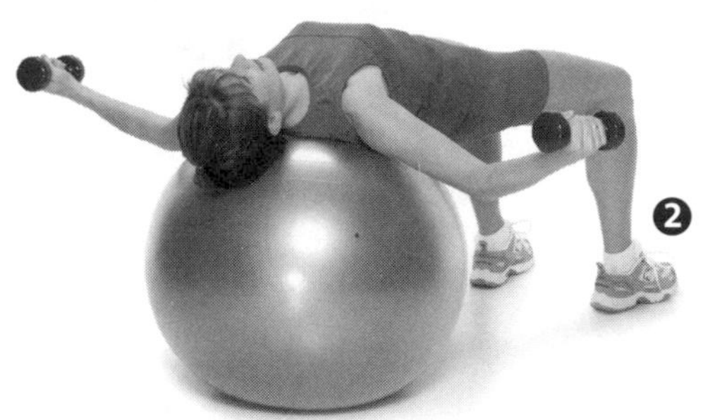

Chest Fly

Starting position: Lie on a stability ball so that it's supporting your head and upper back. Your feet should be flat on the floor and your hips and thighs parallel to the floor. Hold dumbbells above your chest with your palms facing each other and your elbows slightly bent.

Movement: As you inhale, slowly lower your arms out to the sides. Hold for a second and then exhale as you press the dumbbells back up.

Technique: Don't let your buttocks drop toward the floor. Don't lower the dumbbells below shoulder height.

Lying Triceps Extension

Starting position: Lie on a stability ball so that it's supporting your head and upper back. Your feet should be flat on the floor and your hips and thighs parallel to the floor. Hold a dumbbell in each hand over your chest, palms facing each other. Bend your arms so that your elbows are pointing toward the ceiling and the dumbbells are by your ears.

Movement: Exhale as you lift the weights up over your chest without moving your upper arms. Hold for a second and then inhale as you slowly lower.

Technique: Don't let your buttocks drop toward the floor. Don't move your shoulders or arch your back.

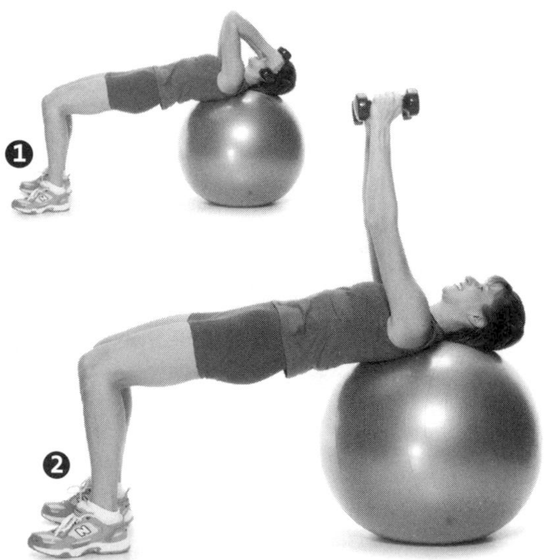

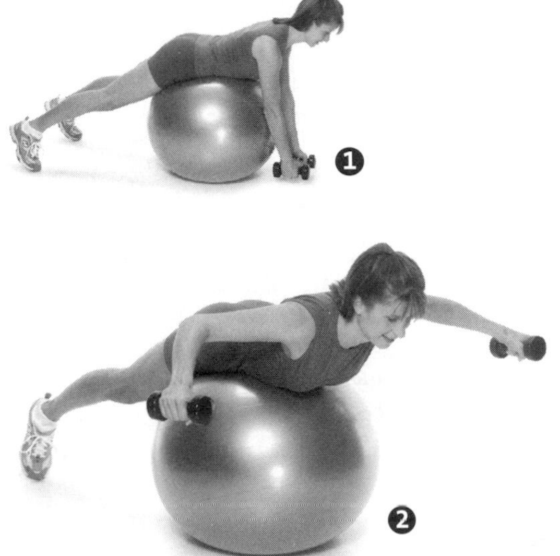

Back Fly

Starting position: While holding a dumbbell in each hand and kneeling facing a stability ball, position your pelvis on the ball and extend your legs. Keep your back flat and let the dumbbells hang at arm's length down in front of the ball, with your palms facing each other and your elbows bent slightly.

Movement: Exhale as you squeeze your shoulder blades together and lift the dumbbells up and out to the sides, pulling your elbows back as far as is comfortably possible. Be sure to keep your back straight. Hold for a second and then inhale as you slowly lower.

Technique: Don't arch your back. Don't lift your torso as you lift the dumbbells.

Back Extension

Starting position: Facing a stability ball, position your pelvis and abs on the ball and extend your legs. Keep your back straight and place your hands behind your head.

Movement: As you exhale, contract your lower-back muscles and lift your upper body so that it forms a straight line with your lower body. Hold for a second and then inhale as you slowly lower.

Technique: Don't lift so high that you arch your back.

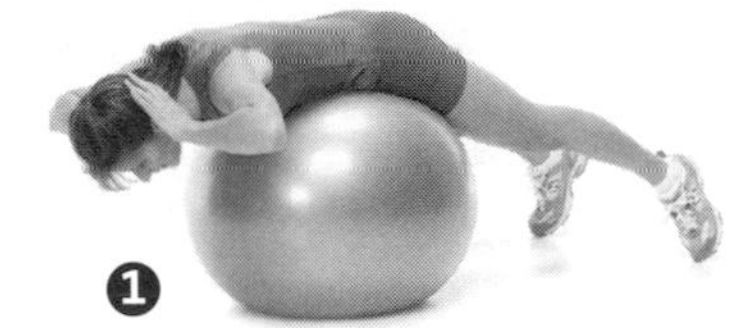

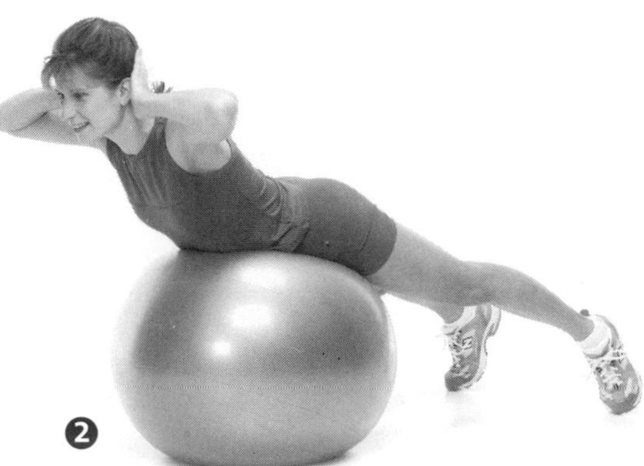

continued

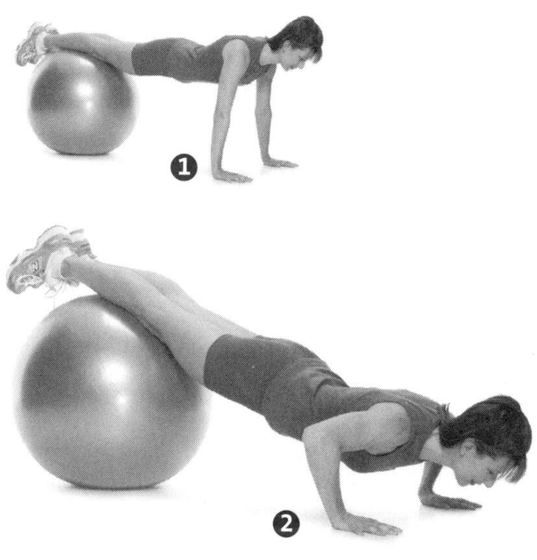

Pushup

Starting position: Kneel facing a stability ball and drape your body over the ball, placing your hands on the floor in front. Walk your hands forward, allowing the ball to roll back until it is supporting your calves and you are balancing on your hands. Your hands should be about shoulder-width apart and directly under your shoulders. Your neck, back, hips, and legs should be in a straight line.

Movement: Inhale as you bend your elbows out to the sides and, while keeping your body in a straight line, lower yourself until your nose nearly touches the floor. Hold for a second and then exhale as you push back up. If you cannot do all the recommended reps in this full pushup position, that's okay. Just drop down onto one or both knees and complete the remaining reps.

Technique: Don't bend at your hips. Don't arch your back.

Ab Crunch

Starting position: Lie on your back on a stability ball so that it supports your back. Your feet should be flat on the floor and your hands behind your head.

Movement: Exhale as you use your abs to slowly raise your head, shoulders, and upper back. Think of shortening the distance between your ribs and pelvis. Hold for a second and then inhale as you slowly lower.

Technique: Don't pull your chin to your chest. Don't arch your back.

More challenging: As you curl up, lift your right foot off the floor, bringing your right knee toward your chest. Alternate legs with each crunch.

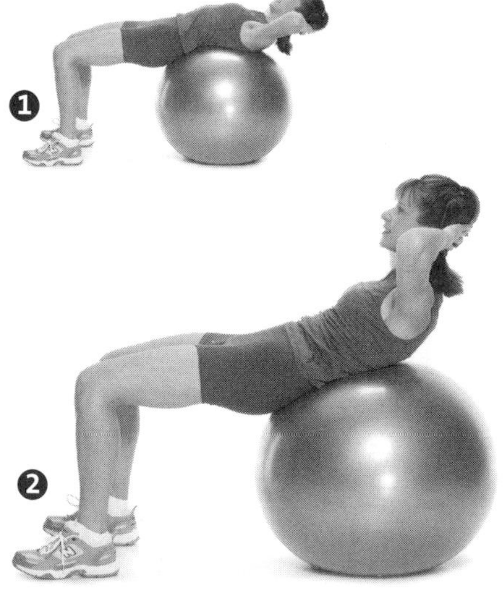

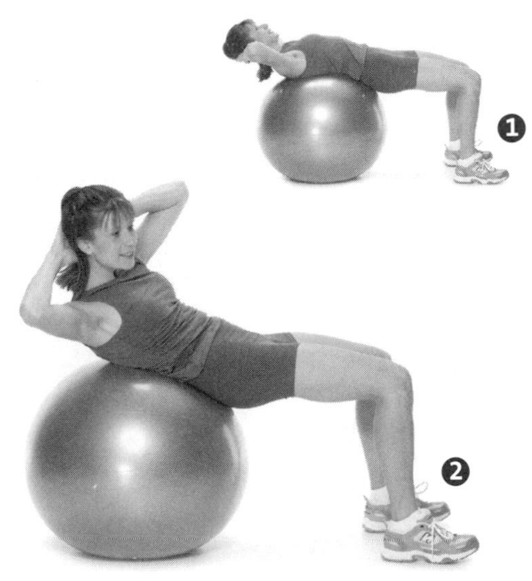

Twisting Crunch

Starting position: Lie on your back on a stability ball so that it supports your back. Your feet should be flat on the floor and your hands behind your head.

Movement: Exhale as you slowly lift your head and left shoulder up, twist to the right, and bring your left shoulder toward your right knee. Hold for a second and then inhale as you slowly lower. Repeat, alternating sides. Do a total of 10 reps, 5 to each side.

Technique: Don't pull your chin to your chest.

Bridge

Starting position: Lie on the floor on your back, extend your legs, and place your heels on top of a stability ball. Your arms should be at your sides, with palms facing up.

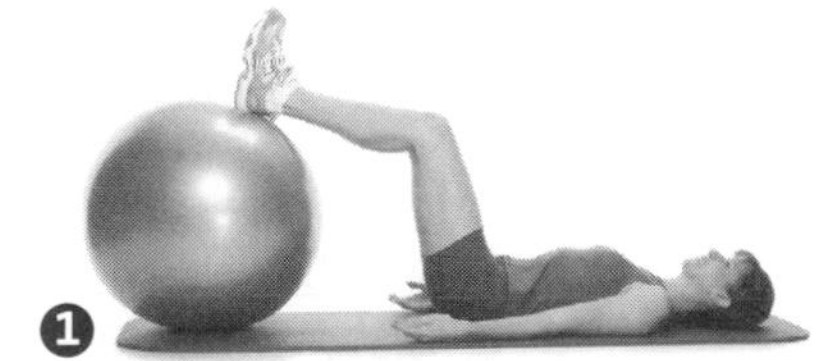

Movement: Exhale as you contract your abs, buttocks, and lower back; press into your heels; and lift your butt, hips, and lower back off the floor to form a straight line, from your upper back to your heels. Hold for three breaths and then relax.

Technique: Don't lift too high—your upper back and shoulders should remain on the floor. Don't bend at your waist or hips. Don't let your knees fall inward or outward.

More challenging: Try lifting one leg off the ball while balancing.

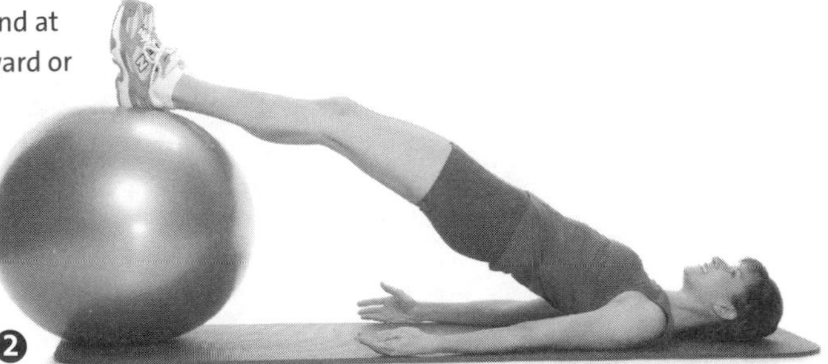

continued

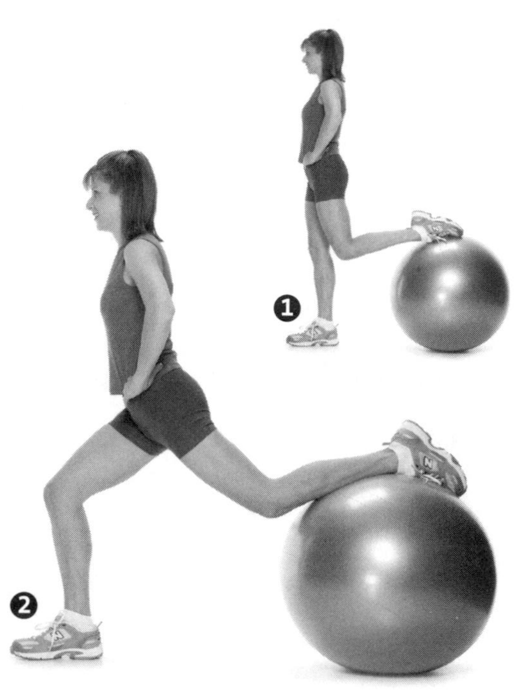

Lunge

Starting position: Stand with your back to a stability ball. Bend your left leg and place the top of your left foot on top of the ball.

Movement: Inhale as you bend your right knee and lower your body. Your left leg will go back, rolling the ball along. Hold for a second and then exhale as you slowly push yourself back up and pull the ball forward. Finish all of your repetitions and then repeat the exercise with your right foot on the ball.

Technique: Don't lean forward. Don't let your front knee move forward over your toes.

That's it!

You now have all the tools

and skills you need

to get firm and stay firm.

Congratulations!

DIET/NUTRITION

American Dietetic Association (ADA)
120 South Riverside Plaza, Suite 2000
Chicago, IL 60606-6995
(800) 877-1600
www.eatright.org

Center for Science in the Public Interest
1875 Connecticut Avenue NW, Suite 300
Washington, DC 20009
(202) 332-9110
www.cspinet.org

USDA Nutrient Database
Nutrient Data Laboratory
Agricultural Research Service
Beltsville Human Nutrition Research Center
10300 Baltimore Avenue
Building 005, Room 107, BARC-West
Beltsville, MD 20705-2350
(301) 504-0630
www.nal.usda.gov/fnic/foodcomp/search/

EXERCISE/PERSONAL TRAINERS

Aerobics and Fitness Association of America
15250 Ventura Boulevard, Suite 200
Sherman Oaks, CA 91403
(877) 968-7263
www.afaa.com

American College of Sports Medicine (ACSM)
PO Box 1440
Indianapolis, IN 46206-1440
(317) 637-9200
www.acsm.org

American Council on Exercise (ACE)
4851 Paramount Drive
San Diego, CA 92123
(858) 279-8227 or (800) 825-3636
www.acefitness.org

The Cooper Institute for Aerobics Research
12330 Preston Road
Dallas, TX 75230
www.cooperinst.org

IDEA Health and Fitness Association
10455 Pacific Center Court
San Diego, CA 92121-4339
(800) 999-4332
www.ideafit.com

The National Strength and Conditioning Association
1885 Bob Johnson Drive
Colorado Springs, CO 80906
(800) 815-6826
www.nsca-lift.org

President's Council on Physical Fitness
Department W
200 Independence Avenue SW, Room 738-H
Washington, DC 20201-0004
(202) 690-9000
www.fitness.gov

HEALTH

U.S. National Library of Medicine
National Institutes of Health
9000 Rockville Pike
Bethesda, MD 20892
(301) 496-4000
www.nlm.nih.gov/medlineplus/

Prevention Magazine
400 South 10th Street
Emmaus, PA 18098
(610) 967-8038
www.prevention.com

INJURIES

American Academy of Orthopaedic Surgeons (AAOS)
6300 North River Road
Rosemont, IL 60018-4262
(847) 823-7186 or (800) 346-2267
www.aaos.org

American Academy of Physical Medicine and Rehabilitation (AAPMR)
One IBM Plaza, Suite 2500
Chicago, IL 60611-3604
(312) 464-9700
www.aapmr.org

American Academy of Podiatric Sports Medicine (AAPSM)
PO Box 723
Rockville, MD 20848-0723
(888) 854-3338
www.aapsm.org

American Physical Therapy Association (APTA)
1111 North Fairfax Street
Alexandria, VA 22314-1488
(703) 684-2782 or (800) 999-2782
www.apta.org

American Podiatric Medical Association (APMA)
9312 Old Georgetown Road
Bethesda, MD 20814
(301) 571-9200 or (800) 275-2762
www.apma.org

PRODUCTS

Fitter International Inc.
3050, 2600 Portland Street SE
Calgary, Alberta
Canada T2G 4M6
(800) 348-8371
www.fitter1.com

Perform Better (M-F Athletic Company)
PO Box 8090
Cranston, RI 02920-0090
(401) 942-9363
(888) 556-7464
www.performbetter.com

SPRI Products, Inc.
1600 Northwind Boulevard
Libertyville, IL 60048
(800) 222-7774
www.spriproducts.com

The Walker's Warehouse
(888) 972-9255
www.walkerswarehouse.com

WEIGHT LOSS

Shape Up America!
c/o WebFront Solutions Corporation
15009 Native Dancer Road
North Potomac, MD 20878
(240) 631-6533
www.shapeup.org

Weight-Control Information Network
1 WIN Way
Bethesda, MD 20892-3665
(202) 828-1025 or (877) 946-4627
www.niddk.nih.gov/health/nutrit/win.htm

INDEX

<u>Underscored</u> page references indicate sidebars and tables. **Boldface** references indicate photographs.

C

D

E

I

M

N

O

P

Q

R

S

T

U

V

W

Y

Conversion Chart

These equivalents have been slightly rounded to make measuring easier.

Volume Measurements

U.S.	Imperial	Metric
¼ tsp	–	1 ml
½ tsp	–	2 ml
1 tsp	–	5 ml
1 Tbsp	–	15 ml
2 Tbsp (1 oz)	1 fl oz	30 ml
¼ cup (2 oz)	2 fl oz	60 ml
⅓ cup (3 oz)	3 fl oz	80 ml
½ cup (4 oz)	4 fl oz	120 ml
⅔ cup (5 oz)	5 fl oz	160 ml
¾ cup (6 oz)	6 fl oz	180 ml
1 cup (8 oz)	8 fl oz	240 ml

Weight Measurements

U.S.	Metric
1 oz	30 g
2 oz	60 g
4 oz (¼ lb)	115 g
5 oz (⅓ lb)	145 g
6 oz	170 g
7 oz	200 g
8 oz (½ lb)	230 g
10 oz	285 g
12 oz (¾ lb)	340 g
14 oz	400 g
16 oz (1 lb)	455 g
2.2 lb	1 kg

Length Measurements

U.S.	Metric
¼"	0.6 cm
½"	1.25 cm
1"	2.5 cm
2"	5 cm
4"	11 cm
6"	15 cm
8"	20 cm
10"	25 cm
12" (1')	30 cm

Pan Sizes

U.S.	Metric
8" cake pan	20 × 4 cm sandwich or cake tin
9" cake pan	23 × 3.5 cm sandwich or cake tin
11" × 7" baking pan	28 × 18 cm baking tin
13" × 9" baking pan	32.5 × 23 cm baking tin
15" × 10" baking pan	38 × 25.5 cm baking tin (Swiss roll tin)
1½ qt baking dish	1.5 liter baking dish
2 qt baking dish	2 liter baking dish
2 qt rectangular baking dish	30 × 19 cm baking dish
9" pie plate	22 × 4 or 23 × 4 cm pie plate
7" or 8" springform pan	18 or 20 cm springform or loose-bottom cake tin
9" × 5" loaf pan	23 × 13 cm or 2 lb narrow loaf tin or pâté tin

Temperatures

Fahrenheit	Centigrade	Gas
140°	60°	–
160°	70°	–
180°	80°	–
225°	105°	¼
250°	120°	½
275°	135°	1
300°	150°	2
325°	160°	3
350°	180°	4
375°	190°	5
400°	200°	6
425°	220°	7
450°	230°	8
475°	245°	9
500°	260°	–